THE SUPERMARKET NUTRITION COUNTER

What's the best way to make sure your family eats balanced meals and healthful snacks? Over 60 percent of Americans look at labels while grocery shopping, but even the new nutrition labels don't always give you all the facts you need. Now, in the most comprehensive supermarket counter ever, nutrition experts Annette B. Natow and Jo-Ann Heslin guide you through the best that supermarkets have to offer. With 16,000 foods in all, *THE SUPERMARKET NUTRITION COUNTER* includes:

- over 250 breads
- over 300 frozen dinners
- over 350 ice creams and frozen desserts
- over 800 supermarket take-out foods
- and much more.

◇

From the psychology of shelving to the truth about how men and women *really* differ—
especially in the supermarket—
THE SUPERMARKET NUTRITION COUNTER has it all!

T·H·E
SUPERMARKET
NUTRITION
·COUNTER·

Annette B. Natow, Ph.D., R.D., and Jo-Ann Heslin, M.A., R.D.

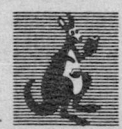

POCKET BOOKS

New York   London   Toronto   Sydney   Tokyo   Singapore

An *Original* Publication of POCKET BOOKS

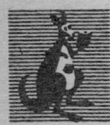

POCKET BOOKS, a division of Simon & Schuster Inc.
1230 Avenue of the Americas, New York, NY 10020

ISBN: 0-671-78328-9

First Pocket Books printing April 1995

10 9 8 7 6 5 4 3 2 1

POCKET and colophon are registered trademarks of
Simon & Schuster Inc.

Cover design by Tom McKeveny

Printed in the U.S.A.

Acknowledgments

Without the tireless cooperation of Steven and Stephen, *The Supermarket Counter* would never have been completed. Our thanks to the National Live Stock and Meat Board and the Food Marketing Institute for providing research material and resources. A special thanks to our editor, Rebecca Todd, and our agent, Nancy Trichter.

"We are all inclined to think the foods which we like are good for us, and appearance and flavor attract or repel very quickly; but as far as real nourishment goes, these things are second hand and the [shopper] must be able to discriminate between real nutritive value and other factors, in order to spend . . . money to the best advantage."

Mary Swartz Rose, Ph.D.
Feeding the Family
The Macmillan Company, 1919

Contents

Sources of Data

Values in this counter have been obtained from the Composition of Foods, United States Department of Agriculture, Agricultural Handbooks: No. 8-1, Dairy and Egg Products; No. 8-2, Spices and Herbs; No. 8-3, Baby Foods; No. 8-4, Fats and Oils; No. 8-5, Poultry Products; No. 8-6, Soups, Sauces and Gravies; No. 8-7, Sausages and Luncheon Meats; No. 8-8, Breakfast Cereals; No. 8-9 Fruit and Fruit Juices; No. 8-10, Pork Products; No. 8-11, Vegetables and Vegetable Products; No. 8-12, Nut and Seed Products; No. 8-13, Beef Products; No. 8-14, Beverages; No. 8-15, Finfish and Shellfish Products; No. 8-16, Legumes and Legume Products; No. 8-17, Lamb, Veal and Game Products; No. 8-18, Baked Products; No. 8-19, Snacks and Sweets; No. 8-20, Cereal Grains and Pasta; No. 8-21, Fast Foods; Supplements 1989, 1990, 1991.

"Nutritive Value of Foods." United States Department of Agriculture, Home and Garden Bulletin No. 72.

J. Davies and J. Dickerson, *Nutrient Content of Food Portions.* Cambridge, UK: The Royal Society of Chemistry, 1991.

G. A. Leveille, M. E. Zabik, K. J. Morgan, *Nutrients in Foods.* Cambridge, MA: The Nutrition Guild, 1983.

Souci, Fachmann, Kraut, *Food Composition and Nutrition Tables.* Stuttgart: Wissenschaftliche Verlagsgesellschaft MbH, 1989.

Information from food labels, manufacturers and processors. The values are based on research conducted through 1994. Manufacturer's ingredients are subject to change, so current values may vary from those listed in the book.

Introduction

It's hard to believe but the average supermarket carries 30,000 separate items and over half of these are foods. No wonder grocery shopping takes so long. And when you try to compare the nutrients in different products to ensure the healthiest menu, it takes even longer. Recent surveys show that over 60 percent of Americans are concerned about the nutritional value in the foods they buy. You want to make good choices but you may not have enough time to spend comparing the labels of five or more pasta sauces, rice mixes or frozen dinners. That's where *The Supermarket Nutrition Counter* lends a hand. Now you have a chance to compare these products before you get near the supermarket.

The Supermarket Nutrition Counter will show you how to navigate the supermarket to find the best choices in each section as you push your cart up and down the aisles. You'll also learn how to interpret the nutrition facts on labels, use cents-off coupons, make use of storage tips to preserve the nutrients in the foods you buy and even how to stock your kitchen so there will always be a quick something to eat.

Fast fact ————————————————————
Nearly 20 percent of the new products introduced in supermarkets are low-fat, low-cholesterol items.

Fast fact ————————————————————
Less than 5 percent of people shop in discount/warehouse food stores, and shopping at warehouse club stores is declining.

TRAVELING THROUGH THE SUPERMARKET

Fast fact _____
In the United States there are 136,000 grocery stores
with $390 billion in sales.

The first step to efficient, healthy shopping is getting to
know the layout of the supermarket where you shop. Grocery
stores tend to be organized in similar layouts and there are
a few tricks to getting the most out of your shopping time.
Wheel your cart around the outside aisles first. You'll be
passing the fresh dairy products, fruits, vegetables, breads
and meat, fish and poultry. These foods are the ones that
are emphasized in the Food Guide Pyramid. Load your basket
with these.

Fast fact _____
**Supermarkets are beginning to use a new strategy
called "Efficient Consumer Response" or ECR. This
system lets stores track consumer patterns more effi-
ciently, electronically. Stores receive orders more
quickly and spend less money on warehousing products. It is estimated that using this procedure will
allow supermarkets to cut their prices by 11 percent.**

Navigating the Supermarket Aisles

Supermarkets are set up to encourage shoppers to buy
more. For instance, milk which is usually bought on every
shopping trip, is placed in the rear of the store to encourage
spontaneous shopping on the way to the dairy case. Market-
ers know we expect to find sale items at the end of the aisle.
Placing not-on-sale items here or at the checkout counter

FOOD GUIDE PYRAMID
A Guide to Daily Food Choices

The Pyramid is an outline of what to eat each day. It's not a rigid prescription, but a general guide that lets you choose a healthful diet that's right for you. The Pyramid calls for eating a variety of foods to get the nutrients you need and at the same time the right amount of calories to maintain a healthy weight.

KEY

These symbols show fats and added sugars in foods.

● Fat (naturally occurring and added)

▼ Sugars (added)

Fats & Sweets
USE SPARINGLY

Milk, Yogurt, & Cheese Group
2-3 SERVINGS

Meat, Poultry, Fish, Dry Beans, Eggs, & Nuts Group
2-3 SERVINGS

Vegetable Group
3-5 SERVINGS

Fruit Group
2-4 SERVINGS

Bread, Cereal, Rice, & Pasta Group.
6-11 SERVINGS

The Food Guide Pyramid emphasizes foods from the five food groups shown in the three lower sections of the Pyramid.

Each of these food groups provides some, but not all, of the nutrients you need. Foods in one group can't replace those in another. No one food group is more important than another—for good health, you need them all.

Source: U.S. DEPARTMENT OF AGRICULTURE and the U.S. DEPARTMENT OF HEALTH AND HUMAN SERVICES

Provided by: the Education Department of the NATIONAL LIVE STOCK AND MEAT BOARD

results in increased sales. Salad dressings placed near the lettuce in the produce section are more likely to be bought than others shelved separately, as are items placed at eye level on store shelves. Studies show that placing a product at eye level can increase sales by 50 percent. Being aware of these practices can start you on the road to savvy shopping.

Fast fact _____

According to a Food Marketing Institute survey, taste, convenience and nutrition are the basic selling points for new food products. In 1992 there were 12,312 new food products introduced. Most of these, 90 percent, were variations of existing products such as new flavors; only 10 percent are truly new items.

Shopping Strategies

Shop with a list whenever you can.

Larger sizes are usually, but not always, a better value. A half gallon of milk costs less than two quart containers, but it's a bargain only if you'll use it up before it spoils.

Prices on store brands can be as much as 50 percent less than the least expensive brand-name competitor, but usually result in savings of 10 to 25 percent. Check this out by comparing the unit cost (price per ounce or per pound) of the store brand and your favorite. Also check out the quality of store brands. You may find them improved over the last time you used them.

Watch out for sale items, especially in the case of produce. You may not be able to use them up before they spoil. Other sale items with freshness dates may be near the end of their shelf life.

Get familiar with the layout of the store you shop in most often. Grocery shoppers spend an average of $1.33

for every minute they remain in the store. Up to a point, the more time spent looking for an item, the more they will buy.

It pays to stoop down to lower shelves when grocery shopping. The high-profit items are at eye level and you'll find the lower mark-up products down below.

Cents-off coupons can save you money if they don't encourage you to buy items you wouldn't ordinarily use. Manufacturers offer cents-off coupons to promote use of their products. If you use them when the supermarket doubles the value or when an item is on sale, you can save even more. You will be seeing more and more of point-of-purchase coupons. Look for them in shelf dispensers or at the checkout counter.

Fast fact _____

Cents-off coupons you get as inserts in newspapers have a redemption rate of 2 to 3 percent. Those distributed in shelf dispensers have redemption rates of 17 percent.

Remember that you pay for convenience. An unsliced loaf of Italian bread costs less than one that is sliced and has a garlic-flavored spread. You may be willing to pay for preparation time saved but, on the other hand, you may prefer to slice and flavor the bread yourself and save money.

Convenience foods like canned vegetables, frozen juice concentrates and packaged mixes for muffins and cakes **can be real time-savers** and save you from having to keep on hand supplies of ingredients you rarely use.

Men and Women in the Supermarket

◇

While male shoppers in the supermarket are still in the minority, their numbers are increasing. A 1993 report by *Progressive Grocer* magazine found 19 percent of the men surveyed said they were the primary grocery shopper, compared with 14 percent in 1988. Other studies report that as many as one-third of the weekend shoppers are men.

Men and women tend to buy different items. Men, especially younger ones, buy beer, cupcakes, ice cream and hot dogs. Women buy more cottage cheese, refrigerated yogurt and salad dressing. Single male shoppers and men who head families grocery shop more times a week than women. They also tend to shop at the last minute and when they are hungry so that they are more susceptible to impulse buying. And men are less likely to use cents-off coupons—30 percent of men compared to 75 percent of women.

FOOD LABELING

In May 1994 the new food labeling law took effect but Americans have always been label conscious. According to a 1994 survey done by the Calorie Control Council, 62 percent of adults said they always try to check nutrition labels of foods to determine the fat content. Almost as many check for calorie content.

Louis W. Sullivan, M.D., then secretary of the Department of Health and Human Services, initiated the food labeling

The New Food Label at a Glance

The new food label will carry an up-to-date, easier-to-use nutrition information guide, to be required on almost all packaged foods (compared to about 60 percent of products up till now). The guide will serve as a key to help in planning a healthy diet.*

Serving sizes are now more consistent across product lines, are stated in both household and metric measures, and reflect the amounts people actually eat.

The list of nutrients covers those most important to the health of today's consumers, most of whom need to worry about getting too much of certain nutrients (fat, for example), rather than too few vitamins or minerals, as in the past.

The label of larger packages may now tell the number of calories per gram of fat, carbohydrate, and protein.

New title signals that the label contains the newly required information.

Calories from fat are now shown on the label to help consumers meet dietary guidelines that recommend people get no more than 30 percent of the calories in their overall diet from fat.

% Daily Value shows how a food fits into the overall daily diet.

Daily Values are also something new. Some are maximums, as with fat (65 grams or less); others are minimums, as with carbohydrate (300 grams or more). The daily values for a 2,000- and 2,500-calorie diet must be listed on the label of larger packages.

Nutrition Facts

Serving Size 1 cup (228g)
Servings Per Container 2

Amount Per Serving

Calories 260   Calories from Fat 120

	% Daily Value*
Total Fat 13g	**20%**
Saturated Fat 5g	**25%**
Cholesterol 30mg	**10%**
Sodium 660mg	**28%**
Total Carbohydrate 31g	**10%**
Dietary Fiber 0g	**0%**
Sugars 5g	
Protein 5g	

Vitamin A 4%	•	Vitamin C 2%
Calcium 15%	•	Iron 4%

* Percent Daily Values are based on a 2,000 calorie diet. Your daily values may be higher or lower depending on your calorie needs:

	Calories:	2,000	2,500
Total Fat	Less than	65g	80g
Sat Fat	Less than	20g	25g
Cholesterol	Less than	300mg	300mg
Sodium	Less than	2,400mg	2,400mg
Total Carbohydrate		300g	375g
Dietary Fiber		25g	30g

Calories per gram:
Fat 9 • Carbohydrate 4 • Protein 4

* This label is only a sample. Exact specifications are in the final rules.
Source: Food and Drug Administration, 1994

reform. "I strongly believe the American consumer should have full access to information that will help them make informed choices about the food they eat. Simply put, the American consumer should be able to read and understand food labels." The new, expanded nutrition label called "Nutrition Facts" is found on almost all packaged foods (see page xxiii).

In a study of reactions to the new label, two-thirds of the shoppers preferred it to the old one. The labels are designed to show how a food fits into the daily diet. They also make it easier to compare one food with another. The amount of calories in a serving (serving size now closely reflects the amounts people actually eat) and the calories from fat are given in numbers. Total fat, cholesterol, sodium, total carbohydrate and dietary fiber are given both as numbers and as percentages of Daily Value (DV).

Daily Values are the label reference numbers. These numbers are set by the government and are based on current nutrition recommendations. The Percent Daily Values are based on a 2,000-calorie diet; values can also be given for an optional 2,500-calorie diet. While these calorie levels cover the average intake of most people, they do not cover everybody. The nutrients listed on the label are the ones that are important for good health; too much of some and too little of others may lead to increased risk for certain diseases. It really isn't necessary to worry about nutrition values for each food you eat or even each meal you eat. What you should aim for most of the time are those foods that give you more carbohydrates, vitamins, minerals and fiber and less sodium, fat, saturated fat and cholesterol.

The Daily Values for total fat, saturated fat, cholesterol and sodium set upper limits on the amount to eat each day to stay healthy. Other DVs help you identify the best levels to aim for each day. This applies to total carbohydrates, fiber, vitamins and minerals.

Loopholes in the Labels

Although the new labeling laws can help guide consumers in making better food choices, they are not perfect. So many issues were involved in formulating labels that accurately represent the nutritional value of different foods that, even with the concerted effort of experts, there remain some gray areas.

Because of an exemption, 2% milk may continue to call itself "low fat" even though it doesn't meet the new FDA definition which limits this designation to 3 grams of fat in a serving. A glass of 2% milk may contain up to 5 grams of fat.

Trans fatty acids are formed when liquid oils are hardened (hydrogenated) to form solid shortenings. These trans fatty acids are found in margarine, chips, crackers, cookies and other processed foods made from hardened fat. Trans fats are included in the "total fat" category on nutrition labels. Under the labeling law, the manufacturer must list the amount of total fat, saturated fat and cholesterol in a food, but not the amount of trans fat. Recent research suggests that trans fat could be responsible for 30,000 deaths from heart disease each year in the U.S. because it raises blood cholesterol the same way saturated fats do. Some experts, however, believe that more studies are needed to clarify the dangers of trans fatty acids.

Fresh meats and poultry are not required to have individual nutrition labels. However, the meat industry is participating in a voluntary program in which supermarkets will display posters showing nutrition information on the most popular cuts.

Rules about the use of the word "healthy" on food labels will not go into effect until 1996. To be labeled as "healthy," foods will have to contain low levels of fat and saturated fat, limited amounts of sodium and cholesterol and at least some amount of a beneficial nutrient, like vitamin C.

Businesses that produce 600,000 or fewer units of food a year are exempt from nutrition labeling rules. These are generally local businesses like a cider mill or small regional bakery. That number will drop to 100,000 units in a few years.

Foods in small packages like Life Savers and snack-size candies don't need nutrition labels but must list a telephone number or address where consumers can get the required information. Also exempt are food products like coffee, tea, some spices and flavorings that contain no significant amounts of any nutrient. Ready-to-eat foods from the deli or bakery prepared on-site and take-out foods also do not need labeling.

What the Label Claims Really Mean

The new FDA-required labels mean you'll no longer have to guess what it means when you see a nutrition claim like *low sodium* or *fat free* on a package. Now these claims can be used only when the food meets strict government definitions.

Label Claim	Label Language Definition*
Calorie Free	• less than 5 calories
Low Calorie	• 40 calories or less
Light or Lite	• ⅓ fewer calories *or* 50% less fat; if more than half the calories are from fat, fat content must be reduced by 50% or more

*Per Reference Amount (standard serving size). Some claims have higher nutrient levels for main dish products and meal products such as frozen entrees and dinners.

Label Claim	Label Language Definition
Light in Sodium	• 50% less sodium than previous standard for the product
Less Sodium or Reduced in Sodium	• 25% less sodium than previous standard for the product
Fat Free	• less than ½ gram fat
Low Fat	• 3 grams or less fat (except for milk, which can contain 5 grams)
Cholesterol Free	• less than 2 milligrams cholesterol and 2 grams or less saturated fat
Low Cholesterol	• 20 milligrams or less cholesterol and 2 grams or less saturated fat
Sodium Free and Salt Free	• Less than 5 milligrams sodium
Very Low Sodium	• 35 milligrams or less sodium
Low Sodium	• 140 milligrams or less sodium
High Fiber	• 5 grams or more fiber
Excellent or High source of a nutrient	• must supply at least 20% of the Daily Value of the nutrient
Good source of a nutrient	• must supply between 10 and 19% of the Daily Value of the nutrient
Lean meat, poultry, seafood, packaged meals	• less than 10 grams of fat, 4 grams of saturated fat, 95 milligrams of cholesterol
Extra lean meat, poultry, seafood, packaged meals	• less than 5 grams of fat, 2 grams of saturated fat and 95 milligrams of cholesterol

Health Claims

In the past you may have seen health claims on labels suggesting that a product could help prevent a specific disease. Today health claims on food labels are regulated. A food must meet certain nutrient levels to make a health claim and only seven types of health claims are allowed—where research supports a link between the nutrient and the disease.

HEALTH CLAIMS ALLOWED ON LABELS

Calcium and Osteoporosis (adult bone loss)
Sodium and High Blood Pressure (hypertension)
Dietary Fat and Cancer
Dietary Saturated Fat and Cholesterol and Risk of Coronary Heart Disease
Fruits and Vegetables and Cancer
Fiber-Containing Grain Products, Fruits and Vegetables and Cancer
Fruits, Vegetables and Grain Products that Contain Fiber and Risk of Coronary Heart Disease

A label may not make a health claim for a specific nutrient in a food if the food also contains other nutrients that would lessen the health benefits. So while a container of skim milk can make a health claim for its calcium content, a container of whole milk cannot, because even though it contains calcium, it also has a lot of fat, which increases the risk for other diseases. Foods that have more than 13 grams of fat, 4 grams of saturated fat, 60 milligrams of cholesterol or 480 milligrams of sodium per serving and have a nutrient claim for a different nutrient must carry the following statement: "See (appropriate panel) for information about (nutrient requiring disclosure) and other nutrients." Because of the complex rules governing putting health claims on labels, experts believe they will not be widely used.

Summing Up: While the new food labels may not be perfect, they are beneficial because so many foods will now be required to display them and serving sizes are now standardized to make comparisons easier. Rather than trying to interpret every fact, concentrate on what is important. The values for carbohydrate, fiber, vitamins A and C, calcium and iron should be high, while the values for total fat, saturated fat, cholesterol and sodium should be low.

Fast fact _____

The American Dietetic Association's National Center for Nutrition and Dietetics has a consumer hotline for food labeling information and materials. Call 800-366-1655.

SECTIONS OF THE SUPERMARKETS

The Bread Box

The experts urge us to eat whole grains. They have all the vitamins, minerals and fiber originally found in grain. Many of these important nutrients are lost when the grains are refined. Some nutrients, vitamins B^1 (thiamin), B^2 (riboflavin), niacin and the mineral iron are added to refined grains, which are then called "enriched." Refined, enriched wheat is the kind usually used to make white bread.

You can't always tell by color whether or not bread is made with whole grains. Some wheat breads look toasty brown but the color is not from whole wheat flour. Caramel (browned sugar), molasses or raisin juice can add rich brown color. The ingredient list on the label will tell you which grains are in the bread. The one listed first is the major grain in the bread, cereal or cracker.

Bread labeled 100 percent whole wheat contains only whole wheat flour. But even when a bread is not 100 percent whole wheat it can still be nutritious. Wheat germ, cracked wheat, oatmeal, sprouted wheat, bran breads and enriched breads are also good sources of nutrients. You may enjoy the flavor of pumpernickel and rye breads which are mixtures of white flour and smaller amounts of whole grains.

What Kinds of Bread Do We Use?

◇

A recent study shows that half of U.S. households use white bread. This is down from three-fourths just 10 years ago. Americans have expanded their tastes in bread:

    49.2% use white bread
    43.8% use whole wheat
    16.4% use 100% whole grain
    16.4% use French/Italian
    12.2% use low-calorie/light
    11.9% use rye/pumpernickel
    10.6% use raisin
    10.5% use sourdough
    9.3% use fiber/high fiber
    8.7% use oat/oat bran

Cereals

Cereals can be hot, cooked in a pan or in the microwave or cold ready-to-eat. They're rich in nutrients, fill you up and are usually low in fat too. If your favorites have a lot of sugar added (you can tell when you see sugar listed as one of the first ingredients), mix it with cereal that contains less sugar.

Note: Some cereals that contain fruit or fruit juice and have more than four grams (one teaspoon) of sugar in a serving may still be good choices. They may look like they're high in sugar but the sugars in the dried fruit or juice are counted in on the label with the added sugar.

Crackers

The cracker shelf is one of the largest and most varied

shelves in the supermarket. For a healthy snack try some of the new reduced-fat varieties. Rice cakes (spicy Mexican style is great), bagel chips, bread sticks, saltines and soda crackers are usually good low-fat choices, but don't forget old-fashioned graham crackers for a sweet treat.

Other Grains

There are many types of delicious grains. Besides regular white, enriched rice, you'll find long grain, short grain, wild rice (not really rice at all), barley, buckwheat (kasha), bulgur, cracked wheat, millet, cornmeal, and quinoa, to name some of the most usual grains available. All can be cooked in an hour or less. If you start soaking them early in the day, you can often cut the cooking time. Package labels give cooking directions.

Summing Up: The Food Pyramid, the new U.S. Department of Agriculture and U.S. Department of Health and Human Services' guide for choosing a good diet (see page xix for the Food Guide Pyramid) recommends eating six to eleven servings from the Bread and Cereal Group each day. A serving is one slice of bread, four crackers, one ounce of ready-to-eat cereal, one half cup of hot cereal, pasta, rice, bulgur or other grains. Studies show that only 5 percent of Americans eat the minimum six grain servings recommended.

The Dairy Case

Choose low-fat or skim milk. Skim milk has all the vitamins and minerals you get in whole milk minus the fat. Whole milk is best for children under two or three. The same holds true for yogurt, with low-fat or fat-free versions best for everyday use.

Milk is 93 percent water so it is easy for bacteria, yeasts and molds to grow in it. That's why milk should be kept cold at all times. Keep the milk container or bottle in the refrigerator. Ultrapasteurized milk is treated at an ultrahigh temperature to kill off the bacteria that cause spoilage and therefore makes milk last longer.

Also in the dairy case is a large selection of reduced-fat cheeses. Try them to see which ones you like best as an alternative to regular cheese, which is high in fat and should be used in smaller amounts.

Summing Up: The Food Guide Pyramid recommends two to three servings from the Milk, Yogurt & Cheese Group each day. Teens, young adults and women who are pregnant

---

Pick Up Some Culture

◇

Bacterial cultures are what causes milk to ferment and makes yogurt yogurt. Research suggests that yogurt containing live bacteria has health benefits. These bacteria seem to boost the immune system helping to prevent colon cancer. Yogurt has also been shown to help prevent diarrhea and canker sores. The types with active cultures are well tolerated by some people who cannot handle the sugar in milk (lactose) and are therefore a good source of calcium. Some yogurt makers pasteurize yogurt after the bacteria is added, killing the cultures and eliminating any possible health benefits.

If you want live cultures, look for a label that states "active yogurt cultures," "live yogurt cultures" or "cultured after pasteurization."

---

or breastfeeding need three servings. The average American has only one serving a day. A serving is one cup of milk, buttermilk or yogurt, one and a half cups light ice cream, one and a half ounces hard cheese or two ounces processed cheese. It takes two cups of cottage cheese to equal the calcium in one cup of milk, so it's not the best milk replacement.

Fruits and Vegetables

Even though fresh fruits and vegetables account for only about 10 percent of grocery sales, surveys show that customers often decide where to shop based on the quality of the produce section. Fruits and vegetables are no longer seasonal. You can now buy almost all kinds year-round. At any one time your supermarket may stock apples from New Zealand, grapes from Chile, melons from Israel and mangoes from Peru.

But remember, buying fruits and vegetables in season means lower prices and better quality. Medium-size fruits are a better buy than larger sizes and you pay a premium price for jumbo because they are scarce.

Prepared produce like precut melons, prewashed salad ingredients, celery or carrot sticks cost much more. A pound of whole carrots may cost as little as 35 cents, the price of precut carrot sticks climbs to almost $2.00 a pound, but the time saved may be well worth the cost.

Note: The Nutrition Facts Panel on dried fruit may lead you to believe that prunes, for example, contain a lot of added sugar. In fact, there is no added sugar. The 11 grams of sugar (almost three teaspoons) in six prunes is all natural sugar. The nutrition label does not distinguish between added sugar and natural sugar. Read the ingredient listing to see if there is any sugar added. When no sugar is listed, all the sugar is natural to the food.

Fruit and vegetable juices are good sources of vitamins and minerals but they do not contain all the fiber from the original fruit. They are available as frozen concentrates, ready to use from the dairy case, and in shelf stable containers (box drinks). Don't confuse pure juice with juice drinks. They are not the same. Pure juice contains 100 percent fruit juice, while juice drinks can contain as little as 10 to 30 percent real juice. In addition these drinks contain water and added sugar.

The federal labeling law requires that the percentage of actual fruit juice or vegetable juice in a drink, punch, ade or cocktail be shown on the label. You will find it on the side nutrition panel of juice packages. Because it is not on the front and it may be in small print, you might have to look carefully to find it, but don't let that stop you. Higher percentages of fruit and vegetable juices mean a healthier beverage, richer in vitamins and minerals with less water and usually fewer sweeteners. Many juice drinks cost the same or even more than pure (100 percent) juice even though sugar and water cost less.

Note: Some 100 percent juice drinks contain a large percentage of apple or grape juice in addition to more exotic juices like guava or papaya that lend their names to the beverage.

Summing Up: The Pyramid Food Guide recommends five or more servings of fruits and vegetables a day. Some surveys show that many Americans may not even eat one. It is much easier to meet this guideline if you stock up on ready-to-use fruits and vegetables when you shop.

A serving of fruit is a half grapefruit, one medium apple, banana or orange, one peach, one pear, two plums, twelve cherries, two raw figs, a half cup cooked or canned fruit, a half cup berries, pineapple or melon chunks, a quarter cup dried fruit or three quarters cup of fruit juice.

A serving of vegetables is one small potato, a half cup of cooked vegetables, one small ear of corn, one cup raw, leafy vegetables, or three quarters cup of vegetable juice.

Fast fact

Potatoes that are sprouting can still be used as long as the potatoes are firm. Simply break off the sprouts and peel before cooking.

Does Sex Really Count?

◇

You may have heard the claim that some eggplants are female and others male. This is determined by the shape of the scarlike depression at the blossom end of the vegetable, opposite the stem end. If the scar is round, the eggplant is male, if it's elongated, the eggplant is female. Don't bother examining your eggplant because experts say gender has no effect on the quality of the vegetable.

Variety in the Salad Bowl

Supermarkets now stock a variety of salad greens, in salad bars, prewashed in bags, or as heads of lettuce. Iceberg lettuce has always been popular because of its crispness but if you want greener, leafier or tastier choices that are more nutrient-rich try arugula, Belgian endive, butterhead, radicchio, romaine, chicory, escarole, spinach or watercress.

Arugula—slender green leaves with a peppery flavor; younger, smaller leaves are milder

Belgian endive—bullet-shaped heads are yellow colored so it really is not a green; it is crisp, mildly sharp and flavorful

Butterhead—includes Boston and Bibb, has soft buttery texture with a mild, sweet flavor

Radicchio—colorful red leaves that look like little red cabbages; not as crisp as endive, which it stars with in tricolored salads

Chicory—also called curly endive, its thin, curly leaves are fairly bitter; can be used raw or cooked

Escarole—leaves are wider and flatter than chicory, slightly bitter but the inner leaves tend to be milder; popular in soups; can be used raw

Romaine—very nutritious green often used in Caesar salads

Watercress—small, dark green leaves with a sharp, peppery flavor; used in salads, sandwiches and as a garnish

Meat Case (and Beans Too)

The meat group in the Food Guide Pyramid includes meat, poultry, fish, dry beans, eggs and nuts. Protein is found in all the foods in this group along with iron and other minerals and vitamins. Animal protein foods also supply vitamin B_{12}, while beans are a good source of fiber.

Four ounces of lean, boneless meat, fish or poultry will give three ounces cooked, about the size of a deck of cards. That's plenty, even though it's less than you usually get in a restaurant.

Poultry is often thought of as low in fat, but some like duck and goose are high in fat and should be eaten only once in a while. While chicken is low in fat, the skin is loaded with it. Research shows that cooking chicken with the skin on keeps the meat moist without adding fat, but always remove and discard the skin before you eat the meat.

Choosing Lower Fat Protein Foods

◇

High-fat option	Low-fat option
Porterhouse steak	Flank steak
Rib roast	Eye round
Regular hamburger	Ground meat, 10% or less fat
Spareribs	Center cut pork loin
Frozen breaded fish	Frozen plain fish
Sardines packed in oil	Sardines in mustard sauce
Tuna packed in oil	Tuna packed in water
Refried beans	Plain beans with salsa
Bluefish, mackerel	Scrod, halibut, tuna
Fried chicken	Baked chicken

Note: Bologna, salami, hot dogs and bacon are high in fat and salt. They also contain nitrites that combine with substances found naturally in some foods and in the stomach to form carcinogens (cancer causing substances) called nitrosamines. Use these kinds of processed meats only once in a while. Nuts and seeds, which are members of the meat group, are good sources of protein but are high in fat. Eat small amounts of these.

The mandatory nutrition labeling requirements established by the labeling act do not apply to fresh meat, including ground beef, poultry and seafood. The meat industry is participating in the voluntary nutrition labeling program in which brochures and posters in supermarkets will offer consumers the same information for fresh meat that is required on packaged foods. In this supplementary material, nutrition information (Nutri-Facts) will be available for 45 commonly consumed meat and poultry cuts and 20 seafood items.

There is a proposal to allow percentages of lean and fat in ground beef to be listed on the package label, provided that nutrition information is available at the point of sale (Nutri-Facts). Nutrition information for three blends of ground beef, ranging from 10 percent to 27 percent fat, will be included in the charts. They will be noted as percent lean and percent fat, so that the ground meat with 10 percent fat will be labeled as 90 percent lean, 10 percent fat. In a survey, four out of ten shoppers chose labels with full descriptions such as Ground Beef 70% Lean/30% Fat.

Fast fact _____
Ham, unlike beef, does not have a lot of marbling. So once the visible fat is trimmed away, you've gotten rid of most of it.

Fast fact _____
The average American ate 14.8 pounds of seafood in 1992. Tuna remained the favorite. The other top nine in order of consumption were shrimp, Alaska pollack (surimi), salmon, cod, catfish, clams, flatfish, crabs, scallops.

Summing Up: The Pyramid Food Guide recommends two to three servings from the Meat, Poultry, Fish, Dry Beans, Eggs & Nuts Group. The average American eats more than two servings from the meat group a day. A serving is equal to three ounces of cooked, lean meat, fish or poultry. One-half cup cooked beans or lentils, two ounces of tofu, two tablespoons of peanut butter, a third cup nuts or one egg can fill in for one ounce of meat.

Why Not Try Tofu?

◇

Ounce for ounce, tofu has just as much protein as meat, is cholesterol free and very low in saturated fat. Because tofu is made from soybeans, it has all the health-giving properties of soy—cholesterol lowering and cancer preventing—that scientists are beginning to learn about.

Tofu can be found in most supermarkets and greengrocers. It is versatile, picking up the flavors of foods it's cooked with. Soft tofu, called silken on the package, can be mashed and used as a substitute for cottage cheese. It can be blended until creamy in a food processor or blender and then substituted for sour cream or mayonnaise in dips. Firm tofu can be sliced and marinated in soy sauce, garlic, sesame oil and ginger (try 2 tablespoons of salt-reduced soy sauce, 1 teaspoon of sesame oil, 1 clove of minced garlic and a sprinkle of ginger) and then stir-fried or, even tastier, broiled for a flavorful meat substitute.

Snacks

Many snacks fall into the fats, oils and sweets food group. This group makes up the tip, the smallest part of the Food Guide Pyramid. Instead of a recommended number of servings, the advice given is to use these foods sparingly. Most of us enjoy high-sugar, high-fat snacks like soda, chips, cookies, cake, ice cream and candy. Considered fun foods, they are often used as a treat or reward, as a cure for boredom as well as a quick way to satisfy hunger. Americans are such eager snackers that over 300 new snack items are introduced every year!

Eating these foods is not the issue, the amount you eat is. Have a snack-size candy bar, not a regular size. Try a coffee cup instead of a soup bowl full of ice cream, an individual bag of chips rather than the giant economy size, a cupcake instead of a large slice of cake.

Choose cookies that snap instead of bend or fruit bars for low-fat choices; air-popped popcorn or pretzels rather than chips. Lower fat versions of your favorite chips are becoming available, look for them.

Americans love candy; we each eat an average of 20 pounds a year! Try some licorice, jelly beans, candy corn or marshmallows. All these are sweet, low-fat treats. Hard candies and lollipops provide long-lasting, low-fat, sweet snacking.

Fast fact _____

Each package of Mars M&M's contains exactly the same percentage of each color: 30 percent brown, 20 percent yellow, 20 percent red, 10 percent orange, 10 percent green, 10 percent tan.

Ice cream should be a sometimes food. While it does contain some calcium, it also has lots of fat, saturated fat and cholesterol. Look for lower fat or fat-free varieties. Or look for lower fat frozen desserts like light ice cream or frozen yogurt. But don't think of light ice cream or frozen yogurt as equivalent to milk or regular yogurt. Most frozen flavors are higher in sugar and fat and lower in calcium. Sorbet and ices are refreshing alternatives, but don't count on them for calcium.

Pastries like pies, Danish pastries, croissants and donuts can be very high in fat. They're all once-in-a-while snacks.

Even muffins, often thought of as a healthy substitute for pastries, can be high in fat. Look for muffins that are labeled low-fat or have a bagel with jelly instead.

Americans drink a lot of soda, $47.3 billion worth a year. This is almost three times the amount spent on milk. One ounce of soda contains about one teaspoon of sugar, so the usual 12 ounces contains 12 teaspoons. Colas and some fruit-flavored sodas often contain caffeine too. Instead of soda, try plain sparkling water (mixed half and half with fruit juice), mineral water or iced tea for a change.

Fast fact

U.S. coffee consumption averaged 26.5 gallons per person in 1992.

Deep Freeze

Frozen fruits and vegetables are a quick and convenient way to add vitamins and minerals to meals. Most of the time, stay away from those that are sauced, buttered and sugared. You can add your own flavorings and toppings, as little or as much as you like, suiting your taste and saving money at the same time. Frozen potatoes are popular, but reading the labels is important because many are high in fat and should be reserved for sometime use.

Instead of complete dinners, use frozen entrees—pasta dishes, pizza, tacos, chicken or fish, pancakes or waffles—convenience foods you can use as the base for a quick meal. Simply add a salad or fresh fruit, some bread and a beverage.

Fast fact

Bird's Eye frozen vegetables got their start back in 1929 when the old Postum Co., now Kraft, acquired quick freezing machinery from a former fur trader, Clarence Birdseye.

Fast fact _____

Frozen dinners have come a long way since they were introduced as TV dinners in 1954. In fact, the name TV dinner is no longer used on the package and the packaging now is microwaveable instead of the original sectioned aluminum tray. The popularity of frozen dinners continues, with sales of more than 1.3 billion dollars in 1993.

SO THAT THERE'S ALWAYS SOMETHING TO EAT

Fast fact _____

In a study of daily activities of over 10,000 people, cooking ranked seventh among the 16 most common activities. It was outranked only by lovemaking, socializing, talking, eating, engaging in sports, and shopping.

Sometimes you just may be too tired to eat out or even take in or order in. Even though there are no leftovers from yesterday, you can easily put together a quick, satisfying meal when you keep your refrigerator and cabinets stocked with foods we used to call staples.

Use the following list for a start, adding your own special favorites. You'll never have to complain again about there being nothing to eat.

FREEZER

Bread: sliced loaf, tortillas or pita
    Made in Minutes: bagel pizza, salad pita, grilled cheese
Vegetables: green peas, mixed vegetables, corn
    Made in Minutes: peas and pasta
Fruit: strawberries, raspberries
    Made in Minutes: fruit cup, topping for angel food cake
Frozen juice and juice drinks
Frozen low-fat yogurt

Meat and Poultry: hamburger or turkey patties, chicken pieces, boneless chicken breast
  Made in Minutes: creamed chicken (use canned cream soup)

REFRIGERATOR

Cheese: your favorite hard cheese, grated cheese
Eggs
Butter or other spread
Vegetables, onions, carrots

CUPBOARD

Canned tomatoes: crushed, stewed, sauce
Pasta, rice
Canned beans: chickpeas, black beans, blackeye peas, baked beans
Oil: olive and another vegetable like corn or canola
Vinegar: try flavored*
Catsup
Soy sauce
Salsa*
Anchovy or sundried tomato paste*
Bread crumbs
Dried fruit: raisins, prunes, apricots
Nuts: walnuts or your favorites
Shelf-stable or evaporated milk
Dried mushrooms*
Spices: cinnamon, ginger, oregano, paprika, curry powder, dried garlic, seasoned pepper
Bouillon cubes
Canned soup: chicken broth, cream soup*
Cereal: Oatmeal and ready-to-eat
Jam or jelly
Sugar
Popcorn, unpopped
Tea
Coffee

*A small amount of these add a punch of flavor

Fast fact _____

You love garlic, know that it's good for you but hate the thought of "garlic breath"? Try chewing on fresh parsley, roasted coffee beans, fresh mint, cardamom or caraway seeds.

Fast fact _____

For a healthful meal, fill three-quarters of your plate with vegetables, beans, lentils, bread, pasta, rice, grains and fruits, and the other quarter fill with lean meat, fish, poultry or protein alternatives like nuts, eggs or tofu.

HANDLING FOOD SAFELY

To keep food at its best in flavor and nutrition and avoid food poisoning, it must be handled and stored carefully. When you're loading your cart in the supermarket, it's a good idea to pick up cold and frozen foods last. Cold food should feel cold and frozen food should be solid. Pack them together in one double bag so they have less chance to thaw out on the way home. And get them home fast. Canned foods should be free of dents, rust, cracks and bulges which can indicate food spoilage. Look for the use-by date on packaged foods and don't buy any that you can't use by this time.

Be sure the temperature of your refrigerator and freezer is kept cold enough. Refrigerators should be at 40°F, as cold as possible without freezing milk or vegetables. The freezer should be at 0°F, keeping the contents frozen hard. Unpack and refrigerate or freeze as soon as you get home. If you can't use meat, poultry or fish within two days, freeze immediately.

Fast fact _____

Forget the myth that dishes prepared with mayonnaise are more likely to spoil in the heat. Foods with mayonnaise are actually safer because of its high acid level.

There is a time limit for storage of all foods. Even canned foods that look like they last forever are best when used within one year. Rotate canned and frozen foods so that the older ones are used up first. You may have noticed that more packaged foods now show a date on their label. Sometimes only a date appears, as on milk and juice containers, other times the statement "best when purchased by (date)" or "sell by (date)" is on condiments, salad dressings and bakery goods. "Use by" is on box drinks, jelly and cereals. Some products have expiration dates which indicate the end of their shelf life. Depending on the product, there is a reasonable time to use it after the sell date before it stales or spoils. Of course, the way the food has been handled before it is sold in the store will affect the length of time it remains usable. It's always best to buy food in a store that has a rapid turnover of products.

A good food rule is, "When in doubt, throw it out." When you see mold on cottage cheese or other soft cheeses, sour cream, yogurt, bread, cake and other baked goods, grains, cooked dried beans or peas or corn on the cob, toss them. Small, moldy spots can be cut away from hard cheese, firm fruits and vegetables like carrots, peppers and cabbage. When you cut the mold away, cut at least one inch around and below the spot. Store the food in a clean container and use it as soon as you can. You can also scoop out tiny spots of mold from jellies. Be careful to scoop out a larger amount around the mold. Pure maple syrup that has become moldy can simply be boiled and used.

The high temperatures of cooking will kill most of the bacteria that cause food-borne illness. Ground meat must be cooked thoroughly, until it is gray, not pink, in the middle, particularly if children, elderly persons or people with compromised immune systems will be eating the meat. Several deaths of children have been reported recently that were due to eating undercooked ground meat from cattle carrying a deadly strain of E. coli bacteria. Thorough cooking of the ground meat will kill the bacteria.

Once cooked, keep the food hot (above 140°F) until it is served. Don't keep cooked foods at room temperature for longer than two hours. Don't cool warm leftovers on the kitchen counter before refrigerating. Thaw perishable foods in the refrigerator or microwave, not at room temperature.

Fast fact

Hot seafood cocktail sauce was found to disinfect the raw oysters it was served on. Horseradish and lemon juice also killed off some bacteria but were not as effective as Tabasco and other hot sauces.

SAFE TIME LIMITS FOR REFRIGERATOR OR FREEZER STORAGE

FOOD	CABINET	REFRIGERATOR	FREEZER
Berries		1–2 days	
Brownie & Cake mixes	9 months		
Chicken, fresh		1–2 days	9 months
Canned foods	12 months		
Dried peas and beans	12 months		
Egg substitutes, opened		3 days	Don't freeze
Eggs		3 weeks	Don't freeze
Fish (cod, sole)		1–2 days	6 months
Fish (salmon)		1–2 days	2–3 months
Flour	6–8 months		
Frozen dinners			3–4 months
Ground meat		1–2 days	3–4 months
Half & half		10 days	
Ham slices		3–4 days	1–2 months
Herbs, dried	6 months		
Hot dogs, luncheon meat, unopened		1 week	1–2 months
Jellies			
unopened	12 months		
opened		3 months	
Mayonnaise			
unopened	2–3 months		
opened		2 months	

FOOD	CABINET	REFRIGERATOR	FREEZER
Meat leftovers		3–4 days	
Milk		5 days	
Pasta	2 years		
Popcorn kernels	2 years		
Potatoes	2–3 months		
Rice, white	2 years		
Salad dressing			
unopened	10–12 months		
opened		3 months	
Salad oil, opened	1–3 months		
Sauce & Gravy mix	6–12 months		
Shrimp			
fresh		1 day	
frozen			12 months
Soups & stews		3–4 days	2–3 months
Spices (basil, cinnamon, thyme, chili powder, parsley flakes, paprika, etc.)	1 year		
Steaks, chops		3–5 days	6–9 months
Sugar			
white	2 years		
brown	4 months		
Syrup	12 months		
Tea bags	18 months		

Food Poisoning

◇

Every year more than 7 million Americans get food poisoning. Symptoms include nausea, vomiting, diarrhea, fever and cramps. They can begin anywhere from 30 minutes to as long as two weeks after the bad food was eaten, but most times symptoms occur within 4 to 48 hours. Sometimes symptoms are very severe. If the person is very young, pregnant, or already ill, call a doctor or go to an emergency room right away.

Fast fact ————————————————————

Although hot dogs are processed meat, they should not be eaten uncooked. A study found that 20 percent of major brand hot dogs contained bacteria that could lead to serious illness in young children, pregnant women, the elderly and people with weakened immune systems. Cooking the hot dogs until they are steaming hot throughout will kill the bacteria.

Safe Handling Instructions for Fresh Meat and Poultry

As of July 1994, the Department of Agriculture required fresh meat and poultry to be labeled with safe handling instructions. The safe handling instruction label was developed to help consumers prevent food-borne illness at home. It covers four safety guidelines: safety, cross-contamination, cooking and handling leftovers.

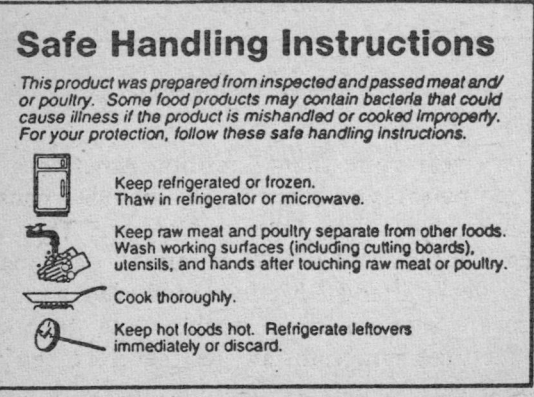

Safe Handling Instructions

This product was prepared from inspected and passed meat and/ or poultry. Some food products may contain bacteria that could cause illness if the product is mishandled or cooked improperly. For your protection, follow these safe handling instructions.

Keep refrigerated or frozen.
Thaw in refrigerator or microwave.

Keep raw meat and poultry separate from other foods. Wash working surfaces (including cutting boards), utensils, and hands after touching raw meat or poultry.

Cook thoroughly.

Keep hot foods hot. Refrigerate leftovers immediately or discard.

USING YOUR SUPERMARKET
NUTRITION COUNTER

Shoppers average just over two trips a week to the supermarket. It doesn't matter if you shop at Safeway, Kroger, A&P, Publix, Associated, Winn-Dixie, Grand Union or Balducci's in New York, this book lists the calories, fat, cholesterol, sodium and fiber of most of the 16,000 foods you'll find there. For the first time, information about these nutrient values is at your fingertips. Now you will find it easy to follow a healthy diet. Before *The Supermarket Nutrition Counter* it was impossible to compare so many foods at one time. For example, when you want to select bread, look up the bread category on page 46. You will find over 250 different breads listed so you can see which one is the best source of carbohydrate and fiber.

The Supermarket Nutrition Counter lists the calories, fat, carbohydrate, sodium, and fiber values. These are key nutrients for good health. Fat and sodium should be limited while carbohydrate and fiber should be increased. The 1990 food labeling act has established guidelines for nutrient intakes. It recommends that a diet of 2,000 calories a day should include at least 300 grams of carbohydrate and 25 grams of dietary fiber and less than 65 grams of total fat and 2400 milligrams of sodium.

In *The Supermarket Nutrition Counter* foods are listed alphabetically. For each group, you will find brand-name foods listed first in alphabetical order, followed by an alphabetical listing of generic foods. The generic listing will help to determine nutrition values for foods when you do not find your favorite brand listed. They also help you to evaluate generic and store brands. Large categories are divided into subcategories such as canned, fresh, frozen and ready-to-use to make it easier to find what you are looking for. Many categories have take-out and home recipe subcategories. Look there for foods you buy at the supermarket that have been prepared there and so do not need to be nutrition labeled. One out of seven shoppers (15 percent) buys take-out foods. *The Supermarket Nutrition Counter* has over eight hundred take-out items for you to choose from to make it easier for you to evaluate these foods.

Most foods are listed alphabetically. But, in some cases, foods are grouped by category. For example, pasta dinners, like spaghetti and meat balls, lasagna and manicotti, are all found under the category PASTA DISHES. Other group categories include:

Fast fact ———————————————————————

Although Orville Redenbacher and Sara Lee are real people, as was the late Duncan Hines, there is no Betty Crocker, Mrs. Paul or Chef Boyardee.

DEFINITIONS

as prep (as prepared): refers to food that has been prepared according to package directions

cooked: refers to food cooked without the addition of fat (oil, butter, margarine, etc.); steaming, poaching, broiling and dry roasting are examples of this type of preparation

generic: describes a food without a brand name

home recipe: describes homemade dishes; those included can be used as guide to the cholesterol and calorie values of similar products you may prepare or take-out food you buy ready-to-eat

lean and fat: describes meat with some fat on its edges that is not cut away before cooking or poultry prepared with skin and fat as purchased

lean only: lean portion, trimmed of all visible fat

shelf stable or **shelf ready:** refers to prepared products found on the supermarket shelf that are ready to be heated and do not require refrigeration

take-out: describes prepared dishes that you purchase ready-to-eat; those included serve as a guide to the sodium and calorie values of similar products you may purchase

trace (tr): value used when a food contains less than one calorie or less than one mg of sodium

ABBREVIATIONS

ave	=	average
diam	=	diameter
frzn	=	frozen
g	=	gram
in	=	inch
lb	=	pound
lg	=	large
med	=	medium
mg	=	milligram
oz	=	ounce
pkg	=	package
pkt	=	packet
prep	=	prepared
pt	=	pint
reg	=	regular
serv	=	serving
sm	=	small
sq	=	square
tbsp	=	tablespoon
tr	=	trace
tsp	=	teaspoon
w/	=	with
w/o	=	without
<	=	less than

EQUIVALENT MEASURES

Dry

3 teaspoons	=	1 tablespoon
4 tablespoons	=	¼ cup
8 tablespoons	=	½ cup
12 tablespoons	=	¾ cup
16 tablespoons	=	1 cup
1000 milligrams	=	1 gram
28 grams	=	1 ounce
4 ounces	=	¼ pound
8 ounces	=	½ pound
12 ounces	=	¾ pound
16 ounces	=	1 pound

Liquid

2 tablespoons	=	1 ounce
2 ounces	=	¼ cup
4 ounces	=	½ cup
6 ounces	=	¾ cup
8 ounces	=	1 cup
2 cups	=	1 pint
2 pints	=	1 quart

NOTE

Discrepancies in figures are due to rounding, product reformulation and reevaluation. Labeling law allows rounding of values. Because most of the data is analysis data, obtained directly from manufacturers—not from labels—in some cases our values may not be exactly the same as label information because they have not been rounded.

All Total Fat, Carbohydrate (CARBO) and Fiber* values are given in grams (g).

All Sodium values are given in milligrams (mg).

A dash (—) indicates data was unavailable.

*All fiber values are dietary fiber. Except for sweets, foods that are high in CARBO (pasta, bread, cereals, fruit, and vegetables) also provide dietary fiber. Animal products—eggs, milk, cheese, meat, fish, poultry—are not sources of fiber. Any fiber values indicated for these foods come from added ingredients.

FOOD	PORTION	CAL	FAT	SOD	CARB	FIB
ABALONE						
FRESH						
fried	3 oz	161	6	502	9	—
raw	3 oz	89	1	255	5	—
ACEROLA						
fresh	1	2	tr	0	tr	—
juice	1 cup	51	1	7	12	—
ADZUKI BEANS						
CANNED						
sweetened	1 cup	702	tr	646	163	—
DRIED						
cooked	1 cup	294	tr	18	57	—
READY-TO-USE						
yokan, sliced	3¼-in slices	112	tr	36	26	—
AKEE						
fresh	3.5 oz	223	20	—	5	—
ALE						
see BEER AND ALE, MALT						
ALFALFA						
sprouts	1 cup	40	tr	2	1	—
sprouts	1 tbsp	1	tr	0	tr	—
ALLIGATOR						
tail, cooked	3.5 oz	143	3	—	1	—
ALLSPICE						
ground	1 tsp	5	tr	1	1	—
ALMONDS						
Almond Butter (Erewhon)	1 tbsp (16 g)	90	8	18	2	—
Almond Butter Natural Raw (Hain)	2 tbsp	190	18	120	3	—
Almond Butter Toasted (Hain)	2 tbsp	220	19	210	3	—
Almonds (Beer Nuts)	1 pkg (1 oz)	180	14	51	7	—
Almonds (Planters)	1 oz	170	15	0	6	—
Blanched Slivered (Dole)	1 oz	170	14	4	5	—
Blanched Whole (Dole)	1 oz	170	14	4	5	—
Chopped Natural (Dole)	1 oz	170	14	4	5	—

FOOD	PORTION	CAL	FAT	SOD	CARB	FIB
Honey Roasted (Planters)	1 oz	170	13	180	9	—
Nutella	1 tbsp (0.5 oz)	85	5	5	9	—
Sliced (Planters)	1 oz	170	15	0	6	—
Sliced Natural (Dole)	1 oz	170	14	4	5	—
Slivered (Planters)	1 oz	170	15	0	6	—
Smoked (Lance)	1 pkg	120	11	130	3	—
Whole Natural (Dole)	1 oz	170	14	4	5	—
almond butter, honey & cinnamon	1 tbsp	96	8	2	4	—
almond butter, w/ salt	1 tbsp	101	9	75	3	—
almond butter, w/o salt	1 tbsp	101	10	2	3	—
almond meal	1 oz	116	5	2	8	—
almond paste	1 oz	127	8	3	12	—
dried, blanched	1 oz	166	15	3	5	—
dried, unblanched	1 oz	167	15	3	6	—
dry roasted, unblanched	1 oz	167	15	3	7	—
dry roasted, unblanched, salted	1 oz	167	15	260	7	—
oil roasted, blanched	1 oz	174	16	3	5	3
oil roasted, blanched, salted	1 oz	174	16	3	5	—
oil roasted, unblanched	1 oz	176	16	3	5	—
toasted, unblanched	1 oz	167	14	3	7	3

AMARANTH
see also CEREAL, COOKIES

FOOD	PORTION	CAL	FAT	SOD	CARB	FIB
Amaranth Cereal With Bananas (Health Valley)	½ cup (1 oz)	110	2	5	20	4
Amaranth Crunch With Raisins (Health Valley)	¼ cup (1 oz)	110	3	10	20	3
Amaranth Flakes 100% Organic (Health Valley)	½ cup (1 oz)	90	tr	5	21	3
Fast Menu Amaranth With Garden Vegetables (Health Valley)	7.5 oz	140	3	140	16	8
Seeds (Arrowhead)	¼ cup (1.6 oz)	170	2	0	29	3
cooked	½ cup	59	tr	14	3	—
uncooked	½ cup	366	6	21	65	—

FOOD	PORTION	CAL	FAT	SOD	CARB	FIB
ANASAZI BEANS						
DRIED						
Arrowhead	¼ cup (1.5 oz)	150	1	0	27	9
Bean Cuisine	½ cup	115	1	5	—	5
ANCHOVY						
CANNED						
in oil	1 can (1.6 oz)	95	4	1651	0	—
in oil	5	42	2	734	0	—
FRESH						
raw	3 oz	62	4	88	0	—
ANGLERFISH						
raw	3.5 oz	72	1	109	0	—
ANISE						
seed	1 tsp	7	tr	tr	1	—
ANTELOPE						
roasted	3 oz	127	2	46	0	—
APPLE						
CANNED						
Apple Sauce						
Mott's	4 oz	88	0	—	—	—
Mott's	6 oz	132	0	—	—	—
Chunky (Mott's)	4 oz	57	0	—	—	—
Chunky (Mott's)	6 oz	86	0	—	—	—
Cinnamon (Mott's)	4 oz	72	0	—	—	—
Cinnamon (Mott's)	6 oz	108	0	—	—	—
Fruit Pak, Cherry (Mott's)	3.75 oz	65	0	—	—	—
Fruit Pak, Peach (Mott's)	3.75 oz	70	0	—	—	—
Fruit Pak, Pineapple (Mott's)	3.75 oz	79	0	—	—	—
Fruit Pak, Strawberry (Mott's)	3.75 oz	70	0	—	—	—
Natural (Mott's)	4 oz	44	0	—	—	—
Natural (Mott's)	6 oz	66	0	—	—	—
Natural Packed w/ Apple Juice (White House)	4 oz	60	0	5	14	1
Regular or Chunky (White House)	4 oz	80	0	5	22	1

FOOD	PORTION	CAL	FAT	SOD	CARB	FIB
Apple Sauce *(cont.)*						
Unsweetened (White House)	4 oz	50	0	0	12	2
100% Gravenstein Sweetened (S&W)	½ cup	90	0	10	24	—
100% Gravenstein Unsweetened (S&W)	½ cup	55	0	5	14	—
Cinnamon (Seneca)	½ cup	90	0	—	—	—
Cinnamon (Tree Top)	½ cup	80	0	0	21	—
Cinnamon (White House)	4 oz	100	0	5	25	1
Diet (S&W)	½ cup	55	0	10	14	—
Natural (Seneca)	½ cup	50	0	—	—	—
Natural (Tree Top)	½ cup	60	0	0	15	—
Original (Tree Top)	½ cup	80	0	0	21	—
Regular (Seneca)	½ cup	90	0	—	—	—
Sweetened (S&W)	½ cup	55	0	10	14	—
Unsweetened (S&W)	½ cup	25	2	5	2	—
Escalloped Apples (White House)	4 oz	120	0	10	28	1
Fried Apples (Luck's)	8 oz	190	0	—	—	—
Sliced (White House)	4 oz	55	0	10	15	1
Spiced Apple Rings (White House)	1 ring	25	0	0	6	tr
applesauce sweetened	½ cup	97	tr	4	25	2
applesauce unsweetened	½ cup	53	tr	2	14	2
sliced sweetened	1 cup	136	1	7	34	—
DRIED						
Mariani	¼ cup	150	0	—	—	—
cooked w/ sugar	½ cup	172	tr	27	29	—
cooked w/o sugar	½ cup	116	tr	26	20	—
rings	10	155	tr	56	42	—
FRESH						
Dole	1	80	1	0	18	5
apple	1	81	tr	1	21	3
w/o skin, sliced	1 cup	62	tr	0	16	2
w/o skin, sliced & cooked	1 cup	91	tr	1	23	—
w/o skin, sliced & microwaved	1 cup	96	tr	1	25	—

FOOD	PORTION	CAL	FAT	SOD	CARB	FIB
FROZEN						
Apple Fritters (Mrs. Paul's)	2	270	9	500	35	—
Escalloped (Stouffer's)	1 cup (6 oz)	180	3	70	37	3
sliced w/o sugar	½ cup	41	tr	3	11	—
JUICE						
Bruce Lite	½ cup	88	0	25	20	—
Hi-C Jammin' Apple	8 fl oz	130	0	30	31	—
Juice Works	6 oz	100	0	—	—	—
Kern's Cinnamon Nectar	6 oz	110	0	0	26	—
Libby's Nectar	6 oz	100	0	25	25	—
Minute Maid Box	8.45 fl oz	120	0	30	29	—
Minute Maid Frozen	8 fl oz	110	0	5	28	—
Minute Maid Juices To Go	1 bottle (10 fl oz)	110	0	30	28	—
Minute Maid Juices To Go	1 bottle (16 fl oz)	160	0	40	40	—
Minute Maid Juices To Go	1 can (11.5 fl oz)	140	0	35	35	—
Minute Maid Naturals	8 fl oz	110	0	30	28	—
Mott's	10 oz	148	0	—	—	—
Mott's	6 oz	88	0	—	—	—
Mott's Natural Style	6 oz	88	0	—	—	—
Ocean Spray	8 fl oz	110	0	35	28	0
S&W 100% Unsweetened	6 oz	85	0	5	20	—
Seneca	6 oz	90	0	—	—	—
Seneca, frzn, as prep	6 oz	90	0	—	—	—
Seneca Natural frzn, as prep	6 oz	90	0	—	—	—
Sippin' Pak 100% Pure	8.45 fl oz	110	0	25	28	—
Sipps Apple	8.45 oz	130	0	—	—	—
Tree Top	6 oz	90	0	10	22	—
Tree Top Cider	6 oz	90	0	10	22	—
Tree Top Cider, frzn, as prep	6 oz	90	0	10	22	—
Tree Top frzn, as prep	6 oz	90	0	10	22	—
Tree Top Sparkling Juice	6 oz	90	0	—	22	—
Tree Top Unfiltered	6 oz	90	0	10	22	—
Tree Top Unfiltered, frzn, as prep	6 oz	90	0	10	22	—
Tree Top w/ Vitamin C	6 oz	90	0	10	22	—

FOOD	PORTION	CAL	FAT	SOD	CARB	FIB
Veryfine 100%	8 oz	107	0	<10	27	—
White House	6 oz	90	0	0	22	0
apple juice	1 cup	116	tr	7	29	tr
frzn, as prep	1 cup	111	tr	17	28	—
frzn, not prep	6 oz	349	1	54	87	—

APRICOTS
CANNED

FOOD	PORTION	CAL	FAT	SOD	CARB	FIB
Halves Unsweetened (S&W)	½ cup	35	0	5	9	—
Halves, Diet (S&W)	½ cup	35	0	5	9	—
Halves, Unpeeled In Heavy Syrup (S&W)	½ cup	110	0	15	28	—
Whole, Peeled Diet (S&W)	½ cup	28	0	5	7	—
Whole, Peeled In Heavy Syrup (S&W)	½ cup	100	0	15	26	—
halves, heavy syrup pack w/ skin	1 cup (9.1 oz)	214	tr	10	55	—
halves, water pack w/ skin	1 cup (8.5 oz)	65	tr	7	16	—
halves, water pack w/o skin	1 cup (8 oz)	51	tr	25	12	—
heavy syrup w/ skin	3 halves	70	tr	3	18	—
juice pack w/ skin	3 halves	40	tr	3	10	—
light syrup w/ skin	3 halves	54	tr	3	14	—
puree, juice pack w/ skin	1 cup (8.7 oz)	119	tr	9	31	—
puree, heavy syrup pack w/ skin	¾ cup (9.1 oz)	214	tr	10	55	—
puree, light pack w/ skin	¾ cup (8.9 oz)	160	tr	10	42	—
puree, water pack w/ skin	¾ cup (8.5 oz)	65	tr	7	16	—
water pack w/ skin	3 halves	22	tr	2	5	—
water pack w/o skin	4 halves	20	tr	10	5	—

DRIED

FOOD	PORTION	CAL	FAT	SOD	CARB	FIB
Mariani	¼ cup	140	0	—	—	—
halves	10	83	tr	3	22	3
halves, cooked w/o sugar	½ cup	106	tr	4	27	—

FRESH

FOOD	PORTION	CAL	FAT	SOD	CARB	FIB
apricots	3	51	tr	1	12	—

FROZEN

FOOD	PORTION	CAL	FAT	SOD	CARB	FIB
sweetened	½ cup	119	tr	5	30	—

FOOD	PORTION	CAL	FAT	SOD	CARB	FIB
JUICE						
Kern's Nectar	6 oz	100	0	10	23	—
Libby's Nectar	6 oz	110	0	0	26	—
S&W Nectar	6 oz	35	0	20	12	—
nectar	1 cup	141	tr	9	36	2
ARROWHEAD						
fresh, boiled	1 med (0.33 oz)	9	tr	2	2	—
ARROWROOT						
flour	1 cup	457	tr	2	113	4
ARTICHOKE						
CANNED						
Hearts Marinated (S&W)	½ cup	225	26	15	6	—
FRESH						
Dole	1 lg	23	tr	65	5	3
boiled	1 med (4 oz)	60	tr	114	13	—
hearts, cooked	½ cup	42	tr	80	9	—
jerusalem, raw, sliced	½ cup	57	tr	—	13	—
FROZEN						
Hearts Deluxe (Birds Eye)	½ cup	30	0	40	7	3
cooked	1 pkg (9 oz)	108	1	127	22	—
ARUGULA						
raw	½ cup	2	tr	3	tr	—
ASPARAGUS						
CANNED						
Cut Spears (Owatonna)	½ cup	20	0	—	—	—
Points, Water Pack (S&W)	½ cup	17	0	10	3	—
Spears, Colossal Fancy (S&W)	½ cup	20	0	320	4	—
Spears, Fancy (S&W)	½ cup	18	0	320	3	—
spears	½ cup	24	1	—	3	—
FRESH						
Dole	5 spears	18	0	0	2	2
cooked	½ cup	22	tr	10	4	—
cooked	4 spears	14	tr	7	3	—
raw	½ cup	16	tr	2	3	—
raw	4 spears	14	tr	1	3	—

FOOD	PORTION	CAL	FAT	SOD	CARB	FIB
FROZEN						
Big Valley	2.7 oz	23	tr	0	4	—
Cut (Birds Eye)	½ cup	23	0	5	4	—
Harvest Fresh Cuts (Green Giant)	½ cup	25	0	60	4	2
Spears (Birds Eye)	½ cup	25	0	0	4	—
cooked	1 pkg (10 oz)	82	1	12	14	—
cooked	4 spears	17	tr	2	3	—

AVOCADO

FOOD	PORTION	CAL	FAT	SOD	CARB	FIB
FRESH						
California	½	153	14	—	—	—
California, mashed	1 cup	407	36	—	—	—
avocado	1	324	31	21	15	—
puree	1 cup	370	35	24	17	—

BABY FOOD

Nutritional guidelines for infants are different from those recommended for older children and adults. Check with a pediatrician for advice on feeding children under the age of 2.

FOOD	PORTION	CAL	FAT	SOD	CARB	FIB
BAKED SELECTIONS						
Gerber						
Chunky Animal Cookies	2 (0.5 oz)	60	2	—	10	—
Chunky Biter Biscuits	1 (0.4 oz)	50	1	—	9	—
Chunky Zwieback Toast	2 (0.5 oz)	70	2	—	10	—
Graduates Animal Crackers Cinnamon	2 (0.2 oz)	30	1	—	5	—
Graduates Arrowroot Cookies	2 (0.4 oz)	50	2	—	8	—
Graduates Pretzels	2 (0.4 oz)	45	0	—	10	—
CEREAL						
Beech-Nut						
Stage 1 Barley	0.5 oz	60	0	10	12	1
Stage 1 Oatmeal	0.5 oz	60	2	15	11	1
Stage 1 Oatmeal & Apples	1 jar (4 oz)	70	0	0	16	1
Stage 1 Rice	0.5 oz	60	0	0	13	0

FOOD	PORTION	CAL	FAT	SOD	CARB	FIB
Stage 2 Mixed	0.5 oz	50	1	10	12	tr
Stage 2 Mixed & Apples	1 jar (4 oz)	70	0	0	16	1
Stage 2 Oatmeal & Chiquita Bananas	0.5 oz	60	1	0	12	1
Stage 2 Rice & Apples	1 jar (4 oz)	70	0	0	16	1
Stage 2 Rice & Chiquita Bananas	0.5 oz	60	0	0	13	0
Stage 2 Rice & Golden Delicious Apples	0.5 oz	60	0	0	14	0
Earth's Best Brown Rice	5 tbsp (0.5 oz)	60	0	0	12	—
Earth's Best Mixed Grain	5 tbsp (0.5 oz)	60	0	0	11	—
Earth's Best Peach, Oatmeal, Banana	1 jar (4.5 fl oz)	60	0	10	12	—
Earth's Best Prunes & Oatmeal	1 jar (4.5 fl oz)	100	0	20	24	—
Gerber						
First Foods Barley	4 tbsp (0.5 oz)	60	1	—	11	—
First Foods Oatmeal	4 tbsp (0.5 oz)	50	1	—	9	—
First Foods Rice	4 tbsp (0.5 oz)	60	1	—	11	—
Second Foods High Protein	4 tbsp (0.5 oz)	50	1	—	6	—
Second Foods Mixed	4 tbsp (0.5 oz)	60	1	—	11	—
Second Foods Mixed With Applesauce & Bananas	1 jar (4 oz)	90	1	—	20	—
Second Foods Mixed With Banana	4 tbsp (0.5 oz)	60	1	—	11	—
Second Foods Oatmeal With Applesauce & Bananas	1 jar (4 oz)	90	1	—	20	—
Second Foods Oatmeal With Banana	4 tbsp (0.5 oz)	60	1	—	10	—
Second Foods Rice With Applesauce & Bananas	1 jar (4 oz)	90	0	—	21	—

FOOD	PORTION	CAL	FAT	SOD	CARB	FIB
Gerber *(cont.)*						
Second Foods Rice With Banana	4 tbsp (0.5 oz)	60	1	—	11	—
Third Foods Mixed With Applesauce & Bananas	1 jar (6 oz)	140	1	—	31	—
Third Foods Oatmeal With Applesauce & Bananas	1 jar (6 oz)	140	1	—	28	—
Third Foods Rice With Mixed Fruit	1 jar (6 oz)	130	0	—	31	—
Tropical Foods Corn Cereal	4 tbsp (0.5 oz)	60	1	—	12	—
Tropical Foods Rice With Mango	4 tbsp (0.5 oz)	50	0	—	12	—
Brown Rice 100% Organic (Health Valley)	1 tbsp (0.5 oz)	60	1	5	10	1
Health Valley Sprouted Baby Cereal 100% Organic	1 tbsp (0.5 oz)	60	1	5	10	—
DESSERT						
Beech-Nut						
Stage 2 Apple & Strawberry Dessert	1 jar (4 oz)	100	0	0	23	1
Stage 2 Apple Yogurt Dessert	1 jar (4 oz)	100	1	25	22	0
Stage 2 Apple, Peach & Strawberry Dessert	1 jar (4 oz)	100	0	0	22	1
Stage 2 Banana Pineapple Dessert	1 jar (4 oz)	100	0	15	23	0
Stage 2 Banana Pudding (Spanish label)	1 jar (4 oz)	110	0	0	26	0
Stage 2 Banana Yogurt Dessert	1 jar (4 oz)	120	2	25	24	0
Stage 2 Cottage Cheese With Pears Dessert	1 jar (4 oz)	120	1	15	24	1
Stage 2 Dutch Apple Dessert	1 jar (4 oz)	100	0	10	22	0
Stage 2 Flan de Banana	1 jar (4 oz)	110	0	0	26	0

FOOD	PORTION	CAL	FAT	SOD	CARB	FIB
Stage 2 Flan de Vanilla	1 jar (4 oz)	120	3	60	23	0
Stage 2 Fruit Dessert	1 jar (4 oz)	80	0	0	19	1
Stage 2 Frutas Islenas Dessert	1 jar (4 oz)	100	0	10	23	0
Stage 2 Guava Tropical Fruit Dessert	1 jar (4 oz)	90	0	10	22	2
Stage 2 Mango Tropical Fruit Dessert	1 jar (4 oz)	110	0	10	26	1
Stage 2 Mixed Fruit Yogurt Dessert	1 jar (4 oz)	100	0	15	21	1
Stage 2 Papaya Tropical Fruit Dessert	1 jar (4 oz)	100	0	10	22	0
Stage 2 Vanilla Custard Pudding	1 jar (4 oz)	120	3	60	23	0
Stage 3 Cottage Cheese With Pears	1 jar (6 oz)	180	2	20	37	1
Stage 3 Fruit Dessert	1 jar (6 oz)	120	0	0	28	2
Stage 3 Mixed Fruit Yogurt Dessert	1 jar (6 oz)	170	0	30	39	1
Stage 3 Vanilla Custard Pudding	1 jar (6 oz)	190	6	85	32	0
Gerber						
Second Foods Banana Apple Dessert	1 jar (4 oz)	80	0	—	19	—
Second Foods Banana Yogurt Dessert	1 jar (4 oz)	90	0	—	21	—
Second Foods Cherry Vanilla Pudding	1 jar (4 oz)	80	0	—	19	—
Second Foods Dutch Apple	1 jar (4 oz)	100	2	—	20	—
Second Foods Fruit Dessert	1 jar (4 oz)	100	0	—	23	—
Second Foods Hawaiian Delight	1 jar (4 oz)	90	0	—	22	—

FOOD	PORTION	CAL	FAT	SOD	CARB	FIB
Gerber *(cont.)*						
Second Foods Mixed Fruit Yogurt Dessert	1 jar (4 oz)	90	0	—	21	—
Second Foods Peach Cobbler	1 jar (4 oz)	90	0	—	21	—
Second Foods Peach Yogurt Dessert	1 jar (4 oz)	90	0	—	21	—
Second Foods Vanilla Custard Pudding	1 jar (4 oz)	100	1	—	21	—
Third Foods Dutch Apple	1 jar (6 oz)	130	2	—	29	—
Third Foods Fruit Dessert	1 jar (6 oz)	120	0	—	30	—
Third Foods Hawaiian Delight	1 jar (6 oz)	150	0	—	35	—
Third Foods Peach Cobbler	1 jar (6 oz)	130	0	—	31	—
Third Foods Vanilla Custard Pudding	1 jar (6 oz)	150	2	—	31	—
Tropical Foods Banana Vanilla Dessert	1 jar (4 oz)	100	1	—	21	—
Tropical Foods Guava With Tapioca	1 jar (4 oz)	80	0	—	21	—
Tropical Foods Mango Banana Passion Fruit	1 jar (4 oz)	80	0	—	20	—
Tropical Foods Mango With Tapioca	1 jar (4 oz)	80	0	—	21	—
Tropical Foods Papaya Pineapple Dessert	1 jar (4 oz)	90	0	—	22	—
Tropical Foods Papaya With Tapioca	1 jar (4 oz)	70	0	—	17	—
Tropical Foods Peaches Mango	1 jar (4 oz)	80	0	—	19	—
Tropical Foods Pineapple Banana Dessert	1 jar (4 oz)	90	0	—	22	—
Tropical Foods Tropical Fruit Medley	1 jar (4 oz)	70	0	—	18	—

FOOD	PORTION	CAL	FAT	SOD	CARB	FIB
DINNER						
Beech-Nut						
Stage 2 Beef & Egg Noodle	1 jar (4 oz)	100	6	50	8	2
Stage 2 Beef Supreme	1 jar (4 oz)	130	9	45	8	1
Stage 2 Chicken & Rice	1 jar (4 oz)	80	3	70	9	1
Stage 2 Chicken Noodle	1 jar (4 oz)	70	4	45	7	2
Stage 2 Chicken Soup	1 jar (4 oz)	90	4	50	8	1
Stage 2 Turkey Supreme	1 jar (4 oz)	90	4	45	9	1
Stage 2 Vegetable Chicken	1 jar (4 oz)	80	4	40	8	1
Stage 2 Vegetable Ham	1 jar (4 oz)	80	3	30	9	1
Stage 2 Vegetable Lamb	1 jar (4 oz)	80	3	55	9	1
Stage 2 Vegetable Beef	1 jar (4 oz)	80	4	45	8	1
Stage 3 Beef & Egg Noodle	1 jar (6 oz)	130	6	50	13	2
Stage 3 Chicken Noodle	1 jar (6 oz)	110	4	55	14	1
Stage 3 Macaroni & Beef	1 jar (6 oz)	130	6	60	14	2
Stage 3 Spaghetti & Beef	1 jar (6 oz)	130	6	70	16	1
Stage 3 Turkey Rice	1 jar (6 oz)	100	3	60	13	2
Stage 3 Vegetable Beef	1 jar (6 oz)	130	6	60	14	2
Stage 3 Vegetable Chicken	1 jar (6 oz)	110	4	55	14	1
Table Time Chicken & Stars	1 bowl (6 oz)	150	6	170	17	1
Table Time Macaroni & Cheese	1 bowl (6 oz)	200	12	320	21	0
Table Time Seashells In Tomato Sauce	1 bowl (6 oz)	150	4	170	25	1
Table Time Spaghetti Rings In Meat Sauce	1 bowl (6 oz)	160	6	180	20	0

FOOD	PORTION	CAL	FAT	SOD	CARB	FIB
Beach-Nut *(cont.)*						
Table Time Turkey Stew With Rice	1 bowl (6 oz)	150	4	200	14	1
Table Time Vegetable Stew With Beef	1 bowl (6 oz)	110	3	170	16	1
Vegetables Stage 2 Turkey Rice	1 jar (4 oz)	70	3	50	8	1
Earth's Best						
Corn, Rice & Cheese Dinner	1 jar (4.5 oz)	120	5	45	13	—
Macaroni & Cheese	1 jar (4.5 oz)	100	4	10	12	—
Pasta Dinner	1 jar (4.5 oz)	90	3	20	13	—
Potato & Green Bean Dinner	1 jar (4.5 oz)	100	3	25	13	—
Rice & Lentil Dinner	1 jar (4.5 oz)	80	2	25	13	—
Summer Vegetable Dinner	1 jar (4.5 oz)	90	3	15	12	—
Gerber						
Second Foods Apples & Chicken	1 jar (4 oz)	70	2	—	12	—
Second Foods Apples & Ham	1 jar (4 oz)	70	1	—	14	—
Second Foods Apples & Turkey	1 jar (4 oz)	80	2	—	13	—
Second Foods Beef Egg Noodle	1 jar (4 oz)	80	3	—	10	—
Second Foods Broccoli & Chicken	1 jar (4 oz)	50	2	—	4	—
Second Foods Carrots & Beef	1 jar (4 oz)	70	3	—	7	—
Second Foods Chicken Noodle	1 jar (4 oz)	70	2	—	11	—
Second Foods Green Beans & Turkey	1 jar (4 oz)	70	2	—	9	—
Second Foods Macaroni Cheese	1 jar (4 oz)	80	3	—	10	—
Second Foods Macaroni Tomato Beef	1 jar (4 oz)	70	2	—	11	—
Second Foods Turkey Rice	1 jar (4 oz)	70	3	—	9	—
Second Foods Vegetable Bacon	1 jar (4 oz)	90	5	—	10	—

FOOD	PORTION	CAL	FAT	SOD	CARB	FIB
Second Foods Vegetable Beef	1 jar (4 oz)	70	3	—	10	—
Second Foods Vegetable Chicken	1 jar (4 oz)	70	2	—	11	—
Second Foods Vegetable Ham	1 jar (4 oz)	70	3	—	10	—
Second Foods Vegetable Turkey	1 jar (4 oz)	60	2	—	9	—
Third Foods Beef Egg Noodle	1 jar (6 oz)	110	4	—	15	—
Third Foods Chicken Noodle	1 jar (6 oz)	100	3	—	15	—
Third Foods Macaroni Tomato Beef	1 jar (6 oz)	110	2	—	19	—
Third Foods Spaghetti Tomato Sauce Beef	1 jar (6 oz)	120	3	—	19	—
Third Foods Turkey Rice	1 jar (6 oz)	100	3	—	14	—
Third Foods Vegetable Chicken	1 jar (6 oz)	100	3	—	15	—
Third Foods Vegetable Bacon	1 jar (6 oz)	130	6	—	17	—
Third Foods Vegetable Beef	1 jar (6 oz)	120	4	—	16	—
Third Foods Vegetable Ham	1 jar (6 oz)	110	4	—	16	—
Third Foods Vegetable Turkey	1 jar (6 oz)	100	3	—	15	—
Chunky Homestyle Noodles & Beef	1 jar (6 oz)	150	6	—	18	—
Chunky Macaroni Alphabets With Beef & Sauce	1 jar (6.3 oz)	140	4	—	20	—
Chunky Noodles & Chicken With Carrots & Peas	1 jar (6 oz)	110	3	—	16	—
Chunky Rice With Beef & Tomato Sauce	1 jar (6.3 oz)	140	4	—	21	—
Chunky Saucy Rice With Chicken	1 jar (6 oz)	120	3	—	19	—

FOOD	PORTION	CAL	FAT	SOD	CARB	FIB
Beach-Nut *(cont.)*						
Chunky Spaghetti Tomato Sauce Beef	1 jar (6.3 oz)	150	4	—	22	—
Chunky Vegetables & Beef	1 jar (6.3 oz)	130	5	—	16	—
Chunky Vegetables & Chicken	1 jar (6.3 oz)	140	5	—	17	—
Chunky Vegetables & Ham	1 jar (6.3 oz)	130	5	—	16	—
Chunky Vegetables & Turkey	1 jar (6.3 oz)	110	3	—	15	—
Graduates Chicken Stew With Noodles	1 bowl (6 oz)	120	4	—	15	—
Graduates Macaroni And Beef In Sauce	1 bowl (6 oz)	150	4	—	20	—
Graduates Spaghetti With Mini Meatballs & Sauce	1 bowl (6 oz)	160	5	—	21	—
Graduates Tomato Sauce With Beef Ravioli	1 bowl (6 oz)	170	4	—	28	—
Graduates Tomato Sauce With Cheese Ravioli	1 bowl (6 oz)	170	4	—	28	—
Graduates Turkey Stew With Rice	1 bowl (6 oz)	100	2	—	13	—
Graduates Vegetable Stew With Beef	1 bowl (6 oz)	130	3	—	15	—
Tropical Foods Beans & Rice	1 jar (4 oz)	60	2	—	9	—
Tropical Foods Chicken & Rice	1 jar (4 oz)	60	2	—	8	—
FRUIT						
Beech-Nut						
Stage 1 Applesauce Golden Delicious	1 jar (2.5 oz)	50	0	0	12	1
Stage 1 Applesauce Golden Delicious	1 jar (4 oz)	70	0	0	15	1
Stage 1 Bananas Chiquita	1 jar (2.5 oz)	70	0	0	16	1
Stage 1 Bananas Chiquita	1 jar (4 oz)	110	0	0	24	1
Stage 1 Chiquita Bananas With Pears & Apples	1 jar (4 oz)	90	0	0	21	1

FOOD	PORTION	CAL	FAT	SOD	CARB	FIB
Stage 1 Peaches Yellow Cling	1 jar (2.5 oz)	45	0	0	11	2
Stage 1 Peaches Yellow Cling	1 jar (4 oz)	70	0	0	14	3
Stage 1 Pears Bartlett	1 jar (4 oz)	70	0	0	18	3
Stage 2 Apples & Apricots	1 jar (4 oz)	70	0	0	17	1
Stage 2 Apples & Blueberries	1 jar (4 oz)	70	0	0	17	1
Stage 2 Apples & Cherries	1 jar (4 oz)	80	0	0	18	1
Stage 2 Apples & Pears	1 jar (4 oz)	80	0	0	19	1
Stage 2 Apples & Bananas	1 jar (4 oz)	60	0	0	14	1
Stage 2 Apples, Pears & Bananas	1 jar (4 oz)	90	0	0	20	1
Stage 2 Apricots With Pears & Apples	1 jar (4 oz)	90	0	0	20	2
Stage 2 Bartlett Pears & Pineapple	1 jar (4 oz)	70	0	0	17	3
Stage 2 Peaches & Bananas	1 jar (4 oz)	70	0	0	15	3
Stage 2 Plums With Apples & Rice	1 jar (4 oz)	90	0	10	18	1
Stage 2 Prunes With Pears	1 jar (4 oz)	110	0	10	24	3
Stage 3 Apples & Bananas	1 jar (6 oz)	90	0	0	21	1
Stage 3 Apples & Cherries	1 jar (6 oz)	110	0	0	26	1
Stage 3 Applesauce	1 jar (6 oz)	100	0	0	23	2
Stage 3 Apricots With Pears & Apples	1 jar (6 oz)	130	0	0	32	—
Stage 3 Bananas Chiquita	1 jar (6 oz)	160	0	0	33	3
Stage 3 Peaches	1 jar (6 oz)	100	0	0	21	4
Stage 3 Pears Bartlett	1 jar (6 oz)	110	0	0	27	5
Earth's Best						
Apples	1 jar (4.5 oz)	70	0	10	17	—
Apples & Apricots	1 jar (4.5 fl oz)	70	0	5	17	—

FOOD	PORTION	CAL	FAT	SOD	CARB	FIB
Earth's Best *(cont.)*						
Apples & Blueberries	1 jar (4.5 fl oz)	70	0	10	17	—
Apples & Plums	1 jar (4.5 fl oz)	70	0	10	17	—
Bananas	1 jar (4.5 oz)	90	0	0	20	—
Pears	1 jar (4.5 fl oz)	60	0	10	14	—
Plums, Bananas & Rice	1 jar (4.5 fl oz)	90	1	10	19	—
Gerber						
First Foods Applesauce	1 jar (2.5 oz)	25	0	—	9	—
First Foods Bananas	1 jar (2.5 oz)	70	0	—	17	—
First Foods Peaches	1 jar (2.5 oz)	30	0	—	7	—
First Foods Pears	1 jar (2.5 oz)	40	0	—	10	—
First Foods Prunes	1 jar (2.5 oz)	70	0	—	17	—
Second Foods Apple Blueberry	1 jar (4 oz)	50	0	—	13	—
Second Foods Applesauce	1 jar (4 oz)	60	0	—	14	—
Second Foods Applesauce Apricot	1 jar (4 oz)	60	0	—	14	—
Second Foods Apricots With Tapioca	1 jar (4 oz)	80	0	—	19	—
Second Foods Banana With Pineapple And Tapioca	1 jar (4 oz)	60	0	—	14	—
Second Foods Banana With Tapioca	1 jar (4 oz)	90	0	—	21	—
Second Foods Peaches	1 jar (4 oz)	70	0	—	17	—
Second Foods Pear Pineapple	1 jar (4 oz)	60	0	—	15	—
Second Foods Pears	1 jar (4 oz)	60	0	—	20	—
Second Foods Plums With Tapioca	1 jar (4 oz)	80	0	—	15	—
Second Foods Prunes With Tapioca	1 jar (4 oz)	90	0	—	21	—
JUICE						
Beech-Nut						
Stage 1 Apple	4 fl oz	60	0	10	15	0
Stage 1 Pear	4 fl oz	60	0	0	15	0
Stage 1 White Grape	4 fl oz	100	0	10	23	0

FOOD	PORTION	CAL	FAT	SOD	CARB	FIB
Stage 2 Apple Banana	4 fl oz	70	0	0	16	0
Stage 2 Apple Cherry	4 fl oz	70	0	10	17	0
Stage 2 Apple Cranberry	4 fl oz	60	0	10	15	0
Stage 2 Apple Grape	4 fl oz	70	0	15	18	0
Stage 2 Juice Plus Grape	4 fl oz	100	0	10	23	0
Stage 2 Mango Nectar (Spanish label)	4 fl oz	80	0	0	18	0
Stage 2 Mixed Fruit	4 fl oz	70	0	10	15	0
Stage 2 Papaya Nectar (Spanish label)	4 fl oz	80	0	10	20	0
Stage 2 Tropical Blend	4 fl oz	90	0	5	15	0
Stage 2 Tropical Blend Nectar (Spanish label)	4 fl oz	90	0	5	19	0
Stage 3 Orange	4 fl oz	60	0	0	15	0
Earth's Best						
Apple	1 bottle (4.2 fl oz)	60	0	20	14	—
Apple Banana	1 bottle (4.2 fl oz)	60	0	20	14	—
Apple Grape	1 bottle (4.2 fl oz)	60	0	15	14	—
Apples & Bananas	1 jar (4.5 fl oz)	80	0	20	18	—
Pear	1 bottle (4.2 fl oz)	60	0	0	15	—
Gerber						
First Foods Apple	4 fl oz	60	0	—	14	—
First Foods Pear	4 fl oz	60	0	—	14	—
First Foods Red Grape	4 fl oz	80	0	—	20	—
First Foods White Grape	4 fl oz	80	0	—	19	—
Second Foods Apple Banana	4 fl oz	60	0	—	15	—
Second Foods Apple Cherry	4 fl oz	60	0	—	14	—
Second Foods Apple Grape	4 fl oz	60	0	—	15	—

FOOD	PORTION	CAL	FAT	SOD	CARB	FIB
Gerber *(cont.)*						
Second Foods Apple Peach	4 fl oz	60	0	—	14	—
Second Foods Apple Plum	4 fl oz	60	0	—	15	—
Second Foods Apple Prune	4 fl oz	60	0	—	16	—
Second Foods Apple With Yogurt	4 fl oz	100	2	—	18	—
Second Foods Banana With Yogurt	4 fl oz	110	2	—	21	—
Second Foods Mixed Fruit	4 fl oz	60	0	—	14	—
Second Foods Mixed Fruit With Yogurt	4 fl oz	100	2	—	18	—
Second Foods Orange	4 fl oz	60	0	—	13	—
Second Foods Pear Peach With Yogurt	4 fl oz	90	1	—	18	—
Third Foods Apple Carrot	4 fl oz	50	0	—	12	—
Third Foods Apple Sweet Potato	4 fl oz	60	0	—	14	—
Third Foods Orange Carrot	4 fl oz	50	0	—	12	—
Third Foods Pineapple Carrot	4 fl oz	60	0	—	13	—
Graduates Apple	4 fl oz	80	0	—	21	—
Graduates Apple Banana	4 fl oz	90	0	—	23	—
Graduates Apple Cherry	4 fl oz	80	0	—	21	—
Graduates Apple Grape	4 fl oz	90	0	—	22	—
Tropical Foods Guava With Mixed Fruit	4 fl oz	70	0	—	18	—
Tropical Foods Mango With Mixed Fruit	4 fl oz	70	0	—	18	—
Tropical Foods Papaya With Mixed Fruit	4 fl oz	70	0	—	18	—

FOOD	PORTION	CAL	FAT	SOD	CARB	FIB
MEAT						
Beech-Nut						
Stage 1 Beef And Broth	1 jar (2.5 oz)	90	6	40	0	0
Stage 1 Chicken And Broth	1 jar (2.5 oz)	70	3	55	0	0
Stage 1 Lamb And Broth	1 jar (2.5 oz)	60	3	50	0	0
Stage 1 Turkey And Broth	1 jar (2.5 oz)	90	6	40	0	0
Stage 1 Veal And Broth	1 jar (2.5 oz)	60	2	50	0	0
Gerber						
Second Foods Beef	1 jar (2.5 oz)	80	4	—	0	—
Second Foods Chicken	1 jar (2.5 oz)	90	6	—	0	—
Second Foods Egg Yolks	1 jar (2.5 oz)	130	11	—	1	—
Second Foods Ham	1 jar (2.5 oz)	90	6	—	0	—
Second Foods Lamb	1 jar (2.5 oz)	80	4	—	0	—
Second Foods Turkey	1 jar (2.5 oz)	80	5	—	0	—
Second Foods Veal	1 jar (2.5 oz)	70	4	—	0	—
Third Foods Beef	1 jar (2.5 oz)	80	4	—	0	—
Third Foods Chicken	1 jar (2.5 oz)	90	6	—	0	—
Third Foods Ham	1 jar (2.5 oz)	90	6	—	0	—
Third Foods Turkey	1 jar (2.5 oz)	90	5	—	0	—
Third Foods Veal	1 jar (2.5 oz)	80	4	—	0	—
Graduates Chicken Sticks	1 jar (2.5 oz)	110	7	—	2	—
Graduates Meat Sticks	1 jar (2.5 oz)	110	7	—	2	—
Graduates Turkey Sticks	1 jar (2.5 oz)	120	8	—	2	—
VEGETABLE						
Beech-Nut						
Stage 1 Butternut Squash	1 jar (2.5 oz)	30	0	10	7	2
Stage 1 Butternut Squash	1 jar (4 oz)	50	0	10	11	3
Stage 1 Carrots Tender Sweet	1 jar (4 oz)	50	0	100	10	4
Stage 1 Carrots Tender Sweet	1 jar (2.5 oz)	30	0	80	7	2

FOOD	PORTION	CAL	FAT	SOD	CARB	FIB
Beach-Nut *(cont.)*						
Stage 1 Green Beans	1 jar (4 oz)	35	0	0	6	3
Stage 1 Green Beans (Spanish label)	1 jar (2.5 oz)	20	0	0	4	2
Stage 1 Peas Tender Sweet	1 jar (2.5 oz)	40	0	0	7	3
Stage 1 Peas Tender Sweet	1 jar (4 oz)	60	0	0	11	5
Stage 1 Sweet Potatoes Tender Golden	1 jar (2.5 oz)	50	0	10	10	0
Stage 1 Sweet Potatoes Tender Golden	1 jar (4 oz)	80	0	10	17	0
Stage 2 Carrots & Peas	1 jar (4 oz)	50	0	25	10	3
Stage 2 Creamed Corn	1 jar (4 oz)	90	0	20	18	2
Stage 2 Garden Vegetables	1 jar (4 oz)	50	0	10	9	3
Stage 2 Mixed Vegetables	1 jar (4 oz)	45	0	10	9	3
Stage 3 Carrots	1 jar (6 oz)	70	0	240	15	5
Stage 3 Green Beans	1 jar (6 oz)	50	0	0	10	4
Stage 3 Sweet Potatoes	1 jar (6 oz)	110	0	15	25	1
Earth's Best						
Carrots	1 jar (4.5 fl oz)	40	0	70	8	—
Carrots & Parsnips	1 jar (4.5 fl oz)	60	0	30	14	—
Corn & Butternut Squash	1 jar (4.5 fl oz)	90	2	0	15	—
Garden Vegetables	1 jar (4.5 fl oz)	70	0	15	15	—
Green Beans & Rice	1 jar (4.5 fl oz)	40	1	15	6	—
Peas & Brown Rice	1 jar (4.5 fl oz)	80	0	10	16	—
Spinach & Potatoes	1 jar (4.5 fl oz)	60	2	25	8	—
Sweet Potatoes	1 jar (4.5 fl oz)	60	1	15	12	—
Winter Squash	1 jar (4.5 fl oz)	50	0	10	12	—
Gerber						
First Foods Carrots	1 jar (2.5 oz)	25	0	—	5	—
First Foods Green Beans	1 jar (2.5 oz)	25	0	—	5	—

FOOD	PORTION	CAL	FAT	SOD	CARB	FIB
First Foods Peas	1 jar (2.5 oz)	30	0	—	6	—
First Foods Squash	1 jar (2.5 oz)	25	0	—	5	—
First Foods Sweet Potatoes	1 jar (2.5 oz)	45	0	—	10	—
Second Foods Beets	1 jar (4 oz)	45	0	—	10	—
Second Foods Carrots	1 jar (4 oz)	30	0	—	7	—
Second Foods Creamed Corn	1 jar (4 oz)	80	1	—	15	—
Second Foods Creamed Spinach	1 jar (4 oz)	50	1	—	8	—
Second Foods Garden Vegetables	1 jar (4 oz)	45	1	—	7	—
Second Foods Green Beans	1 jar (4 oz)	35	0	—	7	—
Second Foods Mixed Vegetables	1 jar (4 oz)	50	1	—	9	—
Second Foods Peas	1 jar (4 oz)	60	1	—	9	—
Second Foods Squash	1 jar (4 oz)	35	0	—	8	—
Second Foods Sweet Potatoes	1 jar (4 oz)	70	0	—	16	—
Third Foods Broccoli Carrots Cheese	1 jar (6 oz)	80	2	—	12	—
Third Foods Carrots	1 jar (6 oz)	50	0	—	11	—
Third Foods Creamed Green Beans	1 jar (6 oz)	80	1	—	16	—
Third Foods Mixed Vegetables	1 jar (6 oz)	70	0	—	15	—
Third Foods Peas	1 jar (6 oz)	80	1	—	14	—
Third Foods Squash	1 jar (6 oz)	60	1	—	12	—
Third Foods Sweet Potatoes	1 jar (6 oz)	100	0	—	24	—
Graduates Carrots	1 jar (4.5 oz)	30	0	—	6	—
Graduates Green Beans	1 jar (4.5 oz)	30	0	—	6	—
Graduates Peas	1 jar (4.5 oz)	60	0	—	11	—
Graduates Potatoes	1 jar (4.5 oz)	50	0	—	11	—

BACON

see also BACON SUBSTITUTES

FOOD	PORTION	CAL	FAT	SOD	CARB	FIB
Armour Lower Salt, cooked	1 strip	30	3	—	—	—
Armour Star, cooked	1 strip	38	3	185	—	—

FOOD	PORTION	CAL	FAT	SOD	CARB	FIB
Hillshire	1 slice	120	12	150	tr	—
Jones, sliced	1 slice	130	13	150	tr	—
Nathan's Beef, cooked	3 slices	100	7	310	tr	—
Oscar Mayer Center Cut, cooked	1 slice	24	2	113	tr	—
Oscar Mayer Lower Salt, cooked	1 strip	33	3	104	tr	—
Oscar Mayer Thick Sliced, cooked	1 slice	58	5	259	tr	—
Oscar Mayer, cooked	1 slice	35	3	138	tr	—
breakfast strips beef, cooked	3 strips (34 g)	153	12	766	tr	—
breakfast strips, cooked	3 strips (34 g)	156	12	—	—	—
cooked	3 strips	109	9	303	tr	—
gammon lean & fat, grilled	4.2 oz	274	15	—	0	0
grilled	2 slices (1.7 oz)	86	4	719	1	—

BACON SUBSTITUTES

FOOD	PORTION	CAL	FAT	SOD	CARB	FIB
Bac'n Pieces (McCormick)	2 tsp	20	tr	140	1	—
Bac-Os	2 tsp (5 g)	25	1	90	2	—
Harvest Direct Bacon Style Bits	3.5 oz	320	15	2000	24	17
Lightlife Fakin' Bacon	3 strips (2 oz)	79	3	233	6	—
Louis Rich Turkey Bacon	1 slice (0.5 oz)	30	3	190	0	0
Morningstar Farms Breakfast Strips	3 strips (25 g)	80	6	350	4	—
Oscar Mayer Bacon Bits	0.25 oz	20	1	138	tr	—
Stripples Worthington	4 strips (33 g)	120	9	460	6	—
bacon substitute	1 strip	25	2	117	1	—

BAGEL
FRESH

FOOD	PORTION	CAL	FAT	SOD	CARB	FIB
cinnamon raisin	1 (3½ in)	194	1	229	39	—
cinnamon raisin, toasted	1 (3½ in)	194	1	229	39	—
egg	1 (3½ in)	197	2	359	38	—
egg, toasted	1 (3½ in)	197	2	358	38	—
oat bran	1 (3½ in)	181	1	360	38	—
oat bran, toasted	1 (3½ in)	181	1	360	38	—

FOOD	PORTION	CAL	FAT	SOD	CARB	FIB
onion	1 (3½ in)	195	1	379	38	2
plain	1 (3½ in)	195	1	379	38	2
plain, toasted	1 (3½ in)	195	1	379	38	2
poppy seed	1 (3½ in)	195	1	379	38	2
FROZEN						
Bagel Sandwich Ham And Cheese (Weight Watchers)	1 (3 oz)	210	6	469	28	—
Cinnamon & Raisin (Sara Lee)	1 (3 oz)	240	2	280	48	—
Cinnamon Raisin (Sara Lee)	1 (2.5 oz)	200	2	230	39	—
Cinnamon'N Raisin (Lender's)	1 (2.5 oz)	200	1	310	40	1
Egg (Lender's)	1 (2 oz)	150	1	360	29	—
Egg (Sara Lee)	1 (2.5 oz)	200	2	360	38	—
Egg (Sara Lee)	1 (3 oz)	250	2	450	48	—
Ham & Cheese On A Bagel (Great Starts)	3 oz	240	8	600	28	—
Oat Bran (Sara Lee)	1 (2.5 oz)	180	1	360	38	—
Oat Bran (Sara Lee)	1 (3 oz)	220	1	450	47	—
Onion (Lender's)	1 (2 oz)	160	1	290	31	1
Onion (Sara Lee)	1 (2.5 oz)	190	1	450	37	—
Onion (Sara Lee)	1 (3 oz)	230	1	560	45	—
Plain (Lender's)	1 (2 oz)	150	1	320	30	—
Plain (Sara Lee)	1 (2.5 oz)	190	1	460	38	—
Plain (Sara Lee)	1 (3 oz)	230	1	580	46	—
Poppy Seed (Sara Lee)	1 (2.5 oz)	190	1	450	37	—
Poppy Seed (Sara Lee)	1 (3 oz)	230	1	560	46	—
Sesame Seed (Sara Lee)	1 (2.5 oz)	190	1	440	37	—
Sesame Seed (Sara Lee)	1 (3 oz)	240	2	550	46	—

BAKING POWDER

Calumet	1 tsp	3	tr	—	—	—
Clabber Girl	1 tsp	0	0	435	—	—
Davis	1 tsp	6	0	450	1	—
baking powder	1 tsp	2	0	488	1	—
low sodium	1 tsp	5	0	4	2	—

BAKING SODA

Arm & Hammer	1 tsp	0	0	1368	0	—
baking soda	1 tsp	0	0	1259	0	—

FOOD	PORTION	CAL	FAT	SOD	CARB	FIB
BALSAM-PEAR						
leafy tips, cooked	½ cup	10	tr	4	2	—
leafy tips, raw	½ cup	7	tr	3	1	—
pods, cooked	½ cup	12	tr	4	3	—
BAMBOO SHOOTS						
CANNED						
Empress Sliced	2 oz	14	0	10	3	—
La Choy	¼ cup	6	tr	2	1	tr
sliced	1 cup	25	1	9	4	—
FRESH						
cooked	½ cup	15	tr	5	2	—
raw	½ cup	21	tr	3	1	—
BANANA						
DRIED						
powder	1 tbsp	21	tr	0	5	—
FRESH						
Chiquita	1 (3.5 oz)	110	0	—	—	—
Dole	1	120	1	0	28	3
banana	1	105	tr	1	27	2
mashed	1 cup	207	1	2	53	4
JUICE						
Libby's Nectar	6 oz	110	0	15	26	—
BARLEY						
Arrowhead	¼ cup (1.7 oz)	170	1	0	37	6
Arrowhead Hulless	¼ cup (1.6 oz)	140	1	0	35	6
Quaker Medium Pearled	¼ cup	172	1	0	36	5
Quaker Quick Pearled	¼ cup	172	1	0	36	5
Scotch Medium Pearled	¼ cup	172	1	0	36	5
Scotch Quick Pearled	¼ cup	172	1	0	36	5
pearled, cooked	½ cup	97	tr	2	30	—
pearled, uncooked	½ cup	352	1	9	78	16
BASIL						
fresh, chopped	2 tbsp	1	tr	0	tr	—
ground	1 tsp	4	tr	tr	1	—
leaves, fresh	5	1	tr	0	tr	—
BASS						
FRESH						
freshwater, raw	3 oz	97	3	59	0	—

FOOD	PORTION	CAL	FAT	SOD	CARB	FIB
sea, cooked	3 oz	105	2	74	0	—
sea, raw	3 oz	82	2	58	0	—
striped, baked	3 oz	105	3	75	0	—

BAY LEAF
crumbled	1 tsp	2	tr	tr	tr	—

BEAN SPROUTS
see also INDIVIDUAL BEAN NAMES
CANNED
La Choy	⅔ cup	8	tr	20	1	tr

BEANS
see also INDIVIDUAL NAMES
CANNED
FOOD	PORTION	CAL	FAT	SOD	CARB	FIB
Baked Beans (Brick Oven)	½ cup	160	2	560	28	—
Baked Beans (Van Camp's)	1 cup	260	2	1020	52	—
Barbecue Beans (Campbell)	½ can (7⅞ oz)	210	4	900	43	—
Barbecue Beans Texas Style (S&W)	½ cup	135	1	550	24	—
Barbeque Baked Beans (B&M)	8 oz	260	6	1000	48	11
Beanee Weenee (Van Camp's)	1 cup	326	7	990	32	7
Big John's Beans 'n Fixin's (Hunt's)	4 oz	170	6	490	26	6
Boston Baked (Health Valley)	7.5 oz	190	tr	300	41	5
Boston Baked No Salt Added (Health Valley)	7.5 oz	190	tr	20	41	5
Brown Sugar Beans (Van Camp's)	1 cup	290	5	640	51	—
Chili (Gebhardt)	4 oz	115	1	580	21	5
Cut Green & Shelled Beans Seasoned w/ Pork (Luck's)	7.25 oz	200	6	—	—	—
Deluxe Baked Beans (Van Camp's)	1 cup	320	4	970	57	—
Fast Menu Honey Baked Organic Beans With Tofu Weiner (Health Valley)	7.5 oz	150	4	140	15	16

FOOD	PORTION	CAL	FAT	SOD	CARB	FIB
Four Bean Salad (Hanover)	½ cup	80	0	—	—	—
Home Style Beans (Campbell)	½ can (8 oz)	220	4	820	48	—
Honey Baked (B&M)	8 oz	240	2	940	50	11
Hot Chili Beans (Campbell)	½ can (7.75 oz)	180	4	870	38	—
Hot N Spicy Baked (B&M)	8 oz	240	3	990	50	12
Maple Baked (B&M)	8 oz	240	2	890	52	11
Maple Baked (Friends)	8 oz	240	2	890	52	11
Maple Sugar Beans (S&W)	½ cup	150	1	586	28	—
Mexe-Beans (Old El Paso)	½ cup	163	1	627	31	13
Mexican Style Chili Beans (Van Camp's)	1 cup	210	2	730	39	—
Mixed Bean Salad Marinated (S&W)	½ cup	90	1	730	17	—
Mixed Beans Seasoned w/ Pork (Luck's)	7.25 oz	200	5	—	—	—
Old Fashioned Beans in Molasses & Brown Sugar Sauce (Campbell)	½ can (8 oz)	230	3	730	49	—
Pork & Beans in Tomato Sauce (Campbell)	½ can (8 oz)	200	3	770	43	—
Pork & Molasses (Libby)	½ cup	140	2	—	—	—
Pork & Tomato Sauce (Libby)	½ cup	140	2	—	—	—
Pork & Tomato Sauce (Seneca)	½ cup	140	2	—	—	—
Pork 'N Beans (S&W)	½ cup	130	2	135	22	—
Pork And Beans (Hunt's)	4 oz	135	1	430	26	8
Pork And Beans (Van Camp's)	1 cup	216	2	1000	41	10
Pork And Beans In Tomato Sauce (Green Giant)	½ cup	90	1	420	21	6
Refried (Casa Fiesta)	3.5 oz	110	2	299	17	—
Refried (Gebhardt)	4 oz	100	2	490	20	7
Refried (Old El Paso)	¼ cup	55	tr	200	8	3

FOOD	PORTION	CAL	FAT	SOD	CARB	FIB
Refried (Rosarita)	4 oz	100	2	480	18	6
Refried Spicy (Old El Paso)	¼ cup	35	1	280	5	2
Refried Vegetarian (Old El Paso)	¼ cup	70	.1	730	15	5
Refried Vegetarian (Rosarita)	4 oz	100	2	480	18	6
Refried With Cheese (Old El Paso)	¼ cup	36	1	280	4	—
Refried With Green Chilies (Old El Paso)	¼ cup	49	tr	252	8	—
Refried With Sausages (Old El Paso)	¼ cup	180	8	300	8	—
Refried Beans & Green Chili (Little Pancho)	½ cup	80	0	330	15	—
Refried Jalapeno (Gebhardt)	4 oz	115	2	270	19	7
Refried Spicy (Rosarita)	4 oz	100	2	500	19	6
Refried With Bacon (Rosarita)	4 oz	110	2	560	20	6
Refried With Green Chilies (Rosarita)	4 oz	90	2	460	18	6
Refried With Nacho Cheese (Rosarita)	4 oz	110	2	490	20	6
Refried With Onions (Rosarita)	4 oz	110	2	490	21	6
Smokey Ranch Beans (S&W)	½ cup	130	2	569	20	—
Spicy (McIlhenny)	1 oz	7	tr	19	1	1
Three Bean Salad (Green Giant)	½ cup	70	tr	470	18	3
Tomato Baked Beans (B&M)	8 oz	230	3	1010	48	—
Vegetarian (Libby)	½ cup	130	1	—	—	—
Vegetarian (Seneca)	½ cup	130	1	—	—	—
Vegetarian Baked Beans (B&M)	8 oz	230	3	370	50	—
Vegetarian Beans (Campbell)	½ can (7.75 oz)	170	1	780	40	—
Vegetarian Beans With Miso (Health Valley)	7.5 oz	180	1	60	38	5
Vegetarian Style (Van Camp's)	1 cup	206	1	950	42	—

FOOD	PORTION	CAL	FAT	SOD	CARB	FIB
baked beans						
plain	½ cup	118	1	504	26	10
vegetarian	½ cup	118	1	504	26	10
with beef	½ cup	161	5	632	22	—
with franks	½ cup	182	8	551	20	9
with pork	½ cup	133	2	522	25	7
with pork & sweet sauce	½ cup	140	2	423	26	7
with pork & tomato sauce	½ cup	123	1	554	24	7
refried beans	½ cup	134	1	534	23	—
FROZEN						
Romano Bean Medley (Hanover)	½ cup	25	0	—	—	—
MIX						
Florentine Beans With Bow Ties (Bean Cuisine)	½ cup	199	7	450	27	—
Pasta & Beans Country French With Gemelli (Bean Cuisine)	½ cup	214	8	369	27	—
TAKE-OUT						
baked beans	½ cup	190	6	532	27	—
barbecue beans	3.5 oz	120	tr	460	26	—
four bean salad	3.5 oz	100	tr	280	20	—
refried beans	½ cup	43	2	104	5	—
three bean salad	¾ cup	230	11	500	31	1

BEAR

simmered	3 oz	220	11	—	0	—

BEAVER

roasted	3 oz	140	6	50	0	—
simmered	3 oz	141	5	39	0	—

BEECHNUTS

dried	1 oz	164	14	—	10	—

BEEF

see also BEEF DISHES, VEAL

Beef is graded according to its marbling, the little flecks of fat in the muscle. Beef graded "Prime" has the highest percentage of fat, followed by "Choice" with less fat and "Select" with the least fat.

FOOD	PORTION	CAL	FAT	SOD	CARB	FIB
CANNED						
Roast Beef (Underwood)	2.08 oz	140	11	360	tr	—
Roast Beef Light (Underwood)	2.08 oz	90	6	210	2	—
Roast Beef Mesquite Smoked (Underwood)	2.08 oz	126	11	300	tr	—
corned beef	1 oz	71	4	—	—	—
corned beef	1 slice (21 g)	53	3	—	—	—
FRESH						

Note that the values for cooked beef may differ slightly from values for raw beef. When meat is cooked some moisture and fat is lost changing the nutrition value slightly. As a rule of thumb it can be assumed that a 4 oz raw portion will equal a 3 oz cooked portion of meat.

FOOD	PORTION	CAL	FAT	SOD	CARB	FIB
Chuck Roast, raw (Dakota Lean)	3 oz	80	2	—	1	—
Eye Round, raw (Dakota Lean)	3 oz	80	2	—	0	—
Filet (Double J)	3.5 oz	130	4	54	—	—
Flank Steak, raw (Dakota Lean)	3 oz	80	1	—	1	—
Ground, raw (Dakota Lean)	3 oz	88	2	—	0	—
NY Strip (Double J)	3.5 oz	133	4	57	—	—
Outside Round, raw (Dakota Lean)	3 oz	80	1	—	0	—
Rib Eye (Double J)	3.5 oz	134	5	55	—	—
Ribeye, raw (Dakota Lean)	3 oz	90	2	—	1	—
Sirloin Tip, raw (Dakota Lean)	3 oz	90	3	—	1	—
Strip Loin, raw (Dakota Lean)	3 oz	90	2	—	1	—
Tenderloin, raw (Dakota Lean)	3 oz	70	1	—	1	—
Top Butt (Double J)	3.5 oz	136	5	55	—	—
Top Round, raw (Dakota Lean)	3 oz	80	1	—	1	—
bottom round, lean & fat trim 0 in, Choice, roasted	3 oz	172	8	56	0	—

FOOD	PORTION	CAL	FAT	SOD	CARB	FIB
bottom round *(cont.)*						
trim 0 in, Select, braised	3 oz	171	6	43	0	—
trim 0 in, Select, roasted	3 oz	150	24	56	0	—
trim 0 in, braised	3 oz	193	26	43	0	—
trim ¼ in, Choice, braised	3 oz	241	15	42	0	—
trim ¼ in, Choice, roasted	3 bz	221	14	53	0	—
trim ¼ in, Select, braised	3 oz	220	13	42	0	—
trim ¼ in, Select, roasted	3 oz	199	11	54	0	—
brisket						
flat half, lean & fat, trim 0 in, braised	3 oz	183	8	53	0	—
flat half, lean & fat, trim ¼ in, braised	3 oz	309	24	48	0	—
point half, lean & fat, trim 0 in, braised	3 oz	304	24	57	0	—
point half, lean & fat, trim ¼ in, braised	3 oz	343	29	55	0	—
whole, lean & fat, trim 0 in, braised	3 oz	247	17	55	0	—
whole, lean & fat, trim ¼ in, braised	3 oz	327	27	52	0	—
chuck						
arm pot roast, lean & fat, trim 0 in, braised	3 oz	238	14	53	0	—
arm pot roast, lean & fat, trim ¼ in, braised	3 oz	282	20	51	0	—
blade roast, lean & fat, trim 0 in, braised	3 oz	284	21	56	0	—
blade roast, lean & fat, trim ¼ in, braised	3 oz	293	22	55	0	—
corned beef brisket, cooked	3 oz	213	16	964	tr	—

FOOD	PORTION	CAL	FAT	SOD	CARB	FIB
eye of round, lean & fat						
trim 0 in, Choice, roasted	3 oz	153	5	53	0	—
trim 0 in, Select, roasted	3 oz	137	4	53	0	—
trim ¼ in, Select, roasted	3 oz	184	10	51	0	—
trim ¼ in, Choice, roasted	3 oz	205	12	50	0	—
flank, lean & fat trim 0 in,						
braised	3 oz	224	14	60	0	—
broiled	3 oz	192	11	69	0	—
ground						
extra lean, broiled medium	3 oz	217	14	59	0	—
extra lean, broiled well-done	3 oz	225	14	70	0	—
extra lean, fried medium	3 oz	216	14	59	0	—
extra lean, fried well-done	3 oz	224	14	69	0	—
extra lean, raw	4 oz	265	19	75	0	—
lean, broiled medium	3 oz	231	16	65	0	—
lean, broiled well-done	3 oz	238	15	76	0	—
low-fat w/ carrageenan, raw	4 oz	160	7	70	tr	—
regular, broiled medium	3 oz	246	18	70	0	—
regular, broiled well-done	3 oz	248	17	79	0	—
porterhouse steak						
lean & fat, trim ¼ in, Choice, broiled	3 oz	260	19	52	0	—
lean only, trim ¼ in, Choice, broiled	3 oz	185	9	56	0	—
rib eye small end, lean & fat, trim 0 in, Choice, broiled	3 oz	261	19	54	0	—
rib large end, lean & fat						
trim 0 in, roasted	3 oz	300	24	55	0	—
trim ¼ in, broiled	3 oz	295	24	54	0	—
trim ¼ in, roasted	3 oz	310	25	54	0	—

FOOD	PORTION	CAL	FAT	SOD	CARB	FIB
rib small end, lean & fat, trim 0 in, broiled	3 oz	252	18	54	0	—
rib small end, lean & fat						
trim ¼ in, broiled	3 oz	285	22	53	0	—
trim ¼ in, roasted	3 oz	295	24	53	0	—
rib whole, lean & fat, trim ¼ in						
Choice, broiled	3 oz	306	25	53	0	—
Choice, roasted	3 oz	320	27	53	0	—
Prime, roasted	3 oz	348	30	54	0	—
Select, broiled	3 oz	274	21	54	0	—
Select, roasted	3 oz	286	23	54	0	—
shank, crosscut, lean & fat, trim ¼ in, Choice, simmered	3 oz	224	12	52	0	—
short loin top loin, lean & fat						
trim 0 in, Choice, broiled	1 steak (5.4 oz)	353	19	104	0	—
trim 0 in, Choice, broiled	3 oz	193	10	57	0	—
trim 0 in, Select, broiled	1 steak (5.4 oz)	309	14	104	0	—
trim ¼ in, Choice, broiled	1 steak (6.3 oz)	536	38	114	0	—
trim ¼ in, Choice, broiled	3 oz	253	18	54	0	—
trim ¼ in, Prime, broiled	1 steak (6.3 oz)	582	43	114	0	—
trim ¼ in, Select, broiled	1 steak (6.3 oz)	473	31	114	0	—
short loin top loin, lean only,						
trim 0 in Choice, broiled	1 steak (5.2 oz)	311	14	101	0	—
trim ¼ in, Choice, broiled	1 steak (5.2 oz)	314	15	100	0	—
shortribs, lean & fat, Choice, braised	3 oz	400	36	43	0	—
t-bone steak, lean & fat, trim ¼ in, Choice, broiled	3 oz	253	18	52	0	—
t-bone steak, lean only, trim ¼ in, Choice, broiled	3 oz	182	9	56	0	—

FOOD	PORTION	CAL	FAT	SOD	CARB	FIB
tenderloin, lean & fat,						
trim ¼ in, Choice, broiled	3 oz	259	19	50	0	—
trim ¼ in, Choice, roasted	3 oz	288	22	55	0	—
trim ¼ in, Prime, broiled	3 oz	270	20	50	0	—
trim ¼ in, Select, roasted	3 oz	275	21	48	0	—
trim 0 in, Select, broiled	3 oz	194	11	52	0	—
trim 0 in, Choice, broiled	3 oz	208	12	52	0	—
tenderloin, lean only						
trim ¼ in, Choice, broiled	3 oz	188	10	54	0	—
trim ¼ in, Select, broiled	3 oz	169	7	54	0	—
trim 0 in, Select, broiled	3 oz	170	7	54	0	—
tip round, lean & fat,						
trim ¼ in, Choice, roasted	3 oz	210	13	53	0	—
trim ¼ in, Prime, roasted	3 oz	233	15	53	0	—
trim ¼ in, Select, roasted	3 oz	191	10	53	0	—
trim 0 in, Choice, roasted	3 oz	170	8	54	0	—
trim 0 in, Select, roasted	3 oz	158	6	55	0	—
top round, lean & fat						
trim ¼ in, Choice, braised	3 oz	221	11	38	0	—
trim ¼ in, Choice, broiled	3 oz	190	9	51	0	—
trim ¼ in, Choice, fried	3 oz	235	13	58	0	—
trim ¼ in, Prime, broiled	3 oz	195	9	51	0	—
trim ¼ in, Select, braised	3 oz	175	7	51	0	—
trim ¼ in, Select, braised	3 oz	199	8	38	0	—

FOOD	PORTION	CAL	FAT	SOD	CARB	FIB
top round (cont.)						
trim 0 in, Choice, braised	3 oz	184	6	38	0	—
trim 0 in, Select, braised	3 oz	170	5	38	0	—
top sirloin, lean & fat						
trim ¼ in, Choice, broiled	3 oz	228	14	53	0	—
trim ¼ in, Choice, fried	3 oz	277	19	59	0	—
trim ¼ in, Select, broiled	3 oz	208	12	54	0	—
trim 0 in, Choice, broiled	3 oz	194	10	55	0	—
trim 0 in, Select, broiled	3 oz	166	6	55	0	—
tripe, raw	4 oz	111	4	52	0	—
FROZEN						
patties, broiled medium	3 oz	240	17	66	0	—
READY-TO-USE						
Roast Beef (Healthy Choice)	1 oz	25	tr	290	tr	—
Roast Beef (Oscar Mayer)	1 slice (.4 oz)	14	tr	55	tr	—
Weight Watchers Deli Thin Oven Roasted Cured	5 slices (⅓ oz)	10	tr	85	tr	—

BEEF DISHES

CANNED						
Beef Stew (Healthy Choice)	½ can (7.5 oz)	140	2	540	16	—
Beef Stew (Wolf Brand)	1 cup	179	8	1043	18	—
Manwich Mexican, as prep	1 sandwich	310	13	690	30	2
Sloppy Joe, as prep (Manwich)	1 sandwich	310	13	620	31	1
FROZEN						
Banquet						
Family Entree Beef Stew	7 oz	140	5	—	18	—

FOOD	PORTION	CAL	FAT	SOD	CARB	FIB
Family Entree Mushroom Gravy & Charbroiled Beef Patties	7 oz	260	18	—	12	—
Family Entree Noodles & Beef w/ Gravy	7 oz	180	6	—	20	—
Family Entree Onion Gravy & Beef Patties	7 oz	260	19	—	13	—
Family Entree Veal Parmagian Patties	7 oz	320	16	—	29	—
Family Entree Gravy & Salisbury Steak	7 oz	260	19	—	11	—
Family Entree Gravy & Sliced Steak	7 oz	140	5	—	8	—
Banquet Entree						
Beef Patties And Mushroom Gravy	7 oz	350	26	1190	12	—
Meatloaf w/ Tomato Sauce	7 oz	330	22	1330	16	—
Salisbury Steak And Gravy	7 oz	300	21	1310	13	—
Chefwich Beef w/ Barbecue Sauce	1	340	10	—	—	—
Ovenstuffs Beef/ Cheddar Deli Melt	1 (4.75 oz)	390	22	820	28	—
Tyson Microwave BBQ Sandwich	1 sandwich	200	3	600	29	—
MIX						
Hamburger Helper						
Beef Noodle, as prep	1 cup	330	15	920	29	—
Beef Romanoff, as prep	1 cup	350	16	1070	31	—
Beef Taco, as prep	1 cup	330	14	970	33	—
Cheddar 'n Bacon, as prep	1 cup	380	19	970	30	—
Cheeseburger Macaroni, as prep	1 cup	370	19	1030	28	—
Cheesy Italian, as prep	1 cup	370	18	1040	29	—
Chili Macaroni, as prep	1 cup	330	14	960	32	—

FOOD	PORTION	CAL	FAT	SOD	CARB	FIB
Hamburger Helper *(cont.)*						
Hamburger Hash, as prep	1 cup	320	15	1020	27	—
Hamburger Pizza Dish, as prep	1 cup	360	14	1010	27	—
Hamburger Stew, as prep	1 cup	300	14	1010	26	—
Lasagne, as prep	1 cup	340	14	910	33	—
Meat Loaf, as prep	5 oz	360	22	710	14	—
Nacho Cheese, as prep	1 cup	360	15	1050	35	—
Pizzabake, as prep	⅙ pkg (4.5 oz)	320	14	840	29	—
Potatoes Stroganoff, as prep	1 cup	330	16	990	26	—
Potatoes Au Gratin, as prep	1 cup	350	18	900	27	—
Rice Oriental, as prep	1 cup	340	14	1120	38	—
Sloppy Joe Bake, as prep	5 oz	340	15	1100	33	—
Spaghetti, as prep	1 cup	340	14	1100	32	—
Stroganoff, as prep	1 cup	390	20	870	30	—
Tacobake, as prep	⅙ pkg (5.75 oz)	320	15	940	31	—
Zesty Italian, as prep	1 cup	340	13	980	35	—
Lipton Microeasy Hearty Beef Stew	¼ pkg	71	1	729	14	—
Lipton Microeasy Homestyle Meatloaf	¼ pkg	87	2	630	15	—
Manwich Seasoning Mix, as prep	1 sandwich	320	13	590	31	2
SHELF STABLE						
Beef Stew (Healthy Choice)	7.5 oz cup	140	2	540	16	—
TAKE-OUT						
bubble & squeak	5 oz	186	13	—	16	3
cornish pasty	1 (8 oz)	847	52	—	79	3
kebab indian	1 (5.4 oz)	553	40	—	2	—
kheena	6.7 oz	781	71	—	1	tr
koftas	5	280	22	—	3	tr
roast beef sandwich plain	1	346	14	792	33	—
roast beef sandwich w/ cheese	1	402	18	1634	27	—

FOOD	PORTION	CAL	FAT	SOD	CARB	FIB
roast beef submarine sandwich w/ tomato, lettuce & mayonnaise	1	411	13	845	44	—
samosa	2 (4 oz)	652	62	—	20	2
shepherds pie	6 oz	196	10	—	15	1
steak & kidney pie w/ top crust	1 slice (5 oz)	400	26	—	23	1
steak sandwich w/ tomato, lettuce, salt & mayonnaise	1	459	14	798	52	—
stew	6 oz	208	13	—	6	1
stew w/ vegetables	1 cup	220	11	292	15	—
stroganoff	¾ cup	260	19	503	43	—
swiss steak	4.6 oz	214	9	139	10	2
toad in the hole	1 (4.7 oz)	383	29	—	23	1

BEEFALO

FOOD	PORTION	CAL	FAT	SOD	CARB	FIB
roasted	3 oz	160	5	70	0	—

BEER AND ALE

FOOD	PORTION	CAL	FAT	SOD	CARB	FIB
Amstel Light	12 oz	95	0	—	—	—
Anheuser Busch Natural Light	12 oz	110	0	—	—	—
Bud Light	12 oz	108	0	—	—	—
Coors	12 oz	132	0	10	30	—
Coors Light	12 oz	101	0	10	13	—
Hamm's	12 oz	137	0	—	12	—
Killian's	12 oz	212	0	10	29	—
Michelob Light	12 oz	134	0	—	—	—
Miller Lite	12 oz	96	0	—	—	—
Molson Light	12 oz	109	0	—	—	—
Old Milwaukee	12 oz	145	0	25	13	—
Old Milwaukee Light	12 oz	122	0	18	9	—
Olympia	12 oz	143	0	—	12	—
Pabst	12 oz	143	0	—	12	—
Piels Light	12 oz	136	0	—	—	—
Schaefer	12 oz	138	0	23	13	—
Schaefer Light	12 oz	111	0	16	8	—
Schlitz	12 oz	145	0	23	13	—
Schlitz Light	12 oz	99	0	9	3	—
Schmidts Light	12 oz	96	0	—	—	—
Signature	12 oz	150	0	21	13	—
Stroh	12 oz	142	0	23	13	—
Stroh Light	12 oz	115	0	11	7	—

FOOD	PORTION	CAL	FAT	SOD	CARB	FIB
Winterfest	12 oz	167	0	11	38	—
ale brown	10 oz	77	0	—	8	0
ale pale	10 oz	88	0	—	12	0
beer light	12 oz can	100	0	10	5	—
beer regular	12 oz can	146	0	19	13	—
lager	10 oz	80	0	—	4	0
stout	10 oz	102	0	—	6	0
NONALCOHOLIC						
Guinness Kaliber	12 oz	43	0	—	—	—
Hamm's	12 oz	55	0	—	12	—
Kingsbury	12 fl oz	60	0	—	—	—
Pabst	12 oz	55	0	—	12	—
Spirit	12 oz	80	0	—	16	—

BEETS
CANNED

FOOD	PORTION	CAL	FAT	SOD	CARB	FIB
Cut (Libby)	½ cup	35	0	—	—	—
Cut (Seneca)	½ cup	35	0	—	—	—
Diced (Libby)	½ cup	35	0	—	—	—
Diced (Seneca)	½ cup	35	0	—	—	—
Diced Tender (S&W)	½ cup	40	0	270	9	—
Harvard (Libby)	½ cup	80	0	—	—	—
Harvard (Seneca)	½ cup	80	0	—	—	—
Julienne French Style (S&W)	½ cup	40	0	270	9	—
Pickled (Libby)	½ cup	35	0	—	—	—
Pickled (Seneca)	½ cup	35	0	—	—	—
Pickled Whole Extra Small (S&W)	½ cup	70	0	215	16	—
Pickled w/ Onions (Libby)	½ cup	80	0	—	—	—
Pickled w/ Onions (Seneca)	½ cup	80	0	—	—	—
Pickled w/ Red Wine Vinegar Sliced (S&W)	½ cup	70	0	215	16	—
Sliced (Libby)	½ cup	35	0	—	—	—
Sliced (Seneca)	½ cup	35	0	—	—	—
Sliced Small Premium (S&W)	½ cup	40	0	270	9	—
Sliced Water Pack (S&W)	½ cup	35	0	40	9	—
Whole (Libby)	½ cup	35	0	—	—	—
Whole (Seneca)	½ cup	35	0	—	—	—

FOOD	PORTION	CAL	FAT	SOD	CARB	FIB
Whole Small (S&W)	½ cup	40	0	270	9	—
harvard	½ cup	89	tr	199	22	—
pickled	½ cup	75	tr	301	19	—
sliced	½ cup	27	tr	—	6	—
FRESH						
greens cooked	½ cup	20	tr	173	4	—
greens raw	½ cup	4	tr	38	1	—
greens raw chopped	½ cup	4	tr	38	1	—
raw sliced	½ cup (2.4 oz)	29	tr	53	7	—
sliced cooked	½ cup (3 oz)	38	tr	65	9	—
whole cooked	2 (3.5 oz)	44	tr	77	10	—
whole raw	2 (5.7 oz)	70	tr	126	16	—
JUICE						
beet juice	3.5 oz	36	0	200	8	—

BEVERAGES

see BEER AND ALE, CHAMPAGNE, COFFEE, DRINK MIXERS, FRUIT DRINKS, MALT, MINERAL WATER/BOTTLED WATER, LIQUOR/LIQUEUR, SODA, TEA/HERBAL TEA, WINE, WINE COOLER

BISCUIT

FOOD	PORTION	CAL	FAT	SOD	CARB	FIB
FROZEN						
Egg, Canadian Bacon & Cheese (Great Starts)	5.2 oz	420	22	1845	37	—
Sausage (Great Starts)	4.7 oz	410	22	1180	36	—
Sausage Biscuit (Weight Watchers)	3 oz	220	11	560	19	—
HOME RECIPE						
buttermilk	1 (2 oz)	212	10	348	27	—
oatcakes	2 (4 oz)	115	5	—	16	1
plain	1 (2 oz)	212	10	348	27	—
MIX						
Biscuit Mix (Arrowhead)	¼ cup (1.2 oz)	120	1	200	23	3
Bisquick	½ cup (57 g)	240	8	700	37	—
Buttermilk Biscuit Mix, not prep (Health Valley)	1 oz	100	1	170	20	3
buttermilk	1 (2 oz)	191	7	544	28	1
plain	1 (2 oz)	191	7	544	28	1
READY-TO-EAT						
Old Fashioned (Arnold)	1	60	3	100	8	—

FOOD	PORTION	CAL	FAT	SOD	CARB	FIB
REFRIGERATED						
1869 Brand Baking Powder	1	100	5	310	12	—
1869 Brand Butter Tastin'	1	100	5	300	12	—
1869 Brand Buttermilk	1	100	5	310	12	—
Ballard Ovenready	1	50	1	180	10	—
Ballard Ovenready Buttermilk	1	50	1	180	10	—
Big Country Southern Style	1	100	4	320	14	—
Hungry Jack						
Butter Tastin' Flaky	1	90	4	280	11	—
Buttermilk Flaky	1	90	4	300	12	—
Buttermilk Fluffy	1	90	4	280	12	—
Extra Rich Buttermilk	1	50	1	180	9	—
Flaky	1	80	4	300	12	—
Honey Tastin' Flaky	1	90	4	290	13	—
Pillsbury						
Butter	1	50	1	180	10	—
Buttermilk	1	50	1	180	10	—
Country	1	50	1	180	10	—
Good'N Buttery Fluffy	1	90	5	270	11	—
Hearty Grains Multi-Grain	1	80	2	230	15	—
Hearty Grains Oatmeal Raisin	1	90	2	210	16	—
Heat N' Eat Big Premium	2	280	15	610	32	—
Tender Layer Buttermilk	1	50	1	170	9	—
Pillsbury Big Country Butter Tastin'	1	100	4	320	14	—
Pillsbury Big Country Buttermilk	1	100	4	320	14	—
Pillsbury Deluxe Heat N' Eat Buttermilk	2	170	5	530	27	—
Roman Meal	2 (2.4 oz)	180	4	456	34	1
Roman Meal Honey Nut Oat Bran	1 (1.5 oz)	131	5	278	21	1
buttermilk	1 (1 oz)	98	4	341	14	—
plain	1 (1 oz)	98	4	341	14	tr

FOOD	PORTION	CAL	FAT	SOD	CARB	FIB
TAKE-OUT						
buttermilk	1	127	6	368	17	—
plain	1 (35 g)	276	34	584	13	—
w/ egg	1	315	20	655	24	—
w/ egg & bacon	1	457	31	999	29	—
w/ egg & sausage	1	582	39	1142	41	—
w/ egg & steak	1	474	28	888	37	—
w/ egg, cheese & bacon	1	477	31	1261	33	—
w/ ham	1	387	18	1433	44	—
w/ sausage	1	485	32	1071	40	—
w/ steak	1	456	26	795	44	—
BISON						
roasted	3 oz	122	2	48	0	—
BLACK BEANS						
CANNED						
Health Valley Fast Menu Organic Black Beans With Tofu Weiners	7.5 oz	150	1	170	20	15
Health Valley Fast Menu Western Black Beans With Garden Vegetable	7.5 oz	160	5	250	14	14
Progresso	½ cup	90	1	350	19	7
DRIED						
Bean Cuisine Black Turtle	½ cup	115	1	5	—	5
cooked	1 cup	227	1	1	41	—
MIX						
Mahatma Black Beans & Rice	1 cup	200	2	850	39	6
Pasta & Beans Black Beans With Fusilli (Bean Cuisine)	½ cup	174	4	453	27	—
BLACKBERRIES						
CANNED						
in heavy syrup	½ cup	118	tr	3	30	—
FRESH						
blackberries	½ cup	37	tr	0	9	3
FROZEN						
unsweetened	1 cup	97	1	2	24	—

FOOD	PORTION	CAL	FAT	SOD	CARB	FIB

BLACKEYE PEAS
CANNED

FOOD	PORTION	CAL	FAT	SOD	CARB	FIB
Seasoned w/ Pork (Luck's)	7.25 oz	200	6	—	—	—
Trappey's	½ cup	90	1	410	17	—
Trappey's Jalapeno w/pork	½ cup	90	1	480	15	—
	½ cup	199	4	840	40	—

DRIED

FOOD	PORTION	CAL	FAT	SOD	CARB	FIB
Hurst Brand	1 cup	233	1	—	—	—
cooked	1 cup	198	1	6	36	16

BLINTZE

FOOD	PORTION	CAL	FAT	SOD	CARB	FIB
Apple Raisin (Golden)	1 (2.25 oz)	80	2	145	16	—
Blueberry (Golden)	1 (2.25 oz)	90	1	150	18	—
Cheese (Golden)	1 (2.25 oz)	80	2	135	13	—
Cherry (Golden)	1 (2.25 oz)	95	1	145	18	—
Potato (Golden)	1 (2.25 oz)	90	4	170	15	—

TAKE-OUT

FOOD	PORTION	CAL	FAT	SOD	CARB	FIB
cheese	2	186	6	268	18	tr

BLUEBERRIES
CANNED

FOOD	PORTION	CAL	FAT	SOD	CARB	FIB
In Heavy Syrup (S&W)	½ cup	111	0	—	30	—
in heavy syrup	1 cup	225	1	9	56	—

FRESH

FOOD	PORTION	CAL	FAT	SOD	CARB	FIB
blueberries	1 cup	82	1	9	20	—

FROZEN

FOOD	PORTION	CAL	FAT	SOD	CARB	FIB
Big Valley	4 oz	60	tr	0	13	—
unsweetened	1 cup	78	1	1	19	—

BLUEFIN

FOOD	PORTION	CAL	FAT	SOD	CARB	FIB
fillet, baked	4.1 oz	186	6	90	0	—

BLUEFISH

FOOD	PORTION	CAL	FAT	SOD	CARB	FIB
fresh, baked	3 oz	135	5	65	0	—

BOAR

FOOD	PORTION	CAL	FAT	SOD	CARB	FIB
wild, roasted	3 oz	136	4	—	0	—

BOK CHOY

FOOD	PORTION	CAL	FAT	SOD	CARB	FIB
Dole, shredded	½ cup	5	tr	23	1	—

BORAGE
FRESH

FOOD	PORTION	CAL	FAT	SOD	CARB	FIB
cooked, chopped	3.5 oz	25	1	88	4	—
raw, chopped	½ cup	9	tr	35	1	—

FOOD	PORTION	CAL	FAT	SOD	CARB	FIB
BOYSENBERRIES						
CANNED						
in heavy syrup	1 cup	226	tr	9	57	—
FROZEN						
Big Valley	3.5 oz	50	tr	0	10	—
unsweetened	1 cup	66	tr	2	16	—
JUICE						
Smucker's	8 oz	120	0	10	30	—
Smucker's Juice Sparkler	10 oz	130	tr	5	31	—
BRAINS						
beef, pan-fried	3 oz	167	13	134	0	—
beef, simmered	3 oz	136	11	102	0	—
lamb, braised	3 oz	124	9	114	0	—
lamb, fried	3 oz	232	19	133	0	—
pork, braised	3 oz	117	8	77	0	—
veal, braised	3 oz	115	8	133	0	—
veal, fried	3 oz	181	14	150	0	—
BRAN						
Fast Menu Oat Bran Pilaf With Garden Vegetables (Health Valley)	7.5 oz	210	7	330	30	15
Oat (Hodgson Mill)	¼ cup (1.3 oz)	120	3	3	23	6
Oat (Roman Mill)	1 oz	94	3	3	13	5
Oat Bran (Arrowhead)	⅓ cup (1.4 oz)	150	3	0	23	7
Oat Bran (Mother's)	⅓ cup	92	2	1	17	4
Quaker Unprocessed Bran	2 tbsp	8	tr	0	4	3
Super Bran (H-O)	⅓ cup	110	2	0	18	3
Toasted Wheat Bran (Kretschmer)	⅓ cup	57	2	2	15	3
Wheat (Hodgson Mill)	¼ cup (0.5 oz)	30	1	0	10	7
Wheat Bran (Arrowhead)	¼ cup (0.6 oz)	30	1	0	7	6
Wheat Bran (Good Shepherd)	1 oz	80	1	5	18	3
corn	⅓ cup	56	tr	2	21	21
oat, cooked	½ cup	44	tr	1	13	—
oat, dry	½ cup	116	3	1	31	7
rice, dry	⅓ cup	88	6	1	14	6
wheat, dry	½ cup	65	1	1	19	13

FOOD	PORTION	CAL	FAT	SOD	CARB	FIB
BRAZIL NUTS						
dried, unblanched	1 oz	186	19	0	4	—
BREAD						
see also BAGEL, BISCUIT, BREADSTICK, CROISSANT, ENGLISH MUFFIN, MUFFIN, ROLL, SCONE						
CANNED						
Brown Bread (B&M)	½-in slice (1.6 oz)	92	0	345	21	4
Brown Bread (Friends)	1 slice (1.6 oz)	92	0	345	21	2
Brown Bread Raisins (B&M)	½-in slice (1.6 oz)	94	0	320	22	4
Brown Bread w/ Raisin (Friends)	1 slice (1.6 oz)	94	0	320	22	2
Brown Bread New England Recipe (S&W)	2 slices	76	0	172	17	—
boston brown	1 slice (1.6 oz)	88	1	284	20	2
HOME RECIPE						
banana	1 slice (2 oz)	195	6	181	33	—
cornbread, as prep w/ 2% milk	1 piece (2.3 oz)	173	5	428	28	—
cornbread, as prep w/ whole milk	1 piece (2.3 oz)	176	5	428	28	—
datenut	½-in slice	92	3	63	15	—
Irish soda bread	1 slice (2 oz)	174	3	239	34	—
pita, whole wheat	6-in pocket	247	1	—	—	—
pumpkin	1 slice (1 oz)	94	4	89	15	—
white, as prep w/ 2% milk	1 slice	81	2	104	14	—
white, as prep w/ nonfat dry milk	1 slice	78	1	95	15	—
white, as prep w/ whole milk	1 slice	82	2	104	14	—
whole wheat	1 slice	71	tr	—	—	—
MIX						
Corn Bread (Ballard)	⅙ bread	140	3	570	25	—
Corn Bread (Dromedary)	1 piece (2 in x 2 in)	130	3	480	20	—
Corn Bread Easy Mix (Aunt Jemima)	⅙ cake	210	7	690	34	1
Cornbread Blue Cornmeal (Zia Foods)	1 piece (1.2 oz)	110	6	—	—	—

FOOD	PORTION	CAL	FAT	SOD	CARB	FIB
cornbread	1 piece (2 oz)	189	6	467	29	1
READY-TO-EAT						
12 Grain Natural (Arnold)	1 slice (0.8 oz)	60	0	100	10	1
7 Grain Hearty Slice (Pepperidge Farm)	2 slices	180	2	340	36	2
9 Grain & Nut (Matthew's)	1 slice	80	3	100	9	2
Augusto Pan De Aqua (Arnold)	1 oz	80	1	150	14	1
Bran'nola Country Oat (Arnold)	1 slice (1.3 oz)	90	3	130	16	3
Bran'nola Country Oat (Brownberry)	1 slice	90	2	166	18	3
Bran'nola Dark Wheat (Arnold)	1 slice (1.3 oz)	90	3	150	15	3
Bran'nola Hearty Wheat (Arnold)	1 slice (1.3 oz)	100	3	160	15	3
Bran'nola Hearty Wheat (Brownberry)	1 slice	88	2	197	17	3
Bran'nola Nutty Grains (Arnold)	1 slice (1.3 oz)	90	2	120	14	3
Bran'nola Nutty Grains (Brownberry)	1 slice	85	2	144	17	3
Bran'nola Original (Arnold)	1 slice (1.3 oz)	90	2	150	16	3
Bran'nola Original (Brownberry)	1 slice	85	1	137	18	3
Brown & Serve Mini Loaf (Roman Meal)	½ loaf (2 oz)	136	2	275	24	1
Butter Crust (Freihofer's)	1 slice	70	1	—	—	—
Canadian Oat (Freihofer's)	1 slice	80	1	—	—	—
Cinnamon (Matthew's)	1 slice	70	1	100	13	2
Cinnamon (Pepperidge Farm)	1 slice	90	3	110	15	2
Cinnamon Chip (Arnold)	1 slice	80	2	90	13	tr
Cinnamon Raisin (Arnold)	1 slice (0.9 oz)	70	1	85	13	1
Club Pullman (Freihofer's)	1 slice	70	1	—	—	—
Country Bran Bakery Light (Arnold)	1 slice (0.8 oz)	40	tr	80	7	3

FOOD	PORTION	CAL	FAT	SOD	CARB	FIB
Cracked Wheat (Pepperidge Farm)	1 slice	70	1	140	13	1
Cracked Wheat (Roman Meal)	1 slice (1.4 oz)	92	2	129	15	2
Cranberry (Arnold)	1 slice (0.9 oz)	70	1	80	14	1
Crunchy Oat 1½ lb Loaf (Pepperidge Farm)	2 slices	190	4	290	34	3
Date Walnut (Pepperidge Farm)	1 slice	90	3	110	14	2
French Fully Baked (Pepperidge Farm)	2 oz	150	2	320	28	1
French Stick Extra Sour (Parisian)	2 oz	150	1	311	27	—
French Stick Francisco (Arnold)	1 slice (1 oz)	70	2	110	12	—
French Stick Savoni (Arnold)	1 oz	80	tr	—	15	1
French Stick Sweet (Parisian)	2 oz	154	2	331	27	—
French Twin (Pepperidge Farm)	1 oz	80	1	160	15	0
French Twin Loaves Franscisco (Arnold)	2 slices (2 oz)	150	2	280	27	—
Golden (Matthew's)	1 slice	70	1	125	14	1
Health Nut (Brownberry)	1 slice	71	3	158	12	3
Hearty Wheat Light (Roman Meal)	1 slice (0.8 oz)	42	tr	102	7	2
Hi-Fibre (Monks' Bread)	1 slice	50	1	110	13	—
Honey Bran (Pepperidge Farm)	1 slice	90	1	160	18	1
Honey Nut Oat Bran (Roman Meal)	1 slice (1 oz)	72	2	129	11	1
Honey Oat Bran (Roman Meal)	1 slice (1 oz)	70	1	132	12	1
Italian (Weight Watchers)	1 slice (0.8 oz)	38	tr	99	7	2
Italian Francisco (Arnold)	1 slice (1 oz)	70	1	110	12	—
Italian Bakery Light (Arnold)	1 slice (0.7 oz)	40	tr	90	7	2
Italian Brown & Serve (Pepperidge Farm)	1 oz	80	1	150	14	0

FOOD	PORTION	CAL	FAT	SOD	CARB	FIB
Italian Light (Wonder)	1 slice	40	0	115	6	3
Italian No Seeds (Freihofer's)	1 slice	70	1	—	—	—
Italian Seeded (Freihofer's)	1 slice	70	1	—	—	—
Italian Sliced (Pepperidge Farm)	1 slice	70	1	125	12	—
Italian Stick Francisco (Arnold)	1 oz	90	1	110	17	—
Lite Diet (Freihofer's)	1 slice	40	0	—	—	—
Malsovit	1 slice	66	1	146	12	4
Multi-Grain (Weight Watchers)	1 slice (0.8 oz)	41	1	98	7	2
Oat (Roman Meal)	1 slice (1 oz)	69	1	100	12	1
Oat (Weight Watchers)	1 slice (0.8 oz)	42	1	102	7	2
Oat Bran (Matthew's)	1 slice	65	0	110	12	2
Oat Bran (Roman Meal)	1 slice (1 oz)	68	1	136	12	1
Oat Bran Light (Roman Meal)	1 slice (0.8 oz)	42	tr	100	7	2
Oatmeal (Pepperidge Farm)	1 slice	70	1	160	12	1
Oatmeal & Bran (Oatmeal Goodness)	1 slice	90	2	—	—	—
Oatmeal & Sunflower Seeds (Oatmeal Goodness)	1 slice	90	2	—	—	—
Oatmeal 1½ lb Loaf (Pepperidge Farm)	1 slice	90	1	200	17	1
Oatmeal Bakery (Arnold)	1 slice	60	1	95	12	2
Oatmeal Bakery Light (Arnold)	1 slice	40	tr	100	8	2
Oatmeal Cinnamon (Oatmeal Goodness)	1 slice	90	2	—	—	—
Oatmeal Light (Pepperidge Farm)	1 slice	45	0	95	9	1
Oatmeal Natural (Brownberry)	1 slice	63	1	144	13	1
Oatmeal Raisin (Arnold)	1 slice (0.9 oz)	60	tr	90	12	2
Oatmeal Soft (Brownberry)	1 slice	48	1	82	10	2
Oatmeal Very Thin Sliced (Pepperidge Farm)	1 slice	40	1	80	8	—

FOOD	PORTION	CAL	FAT	SOD	CARB	FIB
Oatmeal Wheat (Oatmeal Goodness)	1 slice	90	2	—	—	—
Old Fashion (Freihofer's)	1 slice	70	1	—	—	—
Onion Rye (August Bros.)	1 slice	80	1	210	14	1
Pita Oat Bran (Sahara)	½ pocket (1 oz)	66	tr	163	14	2
Pita Wheat (Arnold)	½ pocket (1 oz)	71	0	—	16	—
Pita White (Arnold)	½ pocket (0.5 oz)	71	0	—	16	—
Pita White (Sahara)	½ pocket	78	1	147	16	—
Pita Whole Wheat (Matthew's)	1	210	2	390	45	7
Pumpernickel (Arnold)	1 slice (1.1 oz)	70	1	200	15	1
Pumpernickel (August Bros.)	1 slice	80	1	210	14	1
Pumpernickel (August Bros.)	1 slice (24 oz loaf)	90	1	220	18	1
Pumpernickel Family (Pepperidge Farm)	1 slice	80	1	230	15	2
Pumpernickel Party (Pepperidge Farm)	4 slices	60	1	160	12	1
Raisin (Malsovit)	1 slice	77	1	146	12	3
Raisin (Monks' Bread)	1 slice	70	2	85	10	—
Raisin (Sunmaid)	1 slice	70	tr	85	13	1
Raisin (Weight Watchers)	1 slice (0.9 oz)	55	tr	95	11	1
Raisin Bran (Brownberry)	1 slice	61	1	108	12	2
Raisin Cinnamon (Brownberry)	1 slice	66	1	107	12	1
Raisin Walnut (Brownberry)	1 slice	68	3	96	11	2
Raisin With Cinnamon (Pepperidge Farm)	1 slice	90	2	100	16	1
Rite Diet (Freihofer's)	2 slices	90	1	—	—	—
Round Top (Roman Meal)	1 slice (1 oz)	67	1	142	12	1
Rye (Weight Watchers)	1 slice (0.8 oz)	38	tr	100	7	2
Rye Bakery Soft Light (Arnold)	1 slice (1.1 oz)	40	tr	90	7	2
Rye Bakery Soft Seeded (Arnold)	1 slice (1.1 oz)	70	1	170	14	1
Rye Bakery Soft Unseeded (Arnold)	1 slice (1.1 oz)	70	1	170	14	1

FOOD	PORTION	CAL	FAT	SOD	CARB	FIB
Rye Thin Unseeded (Augusto Bros.)	1 slice	40	—	110	8	1
Rye With Seeds (Augusto Bros.)	1 slice (1 lb loaf)	80	1	210	14	1
Rye Without Seeds (August Bros.)	1 slice	80	1	210	14	1
Rye Dijon (Pepperidge Farm)	1 slice	50	1	180	9	1
Rye Dijon Real Jewish (Arnold)	1 slice	70	tr	210	15	1
Rye Dijon Thick Sliced (Pepperidge Farm)	1 slice	70	1	260	15	2
Rye Dill (Arnold)	1 slice (1.1 oz)	60	1	140	10	1
Rye Family (Pepperidge Farm)	1 slice (32 g)	80	1	220	16	2
Rye N' Pump (Augusto Bros.)	1 slice	90	1	220	18	1
Rye Party (Pepperidge Farm)	4 slices	60	1	250	12	1
Rye Real Jewish Melba Thin (Arnold)	1 slice (0.7 oz)	40	tr	95	9	1
Rye Real Jewish Unseeded (Arnold)	1 slice	80	tr	180	16	1
Rye Seedless Family (Pepperidge Farm)	1 slice	80	1	210	16	2
Rye Soft (Pepperidge Farm)	1 slice	70	1	120	12	—
Rye Soft Pumpernickel (Freihofer's)	1 slice	70	1	—	—	—
Rye Soft Dill & Onion (Freihofer's)	1 slice	70	1	—	—	—
Rye Soft No Seeds (Freihofer's)	1 slice	70	1	—	—	—
Rye Soft Seeded (Freihofer's)	1 slice	70	1	—	—	—
Rye Stub Pullman (Freihofer's)	1 slice	70	1	—	—	—
Rye With Caraway Real Jewish (Arnold)	1 slice	80	tr	180	16	1
Rye With Seeds (August Bros.)	1 slice (24 oz loaf)	90	1	220	18	1
Rye Without Seeds (August Bros.)	1 slice (24 oz loaf)	90	—	220	18	1
Rye Without Seeds Real Jewish (Arnold)	1 slice (1.1 oz)	70	tr	150	15	1

FOOD	PORTION	CAL	FAT	SOD	CARB	FIB
Sandwich (Roman Meal)	1 slice (0.8 oz)	55	1	115	10	1
Sesame Wheat (Pepperidge Farm)	2 slices	190	3	340	36	3
Seven Grain (Roman Meal)	1 slice (1 oz)	67	1	142	12	1
Seven Grain Light (Roman Meal)	1 slice (0.8 oz)	42	1	101	7	3
Sodium Free (Matthew's)	1 slice	70	2	<5	12	2
Sourdough Francisco (Arnold)	1 slice	90	1	250	19	1
Sourdough Light (Roman Meal)	1 slice (0.8 oz)	41	tr	115	7	3
Sourdough Whole Grain Light (Roman Meal)	1 slice (0.8 oz)	40	tr	104	7	3
Sourdough Light (Wonder)	1 slice	40	0	115	6	3
Sprouted Wheat (Pepperidge Farm)	1 slice	70	2	100	11	2
Sun Grain (Roman Meal)	1 slice (1 oz)	70	2	135	11	1
Sunbeam King (Freihofer's)	1 slice	70	1	—	—	—
Sunflower & Bran (Monks' Bread)	1 slice	70	1	80	12	2
The Original (Freihofer's)	1 slice	70	1	—	—	—
Twelve Grain (Roman Meal)	1 slice (1 oz)	70	2	140	11	1
Twelve Grain Light (Roman Meal)	1 slice (0.8 oz)	42	tr	104	7	3
Vienna Light (Pepperidge Farm)	1 slice	45	0	100	10	1
Vienna Thick Sliced (Pepperidge Farm)	1 slice	70	1	125	13	0
Wheat (Freihofer's)	1½ slices	70	1	—	—	—
Wheat (Weight Watchers)	1 slice (0.8 oz)	40	tr	99	7	2
Wheat Light (Roman Meal)	1 slice (0.8 oz)	41	tr	102	7	3
Wheat 1½ lb Loaf (Pepperidge Farm)	1 slice	90	2	190	18	2

FOOD	PORTION	CAL	FAT	SOD	CARB	FIB
Wheat Apple Honey (Brownberry)	1 slice	69	2	148	11	2
Wheat Berry Honey (Arnold)	1 slice (1.1 oz)	80	2	140	13	2
Wheat Brick Oven (Arnold)	1 slice (0.8 oz)	60	2	100	9	2
Wheat Cottage (America's Own)	1 slice	70	1	—	—	—
Wheat Family (Pepperidge Farm)	1 slice	70	1	130	13	2
Wheat Family (Wonder)	1 slice	70	1	150	13	1
Wheat Golden Light (Arnold)	1 slice (0.8 oz)	40	tr	90	7	2
Wheat Light (Pepperidge Farm)	1 slice	45	0	90	9	1
Wheat Light (Wonder)	1 slice	40	0	115	7	2
Wheat Natural (Arnold)	1 slice (1.3 oz)	80	1	180	15	2
Wheat Rite Diet (Freihofer's)	2 slices	90	1	—	—	—
Wheat Small (Freihofer's)	1½ slices	70	1	—	—	—
Wheat Soft (Brownberry)	1 slice	74	2	127	12	1
Wheat Split Top (Freihofer's)	1 slice	70	1	—	—	—
Wheat Stub Pullman (Freihofer's)	1 slice	70	1	—	—	—
Wheat Very Thin Sliced (Pepperidge Farm)	1 slice	35	0	75	7	0
Wheatberry Honey (Roman Meal)	1 slice (1 oz)	67	1	139	12	1
Wheatberry Light (Roman Meal)	1 slice (0.8 oz)	42	tr	102	7	2
White (Freihofer's)	1 slice	70	1	—	—	—
White (Monks' Bread)	1 slice	60	1	95	10	—
White (Weight Watchers)	1 slice (0.8 oz)	40	tr	96	7	2
White (Wonder)	1 slice	70	1	150	13	1
White Light (Roman Meal)	1 slice (0.8 oz)	41	tr	105	7	3
White Light Brick Oven (Arnold)	1 slice (0.8 oz)	40	tr	95	10	2
White Premium Light (Arnold)	1 slice	40	tr	90	7	2

FOOD	PORTION	CAL	FAT	SOD	CARB	FIB
White Thin Sliced Brick Oven (Arnold)	1 slice	40	tr	75	7	tr
White Brick Oven (Arnold)	1 slice (0.8 oz)	60	1	130	11	1
White Cottage (America's Own)	1 slice	70	1	—	—	—
White Country (Arnold)	1 slice (1.3 oz)	100	2	200	18	1
White Country (Pepperidge Farm)	2 slices	190	2	340	38	2
White Extra Fiber Brick Oven (Arnold)	1 slice (0.9 oz)	50	tr	90	10	2
White Large Family Thin Slice (Pepperidge Farm)	1 slice	70	1	150	13	0
White Light (Wonder)	1 slice	40	0	115	7	2
White Sandwich (Pepperidge Farm)	2 slices	130	2	260	24	0
White Split Top (Freihofer's)	1 slice	70	1	—	—	—
White Thin Slice (Pepperidge Farm)	1 slice	80	2	130	14	0
White Toasting (Pepperidge Farm)	1 slice	90	1	200	17	1
White Very Thin Sliced (Pepperidge Farm)	1 slice	40	0	80	8	0
White Whole Special Recipe (Stroehmann)	1 slice	70	1	160	13	—
White Whole Special Recipe Kids (Stroehmann)	1 slice	60	tr	150	12	—
Whole Grain Sourdough (Roman Meal)	1 slice (1 oz)	66	1	141	12	1
Whole Grain 100% (Roman Meal)	1 slice (1.4 oz)	91	1	198	16	2
Whole Wheat (Matthew's)	1 slice	70	1	130	12	2
Whole Wheat 100% (Freihofer's)	1 slice	75	1	—	—	—
Whole Wheat 100% (Roman Meal)	1 slice (1 oz)	64	1	141	11	2
Whole Wheat 100% Light (Roman Meal)	1 slice (0.8 oz)	42	tr	102	7	2

FOOD	PORTION	CAL	FAT	SOD	CARB	FIB
Whole Wheat 100% Light Brick Oven (Arnold)	1 slice (0.8 oz)	40	tr	85	6	3
Whole Wheat 100% Stoneground (Arnold)	1 slice (0.8 oz)	50	1	100	8	2
Whole Wheat 100% Stoneground (Monks' Bread)	1 slice	70	1	110	13	—
Whole Wheat 100% Stoneground (Wonder)	1 slice	80	1	160	13	2
Whole Wheat Thin Slice (Pepperidge Farm)	1 slice	60	1	110	12	2
Wonder Calcium Enriched	1 slice (1 oz)	70	1	150	12	tr
Wonder Light Calcium Enriched Wonder	2 slices (1.6 oz)	80	1	240	18	5
cracked wheat	1 slice	65	1	135	12	1
egg	1 slice (1.4 oz)	115	2	197	19	—
french	1 loaf (1 lb)	1270	18	2633	230	—
french	1 slice (1 oz)	78	1	172	15	1
gluten	1 slice	47	tr	104	8	—
italian	1 loaf (1 lb)	1255	4	2656	256	—
italian	1 slice (1 oz)	81	1	175	15	1
navajo fry	1 (10.5 in diam)	527	15	1112	85	—
navajo fry	1 (5 in diam)	296	9	625	48	—
oat bran	1 slice	71	1	122	12	1
oat bran, reduced calorie	1 slice	46	1	81	10	—
oatmeal	1 slice	73	1	162	13	1
oatmeal, reduced calorie	1 slice	48	1	89	10	—
pita	1 reg (2 oz)	165	1	322	33	1
pita	1 sm (1 oz)	78	tr	152	16	1
pita, whole wheat	1 reg (2 oz)	170	2	340	35	5
pita, whole wheat	1 sm (1 oz)	76	1	151	16	2
protein	1 slice	47	tr	104	8	—
pumpernickel	1 slice	80	1	215	15	2
raisin	1 slice	71	1	101	14	—
rice bran	1 slice	66	1	119	12	—
rye	1 slice	83	1	211	16	2
rye, reduced calorie	1 slice	47	1	93	9	—
seven grain	1 slice	65	1	127	12	2

FOOD	PORTION	CAL	FAT	SOD	CARB	FIB
sourdough	1 slice (1 oz)	78	1	172	15	1
vienna	1 slice (1 oz)	78	1	172	15	1
wheat, reduced calorie	1 slice	46	1	117	10	3
wheat berry	1 slice	65	1	132	12	1
wheat bran	1 slice	89	1	175	17	3
wheat germ	1 slice	74	1	157	14	—
white	1 slice	67	1	135	12	1
white, reduced calorie	1 slice	48	1	104	10	2
white, cubed	1 cup	80	1	154	15	—
white, toasted	1 slice	67	1	136	13	—
whole wheat	1 slice	70	1	149	13	2
REFRIGERATED						
Pillsbury Crusty French Loaf	1-in slice	60	tr	120	11	—
Pillsbury Hearty Grains Country Oatmeal Twists	1	80	2	120	15	—
Pillsbury Hearty Grains Cracked Wheat Twists	1	80	2	120	14	—
Pillsbury Pipin' Hot Wheat Loaf	1-in slice	70	2	170	12	—
Pillsbury Pipin' Hot White Loaf	1-in slice	70	2	170	12	—
Roman Meal Loaf (Roman Meal)	1 slice (1 oz)	85	3	199	13	1
TAKE-OUT						
chapatis, as prep, w/ fat	1 (2.5 oz)	230	9	—	34	5
chapatis, as prep, w/o fat	1 (2.5 oz)	141	1	—	31	5
cornbread	2 in × 2 in (1.4 oz)	107	2	276	18	—
cornstick	1 (1.3 oz)	101	4	195	13	tr
naan	1 (6 oz)	571	21	—	85	4
pappadums, fried	2 (1.5 oz)	81	4	—	9	2
paratha	1 (4.4 oz)	403	18	—	54	5

BREAD COATING

Don's Chuck Wagon Batter

All Purpose Mix (Hodgson Mill)	¼ cup (1 oz)	100	0	580	20	1
Chicken Frying Mix (Hodgson Mill)	¼ cup (1 oz)	95	0	850	21	1

FOOD	PORTION	CAL	FAT	SOD	CARB	FIB
Fish & Chips Mix (Hodgson Mill)	¼ cup (1 oz)	100	0	740	21	1
Fish Mix (Hodgson Mill)	¼ cup (1 oz)	95	0	940	21	1
Mushroom Mix (Hodgson Mill)	¼ cup (1 oz)	95	0	990	21	1
Onion Ring Mix (Hodgson Mill)	¼ cup (1 oz)	100	0	690	21	1
Seafood Seasoned Frying Mix (Hodgson Mill)	¼ cup (1 oz)	95	1	990	21	1
Fryin' Magic (Little Crow)	0.5 oz	43	tr	542	8	—
Golden Dipt Breading Frying Mix	1 oz	90	0	630	20	—
Golden Dipt Chicken Frying Mix	1 oz	90	0	1430	20	—
Golden Dipt Onion Ring Mix	1 oz	100	0	570	22	—
Mrs. Dash Crispy Coating Mix	0.5 oz	63	1	3	10	—
Oven Fry Homestyle Flour Recipe for Chicken	¼ pkg	85	2	971	15	—
Shake 'N Bake						
Extra Crispy Oven Fry For Pork	¼ pkg (1 oz)	120	3	688	21	—
Italian Herb Recipe	¼ pkg (0.5 oz)	77	1	618	14	—
Original Barbecue For Chicken	¼ pkg (0.5 oz)	93	2	841	18	—
Original Barbecue For Pork	¼ pkg (0.5 oz)	38	1	351	7	—
Original Country Mild	¼ pkg (0.5 oz)	76	4	501	10	—
Original For Chicken	¼ pkg (0.5 oz)	75	2	451	14	—
Original For Fish	¼ pkg (0.5 oz)	73	1	406	14	—
Original For Pork	¼ pkg (0.5 oz)	41	1	301	8	—

BREAD MACHINE

MIX

FOOD	PORTION	CAL	FAT	SOD	CARB	FIB
Dromedary Country White	½-in slice (2 oz)	140	1	230	28	1
Pillsbury Cracked Wheat	1/12 pkg (1.3 oz)	130	2	260	25	2

FOOD	PORTION	CAL	FAT	SOD	CARB	FIB
BREADCRUMBS						
4C Salt Free	1 tbsp (0.5 oz)	50	1	0	10	—
4C Seasoned	1 tbsp (0.5 oz)	50	1	270	10	—
4C Toasted	1 tbsp (0.5 oz)	50	1	110	10	—
4C Toasted Salt Free	1 tbsp (0.5 oz)	50	1	0	10	—
Arnold Italian	0.5 oz	50	tr	200	8	tr
Arnold Plain	0.5 oz	50	tr	80	8	tr
Contadina	⅓ cup	100	2	700	19	1
Devonsheer Italian Style	1 oz	104	1	408	20	1
Devonsheer Plain	1 oz	108	1	272	21	1
Friday's Seasoned	1 oz	56	tr	—	—	—
Jaclyn's Organic Whole Wheat Italian Style	0.5 oz	28	1	5	13	—
Jaclyn's Organic Whole Wheat Plain	0.5 oz	28	1	5	13	—
Progresso Italian Style	2 tbsp	60	tr	240	11	—
Progresso Plain	2 tbsp	60	tr	110	11	—
dry	1 cup	426	6	930	78	5
dry seasoned	1 cup (4 oz)	441	3	3180	85	5
fresh	⅔ cup	76	1	153	14	1
BREADFRUIT						
breadfruit	3.5 oz	109	tr	—	—	—
fresh	¼ small	99	tr	2	26	—
seeds, raw	1 oz	54	2	—	8	—
seeds, roasted	1 oz	59	tr	—	11	—
seeds, cooked	1 oz	48	1	—	9	—
BREADNUTTREE SEEDS						
dried	1 oz	104	tr	—	23	—
BREADSTICKS						
Brown & Serve Soft (Roman Meal)	1 (2.7 oz)	181	3	275	32	3
Cheese (Angonoa)	1 oz	110	2	210	20	—
Cheese (Lance)	2	20	0	40	4	—
Deli Garlic Fat Free (Stella D'Oro)	5	60	0	120	12	—
Deli Original Fat Free (Stella D'Oro)	5	60	0	130	12	—
Garlic (Angonoa)	1 oz	120	2	160	21	—
Garlic (J.J. Cassone)	1 (1.6 oz)	150	3	—	26	2
Garlic (Keebler)	2	30	tr	20	6	—
Garlic (Lance)	2	30	0	40	5	—

FOOD	PORTION	CAL	FAT	SOD	CARB	FIB
Garlic (Stella D'Oro)	1	35	1	55	6	—
Grissini Original Fat Free (Stella D'Oro)	3	60	0	130	12	—
Grissini Garlic Fat Free (Stella D'Oro)	3	60	0	120	12	—
Italian (Angonoa)	1 oz	120	2	240	21	—
Low Sodium (Angonoa)	1 oz	120	4	15	19	—
Mini Cheese (Angonoa)	1 oz	110	2	160	20	—
Mini Pizza (Angonoa)	1 oz	120	2	220	21	—
Mini Sesame (Angonoa)	1 oz	120	4	200	17	—
Mini Whole Wheat (Angonoa)	1 oz	120	4	170	17	—
Onion (Angonoa)	1 oz	120	3	150	18	—
Onion (Keebler)	2	30	tr	25	6	—
Onion (Stella D'Oro)	1	40	1	38	6	—
Plain (Keebler)	2	30	tr	30	6	—
Plain (Lance)	2	30	0	50	5	—
Regular (Stella D'Oro)	1	40	1	40	7	—
Regular Sodium Free (Stella D'Oro)	2	80	2	0	14	—
Roman Meal, refrigerated (Roman Meal)	1 (1.4 oz)	117	4	274	18	1
Sesame (Keebler)	2	30	1	30	5	—
Sesame (Lance)	2	30	0	50	4	—
Sesame Low Fat (Stella D'Oro)	2	70	1	90	14	—
Sesame Sodium Free (Stella D'Oro)	1	50	3	0	7	—
Sesame Royale (Angonoa)	1 oz	120	4	200	17	—
Soft Bread Sticks (Pillsbury)	1	100	2	230	17	—
Traditional Garlic Fat Free (Stella D'Oro)	2	70	0	150	15	—
Traditional Original Fat Free (Stella D'Oro)	2	70	0	150	15	—
Wheat (Stella D'Oro)	1	40	1	20	6	—
onion poppyseed, home recipe	1	64	1	69	11	—
plain	1	41	1	66	7	—
plain	1 sm	25	1	66	4	—

FOOD	PORTION	CAL	FAT	SOD	CARB	FIB

BREAKFAST BAR

see also BREAKFAST DRINKS, NUTRITIONAL SUPPLEMENTS

Carnation

Chewy Chocolate Chip	1 (1.26 oz)	150	6	80	22	tr
Chewy Peanut Butter Chocolate Chip	1 (1.26 oz)	140	5	90	21	tr
Chocolate Chunk Granola	1 (1.26 oz)	140	5	65	23	1
Honey & Oats Granola	1 (1.26 oz)	130	4	60	23	1

Nutri-Grain

Apple	1 (1.3 oz)	150	5	65	25	1
Blueberry	1 bar (1.3 oz)	140	4	65	26	1
Raspberry	1 (1.3 oz)	150	5	65	25	1
Strawberry	1 (1.3 oz)	150	5	65	25	1

BREAKFAST DRINKS

see also BREAKFAST BAR, NUTRITIONAL SUPPLEMENTS

Carnation Instant Breakfast

Cafe Mocha	1 can (10 fl oz)	220	3	210	35	0
Cafe Mocha	1 pkg	130	1	100	28	1
Cafe Mocha	1 pkg + skim milk (9 fl oz)	220	1	216	39	1
Classic Chocolate Malt	1 pkg	130	2	130	26	1
Classic Chocolate Malt	1 pkg + skim milk (9 fl oz)	220	1	240	39	1
Creamy Milk Chocolate	1 can (10 fl oz)	220	3	230	37	1
Creamy Milk Chocolate	1 pkg	130	1	100	28	1
Creamy Milk Chocolate	1 pkg + skim milk (9 fl oz)	220	1	240	39	1
Creamy Milk Chocolate	8 fl oz	220	3	220	36	1
French Vanilla	1 pkg	130	0	110	27	0
French Vanilla	1 pkg + skim milk	220	1	240	39	0
Strawberry Creme	1 pkg	130	0	160	28	0
Strawberry Creme	1 pkg + skim milk	220	1	288	39	0

FOOD	PORTION	CAL	FAT	SOD	CARB	FIB
Carnation Instant Breakfast No Sugar Added						
Classic Chocolate	1 pkg	70	2	120	11	1
Classic Chocolate	1 pkg + skim milk (9 fl oz)	160	2	240	24	1
Creamy Milk Chocolate	1 pkg	70	1	90	12	1
Creamy Milk Chococolate	1 pkg + skim milk (9 fl oz)	160	1	216	24	1
French Vanilla	1 pkg	70	0	90	12	0
French Vanilla	1 pkg + skim milk (9 fl oz)	150	1	216	24	0
Strawberry Creme	1 pkg	70	0	90	12	0
Strawberry Creme	1 pkg + skim milk (9 fl oz)	150	1	216	24	0
Instant Breakfast Chocolate, as prep w/ whole milk (Pillsbury)	1 serving	290	9	310	38	—
Instant Breakfast Chocolate Malt, as prep w/ whole milk (Pillsbury)	1 serv	290	9	310	38	—
Instant Breakfast Strawberry, as prep w/ whole milk (Pillsbury)	1 serv	290	9	300	39	—
Instant Breakfast Vanilla, as prep w/ whole milk (Pillsbury)	1 serv	300	9	330	41	—
orange drink powder	3 rounded tsp	93	0	4	24	—
orange drink powder, as prep w/ water	6 oz	86	0	9	22	—

BROAD BEANS
CANNED

broad beans	1 cup	183	1	1161	32	—
DRIED						
cooked	1 cup	186	1	8	33	—
FRESH						
cooked	3.5 oz	56	tr	41	10	—

FOOD	PORTION	CAL	FAT	SOD	CARB	FIB
BROCCOLI						
FRESH						
Dole	1 med spear	40	1	75	4	5
chopped, cooked	½ cup	22	tr	20	4	2
raw, chopped	½ cup	12	tr	12	2	1
FROZEN						
Baby Spears Deluxe (Birds Eye)	⅔ cup	30	0	15	5	3
Big Valley	3.5 oz	25	0	20	5	—
Broccoli With Cheese In Pastry (Pepperidge Farm)	1	230	16	380	18	—
Chopped (Birds Eye)	⅔ cup	25	0	15	5	3
Cuts (Green Giant)	½ cup	12	0	15	3	2
Farm Fresh Spears (Birds Eye)	¾ cup	30	0	25	7	2
Florets (Hanover)	½ cup	30	0	—	—	—
Florets Deluxe (Birds Eye)	½ cup	25	0	20	5	3
Harvest Fresh Cut (Green Giant)	½ cup	16	0	95	3	2
Harvest Fresh Spears (Green Giant)	½ cup	20	0	115	4	2
In Butter Sauce (Green Giant)	½ cup	40	2	350	6	—
In Cheese Sauce (Green Giant)	½ cup	60	2	530	9	2
Mini Spears Select (Green Giant)	4–5 spears	18	0	25	5	3
One Serve Cuts In Butter Sauce (Green Giant)	1 pkg	45	2	10	7	3
One Serve Cuts In Cheese Sauce (Green Giant)	1 pkg	70	3	660	11	3
Polybag Cuts (Birds Eye)	½ cup	25	0	25	4	3
Polybag Deluxe Florets (Birds Eye)	⅔ cup	25	0	15	4	3
Spears (Birds Eye)	⅔ cup	25	0	20	5	3
Valley Combinations Broccoli Fanfare (Green Giant)	½ cup	80	2	340	14	—

FOOD	PORTION	CAL	FAT	SOD	CARB	FIB
With Cheese Sauce (Birds Eye)	½ pkg	110	5	520	9	1
chopped, cooked	½ cup	25	tr	22	5	—
spears, cooked	½ cup	25	tr	22	5	3
spears, cooked	10 oz pkg	69	tr	60	13	4

BROWNIE
FROZEN
FOOD	PORTION	CAL	FAT	SOD	CARB	FIB
Brownie Ala Mode (Weight Watchers)	1	180	4	150	35	—
Chocolate Brownie (Weight Watchers)	1 (1.25 oz)	100	3	150	16	—
Mint Frosted (Weight Watchers)	1 (1.23 oz)	100	5	130	18	—
Monterey Hot Fudge Chocolate Chunk Brownie (Pepperidge Farm)	1	480	26	200	56	—
Newport Hot Fudge Brownie (Pepperidge Farm)	1	400	20	160	50	—

HOME RECIPE
plain	1 (0.8 oz)	112	7	82	12	1
w/nuts	1 (0.8 oz)	95	6	51	11	—

MIX
Brownie With Hot Fudge MicroRave Single (Betty Crocker)	1	350	12	260	55	—
Chewy Recipe Fudge Brownie Mix (Duncan Hines)	1	130	5	—	—	—
Deluxe Family-Size Fudge Brownie (Pillsbury)	2-in sq	150	7	95	20	—
Deluxe Fudge Brownie (Pillsbury)	2-in sq	150	6	100	21	—
Deluxe Fudge Brownie With Walnuts (Pillsbury)	2-in sq	150	8	90	19	—
Estee Brownie Mix	1 (2 in × 2 in)	50	2	5	8	—
Frosted MicroRave (Betty Crocker)	1	180	7	120	21	—
Fudge Family Size (Betty Crocker)	1	150	5	100	22	—

FOOD	PORTION	CAL	FAT	SOD	CARB	FIB
Fudge Light (Betty Crocker)	1	100	1	90	21	—
Fudge MicroRave (Betty Crocker)	1	150	6	110	22	—
Fudge Microwave (Pillsbury)	1	190	9	105	25	—
Fudge Regular Size (Betty Crocker)	1	150	6	105	23	—
Gourmet Truffle Brownie Mix (Duncan Hines)	1	280	13	—	—	—
Gourmet Turtle Brownie Mix (Duncan Hines)	1	240	10	—	—	—
Gourmet Vienna White Brownie Mix (Duncan Hines)	1	240	12	—	—	—
Milk Chocolate Brownie Mix (Duncan Hines)	1	160	7	—	—	—
Original Fudge Brownie Mix (Duncan Hines)	1	160	7	—	—	—
Peanut Butter Chocolate Brownie Mix (Duncan Hines)	1	150	8	—	—	—
Supreme Caramel (Betty Crocker)	1	120	4	115	21	—
Supreme Frosted (Betty Crocker)	1	160	6	120	26	—
Supreme German Chocolate (Betty Crocker)	1	160	7	110	24	—
Supreme Original (Betty Crocker)	1	140	6	80	21	—
Supreme Party (Betty Crocker)	1	160	6	110	26	—
Supreme Walnut (Betty Crocker)	1	140	7	80	18	—
The Ultimate Carmel Fudge Chunk Brownie (Pillsbury)	2-in sq	170	7	105	25	—
The Ultimate Chunky Triple Fudge Brownie (Pillsbury)	2-in sq	170	7	105	25	—

FOOD	PORTION	CAL	FAT	SOD	CARB	FIB
The Ultimate Double Fudge Brownie (Pillsbury)	2-in sq	160	6	105	24	—
The Ultimate Rockey Road Fudge Brownie (Pillsbury)	2-in sq	170	8	95	24	—
Walnut MicroRave (Betty Crocker)	1	160	7	95	21	—
plain	1 (1.2 oz)	139	7	83	20	1
plain, low calorie	1 (0.8 oz)	84	2	21	16	1
READY-TO-EAT						
Brownie (Tastykake)	1 (85 g)	340	14	220	53	5
Brownie Bites (Hostess)	5 (2 oz)	260	14	125	32	2
Brownie Bites Walnut (Hostess)	5 (2 oz)	270	15	140	31	2
Charlotte Fudgey Brownie (Pepperidge Farm)	1	220	11	105	28	2
Fudge (Little Debbie)	1 pkg (2.1 oz)	270	13	170	39	1
Fudge (Little Debbie)	1 pkg (2.5 oz)	310	15	190	44	1
Fudge (Little Debbie)	1 pkg (2.9 oz)	360	17	230	52	1
Fudge (Little Debbie)	1 pkg (3.6 oz)	450	21	280	65	2
Fudge Nut (Frito Lay)	3 oz	360	14	225	56	—
Lance	1 pkg (78 g)	320	12	210	52	—
Tahoe Milk Chocolate Pecan (Pepperidge Farm)	1	210	10	100	30	1
Westport Fudgey Brownies w/ Walnuts (Pepperidge Farm)	1	220	11	105	28	2
plain	1 lg (2 oz)	227	9	175	36	1
plain	1 sm (1 oz)	115	5	88	18	1
w/ nuts	1 (1 oz)	100	4	59	16	—
w/o nuts	1 (2 oz)	243	10	153	39	—

BRUSSELS SPROUTS
FRESH

FOOD	PORTION	CAL	FAT	SOD	CARB	FIB
Dole	½ cup	19	tr	11	4	2
cooked	1 sprout	8	tr	4	2	—
cooked	½ cup	30	tr	17	7	3
raw	1 sprout	8	tr	5	2	1
raw	½ cup	19	tr	11	4	—

FOOD	PORTION	CAL	FAT	SOD	CARB	FIB
FROZEN						
Brussels Sprouts (Birds Eye)	½ cup	35	0	15	7	3
Brussels Sprouts (Hanover)	½ cup	40	0	—	—	—
Green Giant	½ cup	25	0	10	6	2
In Butter Sauce (Green Giant)	½ cup	40	1	280	8	—
Whole (Big Valley)	3.5 oz	30	tr	14	6	—
cooked	½ cup	33	tr	18	6	—
BUCKWHEAT						
Brown Groats Roasted (Wolff's)	1 cup (8 oz)	900	4	—	188	—
Flour (Wolff's)	1 cup (8 oz)	860	5	—	170	—
Kasha Coarse, cooked (Wolff's)	¼ cup (1.6 oz)	170	2	10	35	2
Kasha Fine, cooked (Wolff's)	¼ cup (1.6 oz)	170	2	10	35	2
Kasha Medium, cooked (Wolff's)	¼ cup (1.6 oz)	170	2	10	35	2
Kasha Whole, cooked (Wolff's)	¼ cup (1.6 oz)	170	2	10	35	2
White Grits (Wolff's)	1 cup (8 oz)	840	3	—	173	—
flour, whole groat	1 cup	402	4	—	85	—
groats, roasted, cooked	½ cup	91	tr	4	20	—
groats, roasted, uncooked	½ cup	283	2	9	61	—
BUFFALO						
water, roasted	3 oz	111	2	48	0	—
BULGUR						
Good Shepherd	¼ cup (43 g)	150	1	0	33	1
Hodgson Mill	¼ cup (1.4 oz)	120	1	0	24	1
cooked	½ cup	76	tr	5	17	—
uncooked	½ cup	239	tr	12	53	—
BURBOT (FISH)						
FRESH						
baked	3 oz	98	1	106	0	—
BURDOCK ROOT						
cooked	1 cup	110	tr	5	26	—
raw	1 cup	85	tr	6	20	—

FOOD	PORTION	CAL	FAT	SOD	CARB	FIB

BUTTER

see also BUTTER BLENDS, BUTTER SUBSTITUTES, MARGARINE

REGULAR

FOOD	PORTION	CAL	FAT	SOD	CARB	FIB
Cabot	1 tsp	35	4	41	0	—
Cabot Unsalted	1 tsp	35	4	0	0	—
Crystal Salted	1 tbsp (0.5 oz)	102	11	89	tr	0
Crystal Unsalted	1 tbsp (0.5 oz)	102	11	1	tr	0
Hotel Bar	1 tsp	35	4	35	0	—
Keller's	1 tsp	35	4	35	0	—
Land O'Lakes	1 tbsp (0.5 oz)	100	11	85	0	—
Land O'Lakes Light	1 tbsp	50	6	70	0	—
Land O'Lakes Light Unsalted	1 tbsp	50	6	5	0	—
Land O'Lakes Unsalted	1 tbsp (0.5 oz)	100	11	0	0	—
butter	1 pat	36	4	41	tr	—
butter	1 stick (4 oz)	813	92	937	tr	—
butter oil	1 cup	1795	204	—	0	—
butter oil	1 tbsp	112	13	—	0	—
clarified butter	3.5 oz	876	99	—	0	—

WHIPPED

FOOD	PORTION	CAL	FAT	SOD	CARB	FIB
Land O'Lakes	1 tbsp (0.3 oz)	70	7	55	0	—
Land O'Lakes Unsalted	1 tbsp	60	7	0	0	—
butter	1 pat	27	3	31	tr	—
butter	4 oz	542	61	625	tr	—

BUTTER BEANS

CANNED

FOOD	PORTION	CAL	FAT	SOD	CARB	FIB
Hanover	½ cup	80	0	—	—	—
Hanover In Sauce	½ cup	100	0	—	—	—
Luck's Speckled Seasoned w/ Pork	7.5 oz	230	8	—	—	—
S&W Tender Cooked	½ cup	100	0	440	19	—
Trappey's Large White	½ cup	80	1	410	15	—
Van Camp's	1 cup	162	1	710	30	—

BUTTER BLENDS

see also BUTTER, BUTTER SUBSTITUTES, MARGARINE

REGULAR

FOOD	PORTION	CAL	FAT	SOD	CARB	FIB
Blue Bonnet Better Blend	1 tbsp	90	11	95	0	—
Blue Bonnet Better Blend Unsalted	1 tbsp	90	11	0	0	—
Country Morning Blend (Land O'Lakes)	1 tbsp	100	11	90	0	—

FOOD	PORTION	CAL	FAT	SOD	CARB	FIB
Country Morning Blend Light (Land O'Lakes)	1 tbsp (0.5 oz)	50	6	110	0	—
Country Morning Blend Unsalted (Land O'Lakes)	1 tbsp	100	11	0	0	—
butter blend	1 stick	811	91	1013	1	—
SOFT						
Blue Bonnet Better Blend	1 tbsp	90	11	95	0	—
Country Morning Blend Light Tub (Land O'Lakes)	1 tsp	20	3	30	0	—
Country Morning Blend Light Tub (Land O'Lakes)	1 tbsp (0.5 oz)	50	6	90	0	—
Country Morning Blend Tub (Land O'Lakes)	1 tbsp	100	11	80	0	—
Downey's Cinnamon Honey-Butter	1 tbsp	52	1	5	—	—
Downey's Original Honey-Butter	1 tbsp	52	1	5	—	—
Le Slim Cow	1 tbsp	40	4	15	—	—
Touch of Butter Stick	1 tbsp	90	10	110	0	—
Touch of Butter Tub	1 tbsp	50	6	110	0	—

BUTTER SUBSTITUTES
see also BUTTER BLENDS, MARGARINE

FOOD	PORTION	CAL	FAT	SOD	CARB	FIB
Butter Buds	⅛ oz	12	0	—	—	—
Butter Buds Sprinkles	½ tsp	4	0	—	—	—
Molly McButter	½ tsp (1 g)	3	tr	90	1	—
Molly McButter w/ Bacon	½ tsp (1 g)	4	tr	62	1	—
Molly McButter w/ Cheese	½ tsp (0.9 g)	4	tr	55	tr	—
Molly McButter w/ Sour Cream	½ tsp (1.1 g)	4	tr	69	1	—

BUTTERBUR
CANNED

FOOD	PORTION	CAL	FAT	SOD	CARB	FIB
fuki, chopped	1 cup	3	tr	5	tr	—
FRESH						
fuki, raw	1 cup	13	tr	7	3	—

BUTTERFISH

FOOD	PORTION	CAL	FAT	SOD	CARB	FIB
baked	3 oz	159	9	97	0	—

FOOD	PORTION	CAL	FAT	SOD	CARB	FIB
fillet, baked	1 oz	47	3	29	0	—

BUTTERNUTS
dried	1 oz	174	16	0	3	—

BUTTERSCOTCH
see also CANDY
Nestle Morsels Butterscotch	1 tbsp	80	4	15	10	—

CABBAGE
FRESH
Dole	½ med head	18	0	30	3	2
Dole Napa, shredded	½ cup	6	tr	3	1	tr
chinese pak-choi, raw, shredded	½ cup	5	tr	23	1	—
chinese pak-choi, shredded, cooked	½ cup	10	tr	29	2	—
chinese pe-tsai, raw, shredded	1 cup	12	tr	7	2	—
chinese pe-tsai, shredded, cooked	1 cup	16	tr	11	3	—
danish, raw	1 head (2 lbs)	228	2	164	49	18
danish, raw, shredded	½ cup (1.2 oz)	9	tr	6	2	tr
danish, shredded, cooked	½ cup (2.6 oz)	17	tr	6	3	1
green, raw	1 head (2 lbs)	228	2	164	49	18
green, raw, shredded	½ cup (1.2 oz)	9	tr	6	2	tr
green, shredded, cooked	½ cup (2.6 oz)	17	tr	6	3	1
red, raw, shredded	½ cup	10	tr	4	2	1
red, shredded, cooked	½ cup	16	tr	6	3	—
savoy, raw, shredded	½ cup	10	tr	10	2	—
savoy, shredded, cooked	½ cup	18	tr	17	4	—
HOME RECIPE						
coleslaw w/ dressing	¾ cup	147	11	267	13	—
TAKE-OUT						
coleslaw w/ dressing	½ cup	42	2	14	7	—
stuffed cabbage	1 (6 oz)	373	22	1007	18	—
sweet & sour red cabbage	4 oz	61	3	—	8	3
vinegar & oil coleslaw	3.5 oz	150	9	480	16	—

FOOD	PORTION	CAL	FAT	SOD	CARB	FIB

CAKE

see also BROWNIE, COOKIES, DANISH PASTRY, DOUGHNUTS, PIE

FROSTING/ICING

FOOD	PORTION	CAL	FAT	SOD	CARB	FIB
Butter Pecan Ready-to-Spread (Betty Crocker)	½ tub	170	7	50	26	—
Cake & Cookie Decorator Chocolate (Pillsbury)	1 tbsp	60	2	0	11	—
Cake & Cookie Decorator all colors except chocolate (Pillsbury)	1 tbsp	70	2	0	12	—
Cherry Ready-to-Spread (Betty Crocker)	½ tub	160	6	50	27	—
Chocolate Ready-to-Spread (Betty Crocker)	½ tub	160	7	60	24	—
Chocolate Chip Ready-to-Spread (Betty Crocker)	½ tub	170	7	30	27	—
Chocolate Creamy Frosting (Duncan Hines)	½ pkg	160	7	—	—	—
Chocolate Fudge (Pillsbury)	for ⅛ cake	110	5	65	17	—
Chocolate Fudge, as prep (Betty Crocker)	½ mix	180	6	70	30	—
Chocolate Light Ready-to-Spread (Betty Crocker)	½ tub	130	2	60	28	—
Chocolate With Candy Coated Chocolate Chips Ready-to-Spread (Betty Crocker)	½ tub	160	7	60	24	—
Chocolate With Dinosaurs Ready-to-Spread (Betty Crocker)	½ tub	160	7	60	24	—
Chocolate With Turbo Racers Ready-to-Spread (Betty Crocker)	½ tub	160	7	60	24	—
Coconut Almond Frosting Mix (Pillsbury)	for ½ cake	160	10	85	16	—
Coconut Pecan Frosting Mix (Pillsbury)	for ½ cake	150	7	105	20	—

FOOD	PORTION	CAL	FAT	SOD	CARB	FIB
Coconut Pecan Ready-to-Spread (Betty Crocker)	½ tub	160	9	80	20	—
Coconut Pecan, as prep mix (Betty Crocker)	½ mix	180	8	50	19	—
Cream Cheese Ready-to-Spread (Betty Crocker)	½ tub	170	7	70	26	—
Creamy Milk Chocolate, as prep (Betty Crocker)	½ mix	170	5	40	29	—
Creamy Vanilla, as prep (Betty Crocker)	½ mix	170	5	50	32	—
Dark Dutch Fudge Creamy Frosting (Duncan Hines)	½ pkg	160	7	—	—	—
Dark Dutch Fudge Ready-to-Spread (Betty Crocker)	½ tub	160	7	70	22	—
Fluffy White Frosting Mix (Pillsbury)	for ½ cake	60	0	65	15	—
Frost It Hot Chocolate (Pillsbury)	for ⅙ cake	50	0	50	12	—
Frost It Hot Fluffy White (Pillsbury)	for ⅙ cake	50	0	50	12	—
Frosting Mix, as prep (Estee)	1½ tsp	50	1	0	10	—
Frosting Supreme Caramel Pecan (Pillsbury)	for ½ cake	160	8	70	21	—
Frosting Supreme Chocolate Chip (Pillsbury)	for ½ cake	150	5	70	27	—
Frosting Supreme Chocolate Fudge (Pillsbury)	for ½ cake	150	6	80	24	—
Frosting Supreme Chocolate Mint (Pillsbury)	for ½ cake	150	7	80	24	—
Frosting Supreme Coconut Almond (Pillsbury)	for ½ cake	150	9	60	17	—
Frosting Supreme Coconut Pecan (Pillsbury)	for ½ cake	160	10	60	17	—

FOOD	PORTION	CAL	FAT	SOD	CARB	FIB
Frosting Supreme Cream Cheese (Pillsbury)	for ½ cake	160	6	115	26	—
Frosting Supreme Double Dutch (Pillsbury)	for ½ cake	140	6	45	22	—
Frosting Supreme Lemon (Pillsbury)	for ½ cake	160	6	80	26	—
Frosting Supreme Milk Chocolate (Pillsbury)	for ½ cake	150	6	60	23	—
Frosting Supreme Mocha (Pillsbury)	for ½ cake	150	6	60	24	—
Frosting Supreme Sour Cream Vanilla (Pillsbury)	for ½ cake	160	6	80	27	—
Frosting Supreme Strawberry (Pillsbury)	for ½ cake	160	6	75	26	—
Frosting Supreme Vanilla (Pillsbury)	for ½ cake	160	6	75	26	—
Funfetti Chocolate Fudge (Pillsbury)	½ can	140	6	80	22	—
Funfetti Vanilla Pink (Pillsbury)	½ can	150	6	70	24	—
Funfetti Vanilla White (Pillsbury)	½ can	150	6	70	24	—
Lemon Ready-to-Spread (Betty Crocker)	½ tub	170	6	70	28	—
Milk Chocolate Creamy Frosting (Duncan Hines)	½ pkg	160	7	—	—	—
Milk Chocolate Light Ready-to-Spread (Betty Crocker)	½ tub	140	2	50	29	—
Milk Chocolate Ready-to-Spread (Betty Crocker)	½ tub	160	6	55	25	—
Rainbow Chip Ready-to-Spread (Betty Crocker)	½ tub	170	7	30	27	—
Sour Cream Chocolate Ready-to-Spread (Betty Crocker)	½ tub	160	7	100	23	—

FOOD	PORTION	CAL	FAT	SOD	CARB	FIB
Sour Cream White Ready-to-Spread (Betty Crocker)	½ tub	160	6	50	27	—
Vanilla (Pillsbury)	for ⅙ cake	120	5	60	19	—
Vanilla Creamy Frosting (Duncan Hines)	½ pkg	160	7	—	—	—
Vanilla Light Ready-to-Spread (Betty Crocker)	½ tub	140	2	30	30	—
Vanilla Ready-to-Spread (Betty Crocker)	½ tub	160	6	30	27	—
Vanilla With Teddy Bears Ready-to-Spread (Betty Crocker)	½ tub	160	6	25	27	—
White Fluffy, as prep (Betty Crocker)	½ mix	70	0	40	16	—
FROZEN						
Amhurst Apple Crumb Coffee Cake (Pepperidge Farm)	1	220	11	150	30	—
Apple 'N Spice Bake Dessert Lights (Pepperidge Farm)	1 piece (4.25 oz)	170	2	105	37	—
Apple Crisp (Weight Watchers)	1 (3.5 oz)	190	5	190	40	—
Apple Crisp Light (Sara Lee)	1 (3 oz)	150	2	130	31	—
Apple Turnover (Pepperidge Farm)	1	300	17	210	34	—
Banana Single Layer Iced (Sara Lee)	1 slice (1.7 oz)	170	6	160	28	—
Berkshire Apple Crisp (Pepperidge Farm)	1	250	8	130	43	1
Black Forest Light (Sara Lee)	1 (3.6 oz)	170	5	85	34	—
Black Forest Two Layer (Sara Lee)	1 slice (2.5 oz)	190	8	100	28	—
Blueberry Turnovers (Pepperidge Farm)	1	310	19	230	32	—
Boston Cream Supreme (Pepperidge Farm)	1 piece (2.88 oz)	290	14	190	39	—

FOOD	PORTION	CAL	FAT	SOD	CARB	FIB
Brownie Cheesecake (Weight Watchers)	1 (3.5 oz)	200	5	260	34	—
Butter Pound (Pepperidge Farm)	1 slice (1 oz)	130	7	150	16	—
Carrot Classic (Pepperidge Farm)	1 cake	260	16	280	32	—
Carrot Light (Sara Lee)	1 (2.5 oz)	170	4	75	30	—
Carrot Single Layer Iced (Sara Lee)	1 slice (2.4 oz)	250	13	240	30	—
Carrot w/ Cream Cheese Icing (Pepperidge Farm)	1 slice (1.5 oz)	150	9	160	19	—
Charleston Peach Melba Shortcake (Pepperidge Farm)	1	220	5	170	41	—
Cheese Sweet Roll (Weight Watchers)	1 (2.25 oz)	180	4	—	32	—
Cheesecake Original Strawberry (Sara Lee)	1 slice (3.2 oz)	222	8	171	34	—
Cheesecake Original Cherry (Sara Lee)	1 slice (3.2 oz)	243	8	184	35	—
Cheesecake Original Plain (Sara Lee)	1 slice (2.8 oz)	230	11	153	27	—
Cherries And Cream Cake (Weight Watchers)	1 (3 oz)	150	2	200	30	—
Cherries Supreme Dessert Lights (Pepperidge Farm)	1 piece (3.25 oz)	170	11	35	38	—
Cherry Turnover (Pepperidge Farm)	1	310	19	280	32	—
Chocolate (Weight Watchers)	1 (2.5 oz)	180	5	250	31	—
Chocolate Eclair (Weight Watchers)	1 (2.1 oz)	120	4	110	19	—
Chocolate Free & Light (Sara Lee)	1 slice (1.7 oz)	110	0	140	26	—
Chocolate Fudge Large Layer (Pepperidge Farm)	1 slice (1.63 oz)	180	10	140	23	—
Chocolate Fudge Strip Large Layer (Pepperidge Farm)	1 piece (1.63 oz)	170	9	140	20	—

FOOD	PORTION	CAL	FAT	SOD	CARB	FIB
Chocolate Mousse Cake Dessert Lights (Pepperidge Farm)	1 piece (1.5 oz)	190	9	260	25	—
Chocolate Supreme (Pepperidge Farm)	1 piece (2.88 oz)	16	140	37	—	
Cholesterol Free Pound (Pepperidge Farm)	1 slice (1 oz)	110	6	85	13	—
Cobbler Apple (Pet-Ritz)	⅙ cake (4.33 oz)	290	9	—	50	—
Cobbler Blackberry (Pet-Ritz)	⅙ cake (4.33 oz)	250	10	—	39	—
Cobbler Blueberry (Pet-Ritz)	⅙ cake (4.33 oz)	270	12	—	50	—
Cobbler Cherry (Pet-Ritz)	⅙ cake (4.33 oz)	280	10	—	46	—
Cobbler Peach (Pet-Ritz)	⅙ cake (4.33 oz)	260	10	—	46	—
Cobbler Strawberry (Pet-Ritz)	⅙ cake (4.33 oz)	290	9	—	50	—
Coconut Classic (Pepperidge Farm)	1 cake	230	11	160	31	—
Coconut Large Layer (Pepperidge Farm)	1 slice (1.63 oz)	180	8	120	24	—
Coffee Cake All Butter Butter Streusel (Sara Lee)	1 slice (1.4 oz)	160	7	160	20	—
Coffee Cake All Butter Cheese (Sara Lee)	1 slice (2 oz)	210	11	220	25	—
Coffee Cake All Butter Pecan (Sara Lee)	1 slice (1.4 oz)	160	8	180	19	—
Coffee Cake With Cinnamon Streusel (Weight Watchers)	1 (2.25 oz)	160	4	—	27	—
Devil's Food Large Layer (Pepperidge Farm)	1 slice (1.63 oz)	180	9	135	24	—
Double Chocolate Classic (Pepperidge Farm)	1 cake	250	13	180	31	—
Double Chocolate Light (Sara Lee)	1 (2.5 oz)	150	5	85	23	—
Double Chocolate Three Layer (Sara Lee)	1 slice (2.2 oz)	220	11	130	26	—

FOOD	PORTION	CAL	FAT	SOD	CARB	FIB
Double Fudge (Weight Watchers)	1 piece (2.75 oz)	190	4	150	34	—
Elfin Loaves Apple Cinnamon	1	180	4	260	31	—
Elfin Loaves Banana	1	190	7	260	29	—
Elfin Loaves Blueberry	1	170	4	220	30	—
Elfin Loaves Carrot	1	210	10	170	27	—
French Cheesecake Light (Sara Lee)	1 (3.2 oz)	150	4	90	24	—
French Cheese (Sara Lee)	1 slice (2.9 oz)	250	16	120	23	—
Fruit Squares Apple (Pepperidge Farm)	1	220	12	170	27	—
Fruit Squares Cherry (Pepperidge Farm)	1	230	12	180	28	—
Fudge Golden Classic (Pepperidge Farm)	1 cake	260	14	160	34	—
German Chocolate Classic (Pepperidge Farm)	1 cake	250	13	230	29	—
German Chocolate Large Layer (Pepperidge Farm)	1 slice (1.63 oz)	180	10	170	22	—
Golden Large Layer (Pepperidge Farm)	1 slice (1.63 oz)	180	9	110	24	—
Lemon Cake Supreme Dessert Lights (Pepperidge Farm)	1 piece (2.75 oz)	170	5	100	26	—
Lemon Coconut Classic Cake (Pepperidge Farm)	3 oz	280	13	—	—	—
Lemon Coconut Supreme (Pepperidge Farm)	1 piece (3 oz)	280	13	220	38	—
Lemon Cream Light (Sara Lee)	1 (3.2 oz)	180	6	60	29	—
Lemon Cream Supreme (Pepperidge Farm)	1 piece (1.63 oz)	170	9	120	21	—
Manhattan Strawberry Cheesecake (Pepperidge Farm)	1	300	9	250	49	—
Peach Melba Supreme (Pepperidge Farm)	1 (3.13 oz)	270	7	135	50	—

FOOD	PORTION	CAL	FAT	SOD	CARB	FIB
Peach Parfait Dessert Lights (Pepperidge Farm)	1 piece (4.25 oz)	150	5	70	24	—
Peach Turnover (Pepperidge Farm)	1	310	18	260	34	—
Pineapple Cream Supreme (Pepperidge Farm)	1 piece (2 oz)	190	7	130	28	—
Pound All Butter Family Size (Sara Lee)	1 slice (1 oz)	130	7	85	14	—
Pound All Butter Original (Sara Lee)	1 slice (1 oz)	130	7	85	14	—
Pound Free & Light (Sara Lee)	1 slice (1 oz)	70	0	105	17	—
Raspberry Turnovers (Pepperidge Farm)	1	310	17	260	36	—
Raspberry Vanilla Swirl Dessert Lights (Pepperidge Farm)	1 piece (3.25 oz)	160	5	140	25	—
Strawberry Cheesecake (Weight Watchers)	1 piece (3.9 oz)	180	4	210	28	—
Strawberry Cream Supreme (Pepperidge Farm)	1 piece (2 oz)	190	7	120	30	—
Strawberry Shortcake Dessert Lights (Pepperidge Farm)	1 piece (3 oz)	150	2	65	29	—
Strawberry Shortcake Dessert Lights (Pepperidge Farm)	1 piece (3 oz)	170	5	50	30	1
Strawberry Shortcake Two Layer (Sara Lee)	1 slice (2.5 oz)	190	8	90	26	—
Strawberry Strip Large Layer (Pepperidge Farm)	1 piece (1.5 oz)	160	8	120	21	—
Strawberry Yogurt Dessert Free & Light (Sara Lee)	1 slice 2.2 oz)	120	1	90	26	—
Vanilla Fudge Swirl Classic (Pepperidge Farm)	1 cake	250	11	160	33	—

FOOD	PORTION	CAL	FAT	SOD	CARB	FIB
Vanilla Large Layer (Pepperidge Farm)	1 slice (1.63 oz)	190	8	120	25	—
boston cream pie	⅙ cake (3.2 oz)	323	8	132	40	1
eclair w/ chocolate icing & custard filling	1	205	10	—	—	—
HOME RECIPE						
angelfood	1/12 cake (1.9 oz)	142	tr	96	32	1
boston cream pie	⅙ cake (3.3 oz)	293	12	309	43	1
carrot w/ cream cheese icing	1 cake (10-in diam)	6175	328	4470	775	—
carrot w/ cream cheese icing	1/12 cake (3.9 oz)	484	29	273	52	—
cheesecake	1/12 cake (4.5 oz)	456	9	362	32	—
cheesecake w/ cherry topping	1/12 cake (5 oz)	359	23	254	33	—
chocolate cupcake creme filled w/ frosting	1 (1.8 oz)	188	7	213	30	—
chocolate w/o frosting	1/12 cake (3.3 oz)	340	14	299	51	—
chocolate w/o frosting	2 layers (39.9 oz)	4067	172	3581	608	—
coffeecake creme-filled chocolate frosting	⅙ cake (3.2 oz)	298	10	290	49	2
coffeecake crumb topped cinnamon	1/12 cake (2.1 oz)	240	12	233	30	2
cream puff w/ custard filling	1 (4.6 oz)	336	20	444	30	—
cream puff shell	1 (2.3 oz)	239	17	368	15	—
eclair	1 (3 oz)	262	16	337	24	—
fruitcake	1/36 cake (2.9 oz)	302	10	121	54	3
fruitcake dark	1 cake 7½ in × 2¼ in	5185	228	2123	738	—
gingerbread	⅙ cake (2.6 oz)	264	12	242	36	2
pineapple upside down	⅛ cake (4 oz)	367	14	367	58	—
pound	1 loaf 8½ in × 3½ in	1935	94	1645	265	—
pound cake	1 slice (1 oz)	120	5	96	15	—
sheet cake w/o frosting	1 cake (9-in sq)	2830	108	2331	434	—
sheet cake w/o frosting	⅑ cake	315	12	258	48	—
sheet cake w/ white frosting	1 cake (9-in sq)	4020	129	2488	694	—
sheet cake w/ white frosting	⅑ cake	445	14	275	77	—

FOOD	PORTION	CAL	FAT	SOD	CARB	FIB
shortcake	1 (2.3 oz)	225	9	329	32	—
sponge	1/12 cake (2.2 oz)	140	2	107	27	—
white w/ coconut frosting	1/12 cake (3.9 oz)	399	12	318	71	—
white w/o frosting	1/12 cake (2.6 oz)	264	9	242	42	—
yellow w/o frosting	1/12 cake (2.4 oz)	245	10	233	36	—
yellow w/o frosting	2 layers (28.7 oz)	2947	119	2803	433	—
MIX						
Angel Food Confetti (Betty Crocker)	1/12 cake	150	0	300	34	—
Angel Food Traditional (Betty Crocker)	1/12 cake	130	0	170	30	—
Angel Food Lemon Custard (Betty Crocker)	1/12 cake	150	0	300	34	—
Angel Food White (Betty Crocker)	1/12 cake	150	0	300	34	—
Apple Cinnamon Coffee Cake (Pillsbury)	1/8 cake	240	7	150	40	—
Apple Streusel MicroRave (Betty Crocker)	1/6 cake	240	11	190	33	—
Apple Streusel MicroRave No Cholesterol Recipe (Betty Crocker)	1/6 cake	210	8	200	33	—
Banana Quick Bread (Pillsbury)	1/12 loaf	170	6	200	27	—
Bisquick Reduced Fat	1/2 cup (2 oz)	210	4	660	39	—
Blueberry Nut Quick Bread (Pillsbury)	1/12 loaf	150	4	150	26	—
Butter Chocolate (Betty Crocker)	1/12 cake	280	14	400	35	—
Butter Pecan SuperMoist (Betty Crocker)	1/12 cake	250	11	320	35	—
Butter Pecan No Cholesterol Recipe (Betty Crocker)	1/12 cake	220	7	320	35	—
Butter Recipe (Pillsbury)	1/12 cake	260	12	370	34	—
Butter Recipe Fudge (Duncan Hines)	1/12 cake	270	13	—	—	—

FOOD	PORTION	CAL	FAT	SOD	CARB	FIB
Butter Recipe Golden (Duncan Hines)	1/12 cake	270	13	—	—	—
Butter Yellow (Betty Crocker)	1/12 cake	260	11	340	37	—
Carrot (Betty Crocker)	1/12 cake	250	10	300	36	—
Carrot (Dromedary)	1/12 cake	232	15	292	23	—
Carrot (Estee)	1/10 cake	100	2	65	18	—
Carrot No Cholesterol Recipe (Betty Crocker)	1/12 cake	210	6	300	36	—
Cheese Cake Lite No-Bake (Royal)	1/8 pie	130	3	230	22	—
Cheese Cake Real No-Bake (Royal)	1/8 pie	160	3	250	29	—
Cheesecake (Jell-O)	1/8 cake	277	13	349	36	—
Cheesecake New York Style (Jell-O)	1/8 cake	283	12	421	38	—
Cherry Chip (Betty Crocker)	1/12 cake	190	3	270	37	—
Cherry Nut Quick Bread (Pillsbury)	1/12 loaf	180	5	150	29	—
Chocolate (Estee)	1/10 cake	100	2	100	18	—
Chocolate Chip (Betty Crocker)	1/12 cake	290	15	300	35	—
Chocolate Chip (Pillsbury)	1/12 cake	270	14	290	33	—
Chocolate Chip No Cholesterol Recipe (Betty Crocker)	1/12 cake	220	8	300	35	—
Chocolate Chocolate Chip (Betty Crocker)	1/12 cake	260	12	400	34	—
Chocolate Fudge (Betty Crocker)	1/12 cake	260	12	450	35	—
Chocolate Lite Cake & Frosting Mix (Batter Lite)	1/8 cake	110	2	—	—	—
Chocolate Microwave (Pillsbury)	1/8 cake	210	12	260	23	—
Chocolate Pudding Classic Dessert (Betty Crocker)	1/6 cake	230	5	250	44	—
Chocolate With Chocolate Frosting (Pillsbury)	1/8 cake	300	17	310	35	—

FOOD	PORTION	CAL	FAT	SOD	CARB	FIB
Chocolate With Vanilla Frosting (Pillsbury)	⅛ cake	300	17	300	36	—
Cinnamon Pecan Streusel Microwave (Betty Crocker)	⅙ cake	280	12	220	40	—
Cinnamon Pecan Streusel Microwave No Cholesterol (Betty Crocker)	⅙ cake	230	7	220	40	—
Cobbler Apple Crumb (Dromedary)	⅛ cake	237	6	490	41	—
Cobbler Cherry Crumb (Dromedary)	⅛ cake	231	6	160	42	—
Coffee Cake Easy Mix (Aunt Jemima)	⅛ cake	160	5	290	28	—
Cranberry Quick Bread (Pillsbury)	1/12 loaf	160	4	200	30	—
Dark Dutch Fudge (Duncan Hines)	1/12 cake	280	15	—	—	—
Date Nut (Dromedary)	1/12 cake	183	8	248	26	—
Date Nut Roll (Dromedary)	½-in slice	80	2	160	13	—
Date Quick Bread (Pillsbury)	1/12 loaf	160	2	150	32	—
Devil's Food (Betty Crocker)	1/12 cake	260	12	430	35	—
Devil's Food (Duncan Hines)	1/12 cake	280	15	—	—	—
Devil's Food (Pillsbury)	1/12 cake	270	14	370	32	—
Devil's Food Chocolate Frosting MicroRave (Betty Crocker)	⅙ cake	310	17	250	37	—
Devil's Food No Cholesterol Recipe (Betty Crocker)	1/12 cake	220	7	430	35	—
Devils Food SuperMoist Light (Betty Crocker)	1/12 cake	200	4	340	36	—
Devils Food SuperMoist Light No Cholesterol Recipe (Betty Crocker)	1/12 cake	180	3	370	36	—

FOOD	PORTION	CAL	FAT	SOD	CARB	FIB
Devils Food With Chocolate Frosting MicroRave Single (Betty Crocker)	1	440	18	480	64	—
Double Chocolate Supreme Microwave (Pillsbury)	⅛ cake	330	19	340	39	—
Double Lemon Supreme Microwave (Pillsbury)	⅛ cake	300	15	210	40	—
French Vanilla (Duncan Hines)	1/12 cake	260	11	—	—	—
Fudge Marble (Pillsbury)	1/12 cake	270	12	300	36	—
Fudge Marble (Duncan Hines)	1/12 cake	260	11	—	—	—
German Chocolate (Betty Crocker)	1/12 cake	260	12	420	35	—
German Chocolate (Pillsbury)	1/12 cake	250	11	—	—	—
German Chocolate Frosting MicroRave (Betty Crocker)	⅙ cake	320	18	250	37	—
German Chocolate No Cholesterol Recipe (Betty Crocker)	1/12 cake	220	8	420	35	—
Gingerbread (Dromedary)	1 piece (2 in × 2 in)	100	2	190	19	—
Gingerbread (Pillsbury)	3 in sq	190	4	310	36	—
Gingerbread Classic Dessert (Betty Crocker)	⅑ cake	22	7	330	35	—
Gingerbread Classic Dessert No Cholesterol Recipe (Betty Crocker)	⅑ cake	210	6	330	35	—
Golden Pound Classic Dessert (Betty Crocker)	1/12 cake	200	9	170	28	—
Golden Vanilla (Betty Crocker)	1/12 cake	280	14	270	36	—
Golden Vanilla No Cholesterol Recipe (Betty Crocker)	1/12 cake	220	7	270	36	—

FOOD	PORTION	CAL	FAT	SOD	CARB	FIB
Golden Vanilla Rainbow Chip Frosting MicroRave (Betty Crocker)	⅙ cake	320	18	230	40	—
Lemon (Betty Crocker)	1/12 cake	260	11	280	37	—
Lemon (Estee)	1/10 cake	100	2	67	18	—
Lemon (Pillsbury)	1/12 cake	250	11	290	34	—
Lemon Chiffon Classic Dessert (Betty Crocker)	1/12 cake	200	5	200	36	—
Lemon Microwave (Pillsbury)	⅛ cake	220	13	180	23	—
Lemon No Cholesterol Recipe (Betty Crocker)	1/12 cake	220	7	280	37	—
Lemon Pudding Classic Dessert (Betty Crocker)	⅙ cake	230	5	270	45	—
Lemon Supreme (Duncan Hines)	1/12 cake	260	11	—	—	—
Lemon With Lemon Frosting (Pillsbury)	⅛ cake	300	17	220	37	—
Marble (Betty Crocker)	1/12 cake	260	11	290	36	—
Marble No Cholesterol Recipe (Betty Crocker)	1/12 cake	220	7	290	36	—
Milk Chocolate (Betty Crocker)	1/12 cake	260	12	340	34	—
Milk Chocolate No Cholesterol Recipe (Betty Crocker)	1/12 cake	210	7	340	34	—
Nut Quick Bread (Pillsbury)	1/12 loaf	170	6	190	28	—
Pineapple Supreme (Duncan Hines)	1/12 cake	260	11	—	—	—
Pineapple Upsidedown Classic Dessert (Betty Crocker)	⅙ cake	250	10	210	39	—
Pound (Dromedary)	½-in slice	150	6	160	21	—
Pound (Estee)	1/10 cake	100	2	77	18	—
Rainbow Chip (Betty Crocker)	1/12 cake	250	11	320	35	—
Sour Cream Chocolate (Betty Crocker)	1/12 cake	260	12	430	35	—

FOOD	PORTION	CAL	FAT	SOD	CARB	FIB
Sour Cream Chocolate No Cholesterol Recipe (Betty Crocker)	1/12 cake	220	8	430	35	—
Sour Cream White (Betty Crocker)	1/12 cake	180	3	290	36	—
Spice (Betty Crocker)	1/12 cake	260	11	320	36	—
Spice (Duncan Hines)	1/12 cake	260	11	—	—	—
Spice No Cholesterol Recipe (Betty Crocker)	1/12 cake	220	7	320	36	—
Strawberry (Pillsbury)	1/12 cake	260	11	300	37	—
Strawberry Supreme (Duncan Hines)	1/12 cake	260	11	—	—	—
Streusel Swirl Cinnamon (Pillsbury)	1/16 cake	260	11	200	38	—
Streusel Swirl Cinnamon Microwave (Pillsbury)	1/8 cake	240	11	180	33	—
Streusel Swirl Lemon (Pillsbury)	1/16 cake	270	11	340	39	—
Swiss Chocolate (Duncan Hines)	1/12 cake	280	15	—	—	—
Tunnel of Fudge Bundt (Pillsbury)	1/16 cake	270	12	—	—	—
Tunnel of Fudge Bundt Microwave (Pillsbury)	1/8 cake	290	17	320	36	—
White (Betty Crocker)	1/12 cake	240	9	270	36	—
White (Duncan Hines)	1/12 cake	250	10	—	—	—
White (Estee)	1/10 cake	100	2	67	18	—
White (Pillsbury)	1/12 cake	240	10	290	35	—
White Lite Cake & Frosting Mix (Batter Lite)	1/8 cake	110	2	—	—	—
White No Cholesterol Recipe (Betty Crocker)	1/12 cake	220	7	270	36	—
White SuperMoist Light (Betty Crocker)	1/12 cake	180	3	330	37	—
Whole Wheat Baking Mix (Hain)	1.5 oz	150	1	680	30	5
Yellow (Betty Crocker)	1/12 cake	260	11	300	36	—
Yellow (Duncan Hines)	1/12 cake	260	11	—	—	—
Yellow (Pillsbury)	1/12 cake	260	12	300	36	—

FOOD	PORTION	CAL	FAT	SOD	CARB	FIB
Yellow SuperMoist Light (Betty Crocker)	1/12 cake	200	4	310	37	—
Yellow SuperMoist Light No Cholesterol Recipe (Betty Crocker)	1/12 cake	190	3	330	37	—
Yellow Chocolate Frosting MicroRave (Betty Crocker)	1/6 cake	300	17	220	36	—
Yellow Microwave (Pillsbury)	1/8 cake	220	13	170	23	—
Yellow No Cholesterol Recipe (Betty Crocker)	1/12 cake	220	7	300	36	—
Yellow With Chocolate Frosting (Pillsbury)	1/8 cake	300	17	220	36	—
Yellow With Chocolate Frosting MicroRave Single (Betty Crocker)	1	440	19	500	64	—
angelfood	1/12 cake (1.8 oz)	129	tr	255	29	1
angelfood	10 in cake (20.9 oz)	1535	2	3036	350	9
carrot w/o frosting	1/12 cake (2.5 oz)	239	11	249	33	—
carrot w/o frosting	2 layers (29.6 oz)	2886	133	3001	395	—
cheesecake no-bake	1/8 cake (3.5 oz)	271	13	377	35	2
chocolate pudding type w/o frosting	1/12 cake (2.7 oz)	270	14	402	34	—
chocolate pudding type w/o frosting	2 layers (32.4 oz)	3234	172	4815	409	—
chocolate w/o frosting	1/12 cake (2.3 oz)	198	8	370	32	—
chocolate w/o frosting	2 layers (26.8 oz)	2393	92	4464	384	—
chocolate w/o frosting low sodium	1/10 cake (1.3 oz)	116	3	130	23	—
coffeecake crumb topped cinnamon	1/8 cake (2 oz)	178	5	236	30	2
devil's food w/o frosting	1/12 cake (2.3 oz)	198	8	370	32	—
devil's food w/ chocolate frosting	1 cake (9-in diam)	3755	136	2900	645	—
devil's food w/ chocolate frosting	1/16 cake	235	8	181	40	—
fudge w/o frosting	1/12 cake (2.3 oz)	198	8	370	32	—

FOOD	PORTION	CAL	FAT	SOD	CARB	FIB
german chocolate pudding type w/ coconut nut frosting	1/12 cake (3.9 oz)	404	21	369	55	—
gingerbread	1 cake (8-in sq)	1575	39	1733	291	—
gingerbread	1/6 cake (2.4 oz)	207	7	307	34	2
lemon w/o frosting no sugar low sodium	1/10 cake (1.3 oz)	118	3	83	23	—
marble pudding type w/o frosting	1/12 cake (2.6 oz)	253	12	242	35	—
marble pudding type w/o frosting	2 layers (30.6 oz)	3021	148	2884	412	—
white pudding type w/o frosting	1/12 cake (2.4 oz)	244	10	305	36	—
white pudding type w/o frosting	2 layers (29 oz)	2915	123	3654	427	—
white w/o frosting	1/12 cake (2.2 oz)	190	5	301	34	—
white w/o frosting	2 layers (26 oz)	2265	57	3593	410	—
white w/o frosting no sugar low sodium	1/10 cake (1.3 oz)	118	3	83	23	—
yellow pudding type w/o frosting	1/12 cake (2.6 oz)	257	12	317	35	—
yellow pudding type w/o frosting	2 layers (31 oz)	3084	139	3800	421	—
yellow w/o frosting	1/12 cake (2.2 oz)	202	6	299	34	—
yellow w/o frosting	2 layers (26.5 oz)	2415	71	3580	411	—
yellow w/ chocolate frosting	1 cake (9-in diam)	3895	175	3080	620	—
READY-TO-EAT						
Angel Food Ring (Hostess)	1/8 cake (1.6 oz)	150	3	220	29	0
Apple Puffs (Entenmann's)	1 (3 oz)	280	13	320	39	—
Apple Strudel Old Fashioned (Entenmann's)	1 serving (1.5 oz)	120	5	110	17	—
Cheese Topped Buns (Entenmann's)	1 (2.3 oz)	240	12	240	29	—
Cheesecake La Creame Strawberry (Formagg)	2 oz	115	6	—	—	—
Cheesecake La Creame Amaretto Almond (Formagg)	2 oz	115	6	—	—	—

FOOD	PORTION	CAL	FAT	SOD	CARB	FIB
Cheesecake La Creame Pineapple (Formagg)	2 oz	115	6	—	—	—
Cheesecake La Creame Plain (Formagg)	2 oz	115	6	—	—	—
Cinnamon Buns (Entenmann's)	1 (2.1 oz)	230	10	200	31	—
Cinnamon Filbert Ring (Entenmann's)	1 serving (1.5 oz)	190	12	160	19	—
Coffee Cake Cheese (Entenmann's)	1 serving (1.6 oz)	150	7	140	20	—
Coffee Cake Cheese Filled Crumb (Entenmann's)	1 serving (1.4 oz)	130	6	140	18	—
Coffee Cake Crumb (Entenmann's)	1 serving (1.3 oz)	160	7	160	21	—
Danish Ring (Entenmann's)	1 serving (1.5 oz)	180	10	160	18	—
Danish Ring Pecan (Entenmann's)	1 serving (1.5 oz)	190	12	130	19	—
Danish Ring Walnut (Entenmann's)	1 serving (1.5 oz)	190	12	130	19	—
Danish Twist Lemon (Entenmann's)	1 serving (1.2 oz)	140	7	140	17	—
Danish Twist Raspberry (Entenmann's)	1 serving (1.2 oz)	140	7	120	18	—
Date Nut Loaf (Thomas')	1 oz	90	2	170	18	1
Dessert Shells Chocolate Covered (Dutch Mill)	1 (0.5 oz)	80	5	—	8	0
Devil's Food Cake Fudge Iced (Entenmann's)	1 serving (1.2 oz)	130	5	120	19	—
French Crumb Cake All Butter (Entenmann's)	1 serving (1.6 oz)	180	8	220	26	—
Fruit Cake Holiday (Hostess)	⅙ cake (5.3 oz)	490	14	410	93	3
Louisiana Crunch Cake (Entenmann's)	1 serving (1.7 oz)	180	8	180	27	—
Pound Cake (Hostess)	⅛ cake (3.2 oz)	350	16	360	48	1
Pound Loaf All Butter (Entenmann's)	1 serving (1 oz)	110	5	150	15	—

FOOD	PORTION	CAL	FAT	SOD	CARB	FIB
Pound Loaf Sour Cream (Entenmann's)	1 serving (1 oz)	120	7	90	14	—
Thick Fudge Golden Cake (Entenmann's)	1 serving (1.2 oz)	130	6	120	20	—
angelfood	1 cake (11.9 oz)	876	3	2548	197	5
angelfood	1/12 cake (1 oz)	73	tr	212	16	1
bakewell tart	1 slice (3 oz)	410	27	—	39	2
battenburg cake	1 slice (2 oz)	204	10	—	28	1
cheesecake	1 cake (9-in diam)	3350	213	2464	317	—
cheesecake	1/6 cake (2.8 oz)	256	18	165	20	2
cherry fudge w/ chocolate frosting	1/8 cake (2.5 oz)	187	9	160	27	—
chocolate w/ chocolate frosting	1/8 cake (2.2 oz)	235	11	213	35	2
coffeecake cheese	1/6 cake (2.7 oz)	258	12	257	38	1
coffeecake crumb topped cheese	1/6 cake (2.7 oz)	258	12	257	38	1
coffeecake crumb topped cinnamon	1/9 cake (2.2 oz)	263	15	221	29	2
coffeecake fruit	1/8 cake (1.8 oz)	156	5	192	26	—
crumpets toasted	2 (4 oz)	119	1	—	26	2
eccles cake	1 slice (2 oz)	285	16	—	36	1
eclair	1 (1.4 oz)	149	10	—	15	tr
fruitcake	1 piece (1.5 oz)	139	4	116	27	—
madeira cake	1 slice (1 oz)	98	4	—	15	1
pound	1/10 cake (1 oz)	117	6	119	15	—
pound cake	1 cake (8½ × 3½ × 3 in)	1935	94	1857	257	—
pound cake	1 slice (1 oz)	110	12	108	15	—
sour cream pound	1/10 cake (1 oz)	117	5	120	16	tr
sponge	1/12 cake (1.3 oz)	110	1	93	23	—
strudel apple	1 piece (2½ oz)	195	8	191	29	2
treacle tart	1 slice (2.5 oz)	258	10	—	42	1
vanilla slice	1 slice (2.5 oz)	248	13	—	30	1
white w/ white frosting	1 cake (9-in diam)	4170	148	2827	670	—
white w/ white frosting	1/16 cake	260	9	176	42	—
yellow w/ vanilla frosting	1/8 cake (2.2 oz)	239	9	220	38	—
yellow w/ chocolate frosting	1 cake (9-in diam)	3895	175	3080	620	—
yellow w/ chocolate frosting	1/8 cake (2.2 oz)	242	11	216	36	1

FOOD	PORTION	CAL	FAT	SOD	CARB	FIB
REFRIGERATED						
Apple Turnovers (Pillsbury)	1	170	8	330	23	—
Cheesecake (Baby Watson)	1 slice (3.8 oz)	390	30	330	23	2
Cheesecake Light (Baby Watson)	⅟₁₆ cake (3.9 oz)	280	16	270	24	3
Cherry Turnovers (Pillsbury)	1	170	8	320.	23	—
Coffee Cake Cinnamon Swirl (Pillsbury)	⅛ cake	180	9	170	22	—
Coffee Cake Pecan Streusel (Pillsbury)	⅛ cake	180	9	170	21	—
Pastry Pockets (Pillsbury)	1	240	13	520	25	—
SNACK						
All Butter Pound (Sara Lee)	1	200	11	190	23	—
Apple Delights (Little Debbie)	1 pkg (1.2 oz)	140	5	115	24	1
Apple Light & Fruity (Drake's)	1 (1.2 oz)	90	1	110	20	—
Apple Oatmeal (Lance)	1 pkg (51 g)	200	9	210	35	—
Apple Twist (Hostess)	1 (2.5 oz)	220	4	270	42	tr
Apple-Roos (Little Debbie)	1 pkg (1.5 oz)	150	3	80	32	1
Banana Nut Muffin Loaves (Little Debbie)	1 pkg (1.9 oz)	210	9	210	30	1
Banana Twins (Little Debbie)	1 pkg (2.2 oz)	250	10	180	40	0
Baseball Yellow Cakes (Hostess)	1 (1.6 oz)	160	3	160	32	0
Be My Valentine (Little Debbie)	1 pkg (2.2 oz)	280	14	150	39	1
Blueberry Light & Fruity (Drake's)	1 (1.2 oz)	90	1	95	20	—
Butter Cream Cream Filled Cupcake (Tastykake)	1 (32 g)	120	4	120	20	1
Cherry Cordials (Little Debbie)	1 pkg (1.3 oz)	160	8	100	23	1
Choc-o-Jel (Little Debbie)	1 pkg (1.2 oz)	150	7	95	21	1

FOOD	PORTION	CAL	FAT	SOD	CARB	FIB
Choco-Cakes (Little Debbie)	1 pkg (2.1 oz)	250	13	170	35	1
Choco-Cakes (Little Debbie)	1 pkg (2.2 oz)	240	12	180	35	1
Choco-Diles (Hostess)	1 (1.8 oz)	210	10	160	31	1
Choco Licious (Hostess)	1 (1.5 oz)	170	6	190	28	1
Chocolate (Little Debbie)	1 pkg (3 oz)	360	17	220	52	1
Chocolate Cream Filled Cupcake (Tastykake)	1 (34 g)	130	5	130	21	1
Chocolate Cupcake (Tastykake)	1 (30 g)	100	3	120	19	1
Chocolate Chip (Little Debbie)	1 pkg (2.4 oz)	290	15	190	42	1
Chocolate Fudge Cake (Sara Lee)	1	190	10	125	24	—
Chocolate Twins (Little Debbie)	1 pkg (2.4 oz)	240	9	280	42	1
Christmas Tree Cakes (Little Debbie)	1 pkg (1.5 oz)	190	9	90	27	0
Cinnaminis Original (Hostess)	5 (2.4 oz)	300	17	230	37	2
Cinnamon Raisin Light & Fruity (Drake's)	1 (1.2 oz)	90	1	105	19	—
Cinnamon Roll (Hostess)	1 (2.3 oz)	220	6	260	39	1
Classic Cheesecake (Sara Lee)	1	200	14	150	16	—
Coconut (Little Debbie)	1 pkg (2.1 oz)	270	13	180	38	1
Coconut (Little Debbie)	1 pkg (2.4 oz)	300	14	200	42	0
Coconut Rounds (Little Debbie)	1 pkg (1.2 oz)	140	7	85	22	1
Coffee Cake						
(Drake's)	1 (1.1 oz)	140	6	90	18	—
Apple (Little Debbie)	1 pkg (1.9 oz)	220	7	190	36	1
Apple Cinnamon (Sara Lee)	1	290	13	270	40	—
Apple Streusel (Little Debbie)	1 pkg (2 oz)	220	7	200	37	1
Butter Streusel (Sara Lee)	1	230	12	270	27	—
Chocolate Crumb (Drake's)	1 (2.5 oz)	245	9	206	38	—
Cinnamon Crumb (Drake's)	½ cake (1.3 oz)	150	6	110	22	—

FOOD	PORTION	CAL	FAT	SOD	CARB	FIB
Pecan (Sara Lee)	1	280	16	270	30	—
Small (Drake's)	1 (2 oz)	220	9	160	33	—
Creamies Chocolate (Tastykake)	1	174	7	—	—	—
Creamies Banana Treat (Tastykake)	1	138	3	—	—	—
Creamies Vanilla (Tastykake)	1	182	8	—	—	—
Crumb Cake (Hostess)	1 (1.9 oz)	210	8	135	33	1
Crumb Cake Light (Hostess)	1 (1.8 oz)	150	1	190	35	tr
Cup Cakes Chocolate (Hostess)	1 (1.6 oz)	170	5	160	28	tr
Cup Cakes Orange (Hostess)	1 (1.5 oz)	160	5	160	28	0
Deluxe Carrot Cake (Sara Lee)	1	180	7	200	26	—
Dessert Cups (Hostess)	1 (1 oz)	90	2	170	18	0
Devil Cremes (Little Debbie)	1 pkg (1.6 oz)	190	8	160	28	0
Devil Cremes (Little Debbie)	1 pkg (3.2 oz)	380	17	310	57	1
Devil Dog (Drake's)	1 (1.5 oz)	160	6	135	24	—
Devil Squares (Little Debbie)	1 pkg (2.2 oz)	260	13	180	39	1
Ding Dongs (Hostess)	1 (1.3 oz)	160	9	110	21	tr
Dunking Sticks (Lance)	1 (39 g)	190	10	130	22	—
Easter Basket Cakes (Little Debbie)	1 pkg (2.5 oz)	310	15	180	44	1
Fancy Cakes (Little Debbie)	1 pkg (2.4 oz)	300	15	160	42	0
Fig Cake (Lance)	1 pkg (60 g)	210	3	90	43	—
Fruit Loaf (Hostess)	1 (3.8 oz)	350	10	290	67	2
Fudge Crispy (Little Debbie)	1 pkg (1.1 oz)	170	10	50	20	1
Fudge Round (Little Debbie)	1 pkg (2.5 oz)	290	12	170	49	2
Fudge Round (Little Debbie)	1 pkg (3 oz)	350	14	210	59	2
Fudge Round (Little Debbie)	1 pkg (1.2 oz)	140	5	80	23	1
Funny Bones (Drake's)	1 (1.25 oz)	150	8	110	18	—
Golden Cremes (Little Debbie)	1 pkg (1.5 oz)	170	7	180	25	0

FOOD	PORTION	CAL	FAT	SOD	CARB	FIB
Golden Cremes (Little Debbie)	1 pkg (3 oz)	330	15	350	50	0
Ho Ho's (Hostess)	1 (1 oz)	130	6	75	17	tr
Holiday Cake Chocolate (Little Debbie)	1 pkg (2.4 oz)	290	14	180	43	1
Holiday Cake Vanilla (Little Debbie)	1 pkg (2.5 oz)	310	15	180	44	1
Holiday Cakes (Hostess)	1 (1.6 oz)	160	3	160	32	0
Honey Bun (Little Debbie)	1 pkg (3 oz)	380	23	190	39	4
Honey Bun (Little Debbie)	1 pkg (4 oz)	510	31	250	53	5
Honey Bun Glazed (Hostess)	1 (2.7 oz)	320	19	90	35	2
Honey Bun Iced (Hostess)	1 (3.4 oz)	390	20	220	49	2
Honey Buns (Lance)	1 (85 g)	330	14	210	48	—
Honeybun Glazed (Tastykake)	1 pkg (92 g)	360	20	220	42	4
Honeybun Iced (Tastykake)	1 pkg (92 g)	350	15	250	50	1
Hopper Cakes (Hostess)	1 (1.6 oz)	160	3	160	32	0
Jelly Rolls (Little Debbie)	1 pkg (2.1 oz)	230	7	160	41	0
Junior Chocolate (Tastykake)	1 pkg (94 g)	340	12	220	57	4
Junior Coconut (Tastykake)	1 pkg (94 g)	300	6	300	60	3
Junior Lemon (Tastykake)	1 pkg (94 g)	310	7	330	75	1
Junior Orange (Tastykake)	1 pkg (94 g)	340	9	240	61	1
Kandy Kake Chocolate (Tastykake)	1 (19 g)	80	3	35	13	1
Kandy Kake Coconut (Tastykake)	1 (19 g)	80	4	40	11	1
Kandy Kake Peanut Butter (Tastykake)	1 (19 g)	90	4	40	11	1
Koffee Kake Cream Filled (Tastykake)	1 (29 g)	110	4	80	18	0
Koffee Kake Junior (Tastykake)	1 pkg (71 g)	260	8	210	44	1

FOOD	PORTION	CAL	FAT	SOD	CARB	FIB
Kreme Kup (Tastykake)	1 (25 g)	90	3	115	15	1
Krimpet Butterscotch (Tastykake)	1 (28 g)	100	1	85	19	0
Krimpet Jelly (Tastykake)	1 (28 g)	90	1	80	19	1
Krimpet Strawberry (Tastykake)	1 (28 g)	100	2	85	20	0
Lemon Stix (Little Debbie)	1 pkg (1.5 oz)	210	10	45	30	1
Lil Angels (Hostess)	1 (1 oz)	90	2	130	17	0
Marshmallow Supremes (Little Debbie)	1 pkg (1.1 oz)	130	5	70	22	1
Mint Sprints (Little Debbie)	1 pkg (1.5 oz)	230	13	70	28	1
Nutty Bar (Little Debbie)	1 pkg (2 oz)	290	17	115	34	1
Oatmeal Cake (Lance)	1 (57 g)	240	11	250	35	—
Pastry Pocket Apple (Tastykake)	1 (85 g)	320	18	220	38	—
Pastry Pocket Cheese (Tastykake)	1 (85 g)	330	19	230	38	1
Pastry Pocket Cherry (Tastykake)	1 (85 g)	330	17	230	41	1
Pecan Spinners (Hostess)	1 (1 oz)	110	5	65	15	tr
Pecan Twins (Little Debbie)	1 pkg (2 oz)	220	9	200	32	1
Pecan Twirls (Lance)	1 pkg (57 g)	220	8	190	34	—
Pecan Twirls (Tastykake)	1 (28 g)	110	1	75	17	—
Pop-Tarts						
Apple Cinnamon	1	210	6	170	37	1
Blueberry	1	210	6	210	37	0
Brown Sugar Cinnamon	1	210	8	200	33	0
Cherry	1	210	6	220	37	0
Chocolate Graham	1	210	6	220	37	0
Frosted Brown Sugar Cinnamon	1	210	7	190	34	0
Frosted Cherry	1	210	5	220	37	0
Frosted Chocolate Vanilla Creme	1	200	5	230	37	0
Frosted Chocolate Fudge	1	200	5	220	37	0
Frosted Grape	1	200	5	200	37	0

FOOD	PORTION	CAL	FAT	SOD	CARB	FIB
Pop-Tarts *(cont.)*						
Frosted Raspberry	1	200	5	210	37	0
Frosted Strawberry	1	200	5	190	37	1
Strawberry	1	210	6	200	37	0
Pound Cake (Drake's)	1	110	5	70	16	—
Pumpkin Delights (Little Debbie)	1 pkg (1.1 oz)	130	5	115	21	1
Raisin Cake (Lance)	1 (57 g)	230	10	200	35	—
Ring Ding (Drake's)	1 (1.5 oz)	180	10	115	23	—
Ring Ding Mint (Drake's)	1 (1.5 oz)	190	11	115	22	—
Royale Chocolate Cupcake (Tastykake)	1 (46 g)	170	7	130	28	2
Smiley Faces Cherry (Little Debbie)	1 pkg (1.2 oz)	140	5	115	23	1
Smiley Faces Pumpkin (Little Debbie)	1 pkg (1 oz)	130	5	215	20	1
Snack Cake Chocolate (Little Debbie)	1 pkg (2.5 oz)	300	15	180	43	1
Snack Cake Vanilla (Little Debbie)	1 pkg (2.6 oz)	320	16	180	45	1
Sno Balls (Hostess)	1 (1.6 oz)	160	5	180	29	1
Spice (Little Debbie)	1 pkg (2.5 oz)	300	15	230	43	1
Star Crunch (Little Debbie)	1 pkg (1.1 oz)	140	6	85	21	1
Star Crunch (Little Debbie)	1 pkg (2.6 oz)	330	14	240	51	1
Sunny Doodle (Drake's)	1 (1 oz)	100	3	100	16	—
Suzy Q's (Hostess)	1 (2 oz)	220	9	270	35	2
Suzy Q's Banana (Hostess)	1 (2 oz)	220	10	280	32	tr
Swirls Caramel Pecan (Hostess)	1 (2 oz)	140	15	55	25	1
Swiss Rolls (Little Debbie)	1 pkg (2.1 oz)	250	12	160	38	1
Swiss Rolls (Little Debbie)	1 pkg (2.7 oz)	320	15	210	47	1
Swiss Rolls (Little Debbie)	1 pkg (3.2 oz)	380	18	250	57	1
Tasty Too Chocolate Cream Filled Cupcake (Tastykake)	1 (32 g)	100	1	115	21	1
Tasty Too Vanilla Cream Filled Cupcake (Tastykake)	1 (32 g)	100	1	120	21	1

FOOD	PORTION	CAL	FAT	SOD	CARB	FIB
Tasty Twists (Tastykake)	1 (4 g)	18	1	—	3	—
Teddy Berries (Little Debbie)	1 pkg (1.2 oz)	130	4	105	23	1
Tiger Tails (Hostess)	1 (1.5 oz)	160	6	150	26	tr
Toast-R-Cakes BlueBerry	1	110	3	158	18	—
Toast-R-Cakes Bran	1	103	3	163	18	—
Toast-R-Cakes Corn	1	120	4	142	19	—
Toaster Tart Apple Cinnamon (Pepperidge Farm)	1	170	7	120	25	—
Toaster Tart Cheese (Pepperidge Farm)	1	190	10	180	22	—
Toaster Tart Strawberry (Pepperidge Farm)	1	190	7	120	28	—
Toastettes (Nabisco)						
Apple	1	290	5	170	36	1
Blueberry	1	190	5	200	35	1
Cherry	1	190	5	200	35	1
Frosted Apple	1	190	5	170	35	—
Frosted Blueberry	1	190	0	200	35	1
Frosted Brown Sugar Cinnamon	1	190	5	180	35	1
Frosted Cherry	1	190	5	200	35	1
Frosted Fruit Punch	1	190	5	200	35	1
Frosted Fudge	1	200	5	280	34	1
Frosted Strawberry	1	190	5	200	35	1
Strawberry	1	190	5	200	35	1
Twinkies (Hostess)	1 (1.4 oz)	140	4	180	25	0
Banana	2 (2.7 oz)	300	13	370	42	tr
Devil Food	2 (2.7 oz)	300	12	360	47	2
Lights	1 (1.4 oz)	120	2	200	24	0
Strawberry Fruit 'n Creme	1 (1.6 oz)	150	3	200	30	tr
Vanilla (Little Debbie)	1 pkg (3 oz)	370	18	210	53	0
Vanilla Cremes (Little Debbie)	1 pkg (1.4 oz)	170	7	125	25	0
Yankee Doodle (Drake's)	1 (1 oz)	100	4	110	16	—
Yodel's (Drake's)	1 (1 oz)	150	9	65	16	—
Zebra Cakes (Little Debbie)	1 pkg (2.6 oz)	150	16	180	45	1
devil's food cupcake w/ chocolate frosting	1	120	4	92	20	—

FOOD	PORTION	CAL	FAT	SOD	CARB	FIB
devil's food w/ creme filling	1 (1 oz)	105	4	105	17	—
sponge w/ creme filling	1 (1.5 oz)	155	5	155	27	—
toaster pastry, apple	1 (1.75 oz)	204	5	218	37	—
toaster pastry, blueberry	1 (1.75 oz)	204	5	218	37	—
toaster pastry, brown sugar cinnamon	1 (1.75 oz)	206	7	212	34	—
toaster pastry, strawberry	1 (1.75 oz)	204	5	218	37	—
TAKE-OUT						
baklava	1 oz	126	9	78	10	1
strudel	1 piece (4.1 oz)	272	8	142	50	3
trifle w/ cream	6 oz	291	16	—	34	1

CANADIAN BACON

FOOD	PORTION	CAL	FAT	SOD	CARB	FIB
Jones	1 slice	30	1	160	tr	—
Oscar Mayer	1 slice	28	1	305	tr	—
unheated	2 slices (1.9 oz)	89	4	799	1	—

CANDY
see also MARSHMALLOW

FOOD	PORTION	CAL	FAT	SOD	CARB	FIB
100 Grand (Nestle)	1 bar (1.5 oz)	200	8	75	30	tr
3 Musketeers	1 (2.1 oz)	260	8	110	46	1
3 Musketeers	2 bars fun size (1.1 oz)	140	5	60	25	0
5th Avenue	1 (2.1 oz)	290	13	140	39	—
After Eight Dark Chocolate Wafer Thin Mints (Rowntree)	1	35	1	0	6	—
Almond Butter Dome (Godiva)	3 pieces (1.5 oz)	240	17	20	19	0
Almond Joy	1 (1.76 oz)	250	14	70	28	—
Areo Bar (Nestle)	1 bar (1.45 oz)	210	13	20	26	2
Baby Ruth (Nestle)	1 bar (2.1 oz)	280	12	135	38	2
Baby Ruth Fun Size (Nestle)	2 pieces	200	9	95	27	1
Bar None	1 (1.5 oz)	240	14	50	23	—
Bit-O-Honey	1.7 oz	200	4	125	39	—
Bouchee Au Chocolat (Godiva)	1 piece (1.5 oz)	210	11	40	25	0
Bouchee Ivory Raspberry (Godiva)	1 piece (1 oz)	160	9	25	17	0

FOOD	PORTION	CAL	FAT	SOD	CARB	FIB
Breath Savers Sugar Free						
Cinnamon	1 candy	2	0	0	1	0
Peppermint	1 candy	2	0	0	0	0
Spearmint	1 candy	2	0	0	1	0
Wintergreen	1 candy	2	0	0	1	0
Buncha Crunch (Nestle)	1 pkg (1.4 oz)	90	10	95	26	tr
Butter Mints (Kraft)	1	8	0	0	2	—
Butterfinger (Nestle)	1 bar (2.1 oz)	280	11	120	41	1
Butterfinger BB's (Nestle)	1 pkg (1.7 oz)	230	10	90	34	1
Butterfinger Fun Size (Nestle)	2 bars (1.6 oz)	200	8	85	30	1
Butterscotch Discs (Brock)	3 pieces (0.6 oz)	70	0	80	17	—
Candy Corn (Brock)	21 pieces (1.4 oz)	150	0	85	37	—
Candy Rolls (Brock)	2 rolls (0.5 oz)	50	0	0	12	—
Caramel Dots (Brock)	3 pieces (1.3 oz)	140	3	50	25	tr
Caramello	1 (1.6 oz)	220	11	60	28	—
Caramels (Kraft)	1	30	1	25	6	—
Caramels Chocolate (Estee)	1	30	1	15	5	—
Caramels Vanilla (Estee)	1	30	1	15	5	—
Caroby Almond Bar (Natural Touch)	4 sections (28 g)	150	10	50	12	—
Caroby Milk Bar (Natural Touch)	4 sections (28 g)	150	9	55	13	—
Caroby Milk Free Bar (Natural Touch)	4 sections (28 g)	160	11	25	11	—
Caroby Mint Bar (Natural Touch)	4 sections (28 g)	150	9	55	13	—
Certs	1 piece (1.67 g)	6	0	—	2	—
Certs Sugar Free	1 piece (1.67 g)	7	0	—	2	—
Certs Mini Sugar Free Certs	1 piece (0.365 g)	1	0	—	tr	—
Charleston Chew (Cambridge)	1 pkg (1.9 oz)	230	7	—	—	—
Charleston Chew! Chocolate (Pearson's)	½ bar	120	3	—	—	—

FOOD	PORTION	CAL	FAT	SOD	CARB	FIB
Charleston Chew! Strawberry (Pearson's)	½ bar	120	3	—	—	—
Charleston Chew! Vanilla (Pearson's)	½ bar	120	3	—	—	—
Charms Blow Pop	1 (0.7 oz)	80	0	—	—	—
Charms Pop	1 (0.6 oz)	70	0	—	—	—
Chocolate Covered Cherries Dark Chocolate (Cellas)	2 pieces (1 oz)	100	4	—	—	—
Chocolate Covered Cherries Milk Chocolate (Cellas)	2 pieces (1 oz)	110	4	15	18	2
Chocolate Fudgies (Kraft)	1	35	1	25	6	—
Chocolate Bar (Estee)						
Almond	2 squares	60	4	10	4	—
Coconut	2 squares	60	4	10	4	—
Fruit & Nut	2 squares	60	4	10	4	—
Peanut	2 squares	60	4	10	4	—
Chocolate Coated Raisins (Estee)	10 pieces	30	1	10	5	—
Chocolaty Peanut Bar (Lance)	1 (57 g)	320	18	40	29	—
Chunky (Nestle)	1 bar (1.4 oz)	200	11	20	22	2
Cinnamon Discs (Brock)	3 pieces (0.6 oz)	70	0	5	17	—
Circus Peanuts (Brock)	11 pieces (2.5 oz)	260	0	25	65	—
Clorets Mints (Clorets)	1 piece (1.67 g)	6	0	—	2	—
Coconut Mountains (Brock)	4 pieces (1.4 oz)	170	6	80	29	—
Crunch Fun Size (Nestle)	4 bars (1.5 oz)	200	10	55	25	1
Crunch 'N Munch (Franklin)						
Candied	1.25 oz	170	7	200	28	1
Caramel	1.25 oz	160	5	130	28	1
Maple Walnut	1.25 oz	160	6	180	28	1
Toffee	1.25 oz	160	5	210	28	1
Crunch Chocolate Bar (Estee)	2 squares	45	3	20	4	—
Dark Chocolate Bar (Estee)	2 squares	60	5	0	5	—

FOOD	PORTION	CAL	FAT	SOD	CARB	FIB
Dark Chocolate Mint Bar (Estee)	2 squares	60	5	0	5	—
Dove						
Dark Chocolate	1 bar (1.3 oz)	200	12	0	22	2
Dark Chocolate	¼ bar (1.5 oz)	230	14	0	26	3
Dark Chocolate Miniatures	7 (1.5 oz)	230	14	0	26	2
Milk Chocolate	¼ bar (1.5 oz)	230	13	30	25	1
Milk Chocolate	1 bar (1.3 oz)	200	7	25	22	1
Milk Chocolate Miniatures	7 (1.5 oz)	230	13	30	25	1
Estee-ets (Estee)	5 pieces	35	2	10	4	—
Fruit & Nut Bar (Cadbury)	1 oz	150	8	—	—	—
Fruit And Nut Mix (Estee)	4 pieces	35	2	10	3	—
Fruit Basket (Brock)	3 pieces (0.6 oz)	60	0	0	15	—
Fruit Kisses (Brock)	3 pieces (0.6 oz)	70	0	5	17	—
Glitters (Brock)	2 pieces (0.5 oz)	50	0	15	13	—
Gold Ballotin (Godiva)	3 pieces (1.5 oz)	210	10	15	27	0
Golden Almond	½ bar	260	17	35	20	—
Golden III	½ bar	250	15	40	26	—
Goobers (Nestle)	1 pkg (1.38 oz)	210	13	20	19	3
Gum Drops (Estee)	4 pieces	25	0	0	6	—
Gummy Bears (Brock)	5 pieces (1.4 oz)	130	0	15	30	—
Gummy Bears (Estee)	3 pieces	20	0	0	4	—
Gummy Squirms (Brock)	5 pieces (1.3 oz)	120	0	15	28	—
Hard Candy (Estee)	2	25	0	0	6	—
Hershey Bar	1 (1.55 oz)	240	14	40	25	—
Hershey Bar With Almonds	1 (1.45 oz)	230	14	55	20	—
Hershey's Kisses	9 pieces (1.46 oz)	220	13	35	23	—
Jelly Beans (Brock)	12 pieces (1.4 oz)	140	0	15	36	—
Jelly Beans (Just Born)	1 oz	108	tr	—	—	—
Junior Mints	12 pieces	120	3	—	—	—

FOOD	PORTION	CAL	FAT	SOD	CARB	FIB
Junior Mints (Cambridge)	1 pkg (1.6 oz)	190	4	—	—	—
Just Born Sugar Coated	1.5 oz	148	tr	—	—	—
Just Born Toasted Coconut	1.38 oz	140	2	—	—	—
Kit Kat Wafer	1 (1.625 oz)	250	13	60	29	—
Krackel	1 (1.55 oz)	230	13	80	27	—
Laffy Taffy (Beich's)						
Apple Chews	1 oz	110	1	55	26	—
Banana Chews	1 oz	110	1	55	26	—
Grape Chews	1 oz	110	1	60	26	—
Passion Punch Chews	1 oz	110	1	50	26	—
Strawberry Chews	1 oz	110	1	55	26	—
Sweet & Sour Cherry Chews	1 oz	110	1	55	26	—
Watermelon Chews	1 oz	110	1	55	26	—
Lemon Drops (Brock)	3 pieces (0.5 oz)	60	0	5	14	—
Life Savers Lollipops All Flavors	1	45	0	—	—	—
Life Savers Sugar Free	1 piece	8	0	—	—	—
Life Savers Holes						
Sunshine Fruits	1 candy	2	0	0	1	0
Tangerine	1 candy	2	0	0	1	0
Life Savers						
Christmas Lollipops	1	40	0	0	10	—
Easter Pops	1	40	0	0	10	—
Fancy Fruits	1 candy	8	0	0	2	—
Fruit Juicers Citrus Fruits	1 candy	8	0	0	2	0
Fruit Juicers Easter Egg-Sortments	1 candy	10	0	0	2	0
Fruit Juicers Fruit Punch	1 candy	8	0	0	2	0
Fruit Juicers Grape	1 candy	8	0	0	2	0
Fruit Juicers Lollipops	1	40	0	0	10	0
Fruit Juicers Mixed Berries	1 candy	8	0	0	2	0
Fruit Juicers Strawberry	1 candy	8	0	0	2	0
Gummi Savers Grape	1 candy	12	0	0	3	0

FOOD	PORTION	CAL	FAT	SOD	CARB	FIB
Gummi Savers Mixed Berry	1 candy	12	0	0	3	0
Sunshine Fruits	1 candy	8	0	0	2	—
Tropical Fruits	1 candy	8	0	0	2	—
Valentine Pops	1	40	0	0	10	—
Wild Cherry	1 candy	8	0	0	2	—
Lollipops (Estee)	1	25	0	0	6	—
Lollipops Sugar Free (Louis Sherry)	1	18	0	—	—	—
M&M's						
Almond	1 pkg (1.3 oz)	200	11	20	21	2
Almond	1.5 oz	220	12	20	24	2
Mint	1 pkg (1.7 oz)	230	10	35	34	1
Mint	1.5 oz	200	9	30	30	1
Peanut	1 fun size (0.7 oz)	110	5	10	13	1
Peanut	1 pkg (1.7 oz)	250	13	25	30	2
Peanut	1.5 oz	220	11	20	25	2
Peanut	½ bag king size (1.6 oz)	240	12	25	28	2
Peanut Butter	1 fun size (0.7 oz)	110	6	45	12	1
Peanut Butter	1 pkg (1.6 oz)	240	13	100	27	2
Peanut Butter	1.5 oz	220	11	90	25	2
Plain	1 pkg (1.7 oz)	230	10	35	34	1
Plain	1 pkg fun size (0.7 oz)	100	5	15	15	0
Plain	1.5 oz	200	9	30	30	1
Plain	½ pkg king size (1.6 oz)	220	9	30	32	1
Semisweet	0.5 oz	70	4	0	9	1
Mars	1 bar (1.8 oz)	240	13	85	31	1
Mars Almond Bar	2 fun size (1.3 oz)	190	10	65	23	1
Milk Chocolate Bar (Estee)	2 squares	60	4	10	4	—
Milky Way	1 bar (2.1 oz)	280	11	90	43	0
Milky Way	2 fun size (1.4 oz)	180	7	60	28	0
Milky Way Miniature	5 (1.5 oz)	190	7	65	30	0
Milky Way Dark	1 bar (1.8 oz)	220	8	85	36	1
Milky Way Dark	1 fun size (0.7 oz)	90	3	35	14	0
Mounds	1 (1.9 oz)	260	14	85	31	—
Mr. Goodbar	1 (1.75 oz)	290	19	20	23	—

FOOD	PORTION	CAL	FAT	SOD	CARB	FIB
Munch Bar	1 (1.4 oz)	230	15	150	17	2
NECCO Mint	1 piece	12	tr	—	—	—
Nestle Milk Chocolate	1 bar (1.45 oz)	220	13	30	23	2
Nestle Crunch	1 bar (1.55 oz)	230	12	60	28	1
Nips						
Butter Rum (Pearson's)	2 pieces (0.5 oz)	60	2	35	12	—
Caramel (Pearson's)	2 pieces (0.5 oz)	60	2	40	12	—
Chocolate Parfait (Pearson's)	2 pieces (0.5 oz)	60	2	35	11	—
Chocolate Mint (Pearson's)	2 pieces (0.5 oz)	60	2	40	11	—
Licorice (Pearson's)	2 pieces (0.5 oz)	60	2	40	12	—
Peanut Butter Parfait (Pearson's)	2 pieces (0.5 oz)	60	2	40	11	—
Oh Henry! (Nestle)	1 bar (1.8 oz)	230	9	125	32	2
Orange Slices (Brock)	4 pieces (1.5 oz)	140	0	20	36	—
PB Max	2 (1.6 oz)	240	15	160	22	1
PB Max	2 fun size (1.2 oz)	180	12	115	16	1
Party Mints (Brock)	9 pieces (0.5 oz)	60	0	0	15	—
Party Mints (Kraft)	1	8	0	0	2	—
Peanut Bar (Lance)	1 pkg (50 g)	260	14	80	24	—
Peanut Brittle (Estee)	¼ oz	35	1	30	5	—
Peanut Brittle (Kraft)	1 oz	130	5	135	20	—
Peanut Butter Crunch (Brock)	3 pieces (0.6 oz)	80	2	45	15	—
Peanut Butter Cups (Estee)	1	40	3	20	3	—
Peanut Chews (Goldenberg's)	4 pieces (1.7 oz)	215	7	45	32	—
Pez	1 roll (0.3 oz)	35	0	0	9	—
Pez	1 roll (0.3 oz)	30	0	0	8	—
Pom Pom (Cambridge)	1 pkg (1.6 oz)	200	6	—	—	—
Pops Assorted (Brock)	2 (0.5 oz)	60	0	5	15	—
Popscotch (Lance)	1 pkg (35 g)	160	6	120	24	—
Raisinets (Nestle)	1 pkg (1.58 oz)	200	8	15	31	2
Reese's Peanut Butter Cups	1 (1.8 oz)	280	17	180	26	—
Reese's Pieces	1.85 oz	260	11	90	32	—

FOOD	PORTION	CAL	FAT	SOD	CARB	FIB
Rolo Carmels in Milk Chocolate	8 pieces (1.93 oz)	270	12	110	37	—
Skittles	1 pkg (2.2 oz)	250	3	10	55	0
Skittles	1.5 oz	170	2	5	38	0
Original	2 pkg fun size (1.4 oz)	160	2	5	36	0
Tart-N-Tangy	1 bag (2.2 oz)	250	3	10	55	0
Tart-N-Tangy	1.5 oz	170	2	5	38	0
Tart-N-Tangy	2 bags fun size (1.4 oz)	160	2	5	36	0
Tropical	1 bag (2.2 oz)	250	3	10	55	0
Tropical	1.5 oz	170	2	5	38	0
Tropical	2 bags fun size (1.4 oz)	160	2	5	36	0
Wild Berry	1 bag (2.2 oz)	250	3	10	55	0
Wild Berry	1.5 oz	170	2	5	38	0
Wild Berry	2 bags fun size (1.4 oz)	160	2	5	36	0
Skor Toffee Bar	1 (1.4 oz)	220	14	125	22	—
Snickers	1 bar (2.1 oz)	280	14	150	36	1
Snickers	2 bars fun size (1.4 oz)	190	9	100	24	1
Snickers Miniatures	4 (1.3 oz)	170	8	90	22	1
Snickers Peanut Butter	1 bar (2 oz)	310	20	150	28	1
Sno Caps (Nestle)	1 pkg (2.3 oz)	300	13	0	48	3
Solitaires With Almonds	½ bag	260	17	25	20	—
Sour Balls (Brock)	3 pieces (0.6 oz)	70	0	5	17	—
Sour Sharks (Brock)	23 pieces (2.5 oz)	30	3	45	60	—
Spearmint Starlights (Brock)	3 pieces (0.6 oz)	60	0	5	16	—
Special Dark Sweet Chocolate Bar (Hershey)	1 (1.45)	220	12	5	25	—
Spice Drops (Brock)	12 pieces (1.4 oz)	130	0	20	33	—
Starburst						
California Fruits	1 stick (2.1 oz)	240	5	35	48	0
California Fruits	8 pieces (1.4 oz)	160	4	20	33	0
Strawberry Fruits	1 stick (2.1 oz)	240	5	35	48	0
Strawberry Fruits	8 pieces (1.4 oz)	160	3	20	33	0

FOOD	PORTION	CAL	FAT	SOD	CARB	FIB
Starburst *(cont.)*						
Tropical Fruits	1 stick (2.1 oz)	240	5	35	48	0
Tropical Fruits	8 pieces (1.4 oz)	160	3	20	33	0
Starlight Mints (Brock)	3 pieces (0.6 oz)	60	0	5	16	—
Sugar Babies (Cambridge)	1 pkg (1.7 oz)	190	2	—	—	—
Sugar Babies (Tidbits)	1 pkg	180	2	—	—	—
Sugar Daddy	1 pop	150	1	—	—	—
Sugar Daddy (Cambridge)	1 pkg (1.7 oz)	200	3	—	—	—
Swedish Fish Red	19 pieces (1.4 oz)	150	1	20	35	—
Symphony Almond/Butterchips	1 (1.4 oz)	220	14	40	20	—
Symphony Milk Chocolate	1 (1.4 oz)	220	13	35	22	—
Toffee (Brock)	6 pieces (1.5 oz)	170	5	45	31	—
Tootsie Roll	1 (1 oz)	110	2	—	—	—
Tootsie Roll Dots	12 (1.5 oz)	160	0	—	—	—
Tootsie Roll Midgees	6 (1.4 oz)	160	3	—	—	—
Tootsie Roll Pop	1 (0.6 oz)	60	0	—	—	—
Truffle Amaretto di Saronno (Godiva)	2 pieces (1.5 oz)	210	12	25	24	0
Truffle Deluxe Liqueur (Godiva)	2 pieces (1.5 oz)	210	13	25	23	0
Turtles Pecan Caramel Candy (Nestle)	2 pieces (1.2 oz)	160	9	30	20	1
Twix						
Caramel	1 (1 oz)	140	7	60	19	0
Caramel	1 fun size (0.6 oz)	80	4	30	10	0
Caramel	2 (1 pkg, 2 oz)	280	14	115	37	0
Cookies-N-Creme	1 (0.8 oz)	130	8	45	13	0
Fudge N Crunchy	1 (0.7 oz)	110	6	35	12	1
Peanut Butter	1 (0.9 oz)	130	8	70	13	1
Twizzlers (Y&S Candies)	4 pieces (1.4 oz)	130	1	95	30	—
Velamints	1 mint	9	0	—	—	—
Velamints Cocoamint	1 mint	8	0	—	—	—
Whatchamacallit	1 (1.8 oz)	260	13	130	30	—
Y&S Bites Cherry	1 oz	100	1	85	23	—

FOOD	PORTION	CAL	FAT	SOD	CARB	FIB
York Peppermint Pattie	1 (1.5 oz)	180	4	20	34	—
boiled sweets	¼ lb	327	0	—	87	0
candied cherries	1 (4 g)	12	tr	—	3	—
candied citron	1 oz	89	tr	82	23	—
candied lemon peel	1 oz	90	tr	14	23	—
candied orange peel	1 oz	90	tr	14	23	—
candied pineapple slice	1 slice (2 oz)	179	tr	—	45	—
candy corn	1 oz	105	0	57	27	—
caramels chocolate	1 oz	115	3	64	22	—
caramels plain	1 oz	115	3	64	22	—
chocolate	1 oz	145	9	23	16	—
chocolate crisp	1 oz	140	7	46	18	—
chocolate w/ almonds	1 oz	150	10	23	15	—
chocolate w/ peanuts	1 oz	155	11	19	13	—
dark chocolate	1 oz	150	10	5	16	—
fruit pastilles	1 tube (1.4 oz)	101	0	—	25	—
fudge chocolate	1 oz	115	3	54	21	—
fudge vanilla	1 oz	115	3	54	21	—
gum drops	1 oz	100	tr	10	25	—
hard candy	1 oz	110	0	7	28	—
jelly beans	1 oz	105	tr	7	26	—
marzipan	3.5 oz	497	25	5	57	—
mint fondant	1 oz	105	0	57	27	—
nougat nut cream	3.5 oz	342	31	—	58	—

CANTALOUPE

Chiquita	1 cup	70	0	—	—	—
Dole	¼	50	0	35	11	0
cubed	1 cup	57	tr	14	13	1
half	½	94	1	23	22	2

CARAMBOLA

fresh	1	42	tr	2	10	—

CARAWAY

seed	1 tsp	7	tr	tr	1	—

CARDAMOM

ground	1 tsp	6	tr	tr	1	—

CARDOON

fresh, cooked	3.5 oz	22	tr	176	5	—
raw, shredded	½ cup	36	tr	151	4	—

CARIBOU

roasted	3 oz	142	4	51	0	—

FOOD	PORTION	CAL	FAT	SOD	CARB	FIB
CARISSA						
fresh	1	12	tr	1	3	—
CAROB						
carob mix	3 tsp	45	0	12	11	—
carob mix, as prep w/ whole milk	9 oz	195	8	132	23	—
flour	1 cup	185	1	36	92	—
flour	1 tbsp	14	tr	3	7	—
CARP						
FRESH						
cooked	1 fillet (6 oz)	276	12	107	0	—
cooked	3 oz	138	6	54	0	—
raw	3 oz	108	5	42	0	—
roe, raw	3.5 oz	130	2	—	2	—
CARROTS						
CANNED						
Diced (Libby)	½ cup	20	0	—	—	—
Diced (Seneca)	½ cup	20	0	—	—	—
Diced Fancy (S&W)	½ cup	30	0	240	7	—
Julienne French Style Fancy (S&W)	½ cup	30	240	7	—	
Sliced (Libby)	½ cup	20	0	—	—	—
Sliced (Seneca)	½ cup	20	0	—	—	—
Sliced Fancy (S&W)	½ cup	30	0	240	7	—
Sliced Water Pack (S&W)	½ cup	30	0	50	7	—
Whole Tiny Fancy (S&W)	½ cup	30	0	240	7	—
slices	½ cup	17	tr	176	4	1
slices, low sodium	½ cup	17	tr	31	4	1
FRESH						
Dole	1 med	40	1	40	8	1
baby raw	1 (0.5 oz)	6	tr	5	1	—
raw	1 (2.5 oz)	31	tr	25	7	2
raw, shredded	½ cup	24	tr	19	6	2
slices, cooked	½ cup	35	tr	52	8	—
FROZEN						
Baby Whole Deluxe (Birds Eye)	½ cup	40	0	45	9	2
Crinkle Cut (Big Valley)	3.5 oz	40	tr	40	9	—
Crinkle Sliced (Hanover)	½ cup	35	0	—	—	—

FOOD	PORTION	CAL	FAT	SOD	CARB	FIB
Harvest Fresh Baby (Green Giant)	½ cup	18	0	75	5	2
Polybag Sliced (Birds Eye)	¾ cup	35	0	40	8	1
Whole (Big Valley)	3.5 oz	40	tr	40	9	—
slices, cooked	½ cup	26	tr	43	6	—
JUICE						
Hain	6 fl oz	80	0	170	17	—
Hollywood	6 fl oz	80	0	170	17	2
canned	6 oz	73	tr	54	17	—

CASABA

FOOD	PORTION	CAL	FAT	SOD	CARB	FIB
cubed	1 cup	45	tr	20	11	—
fresh	⅒	43	tr	20	10	—

CASHEWS

FOOD	PORTION	CAL	FAT	SOD	CARB	FIB
Cashew Butter Raw (Hain)	2 tbsp	190	15	125	8	—
Cashew Butter Raw Unsalted (Hain)	2 tbsp	210	9	170	8	—
Cashew Butter Toasted (Hain)	2 tbsp	210	17	190	7	—
Cashews (Beer Nuts)	1 pkg (1 oz)	170	13	65	8	—
Fancy (Planters)	1 oz	170	14	110	8	—
Frito Lay	1 oz	170	14	115	9	—
Honey Roasted (Eagle)	1 oz	170	12	130	9	—
Honey Roasted (Planters)	1 oz	170	12	140	11	1
Lance	1 pkg (32 g)	190	15	95	8	—
Low Salt (Eagle)	1 oz	170	14	110	7	—
Unsalted Halves (Planters)	1 oz	170	14	0	8	—
Whole Salted (Guy's)	1 oz	170	14	140	5	—
cashew butter w/o salt	1 tbsp	94	8	2	4	—
dry roasted	1 oz	163	13	4	9	—
dry roasted, salted	1 oz	163	13	213	9	—
oil roasted	1 oz	163	14	5	8	—
oil roasted, salted	1 oz	163	14	209	8	—

CASSAVA

FOOD	PORTION	CAL	FAT	SOD	CARB	FIB
raw	3.5 oz	120	tr	8	27	—

CATFISH

FRESH

FOOD	PORTION	CAL	FAT	SOD	CARB	FIB
channel, breaded & fried	3 oz	194	11	238	7	—

FOOD	PORTION	CAL	FAT	SOD	CARB	FIB
channel, raw	3 oz	99	4	54	0	—

CATSUP
Estee	1 tbsp	6	0	20	1	—
Hain Natural	1 tbsp	16	0	155	4	—
Hain Natural No Salt Added	1 tbsp	16	0	5	4	—
Heinz	1 tbsp	16	0	200	4	—
Heinz Hot	1 tbsp	14	0	185	3	—
Heinz Lite	1 tbsp	8	0	115	2	—
Hunt's	1 tbsp	15	tr	160	4	tr
Hunt's No Salt Added	1 tbsp	20	tr	0	5	tr
McIlhenny	1 tbsp (0.6 oz)	23	tr	128	5	tr
McIlhenny Spicy Ketchup	1 tbsp (0.6 oz)	23	tr	128	5	tr
Smucker's	1 tsp	8	0	0	2	—
Weight Watchers	2 tsp	8	0	110	2	—
catsup	1 pkt (0.2 oz)	6	tr	71	2	tr
catsup	1 tbsp	16	tr	178	4	tr
low sodium	1 tbsp	16	tr	3	4	tr

CAULIFLOWER
FRESH
Dole	⅙ med head	18	0	45	3	2
cooked	½ cup (2.2 oz)	14	tr	9	3	1
flowerets, cooked	3 (2 oz)	12	tr	8	2	1
flowerets, raw	3 (2 oz)	14	tr	17	3	1
raw	½ cup (1.8 oz)	13	tr	15	3	1

FROZEN
Big Valley	3.3 oz	25	0	15	5	—
Birds Eye	⅔ cup	25	0	20	5	2
cauliflower (Hanover)	½ cup	20	0	—	—	—
Cuts (Green Giant)	½ cup	12	0	25	3	1
Florets (Hanover)	½ cup	20	0	—	—	—
In Cheese Sauce (Green Giant)	½ cup	60	2	500	10	2
One Serve In Cheese Sauce (Green Giant)	1 pkg	80	3	690	14	2
Polybag (Birds Eye)	½ cup	20	0	15	4	—
With Cheese Sauce (Birds Eye)	½ pkg	90	5	480	8	1
Cooked	½ cup	17	tr	16	3	—

JARRED
Hot & Spicy (Vlasic)	1 oz	4	0	435	1	—
Sweet (Vlasic)	1 oz	35	0	225	9	—

FOOD	PORTION	CAL	FAT	SOD	CARB	FIB
CAVIAR						
black granular	1 oz	71	5	420	1	—
black granular	1 tbsp	40	3	240	1	—
red granular	1 oz	71	5	420	1	—
red granular	1 tbsp	40	3	240	1	—
CELERIAC						
fresh, cooked	3.5 oz	25	tr	61	6	—
raw	½ cup	31	tr	78	7	—
CELERY						
DRIED						
seed	1 tsp	8	tr	3	1	—
FRESH						
Dole	2 med stalks	20	0	140	2	4
diced, cooked	½ cup	13	tr	68	3	—
raw	1 stalk (1.3 oz)	6	tr	35	1	1
raw, diced	½ cup	10	tr	52	2	1
CELTUCE						
raw	3.5 oz	22	tr	11	4	—
CEREAL						
COOKED						
4 Grain + Flax (Arrowhead)	¼ cup (1.6 oz)	150	2	0	28	6
5-Bran Kashi (Kashi)	2.5 oz	281	6	13	47	16
7 Grain (Arrowhead)	⅓ cup (1.4 oz)	140	2	0	25	5
Apple Cinnamon (Roman Meal)	1.2 oz	105	2	6	18	6
Barley Plus (Erewhon)	1 oz	110	1	0	22	1
Bear Mush (Arrowhead)	¼ cup (1.6 oz)	160	1	0	33	2
Brown Rice Cream (Erewhon)	1 oz	110	1	20	23	—
Coco Wheat (Little Crow)	3 tbsp (36 g)	130	1	12	28	4
Corn Flakes (Ralston)	1 ¼ cup (1.1 oz)	120	0	280	27	1
Cream of Rye (Roman Meal)	1.3 oz	111	1	2	20	5
Cream of Rice (Nabisco)	1 oz	100	0	0	23	—
Cream of Wheat Instant (Nabisco)	1 oz	100	tr	0	22	1

FOOD	PORTION	CAL	FAT	SOD	CARB	FIB
Cream of Wheat Quick (Nabisco)	1 oz	100	tr	80	22	tr
Cream of Wheat Regular (Nabisco)	1 oz	100	0	0	22	1
Enriched White Hominy Grits Quick (Quaker)	3 tbsp	101	tr	1	22	1
Enriched White Hominy Grits Regular (Aunt Jemima)	3 tbsp	101	tr	1	22	1
Enriched Yellow Hominy Quick Grits (Quaker)	3 tbsp	101	tr	1	22	1
Farina (Pillsbury)	⅔ cup	80	tr	170	17	—
Farina Instant (H-O)	1 pkg	110	0	235	22	3
Farina, not prep (H-O)	3 tbsp	120	0	0	26	3
Hominy Quick Grits, uncooked (Albers)	¼ cup	140	1	0	31	1
Instant Grits White Hominy (Quaker)	1 pkg	79	tr	440	18	1
Instant Grits With Imitation Bacon Bits (Quaker)	1 pkg	101	tr	590	22	2
Instant Grits With Imitation Ham Bits (Quaker)	1 pkg	99	tr	800	21	2
Instant Grits with Real Cheddar Cheese (Quaker)	1 pkg	104	1	497	22	1
Irish Oatmeal (McCann's)	1 oz	110	2	0	20	3
Kashi	2 oz	177	1	5	38	5
Maltex	1 oz	105	1	0	21	3
Maypo (30 Second)	1 oz	100	1	0	19	2
Maypo (Vermont Style)	1 oz	105	1	0	20	2
Maypo (With Oat Bran)	1 oz	130	2	1	26	4
Mix'n Eat Cream of Wheat Brown Sugar Cinnamon (Nabisco)	1 pkg (1.25 oz)	130	0	230	29	1
Mix'n Eat Cream of Wheat Apple And Cinnamon (Nabisco)	1 pkg (1.25 oz)	130	0	250	29	1
Mix'n Eat Cream of Wheat Maple Brown Sugar (Nabisco)	1 pkg (1.25 oz)	130	0	180	29	1

FOOD	PORTION	CAL	FAT	SOD	CARB	FIB
Mix'n Eat Cream of Wheat Our Original (Nabisco)	1 pkg (1.25 oz)	100	0	170	21	1
Oat Bran (Quaker)	½ cup	92	2	1	17	4
Oat Bran Natural Apples & Cinnamon (Health Valley)	¼ cup (1 oz)	100	tr	10	19	4
Oat Bran Natural Raisins & Spice (Health Valley)	¼ cup	100	tr	10	19	4
Oat Bran With Toasted Wheat Germ (Erewhon)	1 oz	115	2	15	18	3
Oat Flakes Rolled (Arrowhead)	⅓ cup (1.2 oz)	130	3	0	23	4
Oat Groats (Arrowhead)	¼ cup (1.5 oz)	160	3	0	29	4
Oatmeal Cinnamon Graham Cookie (Quaker)	1 pkg (1.4 oz)	140	2	170	29	3
Oatmeal Radical Raspberry (Quaker)	1 pkg (1.4 oz)	150	3	170	28	3
Oatmeal Strawberries 'N Stuff (Quaker)	1 pkg (1.4 oz)	140	2	170	30	3
Oatmeal Instant						
H-O	1 pkg	110	2	230	18	3
H-O	½ cup	130	2	<5	22	3
Apple Cinnamon (Erewhon)	1.25 oz	145	3	100	25	—
Apple Cinnamon (H-O)	1 pkg	130	2	220	26	3
Apple Raisin (Erewhon)	1.3 oz	150	3	100	27	—
Apples & Cinnamon (Quaker)	1 pkg	118	2	128	26	3
Cinnamon & Spice (Quaker)	1 pkg	164	2	322	35	3
Dates & Walnuts (Erewhon)	1.2 oz	130	3	60	24	3
Extra Fortified Apples & Spice (Quaker)	1 pkg	133	2	191	27	3
Extra Fortified Raisins & Cinnamon (Quaker)	1 pkg	129	2	119	27	3

FOOD	PORTION	CAL	FAT	SOD	CARB	FIB
Oatmeal Instant *(cont.)*						
Extra Fortified Regular (Quaker)	1 pkg	95	2	219	18	3
Maple & Brown Sugar (Quaker)	1 pkg	152	2	320	32	3
Maple Brown Sugar (H-O)	1 pkg	160	2	285	32	3
Maple Spice (Erewhon)	1.2 oz	140	3	100	24	—
Original (Arrowhead)	1 oz	100	0	15	22	—
Peaches & Cream Flavors (Quaker)	1 pkg	129	2	179	26	2
Raisin & Spice (H-O)	1 pkg	150	2	140	32	3
Raisin & Spice (Quaker)	1 pkg	149	2	266	32	3
Raisin, Dates & Walnuts (Quaker)	1 pkg	141	4	216	25	2
Regular (Quaker)	1 pkg	94	2	270	18	3
Strawberries & Cream Flavors (Quaker)	1 pkg	129	2	204	27	2
Sweet 'n Mellow (H-O)	1 pkg	150	2	270	30	3
With Added Oat Bran (Erewhon)	1.25 oz	125	3	0	23	4
Oats 'n Fiber (H-O)	1 pkg	110	2	140	18	3
Oats 'n Fiber (H-O)	½ cup	100	2	5	15	3
Oats 'n Fiber Apple & Bran (H-O)	1 pkg	130	2	140	26	3
Oats 'n Fiber Raisin & Bran (H-O)	1 pkg	150	2	140	32	3
Oats Gourmet (H-O)	⅓ cup	100	2	0	18	3
Oats Old Fashion (Quaker)	⅔ cup	99	2	1	19	3
Oats Quick (H-O)	½ cup	130	2	<5	22	3
Oats Quick (Quaker)	⅔ cup	99	2	1	19	3
Oats, Wheat, Dates, Raisins, Almonds (Roman Meal)	1.3 oz	129	2	3	24	3
Oats, Wheat, Honey, Coconuts, Almonds (Roman Meal)	1.3 oz	155	5	8	22	3
Original (Roman Meal)	1 oz	83	1	tr	15	5
Original With Oats (Roman Meal)	1.2 oz	108	1	1	19	5

FOOD	PORTION	CAL	FAT	SOD	CARB	FIB
Rice & Shine (Arrowhead)	¼ cup (1.5 oz)	150	1	0	32	2
Spelt (Good Shepherd)	1 oz	90	tr	0	20	3
Wheat Flakes Rolled (Arrowhead)	⅓ cup (1.2 oz)	110	1	0	24	5
Wheatena	⅓ cup (1.4 oz)	150	1	0	32	5
Whole Wheat Hot Natural Cereal (Quaker)	⅔ cup	92	1	1	21	2
corn grits, instant	1 pkg (0.8 oz)	82	tr	344	18	—
corn grits, quick	1 cup	146	1	0	31	—
corn grits, quick, not prep	1 cup	579	2	1	124	—
corn grits, quick, not prep	1 tbsp	36	tr	0	8	—
corn grits, regular	1 cup	146	1	0	31	—
corn grits, regular, not prep	1 cup	579	2	1	124	—
farina	¾ cup	87	tr	1	19	3
farina, not prep	1 tbsp	40	0	0	9	tr
oatmeal	1 cup	145	2	1	25	—
oatmeal, instant, cooked w/o salt	1 cup	145	2	2	25	—
oatmeal, not prep	1 cup	311	5	3	54	9
oatmeal, quick, cooked w/o salt	1 cup	145	2	2	25	—
oatmeal, regular, cooked w/o salt	1 cup	145	2	2	25	—
READY-TO-EAT						
100% Bran (Nabisco)	½ cup (1 oz)	70	2	130	21	10
100% Natural Bran With Apples & Cinnamon (Health Valley)	¼ cup (1 oz)	100	1	10	22	5
All-Bran (Kellogg's)	⅓ cup (1 oz)	70	1	260	21	9
All-Bran With Extra Fiber (Kellogg's)	½ cup (1 oz)	50	1	140	22	14
Almond Delight (Ralston)	1 cup (1.8 oz)	210	3	410	41	4
Alpha-Bits (Post)	1 cup (1 oz)	111	1	176	24	1
Alpha-Bits Marshmallow Sweetened Letter Shaped Oats (Post)	1 cup	110	1	152	25	1

FOOD	PORTION	CAL	FAT	SOD	CARB	FIB
Amaranth Flakes (Arrowhead)	1 cup (1.2 oz)	130	2	0	25	3
Apple Cinnamon Natural (Grist Mill)	½ cup (1.9 oz)	260	10	20	36	3
Apple Cinnamon Square (Kellogg's)	½ cup (1 oz)	90	1	5	23	2
Apple Corns (Arrowhead)	1 cup (1.5 oz)	150	2	110	35	4
Apple Jacks (Kellogg's)	1 cup (1 oz)	110	0	125	26	1
Apple Raisin Crisp (Kellogg's)	⅔ cup (1.3 oz)	130	0	230	32	3
Aztec (Erewhon)	1 oz	100	0	85	24	1
Basic 4 (General Mills)	¾ cup	130	2	290	28	2
Blue Corn Flakes 100% Organic (Health Valley)	½ cup (1 oz)	90	tr	10	19	3
Blueberry Squares (Kellogg's)	½ cup (1 oz)	90	tr	5	23	3
Body Buddies Natural Fruit (General Mills)	1 cup (1 oz)	110	1	280	24	—
Booberry (General Mills)	1 cup (1 oz)	110	1	210	24	—
Bran (Grist Mill)	½ cup (1.9 oz)	250	8	40	37	11
Bran Buds (Kellogg's)	⅓ cup (1 oz)	70	1	200	23	11
Bran Cereal With Dates 100% Organic (Health Valley)	¼ cup (1 oz)	100	1	5	20	5
Bran Cereal With Raisins 100% Organic (Health Valley)	¼ cup (1 oz)	100	1	5	20	5
Bran Flakes (Arrowhead)	1 cup (1 oz)	100	1	80	22	4
Bran Flakes (Kellogg's)	⅔ cup (1 oz)	90	tr	220	23	5
Bran Flakes (Ralston)	¾ cup (1.1 oz)	110	1	220	24	5
Cap'n Crunch (Quaker)	¾ cup	113	2	241	24	1
Cap'n Crunch's Crunchberries (Quaker)	¾ cup	113	2	247	24	1
Cap'n Crunch's Peanut Butter Crunch (Quaker)	¾ cup	119	3	281	22	1
Cheerios (General Mills)	1¼ cup (1 oz)	110	2	290	20	2
Cheerios Apple Cinnamon (General Mills)	¾ cup (1 oz)	110	2	180	22	2
Cheerios Honey Nut (General Mills)	¾ cup (1 oz)	110	1	250	23	2
Cheerios-to-Go (General Mills)	1 pkg (0.75 oz)	80	2	220	15	2

FOOD	PORTION	CAL	FAT	SOD	CARB	FIB
Cheerios-to-Go Apple Cinnamon (General Mills)	1 pkg (1 oz)	110	2	180	22	2
Cheerios-to-Go Honey Nut (General Mills)	1 pkg (1 oz)	110	1	250	23	2
Chex Corn (Ralston)	1¼ cup (1 oz)	110	0	270	26	1
Chex Double (Ralston)	1¼ cup (1 oz)	120	0	230	27	0
Chex Graham (Ralston)	1 cup (1.8 oz)	210	2	340	45	1
Chex Multi-Bran (Ralston)	1¼ cup (2 oz)	220	2	320	46	7
Chex Rice (Ralston)	1 cup (1.1 oz)	120	0	230	27	0
Chex Wheat (Ralston)	¾ cup (1.8 oz)	190	1	390	41	5
Cinnamon Mini Buns (Kellogg's)	¾ cup (1 oz)	110	1	200	25	1
Cinnamon Toast Crunch (General Mills)	¾ cup (1 oz)	120	3	210	22	1
Clusters (General Mills)	½ cup (1 oz)	110	2	140	22	2
Cocoa Crispy Rice (Ralston)	1 cup (1.8 oz)	200	1	340	45	tr
Cocoa Crunchies (Ralston)	¾ cup (1.1 oz)	120	1	170	26	0
Cocoa Krispies (Kellogg's)	¾ cup (1 oz)	110	0	190	25	0
Cocoa Pebbles (Post)	⅞ cup (1 oz)	113	1	160	25	tr
Cocoa Puffs (General Mills)	1 cup (1 oz)	110	1	180	25	—
Coconut (Heartland)	1 oz	130	5	80	18	2
Common Sense Oat Bran (Kellogg's)	¾ cup (1 oz)	100	1	250	22	3
Common Sense Oat Bran With Raisins (Kellogg's)	¾ cup (1.3 oz)	130	1	250	29	3
Cookie Crisp (Ralston)	1 cup (1 oz)	120	2	110	25	0
Corn Flakes (Kellogg's)	1 cup (1 oz)	100	0	290	24	1
Corn Pops (Kellogg's)	1 cup (1 oz)	110	0	90	26	1
Count Chocula (General Mills)	1 cup (1 oz)	110	1	210	24	—
Country Corn Flakes (General Mills)	1 cup (1 oz)	110	1	260	24	—
Cracklin' Oat Bran (Kellogg's)	½ cup (1 oz)	110	3	140	21	4
Crisp Crunch (Ralston)	¾ cup (1.1 oz)	120	1	240	26	tr
Crisp Rice (Ralston)	1¼ cup (1.2 oz)	130	0	330	28	0
Crispix (Kellogg's)	1 cup (1 oz)	110	0	220	25	1

FOOD	PORTION	CAL	FAT	SOD	CARB	FIB
Crispy Brown Rice (Erewhon)	1 oz	110	1	185	24	4
Crispy Critters (Post)	1 cup (1 oz)	110	0	232	24	1
Crispy Wheats 'N Raisins (General Mills)	¾ cup (1 oz)	100	1	140	23	2
Crunchy Bran (Quaker)	⅔ cup	89	1	316	23	5
Crunchy Not Oh!s (Quaker)	1 cup	127	4	164	22	1
Double Dip Crunch (Kellogg's)	⅔ cup (1 oz)	110	0	150	26	0
Fiber 7 Flakes 100% Organic (Health Valley)	½ cup (1 oz)	90	tr	0	20	5
Fiber 7 Flakes With Raisins 100% Organic (Health Valley)	½ cup (1 oz)	90	tr	0	20	5
Fiber One (General Mills)	½ cup (1 oz)	60	1	140	23	13
Frankenberry (General Mills)	1 cup (1 oz)	110	1	210	24	—
Froot Loops (Kellogg's)	1 cup (1 oz)	110	1	125	25	1
Frosted Mini-Wheats (Kellogg's)	4 biscuits (1 oz)	100	0	0	24	3
Frosted Mini-Wheats Bite Size (Kellogg's)	½ cup (1 oz)	100	0	0	24	3
Frosted Bran (Kellogg's)	⅔ cup (1 oz)	100	0	190	25	3
Frosted Flakes (Kellogg's)	¾ cup (1 oz)	110	0	190	26	0
Frosted Flakes (Ralston)	¾ cup (1.1 oz)	120	0	180	28	1
Frosted Krispies (Kellogg's)	¾ cup (1 oz)	110	0	220	26	0
Fruit & Fibre Dates, Raisins, Walnuts With Oat Clusters (Post)	⅔ cup	120	2	167	27	5
Fruit & Fibre Tropical Fruit With Oat Clusters (Post)	⅔ cup	125	3	167	27	5
Fruit & Fitness (Health Valley)	1 cup (2 oz)	220	4	5	37	11
Fruit 'n Wheat (Erewhon)	1 oz	100	1	75	21	3
Fruit Lites Corn (Healthy Valley)	½ cup (0.5 oz)	45	0	2	10	tr
Fruit Lites Rice (Health Valley)	½ cup (0.5 oz)	45	1	2	11	tr

FOOD	PORTION	CAL	FAT	SOD	CARB	FIB
Fruit Lites Wheat (Health Valley)	½ cup (0.5 oz)	45	1	2	11	2
Fruit Rings (Ralston)	¾ cup (0.9 oz)	100	1	115	23	0
Fruit Wheats Apple (Nabisco)	1 oz	90	0	15	23	3
Fruitful Bran (Kellogg's)	2/3 cup (1.4 oz)	120	0	240	31	5
Fruity Marshmallow Krispies (Kellogg's)	1¼ cup (1.3 oz)	140	0	210	32	0
Fruity Pebbles (Post)	⅞ cup	113	1	156	25	1
Fruity Yummy Mummy (General Mills)	1 cup (1 oz)	110	1	160	24	—
Golden Grahams (General Mills)	¾ cup (1 oz)	110	1	280	24	—
Grape-Nuts (Post)	¼ cup (1 oz)	105	0	170	23	3
Grape-Nuts Raisin (Post)	¼ cup (1 oz)	102	0	141	23	2
Healthy Crunch Almond Date (Health Valley)	¼ cup (1 oz)	110	3	5	18	4
Healthy Crunch Apple Cinnamon (Health Valley)	¼ cup (1 oz)	110	3	10	18	4
Healthy O's 100% Organic (Health Valley)	¾ cup (1 oz)	90	1	1	18	3
Honey Bunches Of Oats Honey Roasted (Post)	⅔ cup (1 oz)	111	2	176	23	2
Honey Bunches of Oats With Almonds (Post)	⅔ cup (1 oz)	115	3	157	22	2
Honey Graham Ohs! (Quaker)	1 cup	122	3	217	23	1
Honeycomb (Post)	1⅓ cups (1 oz)	110	0	172	26	1
Just Right With Crunchy Nuggets (Kellogg's)	⅔ cup (1 oz)	110	1	170	24	1
Just Right With Raisins, Dates & Nuts (Kellogg's)	¾ cup (1.3 oz)	140	1	170	31	2
Kaboom (General Mills)	1 cup (1 oz)	110	1	270	23	—
Kamut Flakes (Arrowhead)	1 cup (1.1 oz)	120	1	65	25	3
Kashi Brittles Sesame/ Maple (Kashi)	3.5 oz	473	19	85	65	—

FOOD	PORTION	CAL	FAT	SOD	CARB	FIB
Kashi Puffed (Kashi)	0.75 oz	74	1	2	16	2
Kenmei (Kellogg's)	¾ cup (1 oz)	110	1	230	24	1
King Vitaman (Quaker)	1½ cup	110	1	280	23	1
Kix (General Mills)	1½ cup (1 oz)	110	1	260	24	—
Life (Quaker)	⅔ cup	101	2	186	19	3
Life Cinnamon (Quaker)	⅔ cup	101	2	182	19	3
Lites Puffed Corn (Health Valley)	½ cup (1 oz)	50	0	0	11	tr
Lites Puffed Rice (Health Valley)	½ cup (1 oz)	50	0	0	12	tr
Lites Puffed Wheat (Health Valley)	½ cup (1 oz)	50	0	0	11	1
Lucky Charms (General Mills)	1 cup (1 oz)	110	1	240	24	—
Magic Stair (Ralston)	¾ cup (1.1 oz)	120	1	160	26	tr
Maple Corns (Arrowhead)	1 cup (1.9 oz)	190	3	140	43	6
Millet Rice Flakes Wheat Free (Good Shepherd)	1 oz	95	1	30	19	1
Muesli (Little Debbie)	1.9 oz	210	2	70	44	3
Muesli (Ralston)						
Blueberry	1 cup (1.9 oz)	200	3	170	41	4
Cranberry	¾ cup (1.9 oz)	200	3	180	40	4
Peach	¾ cup (1.9 oz)	200	3	170	39	4
Raspberry	¾ cup (2 oz)	220	3	170	44	4
Strawberry	1 cup (1.9 oz)	210	3	170	41	4
Mueslix Crispy Blend (Kellogg's)	⅔ cup (1.5 oz)	150	2	150	33	3
Mueslix Golden Crunch (Kellogg's)	½ cup (1.2 oz)	120	2	170	25	3
Multi Grain Flakes (Arrowhead)	1 cup (1.2 oz)	140	2	130	29	3
Multi Vitamin Whole Grain Flakes (Ralston)	1 cup (1.1 oz)	120	1	300	25	3
Natural Bran Flakes (Post)	⅔ cup (1 oz)	88	0	205	23	6
Nature O's (Arrowhead)	1 cup (1.1 oz)	130	2	5	24	3
Nut & Honey Crunch (Kellogg's)	⅔ cup (1 oz)	120	1	190	24	0
Nut & Honey Crunch O's (Kellogg's)	⅔ cup (1 oz)	110	2	190	22	2

FOOD	PORTION	CAL	FAT	SOD	CARB	FIB
Nutri-Grain (Kellogg's)						
Almond Raisin	⅔ cup (1.4 oz)	140	2	220	31	3
Nuggets	¼ cup (1 oz)	90	0	180	23	3
Raisin Bran	1 cup (1.4 oz)	130	1	200	31	5
Wheat	⅔ cup (1 oz)	90	0	170	23	3
Nutty Nuggets (Ralston)	½ cup (1.7 oz)	180	2	220	38	5
Oat & Honey Natural (Grist Mill)	½ cup (1.9 oz)	270	12	10	34	4
Oat Bran Flakes (Arrowhead)	1 cup (1.2 oz)	110	2	60	22	4
Oat Bran Flakes 100% Organic (Health Valley)	½ cup (1 oz)	100	tr	0	20	4
Oat Bran Flakes Almonds/Dates 100% Organic (Health Valley)	½ cup (1 oz)	100	tr	0	20	4
Oat Bran Flakes With Raisins 100% Organic (Health Valley)	½ cup (1 oz)	100	tr	0	20	4
Oat Bran O's 100% Organic (Health Valley)	½ cup (1 oz)	110	tr	0	20	3
Oat Bran O's Fruit & Nuts (Health Valley)	½ cup (1 oz)	110	3	0	19	3
Oat Flakes (Post)	⅔ cup (1 oz)	107	1	127	22	2
Oat, Honey & Raisin Natural (Grist Mill)	¼ cup (1.9 oz)	260	10	10	35	4
Oat Squares (Quaker)	½ cup	105	2	159	21	2
Oatbake Honey Bran (Kellogg's)	⅓ cup (1 oz)	110	3	190	21	3
Oatbake Raisin Nut (Kellogg's)	⅓ cup (1 oz)	110	3	190	21	3
Oatmeal Crisp (General Mills)	½ cup (1 oz)	110	2	180	22	1
Oatmeal Raisin Crisp (General Mills)	½ cup (1.2 oz)	130	2	170	25	2
Orangeola Almonds & Dates (Health Valley)	¼ cup	110	3	5	18	4
Orangeola Bananas & Hawaiian Fruit (Health Valley)	¼ cup (1 oz)	120	4	10	20	4
Plain (Heartland)	1 oz	130	4	80	18	2
Popeye Sweet Crunch (Quaker)	1 cup	113	2	254	24	1
Poppets (US Mills)	1 oz	110	1	10	24	1

FOOD	PORTION	CAL	FAT	SOD	CARB	FIB
Post Toasties (Corn Flakes)	1¼ cup (1 oz)	111	0	310	24	1
Product 19 (Kellogg's)	1 cup (1 oz)	100	0	320	24	1
Puffed Corn (Arrowhead)	1 cup (0.8 oz)	80	0	0	16	1
Puffed Kamut (Arrowhead)	1 cup (0.6 oz)	50	0	0	11	2
Puffed Millet (Arrowhead)	1 cup (0.9 oz)	90	1	0	19	1
Puffed Rice (Arrowhead)	1 cup (0.8 oz)	90	0	0	19	1
Puffed Rice (Quaker)	1 cup	54	tr	1	13	tr
Puffed Wheat (Arrowhead)	1 cup (0.9)	90	1	0	20	2
Puffed Wheat (Quaker)	1 cup	50	tr	1	11	1
Quaker 100% (Natural)	¼ cup	127	6	14	18	2
Quaker 100% Natural Apples & Cinnamon	¼ cup	126	5	13	19	2
Quaker 100% Natural Raisins & Date	¼ cup	123	5	14	18	2
Raisin (Heartland)	1 oz	130	4	80	18	2
Raisin Bran (Erewhon)	1 oz	100	0	80	22	3
Raisin Bran (Kellogg's)	¾ cup (1.4 oz)	120	1	220	32	5
Raisin Bran (Post)	⅔ cup (40 g)	122	1	198	32	6
Raisin Bran (Ralston)	¾ cup (1.9 oz)	190	1	290	41	6
Raisin Bran Flakes 100% Organic (Health Valley)	½ cup (1 oz)	100	tr	5	21	6
Raisin Nut Bran (General Mills)	½ cup (1 oz)	110	3	140	20	3
Raisin Squares (Kellogg's)	½ cup (1 oz)	90	tr	0	23	2
Real Oat Bran Almond Crunch (Health Valley)	¼ cup (1 oz)	110	3	2	17	4
Real Oat Bran Hawaiian Fruit (Health Valley)	¼ cup (1 oz)	130	3	2	22	5
Real Oat Bran Raisin Nut (Health Valley)	¼ cup (1 oz)	130	3	2	21	5
Rice Bran O's (Health Valley)	½ cup	110	1	5	22	2
Rice Bran With Almonds & Dates (Health Valley)	½ cup (1 oz)	110	3	2	19	2
Rice Krispies (Kellogg's)	1 cup (1 oz)	110	0	290	25	0

FOOD	PORTION	CAL	FAT	SOD	CARB	FIB
Rice Krispies Treats (Kellogg's)	¾ cup (1 oz)	110	1	160	24	0
Ruskets Biscuits (LaLoma)	2 biscuits (30 g)	110	0	95	22	—
S'Mores Grahams (General Mills)	¾ cup (1 oz)	120	2	250	24	—
Shredded Wheat (Quaker)	2 biscuits	132	1	1	32	4
Shredded Wheat (Sunshine)	1 buscuit	90	1	0	19	—
Shredded Wheat 'n Bran (Nabisco)	⅔ cup (1 oz)	90	1	0	23	4
Shredded Wheat Bite Size (Sunshine)	⅔ cup	110	1	0	22	—
Shredded Wheat Spoon Size (Nabisco)	⅔ cup (1 oz)	90	1	0	23	3
Shredded Wheat With Oat Bran (Nabisco)	⅔ cup (1 oz)	100	1	0	22	4
Smacks (Kellogg's)	¾ cup (1 oz)	110	1	70	25	1
Special K (Kellogg's)	1 cup (1 oz)	100	0	230	20	1
Spelt Flakes (Arrowhead)	1 cup (1.1 oz)	100	1	60	22	3
Spelt Flakes (Good Shepherd)	1 oz	100	6	80	21	2
Sprouts 7 Bananas & Hawaiian Fruit (Health Valley)	¼ cup (1 oz)	90	1	5	16	4
Sprouts 7 Raisin (Health Valley)	¼ cup	90	1	5	16	5
Strawberry Squares (Kellogg's)	½ cup (1 oz)	90	tr	5	23	3
Super Golden Crisp (Post)	⅞ cup (1 oz)	104	0	44	26	tr
Super-O's (Erewhon)	1 oz	110	0	5	24	4
Swiss Breakfast Raisin Nut (Health Valley)	¼ cup (1 oz)	100	3	10	19	3
Swiss Breakfast Tropical Fruit (Health Valley)	¼ cup (1 oz)	100	3	10	19	3
Tasteeos (Ralston)	1¼ cup (1.1 oz)	130	3	260	22	3
Tasteeos Apple Cinnamon (Ralston)	1 cup (1.2 oz)	130	2	150	27	1
Tasteeos Honey Nut (Ralston)	1 cup (1.2 oz)	130	2	250	28	1

FOOD	PORTION	CAL	FAT	SOD	CARB	FIB
Team (Nabisco)	1 cup	110	1	180	24	—
Total (General Mills)	1 cup (1 oz)	100	1	200	22	3
Total Corn Flakes (General Mills)	1 cup (1 oz)	110	tr	200	24	—
Total Raisin Bran (General Mills)	1 cup (1.5 oz)	140	1	190	33	4
Triples (General Mills)	¾ cup (1 oz)	110	1	250	24	—
Trix (General Mills)	1 cup (1 oz)	110	1	140	25	—
Uncle Sam Cereal (US Mills)	1 oz	110	1	65	20	7
Weetabix	2 (1.3 oz)	142	1	—	31	3
Wheat Flakes (Erewhon)	1 oz	100	0	75	22	4
Wheaties (General Mills)	1 cup (1 oz)	100	1	200	23	3
all bran	½ cup (1 oz)	76	1	196	21	—
bran flakes	¾ cup (1 oz)	90	1	264	22	—
corn flakes	1¼ cup (1 oz)	110	tr	351	24	—
corn flakes, low sodium	1 cup	100	tr	3	22	—
crispy rice	1 cup	111	tr	205	25	—
fortified oat flakes	1 cup	177	1	429	35	—
puffed rice	1 cup	57	tr	0	13	—
puffed wheat	1 cup	44	tr	0	10	—
shredded wheat	1 biscuit	83	tr	0	19	—
sugar-coated corn flakes	¾ cup (1 oz)	110	1	230	26	—

CHAMPAGNE

FOOD	PORTION	CAL	FAT	SOD	CARB	FIB
Andre Blush	1 fl oz	22	0	1	1	—
Andre Brut	1 fl oz	21	0	1	1	—
Andre Cold Duck	1 fl oz	25	0	1	2	—
Andre Extra Dry	1 fl oz	23	0	1	1	—
Ballatore Gran Spumante Ballatore	1 fl oz	23	0	2	2	—
Eden Roc Brut	1 fl oz	21	0	1	1	—
Eden Roc Brut Rosé	1 fl oz	22	0	1	2	—
Eden Roc Extra Dry	1 fl oz	21	0	1	1	—
Tott's Blanc de Noir	1 fl oz	22	0	1	2	—
Tott's Brut	1 fl oz	20	0	1	tr	—
Tott's Extra Dry	1 fl oz	21	0	1	1	—

CHAYOTE

FOOD	PORTION	CAL	FAT	SOD	CARB	FIB
fresh, cooked	1 cup	38	1	1	8	—
raw	1 (7 oz)	49	1	8	11	—
raw, cut up	1 cup	32	tr	198	7	—

FOOD	PORTION	CAL	FAT	SOD	CARB	FIB

CHEESE

see also cheese dishes, cheese substitutes, cottage cheese, cream cheese

NATURAL

FOOD	PORTION	CAL	FAT	SOD	CARB	FIB
Asiago (Frigo)	1 oz	110	9	400	1	—
Baby Swiss (Cracker Barrel)	1 oz	110	9	65	0	—
Babybel (Laughing Cow)	1 oz	90	7	230	0	0
Babybel Mini (Laughing Cow)	1 (0.7 oz)	70	6	170	0	0
Babybel Mini Light (Laughing Cow)	1 (0.7 oz)	45	3	180	0	0
Blue (Frigo)	1 oz	100	8	400	1	—
Blue (Kraft)	1 oz	100	9	330	1	—
Blue (Sargento)	1 oz	100	8	396	1	—
Bonbel (Laughing Cow)	1 oz	100	8	230	0	0
Bonbel Mini (Laughing Cow)	1 (0.7 oz)	70	6	170	0	0
Breakfast (Marin French Cheese)	1 oz	86	7	—	1	—
Brick (Kraft)	1 oz	110	9	180	0	—
Brick (Land O'Lakes)	1 oz	110	8	160	1	—
Brie (Marin French Cheese)	1 oz	86	7	—	1	—
Brie (Sargento)	1 oz	95	8	178	tr	—
Bruger Cheese (Sargento)	1 oz	106	8	406	tr	—
Cajun (Sargento)	1 oz	110	9	164	tr	—
Camembert (Marin French Cheese)	1 oz	86	7	—	1	—
Camembert (Sargento)	1 oz	85	7	239	tr	—
Cheda-Jack Reduced Fat Low Sodium (Dorman)	1 oz	80	5	140	1	—
Chedarella (Land O'Lakes)	1 oz	100	8	180	tr	—
Cheddar						
(Armour)	1 oz	110	9	—	—	—
(Cabot)	1 oz	110	9	175	0	—
(Dorman)	1 oz	110	9	200	1	—
(Frigo)	1 oz	110	9	200	1	—
(Kraft)	1 oz	110	9	180	1	—
(Land O'Lakes)	1 oz	110	9	180	tr	—
(Sargento)	1 oz	114	9	176	tr	—
Curds Snack (Heluva Good Cheese)	1 oz	113	9	179	1	0

FOOD	PORTION	CAL	FAT	SOD	CARB	FIB
Cheddar *(cont.)*						
Extra-Sharp (Heluva Good Cheese)	1 oz	110	9	180	1	0
Extra-Sharp Premium (Father Time)	1 oz	110	9	180	1	0
Mild (Heluva Good Cheese)	1 oz	110	9	180	1	0
Mild Reduced Fat (Heluva Good Cheese)	1 oz	80	6	200	1	0
Reduced Fat (Alpine Lace)	1 piece (1 oz)	80	5	95	1	0
Sharp (Heluva Good Cheese)	1 oz	110	9	180	1	0
Shredded (Heluva Good Cheese)	¼ cup (1 oz)	110	9	180	1	0
Very Low Sodium (Heluva Good Cheese)	1 oz	110	9	140	0	0
Cheddar Light (Bristol Gold)	1 oz	70	4	150	3	—
Cheddar Light With Simplesse (White Clover)	1 oz	80	4	160	tr	—
Cheddar Lite (Frigo)	1 oz	80	5	190	1	—
Cheddar Lower Salt (Armour)	1 oz	110	9	106	—	—
Cheddar Mild						
MooTown Snackers Light (Sargento)	1 stick	70	5	140	tr	—
Preferred Light (Sargento)	1 oz	90	5	180	3	—
Reduced Fat Light (Kraft)	1 oz	80	5	220	0	—
Shredded (Weight Watchers)	1 oz	80	5	150	1	—
Shredded Preferred Light (Sargento)	1 oz	90	5	180	3	—
White (Weight Watchers)	1 oz	80	5	150	1	—
Yellow (Weight Watchers)	1 oz	80	5	150	1	—
Cheddar Mild Low Sodium White (Weight Watchers)	1 oz	80	5	70	1	—

FOOD	PORTION	CAL	FAT	SOD	CARB	FIB
Cheddar Mild Low Sodium Yellow (Weight Watchers)	1 oz	80	5	70	1	—
Cheddar New York (Sargento)	1 oz	114	9	176	tr	—
Cheddar Reduced Fat Low Sodium (Dorman)	1 oz	80	5	140	1	—
Cheddar Sharp						
Light Reduced Fat White (Cracker Barrel)	1 oz	80	5	220	1	—
Nut Log (Sargento)	1 oz	97	7	252	3	—
Reduced Fat Light (Kraft)	1 oz	80	5	220	1	—
White (Weight Watchers)	1 oz	80	5	150	1	—
Yellow (Weight Watchers)	1 oz	80	5	150	1	—
Cheddar Shredded (Polly-O)	1 oz	110	9	—	—	—
Cheddar White						
Extra-Sharp (Heluva Good Cheese)	1 oz	110	9	180	1	0
Mild (Heluva Good Cheese)	1 oz	110	9	180	1	0
Sharp (Heluva Good Cheese)	1 oz	110	9	180	1	0
Shredded (Heluva Good Cheese)	¼ cup (1 oz)	110	9	180	1	0
Very Low Sodium (Heluva Good Cheese)	1 oz	110	9	140	0	0
Chevre (Brier Run)	1 oz	61	5	70	—	—
Colby						
(Dorman)	1 oz	110	9	190	1	—
(Heluva Good Cheese)	1 oz	117	9	186	0	0
(Kraft)	1 oz	110	9	180	1	—
(Land O'Lakes)	1 oz	110	9	170	1	—
(Sargento)	1 oz	112	9	171	1	—
Colby (Weight Watchers)	1 oz	80	5	150	1	—
Colby Reduced Fat (Alpine Lace)	1 piece (1 oz)	80	5	115	1	0
Reduced Fat Light (Kraft)	1 oz	80	5	220	0	—

FOOD	PORTION	CAL	FAT	SOD	CARB	FIB
Colby And Monterey Jack Shredded Reduced Fat Light (Kraft)	1 oz	80	5	220	1	—
Colby Light With Simplesse (White Clover)	1 oz	80	4	180	tr	—
Colby Lower Salt (Armour)	1 oz	110	9	—	—	—
Colby-Jack (Heluva Good Cheese)	1 oz	110	9	200	0	0
Colby-Jack (Sargento)	1 oz	109	9	162	tr	—
Edam						
(Dorman)	1 oz	100	8	200	1	—
(Holland Farm)	1 oz	97	8	—	—	—
(Kraft)	1 oz	90	7	310	0	—
(Land O'Lakes)	1 oz	110	8	270	tr	—
(MayBud)	1 oz	100	8	210	1	0
(Sargento)	1 oz	101	8	274	tr	—
Farmer (Friendship)	2 tbsp (1 oz)	50	3	120	0	0
Farmer (Holland Farm)	1 oz	102	8	—	—	—
Farmer No Salt Added (Friendship)	2 tbsp (1 oz)	50	3	10	0	0
Farmer's MooTown Snackers Light (Sargento)	1 stick	70	4	140	tr	—
Farmer's Preferred Light (Sargento)	1 oz	80	5	180	1	—
Farmer's Shredded Preferred Light (Sargento)	1 oz	80	5	180	1	—
Feta						
(Churney)	1 oz	80	6	320	tr	0
(Frigo)	1 oz	100	8	400	1	—
(Sargento)	1 oz	75	6	316	1	—
Finland Swiss (Sargento)	1 oz	107	8	74	1	—
Fior di Latte (Polly-O)	1 oz	80	6	—	—	—
Fontina (Sargento)	1 oz	110	9	—	tr	—
French Onion Light (Bristol Gold)	1 oz	70	4	150	3	—
Fruit Moos						
Apricot (Dannon)	3.5 oz	150	8	40	16	—
Banana	3.5 oz	150	8	40	16	—
Raspberry	3.5 oz	150	8	40	16	—
Strawberry	3.5 oz	150	8	40	16	—

FOOD	PORTION	CAL	FAT	SOD	CARB	FIB
Garlic & Herb Light (Bristol Gold)	1 oz	70	4	150	3	—
Gjetost (Sargento)	1 oz	132	8	170	12	—
Gouda						
(Dorman)	1 oz	100	8	210	1	—
(Holland Farm)	1 oz	103	8	—	—	—
(Kraft)	1 oz	110	9	200	0	—
(Land O'Lakes)	1 oz	110	8	230	1	—
(MayBud)	1 oz	100	8	210	1	0
(Sargento)	1 oz	101	8	232	1	—
Gouda Mini (Laughing Cow)	1 (0.7 oz)	80	6	170	0	0
Gouda Round (MayBud)	1 oz	100	8	210	1	0
Gourmet Parm (Sargento)	1 tbsp	20	1	95	tr	—
Havarti (Casino)	1 oz	120	11	140	0	—
Havarti (Sargento)	1 oz	118	11	200	tr	—
Hoop (Friendship)	2 tbsp (1 oz)	20	0	10	0	0
Horseradish Light (Bristol Gold)	1 oz	70	4	150	3	—
Impastata (Frigo)	1 oz	60	5	50	1	—
Italian Style Grated Cheeses (Sargento)	1 oz	108	8	106	1	—
Jarlsberg (Sargento)	1 oz	100	7	130	1	—
Limburger (Sargento)	1 oz	93	8	227	tr	—
Limburger Little Gem Size (Mohawk Valley)	1 oz	90	8	250	0	—
Monterey Jack						
(Armour)	1 oz	110	9	—	—	—
(Cabot)	1 oz	80	5	200	1	—
(Dorman)	1 oz	100	8	180	1	—
(Heluva Good Cheese)	1 oz	100	8	180	0	0
(Holland Farm)	1 oz	102	9	—	—	—
(Kraft)	1 oz	110	9	190	0	—
(Land O'Lakes)	1 oz	110	9	150	tr	—
(Sargento)	1 oz	106	9	152	tr	—
(Weight Watchers)	1 oz	80	5	150	1	—
Hot Pepper (Land O'Lakes)	1 oz	110	7	150	tr	—
Light With Simplesse (White Clover)	1 oz	70	4	190	tr	—
Lower Salt (Armour)	1 oz	110	9	111	—	—
Reduced Fat (Alpine Lace)	1 piece (1 oz)	70	5	170	1	0

FOOD	PORTION	CAL	FAT	SOD	CARB	FIB
Monterey Jack *(cont.)*						
Reduced Fat Light (Kraft)	1 oz	80	5	220	0	—
Shredded (Heluva Good Cheese)	¼ cup (1 oz)	100	8	170	1	0
With Caraway Seeds (Kraft)	1 oz	100	8	180	1	—
With Jalapeno Peppers (Kraft)	1 oz	110	9	190	1	—
With Jalapenos (Heluva Good Cheese)	1 oz	100	8	180	0	0
With Peppers Reduced Fat Light (Kraft)	1 oz	80	5	220	1	—
Monterey Reduced Fat Low Sodium (Dorman)	1 oz	80	5	140	1	—
Mozzarella						
(Weight Watchers)	1 oz	70	4	150	1	—
Low Moisture Part Skim (Alpine Lace)	1 piece (1 oz)	70	5	75	1	0
Part Skim Low Moisture Shredded (Heluva Good Cheese)	¼ cup (1 oz)	80	5	170	1	0
Preferred Light (Sargento)	1 oz	60	3	150	1	—
Reduced Fat Light (Kraft)	1 oz	80	4	200	1	—
Reduced Fat Low Sodium (Dorman)	1 oz	80	4	140	1	—
Shredded (Weight Watchers)	1 oz	80	5	150	1	—
Shredded Preferred Light (Sargento)	1 oz	60	3	150	1	—
Smoked (Polly-O)	1 oz	85	7	—	—	—
Whole Milk (Heluva Good Cheese)	1 oz	80	6	220	tr	0
Mozzarella Lite						
Low Moisture Whole Milk (Frigo)	1 oz	60	2	140	1	—
Sandwich Slices (Polly-O)	1 oz	70	4	—	—	—
Mozzarella Low Moisture						
(Kraft)	1 oz	90	7	190	1	—
Part Skim (Frigo)	1 oz	80	5	190	1	—
Part Skim (Kraft)	1 oz	80	5	200	1	—

FOOD	PORTION	CAL	FAT	SOD	CARB	FIB
Part Skim (Sargento)	1 oz	79	5	150	1	—
Whole Milk (Frigo)	1 oz	90	7	190	1	—
Mozzarella Part Skim						
(Dorman)	1 oz	90	7	190	1	—
(Polly-O)	1 oz	80	5	—	—	—
(Land O'Lakes)	1 oz	80	5	150	1	—
Shredded (Polly-O)	1 oz	80	6	—	—	—
Mozzarella Whole Milk						
(Polly-O)	1 oz	90	6	—	—	—
(Sargento)	1 oz	90	7	118	1	—
Sandwich Slices (Polly-O)	1 oz	90	6	—	—	—
Shredded (Polly-O)	1 oz	90	6	—	—	—
Muenster						
(Alpine Lace)	1 piece (1 oz)	100	9	85	1	0
(Dorman)	1 oz	110	9	190	0	—
(Heluva Good Cheese)	1 oz	100	8	180	0	0
(Holland Farm)	1 oz	102	9	—	—	—
(Land O'Lakes)	1 oz	100	9	180	tr	—
Muenster Light With Simplesse (White Clover)	1 oz	70	4	190	tr	—
Muenster Low Sodium (Dorman)	1 oz	110	9	95	0	—
Muenster Red Rind (Sargento)	1 oz	104	9	180	tr	—
Muenster Reduced Fat Low Sodium (Dorman)	1 oz	80	5	140	tr	—
Naturally Slender (Northfield)	1 oz	90	7	—	—	—
Parmazest (Frigo)	1 oz	120	7	410	5	—
Parmesan (Dorman)	1 oz	110	7	350	1	—
Parmesan & Romano Dry Grated (Frigo)	1 oz	130	9	510	1	—
Parmesan & Romano Grated (Frigo)	1 oz	110	7	350	1	—
Parmesan & Romano Grated (Sargento)	1 oz	111	7	397	1	—
Parmesan Dry Grated (Frigo)	1 oz	130	9	510	1	—
Parmesan Fresh (Sargento)	1 oz	111	7	454	1	—
Parmesan Grated						
(Frigo)	1 oz	110	7	350	1	—
(Kraft)	1 oz	130	9	430	1	—

FOOD	PORTION	CAL	FAT	SOD	CARB	FIB
Parmesan Grated *(cont.)*						
(Polly-O)	1 oz	130	9	—	—	—
(Progresso)	1 tbsp	23	2	95	tr	0
(Sargento)	1 oz	129	9	528	1	—
Parmesan Natural (Kraft)	1 oz	100	7	290	1	—
Parmesan Shreds (DiGiorno)	2 tsp (5 g)	20	2	75	0	0
Parmesan Whole (Frigo)	1 oz	110	7	350	1	—
Pizza Shredded (Frigo)	1 oz	65	3	150	1	—
Port Wine Cup Cheese (Weight Watchers)	1½ tbsp (1 oz)	70	3	190	7	—
Port Wine Nut Log (Sargento)	1 oz	97	7	252	3	—
Provolone						
(Dorman)	1 oz	90	7	290	1	—
(Frigo)	1 oz	100	7	230	1	—
(Kraft)	1 oz	100	7	260	1	—
(Land O'Lakes)	1 oz	100	8	250	1	—
(Sargento)	1 oz	100	8	248	1	—
Provolone Reduced Fat (Alpine Lace)	1 piece (1 oz)	70	5	120	1	0
Provolone Reduced Fat Low Sodium (Dorman)	1 oz	80	4	140	1	—
Provolone Lite (Frigo)	1 oz	70	4	205	1	—
Quark (Brier Run)	1 oz	34	3	15	—	—
Queso Blanco (Sargento)	1 oz	104	9	178	tr	—
Queso de Papa (Sargento)	1 oz	114	9	176	tr	—
Ricotta Lite (Polly-O)	2 oz	80	4	—	—	—
Ricotta Lite (Sargento)	1 oz	24	1	23	2	—
Ricotta Low Fat Low Salt (Frigo)	1 oz	30	1	10	1	—
Ricotta Part Skim						
(Frigo)	1 oz	40	3	30	1	—
(Polly-O)	2 oz	90	6	—	—	—
(Sargento)	1 oz	32	2	27	1	—
Ricotta Part Skim No Salt (Polly-O)	2 oz	90	6	—	—	—
Ricotta Whole Milk (Frigo)	1 oz	60	5	40	1	—
Ricotta Whole Milk (Polly-O)	2 oz	100	7	—	—	—

FOOD	PORTION	CAL	FAT	SOD	CARB	FIB
Ricotta Whole Milk No Salt (Polly-O)	2 oz	100	7	—	—	—
Romano (Dorman)	1 oz	100	7	350	1	—
Romano (Sargento)	1 oz	110	8	340	1	—
Romano Dry Grated (Frigo)	1 oz	130	9	510	1	—
Romano Grated						
(Casino)	1 oz	130	9	350	1	—
(Frigo)	1 oz	110	8	350	1	—
(Polly-O)	1 oz	130	10	—	—	—
(Progresso)	1 tbsp	23	2	70	tr	0
Romano Natural (Casino)	1 oz	100	7	250	1	—
Romano Whole (Frigo)	1 oz	110	8	350	1	—
Schloss (Marin French Cheese)	1 oz	86	7	—	1	—
Sharp Cheddar Cup Cheese (Weight Watchers)	1½ tbsp (1 oz)	70	3	190	7	—
Sheep's Milk (Hollow Road Farms)	1 oz	45	3	65	1	—
Smoke Light (Bristol Gold)	1 oz	70	4	150	3	—
Smokestick (Sargento)	1 oz	103	7	388	1	—
String						
(Frigo)	1 oz	80	5	190	1	—
(Polly-O)	1 oz	90	6	—	—	—
(Sargento)	1 oz	79	5	150	1	—
String Lite (Frigo)	1 oz	60	2	140	1	—
String MooTown Snackers Light (Sargento)	1 stick	40	2	125	tr	—
String Smoked (Sargento)	1 oz	79	5	150	1	—
String With Jalapeno Peppers (Kraft)	1 oz	80	5	230	1	—
Swiss						
(Casino)	1 oz	110	8	35	1	—
(Dorman)	1 oz	100	8	80	0	—
(Frigo)	1 oz	110	8	80	1	—
(Heluva Good Cheese)	1 oz	112	8	62	0	0
(Kraft)	1 oz	110	8	40	1	—
(Land O'Lakes)	1 oz	110	8	75	1	—
(Sargento)	1 oz	107	8	74	1	—
Reduced Fat (Alpine Lace)	1 piece (1 oz)	90	6	35	1	0

FOOD	PORTION	CAL	FAT	SOD	CARB	FIB
Swiss Aged (Kraft)	1 oz	110	8	45	1	—
Swiss Almond Nut Log (Sargento)	1 oz	94	7	349	2	—
Swiss No Salt Added (Dorman)	1 oz	100	8	10	tr	—
Swiss Reduced Fat Light (Kraft)	1 oz	90	5	70	1	—
Swiss Reduced Fat Low Sodium (Dorman)	1 oz	90	5	60	tr	—
Swiss Very Low (Kraft)	1 oz	110	8	10	1	—
Swiss Wafer Thin Preferred Light (Sargento)	1 oz	80	4	75	1	—
Taco (Sargento)	1 oz	109	9	162	tr	—
Taco Shredded (Frigo)	1 oz	110	9	200	1	—
Taco Shredded (Kraft)	1 oz	110	9	190	1	—
Tilsiter (Sargento)	1 oz	96	7	213	1	—
Tybo Red Wax (Sargento)	1 oz	98	7	200	tr	—
Vitalait (Cabot)	1 oz	70	4	170	1	—
Vitalait Jalapeno (Cabot)	1 oz	70	4	170	1	—
Washed Curd Cheese (Heluva Good Cheese)	1 oz	110	9	170	1	0
Wine Light (Bristol Gold)	1 oz	70	4	150	3	—
bel paese	3.5 oz	391	30	—	0	—
blue	1 oz	100	8	396	1	—
blue, crumbled	1 cup	477	39	1884	3	—
brick	1 oz	105	8	159	1	—
brie	1 oz	95	8	178	tr	—
caerphilly	1.4 oz	150	13	—	0	0
camembert	1 oz	85	7	239	tr	—
camembert	1 wedge (1.33 oz)	114	9	320	tr	—
caraway	1 oz	107	8	196	1	—
cheddar	1 oz	114	9	176	tr	—
cheddar, reduced fat	1.4 oz	104	6	—	0	0
cheddar, shredded	1 cup	455	37	701	1	—
cheshire	1 oz	110	9	198	1	—
cheshire, reduced fat	1.4 oz	108	6	—	tr	0
colby	1 oz	112	9	171	1	—
derby	1.4 oz	161	14	—	0	0
double gloucester	1.4 oz	162	14	—	0	0
edam	1 oz	101	8	274	tr	—
edam, reduced fat	1.4 oz	92	4	—	tr	0
emmentaler	3.5 oz	403	30	450	tr	—
feta	1 oz	75	6	316	1	—
fontina	1 oz	110	9	—	tr	—

FOOD	PORTION	CAL	FAT	SOD	CARB	FIB
fromage frais	1.6 oz	51	3	—	3	0
gjetost	1 oz	132	8	170	12	—
goat hard	1 oz	128	10	98	1	—
goat, semisoft	1 oz	103	8	146	1	—
goat, soft	1 oz	76	6	104	tr	—
gorgonzola	3.5 oz	376	31	—	1	—
gouda	1 oz	101	8	232	1	—
gruyere	1 oz	117	9	95	tr	—
lancashire	1.4 oz	149	12	—	0	0
leicester	1.4 oz	160	14	—	0	0
limburger	1 oz	93	8	227	tr	—
lymeswold	1.4 oz	170	16	—	tr	0
monterey	1 oz	106	9	152	tr	—
mozzarella	1 lb	1276	98	1692	10	—
mozzarella	1 oz	80	6	106	1	—
mozzarella, low moisture	1 oz	90	7	118	1	—
mozzarella, low moisture, part skim	1 oz	79	5	150	1	—
mozzarella, part skim	1 oz	72	5	132	1	—
muenster	1 oz	104	9	178	tr	—
parmesan, grated	1 oz	129	9	528	1	—
parmesan, grated	1 tbsp	23	2	93	tr	—
parmesan, hard	1 oz	111	7	454	1	—
port du salut	1 oz	100	8	151	tr	—
provolone	1 oz	100	8	248	1	—
quark, 20% fat	3.5 oz	116	5	35	3	—
quark, 40% fat	3.5 oz	167	11	34	3	—
quark, made w/ skim milk	3.5 oz	78	tr	40	4	—
ricotta	1 cup	428	32	207	7	—
ricotta	½ cup	216	16	104	4	—
ricotta, part skim	1 cup	340	19	307	13	—
ricotta, part skim	½ cup	171	10	155	6	—
romadur, 40% fat	3.5 oz	289	20	—	tr	—
romano	1 oz	110	8	340	1	—
roquefort	1 oz	105	9	513	1	—
stilton, blue	1.4 oz	164	14	—	0	0
stilton, white	1.4 oz	145	13	—	0	0
swiss	1 oz	107	8	74	1	—
tilsit	1 oz	96	7	213	1	—
wensleydale	1.4 oz	151	13	—	0	0
yogurt cheese	1 oz	20	0	—	—	—
PROCESSED						
Alpine Lace						
American	1 piece (1 oz)	80	6	200	2	0

FOOD	PORTION	CAL	FAT	SOD	CARB	FIB
Alpine Lace *(cont.)*						
American Fat Free	1 piece (1 oz)	45	0	280	2	0
Cheddar Fat Free	1 piece (1 oz)	45	0	280	2	0
Mozzarella Fat Free	1 piece (1 oz)	45	0	280	2	0
Borden						
American Slices	1 oz	110	9	490	1	—
American Very Sharp	1 oz	110	9	490	1	—
Lite Line Mozzarella	1 oz	50	2	—	—	—
Lite Line Sharp Cheddar	1 oz	50	2	—	—	—
Lite Line Swiss	1 oz	50	2	—	—	—
Swiss Slices	1 oz	100	8	380	1	—
Cheez Whiz	1 oz	80	6	470	2	—
Mild Mexican	1 oz	80	6	430	2	—
With Jalapeno Peppers	1 oz	80	6	430	2	—
Churney Diet Snack						
Cheddar Flavored	1 oz	70	3	—	—	—
Port Wine Flavored	1 oz	70	3	—	—	—
Cracker Barrel						
Cheese Ball Sharp Cheddar With Almonds	1 oz	100	7	250	4	—
Cheese Log Port Wine With Almonds	1 oz	90	6	260	4	—
Cheese Log Sharp Cheddar With Almonds	1 oz	90	6	250	4	—
Cheese Log Smokey Cheddar With Almonds	1 oz	90	6	250	4	—
Extra Sharp Cheddar	1 oz	90	7	240	3	—
Port Wine Cheddar	1 oz	100	7	230	3	—
Sharp Cheddar	1 oz	100	7	230	4	—
With Bacon	1 oz	90	7	280	3	—
Dorman's Lo-Chol						
Cheddar	1 oz	100	7	140	1	—
Colby	1 oz	100	7	140	1	—
Mozzarella	1 oz	90	6	140	1	—
Muenster	1 oz	100	7	140	1	—
Swiss	1 oz	100	7	140	1	—
Easy Cheese Sharp Cheddar Spread	1 oz	80	6	340	2	—
Formagg						
American Swiss Slices	0.75 oz	70	5	—	—	—
American White Slices	0.75 oz	70	5	—	—	—

FOOD	PORTION	CAL	FAT	SOD	CARB	FIB
American Yellow Slices	0.75 oz	70	5	—	—	—
Cheddar	1 oz	70	5	—	—	—
Monterey Jack	1 oz	70	5	—	—	—
Monterey Jack Jalapeno Flavored	1 oz	70	5	—	—	—
Mozzarella	1 oz	70	5	—	—	—
Pizza Topper	1 oz	70	5	—	—	—
Provolone	1 oz	70	5	—	—	—
Ricotta	1 oz	130	5	—	—	—
Shredded Cheddar	1 oz	70	5	—	—	—
Shredded Mozzarella	1 oz	70	5	—	—	—
Shredded Parmesan	1 oz	70	4	—	—	—
Shredded Provolone	1 oz	70	5	—	—	—
Shredded Salad Topping	1 oz	70	5	—	—	—
Shredded Swiss	1 oz	70	5	—	—	—
Swiss	1 oz	70	5	—	—	—
Formagg Grated Italian Pasta Topping	1 oz	100	7	—	—	—
Frigo Imitation Cheddar	1 oz	90	7	280	1	—
Frigo Imitation Mozzarella	1 oz	90	7	240	1	—
Harvest Moon American	1 oz	70	4	420	2	—
Heluva Good Cheese						
American	1 slice (0.7)	45	5	390	2	0
Cheddar Sharp Cold Pack	2 tbsp (1 oz)	90	7	210	3	0
Cheddar Sharp With Bacon Cold Pack	2 tbsp (1 oz)	90	7	210	3	0
Cheddar Sharp With Horseradish Cold Pack	2 tbsp (1 oz)	90	7	210	3	0
Cheddar Sharp With Jalapenos Cold Pack	2 tbsp (1 oz)	90	7	210	3	0
Cheddar Sharp With Port Wine Cold Pack	2 tbsp (1 oz)	90	7	210	3	0
Hoffman						
American Yellow	1 oz	110	9	400	1	0
Hot Pepper	1 oz	90	7	460	2	0
Super Sharp	1 oz	110	9	380	1	0
Kraft						
American Cheese Spread	1 oz	80	6	470	2	—
American Grated	1 oz	130	7	740	8	—

FOOD	PORTION	CAL	FAT	SOD	CARB	FIB
Kraft *(cont.)*						
Cheese Food With Jalapeno Peppers	1 oz	90	7	390	2	—
Cheese Spread With Bacon	1 oz	80	7	560	1	—
Cheese With Garlic	1 oz	90	7	370	2	—
Jalapeno Pepper Spread	1 oz	70	5	95	3	—
Jalapeno Spread	1 oz	80	6	470	2	—
Olives & Pimento Spread	1 oz	60	5	160	2	—
Pimento Spread	1 oz	70	5	120	3	—
Pineapple Spread	1 oz	70	5	75	4	—
Singles American	1 oz	90	7	390	2	—
Singles Cheez 'n Bacon	1 oz	90	7	400	2	—
Singles Free	1 oz	45	5	420	4	—
Singles Jalapeno	1 oz	90	7	450	2	—
Singles Light	1 oz	70	4	410	2	—
Singles Light American	1 oz	70	4	70	2	—
Singles Light Swiss	1 oz	70	3	350	2	—
Singles Monterey Jack	1 oz	90	7	390	2	—
Singles Pimento	1 oz	90	7	390	2	—
Singles Sharp	1 oz	100	8	400	1	—
Singles Swiss	1 oz	90	7	440	2	—
Singles White American	1 oz	90	7	400	2	—
Kraft Deluxe						
American Cheese	1 oz	110	9	450	1	—
Pimento Cheese	1 oz	100	8	440	1	—
Swiss Cheese	1 oz	90	7	420	1	—
Kraft Singles Light Sharp Cheddar	1 oz	70	4	380	2	—
Lactaid American	3.5 oz	328	25	1189	7	0
Land O'Lakes						
American	1 oz	110	9	450	1	—
American & Swiss	1 oz	100	8	400	1	—
Cheddar & Bacon	1 oz	110	9	350	1	—
Extra Sharp Cheddar	1 oz	100	9	370	1	—
Golden Velvet Cheese Spread	1 oz	80	6	370	2	—
Italian Herb Cheese Food	1 oz	90	7	430	2	—

FOOD	PORTION	CAL	FAT	SOD	CARB	FIB
Jalapeno Cheese Food	1 oz	90	7	400	2	—
Jalapeno Jack	1 oz	90	8	430	1	—
Onion Cheese Food	1 oz	90	7	70	2	—
Pepperoni Cheese Food	1 oz	90	7	430	1	—
Salami Cheese Food	1 oz	90	7	410	2	—
Sharp American	1 oz	100	9	360	1	—
Laughing Cow						
Assorted Wedge	1 (1 oz)	70	6	370	1	0
Cheesebits	6 pieces (1 oz)	70	6	370	1	0
Original Wedge	1 (1 oz)	70	6	370	1	0
Wedge Light	1 (1 oz)	50	3	370	1	0
Light n' Lively						
Singles American	1 oz	70	4	420	2	—
Singles American White	1 oz	70	4	410	2	—
Singles Sharp Cheddar	1 oz	70	4	380	2	—
Singles Swiss	1 oz	70	3	350	2	—
Lunch Wagon Sandwich Slices	1 oz	90	7	370	2	—
Michael's						
Country Gourmet Spread French Onion	1 oz	48	5	—	—	—
Country Gourmet Spread Garden Vegetable	1 oz	48	5	—	—	—
Country Gourmet Spread Garlic & Herbs	1 oz	48	5	—	—	—
Mohawk Valley Limburger Cheese Spread	1 oz	70	6	420	0	—
Nippy Cheese Food	1 oz	90	7	380	2	—
Old English Sharp American	1 oz	110	9	440	1	—
Old English Sharp Cheese Spread	1 oz	90	7	480	1	—
Price's						
Cheese & Bacon Spread	2 tbsp (1.1 oz)	90	7	340	2	0
Jalapeno Nacho Dip Hot	2 tbsp (1.1 oz)	80	7	370	2	0
Jalapeno Nacho Dip Mild	2 tbsp (1.1 oz)	80	7	370	2	0

FOOD	PORTION	CAL	FAT	SOD	CARB	FIB
Price's *(cont.)*						
Pimiento Cheese Spread	2 tbsp (1.1 oz)	80	7	320	2	0
Pimiento Cheese Spread Light	2 tbsp (1.1 oz)	60	4	260	3	0
Vegetable Garden	2 tbsp (1.1 oz)	70	5	290	3	0
Roka Blue Spread	1 oz	70	6	270	2	—
Rondele Soft Spreadable Garlic & Herbs	2 tbsp (1 oz)	100	9	180	1	0
Rondele Light Soft Spreadable Garlic & Herb Rondele	2 tbsp (0.9 oz)	60	4	190	2	0
Sargento						
American Hot Pepper	1 oz	106	9	406	tr	—
American Sharp Spread	1 oz	106	9	406	tr	—
American w/ Pimento	1 oz	106	9	405	tr	—
Brick	1 oz	95	9	431	1	—
Imitation Cheddar	1 oz	85	6	350	tr	—
Imitation Mozzarella	1 oz	80	6	310	tr	—
Swiss	1 oz	95	7	388	1	—
Smart Beat						
American	1 slice (0.6 oz)	35	2	180	2	—
Low Sodium	1 slice (0.6 oz)	35	2	90	2	—
Sharp	1 slice (0.6 oz)	35	2	210	2	—
Spreadery						
Medium Cheddar	1 oz	70	4	250	3	—
Mild Mexican With Jalapeno Peppers	1 oz	70	4	260	3	—
Nacho	1 oz	70	4	240	3	—
Port Wine	1 oz	70	4	250	3	—
Sharp Cheddar	1 oz	70	4	240	3	—
Vermont White Cheddar	1 oz	70	4	230	3	—
Squeez-A-Snak						
Garlic	1 oz	80	7	430	1	—
Hickory Smoke	1 oz	80	7	440	1	—
Sharp	1 oz	80	7	440	1	—
With Bacon	1 oz	90	7	500	1	—
With Jalapeno Pepper	1 oz	80	6	510	1	—
Velveeta						
Light Singles	1 oz	70	4	470	3	—

FOOD	PORTION	CAL	FAT	SOD	CARB	FIB
Mexican Hot	1 oz	80	6	520	3	—
Mexican Mild	1 oz	80	6	440	3	—
Pimento	1 oz	80	6	400	3	—
Shredded	1 oz	100	7	210	3	—
Shredded Hot Mexican With Jalapeno Peppers	1 oz	100	7	430	3	—
Shredded Mild Mexican With Jalapeno Peppers	1 oz	100	7	420	3	—
Slices	1 oz	90	6	400	3	—
Spread	1 oz	80	6	430	3	—
Weight Watchers						
American Slices Low Sodium Yellow	2 slices (0.66 oz)	35	1	80	2	—
American Slices Low Sodium White	2 slices (0.66 oz)	35	1	80	2	—
American Slices White	2 slices (0.66 oz)	35	1	270	1	—
American Slices Yellow	2 slices (0.66 oz)	35	1	270	1	—
Sharp Cheddar Slices	2 slices (0.66 oz)	35	1	270	2	—
Swiss Slices	2 slices (0.66 oz)	35	1	270	2	—
WisPride						
Chunk	1 oz	110	8	180	4	0
Garlic & Herb Cup	2 tbsp (1.1 oz)	100	7	270	4	0
Hickory Smoked Cup	2 tbsp (1.1 oz)	100	7	230	4	0
Port Wine Ball	2 tbsp (1.1 oz)	100	8	190	4	0
Port Wine Cup	2 tbsp (1.1 oz)	100	7	230	4	0
Port Wine Light Cup	2 tbsp (1.1 oz)	80	3	200	5	0
Sharp Ball	2 tbsp (1.1 oz)	100	8	190	4	0
Sharp Cup	2 tbsp (1.1 oz)	100	7	230	4	0
Sharp Cheddar Ball	2 tbsp (1.1 oz)	100	8	190	4	0
Sharp Light Cup	2 tbsp (1.1 oz)	80	3	200	5	0
Swiss Ball	2 tbsp (1.1 oz)	110	8	125	5	0
american	1 oz	93	7	337	2	—
american cheese food	1 pkg (8 oz)	745	56	2700	17	—
american cheese spread	1 jar (5 oz)	412	30	1910	12	—
american cheese spread	1 oz	82	6	381	2	—
american cold pack	1 pkg (8 oz)	752	56	2193	19	—
pimento	1 oz	106	9	405	tr	—
swiss	1 oz	95	7	388	1	—
swiss cheese food	1 pkg (8 oz)	734	55	3523	10	—

FOOD	PORTION	CAL	FAT	SOD	CARB	FIB

CHEESE DISHES
FROZEN

Welsh Rarebit (Stouffer's)	¼ cup (1.1 oz)	120	9	280	5	—
Mozzarella Cheese Nuggets (Banquet)	2.5 oz	230	12	510	15	—

HOME RECIPE

Welsh rarebit, as prep w/ 1 white toast	1 slice	228	16	—	14	1

TAKE-OUT

cheese omelette, as prep w/ 2 eggs	1 (6.8 oz)	519	44	—	tr	0
fondue	½ cup	303	18	194	5	—
macaroni & cheese	6.3 oz	320	19	—	25	1

CHEESE SUBSTITUTES

Borden Taco-Mate	1 oz	100	7	360	2	—
Cheese Two	1 oz	90	7	360	2	—
Georgio's Imitation Cheddar Shredded	¼ cup (1 oz)	90	7	450	1	0
Georgio's Imitation Mozzarella Shredded	¼ cup (1 oz)	90	7	350	1	0
Golden Image American	1 oz	90	6	360	2	—
Golden Image Colby	1 oz	110	9	190	1	—
Golden Image Mild Cheddar	1 oz	110	9	190	0	—
mozzarella	1 oz	70	3	194	7	—

CHERIMOYA

fresh	1	515	2	—	131	—

CHERRIES
CANNED

sour in heavy syrup	½ cup	232	tr	18	60	—
sour in light syrup	½ cup	189	tr	18	49	—
sour, water packed	1 cup	87	tr	17	22	—
sweet, in heavy syrup	½ cup	107	tr	3	27	—
sweet, in light syrup	½ cup	85	tr	3	22	—
sweet, juice pack	½ cup	68	tr	3	17	—
sweet, water pack	½ cup	57	tr	2	15	—

DRIED

Bing (Chukar)	2 oz	160	1	3	35	—
Rainer (Chukar)	2 oz	160	1	3	35	—
Tart (Chukar)	2 oz	170	0	10	43	—
Tart 'n Sweet (Chukar)	2 oz	180	0	10	43	—

FOOD	PORTION	CAL	FAT	SOD	CARB	FIB
FRESH						
Dole	1 cup	90	1	0	19	3
sour	1 cup	51	tr	3	13	—
sweet	10	49	1	0	11	—
FROZEN						
Dark Sweet (Big Valley)	4 oz	60	tr	0	14	—
sour, unsweetened	1 cup	72	1	1	17	—
sweet, sweetened	1 cup	232	tr	3	58	—
JUICE						
Dole Pure & Light	6 oz	90	tr	10	22	—
Hi-C	8 fl oz	130	0	30	33	—
Hi-C Box	8.45 fl oz	140	0	30	35	—
Juice Works Cherry	6 oz	100	0	—	—	—
Juicy Juice	6 fl oz	90	0	10	23	—
Kool-Aid	8 oz	98	0	—	25	—
Kool-Aid Black Cherry	8 oz	98	0	—	25	—
Kool-Aid Sugar Free	8 oz	3	0	3	0	—
Kool-Aid Koolers	1 (8.45 oz)	142	0	3	38	—
Sipps Wild Cherry	8.45 oz	130	0	—	—	—
Smucker's Black Cherry	8 oz	130	0	10	31	—
Smucker's Black Cherry Sparkler	10 oz	120	tr	5	30	—
Tang Fruit Box	8.45 oz	121	0	2	32	—
Wylers Drink Mix Unsweetened Cherry	8 oz	2	0	15	1	—
Wylers Drink Mix Wild Cherry	8 oz	81	0	tr	21	—

CHERVIL
FOOD	PORTION	CAL	FAT	SOD	CARB	FIB
seed	1 tsp	1	tr	tr	tr	—

CHESTNUTS
FOOD	PORTION	CAL	FAT	SOD	CARB	FIB
chinese, cooked	1 oz	44	tr	1	10	—
chinese, dried	1 oz	103	tr	2	23	—
chinese, raw	1 oz	64	tr	1	14	—
chinese, roasted	1 oz	68	tr	1	15	—
cooked	1 oz	37	tr	8	8	—
dried, peeled	1 oz	105	1	11	22	—
japanese, cooked	1 oz	16	tr	1	4	—
japanese, dried	1 oz	102	tr	10	23	—
japanese, raw	1 oz	44	tr	4	10	—
japanese, roasted	1 oz	57	tr	—	13	—
raw, peeled	1 oz	56	tr	1	13	—
roasted	1 cup	350	3	3	76	—
roasted	1 oz	70	1	1	15	—

FOOD	PORTION	CAL	FAT	SOD	CARB	FIB
CHEWING GUM						
Beech-Nut Cinnamon	1 piece	10	0	0	2	—
Beech-Nut Fruit	1 piece	10	0	0	2	—
Beech-Nut Peppermint	1 piece	10	0	0	2	—
Beech-Nut Spearmint	1 piece	10	0	0	2	—
Big Red	1 stick	10	tr	0	2	—
Brock Bubble Gum	1 piece (0.2 oz)	20	0	0	4	—
Bubbicious Bubblicious	1 piece (7.9 g)	25	0	—	6	—
Bubble Yum Fruit Juice Variety	1 piece	20	0	0	7	1
Bubble Yum Luscious Lime	1 piece	25	0	0	7	1
Care*Free Sugarless All Flavors	1 piece	8	0	—	—	—
Care*Free Sugarless Bubble Gum All Flavors	1 piece	10	0	—	—	—
Chiclets	1 piece (1.59 g)	6	0	—	2	—
Chiclets Tiny Size	8 pieces (0.13g)	tr	0	—	tr	—
Clorets	1 piece (1.59 g)	6	0	—	2	—
Dentyne	1 piece (1.88 g)	6	0	—	1	—
Dentyne Cinn-A-Burst	1 piece (3.2 g)	9	0	—	2	—
Dentyne Sugar Free	1 piece (1.88 g)	5	0	—	1	—
Extra Sugar Free Cinnamon	1 piece	8	tr	0	tr	—
Extra Sugar Free Spearmint & Peppermint	1 stick	8	tr	0	tr	—
Extra Sugar Free Winter Fresh	1 piece	8	tr	0	tr	—
Freedent Spearmint, Peppermint & Cinnamon	1 stick	10	tr	0	3	—
Freshen-Up	1 piece (4.2 g)	13	0	—	3	—
Fruit Stripe	1 piece	8	0	0	3	1
Fruit Stripe Bubble Gum	1 piece	8	0	0	2	—
Fruit Stripe Variety Pack	1 piece	8	0	0	2	0
Hubba Bubba Bubble Gum						
Cola	1 piece	23	tr	0	6	—
Original	1 piece	23	tr	0	6	—
Strawberry Grape Raspberry	1 piece	23	tr	0	6	—
Sugarfree Grape	1 piece	13	tr	0	tr	—
Sugarfree Original	1 piece	14	tr	0	tr	—

FOOD	PORTION	CAL	FAT	SOD	CARB	FIB
Juicy Fruit	1 stick	10	tr	0	2	—
Swell Bubble Gum	1 piece (3 g)	10	0	0	2	—
Trident	1 piece (1.88 g)	5	0	—	1	—
Trident Soft Bubble Gum	1 piece (3.3 g)	9	0	—	2	—
Wrigley's Doublemint	1 piece	10	tr	0	2	—
Wrigley's Spearmint	1 stick	10	tr	0	2	—

CHIA SEEDS

dried	1 oz	134	7	—	14	—

CHICKEN

see also CHICKEN DISHES, CHICKEN SUBSTITUTES, DINNER, HOT DOGS

CANNED

FOOD	PORTION	CAL	FAT	SOD	CARB	FIB
Chunk Style Mixin' Chicken (Swanson)	2.5 oz	130	8	230	1	—
Chunky (Underwood)	2.08 oz	150	9	440	2	—
Chunky Light (Underwood)	2.08 oz	80	3	330	2	—
Smoky (Underwood)	2.08 oz	150	8	290	10	—
White (Swanson)	2.5 oz	100	4	235	0	—
White & Dark (Swanson)	2.5 oz	100	4	240	0	—
chicken spread	1 oz	55	3	—	2	—
chicken spread	1 tbsp	25	2	—	1	—
chicken spread barbeque flavor	1 oz	55	3	—	2	—
w/ broth	1 can (5 oz)	234	11	714	0	—
w/ broth	½ can (2.5 oz)	117	6	357	0	—
FRESH						
Breast (Tyson)	3 oz	116	2	63	0	—
Breast Oven Stuffer Roaster w/ Skin, cooked (Perdue)	1 oz	42	2	11	0	—
Breast Quarters Fresh Young w/ Skin, cooked (Perdue)	1 oz	48	3	14	0	—
Breast Skinless & Boneless Oven Stuffer Roaster, cooked (Perdue)	1 oz	31	tr	9	0	—
Breast Skinless Boneless, cooked (Perdue)	1 oz	30	tr	10	0	—
Breast Split Fresh Young w/ Skin, cooked (Perdue)	1 oz	45	3	12	0	—

FOOD	PORTION	CAL	FAT	SOD	CARB	FIB
Breast Tender Skinless & Boneless, cooked (Perdue)	1 oz	29	tr	14	0	—
Breast Thin-Sliced Skinless & Boneless Oven Stuffer, cooked (Perdue)	1 oz	31	tr	9	0	—
Breast Whole Fresh Young w/ Skin, cooked (Perdue)	1 oz	45	3	12	0	—
Breast Whole Oven Stuffer Meat Only, cooked (Perdue)	3 oz	169	—	—	—	—
Cornish Hen (Tyson)	3.5 oz	250	15	80	1	—
Cornish Hen White Meat w/ Skin, cooked (Perdue)	1 oz	42	3	12	0	—
Cornish Hen Dark Meat w/ Skin, cooked (Perdue)	1 oz	43	3	10	0	—
Drumstick (Tyson)	3 oz	131	4	81	0	—
Drumsticks Fresh Young w/ Skin, cooked (Perdue)	1 oz	42	2	21	0	—
Drumsticks Oven Stuffer Roaster w/ Skin, cooked (Perdue)	1 oz	41	2	16	0	—
Ground Fresh Young, cooked (Perdue)	1 oz	49	3	14	0	—
Leg Quarters Fresh Young w/ Skin, cooked (Perdue)	1 oz	49	4	15	0	—
Legs Fresh Young w/ Skin, cooked (Perdue)	1 oz	51	4	16	0	—
Soup & Stew Baking Hen Dark Meat w/ Skin, cooked (Perdue)	1 oz	41	3	9	0	—
Soup & Stew Baking Hen White Meat w/ Skin, cooked (Perdue)	1 oz	41	2	11	0	—
Thigh (Tyson)	3 oz	152	7	75	0	—
Thighs Fresh Young w/ Skin, cooked (Perdue)	1 oz	57	4	15	0	—

FOOD	PORTION	CAL	FAT	SOD	CARB	FIB
Thighs Skinless & Boneless Oven Stuffer Roaster, cooked (Perdue)	1 oz	34	2	13	0	—
Thighs Skinless & Boneless, cooked (Perdue)	1 oz	30	2	10	0	—
Whole (Tyson)	3 oz	134	4	73	0	—
Whole Fresh Young Dark Meat w/ Skin, cooked (Perdue)	1 oz	47	3	12	0	—
Whole Fresh Young White Meat w/ Skin, cooked (Perdue)	1 oz	43	2	11	0	—
Whole Oven Stuffer Roaster Dark Meat w/ Skin, cooked (Perdue)	1 oz	49	3	16	0	—
Whole Oven Stuffer Roaster White Meat w/ Skin, cooked (Perdue)	1 oz	44	2	12	0	—
Wing (Tyson)	3 oz	147	6	78	0	—
Wing Drumettes Fresh Young w/ Skin, cooked (Perdue)	1 oz	50	3	13	0	—
Wingettes Oven Stuffer Roaster w/ Skin, cooked (Perdue)	1 oz	52	3	17	0	—
Wings Fresh Young w/ Skin, cooked (Perdue)	1 oz	54	4	19	0	—
broiler/fryer						
back w/ skin, batter dipped & fried	½ back (2.5 oz)	238	16	228	7	—
back w/ skin, floured & fried	1.5 oz	146	9	40	3	—
back w/ skin, roasted	1 oz	96	7	28	0	—
back w/ skin, stewed	½ back (2.1 oz)	158	11	39	0	—
back w/o skin, fried	½ back (2 oz)	167	9	58	3	—
breast w/ skin, batter dipped & fried	½ breast (4.9 oz)	364	18	385	13	—
breast w/ skin, batter dipped & fried	2.9 oz	218	11	231	8	—
breast w/ skin, roasted	½ breast (3.4 oz)	193	8	69	0	—

FOOD	PORTION	CAL	FAT	SOD	CARB	FIB
broiler/fryer *(cont.)*						
breast w/ skin, roasted	2 oz	115	5	41	0	—
breast w/ skin, stewed	½ breast (3.9 oz)	202	8	68	0	—
breast w/o skin, fried	½ breast (3 oz)	161	4	68	tr	—
breast w/o skin, roasted	½ breast (3 oz)	142	3	63	0	—
breast w/o skin, stewed	2 oz	86	2	36	0	—
dark meat w/ skin, batter dipped & fried	5.9 oz	497	31	493	16	—
dark meat w/ skin, floured & fried	3.9 oz	313	19	98	4	—
dark meat w/ skin, roasted	3.5 oz	256	16	88	0	—
dark meat w/ skin, stewed	3.9 oz	256	16	77	0	—
dark meat w/o skin, fried	1 cup (5 oz)	334	16	136	4	—
dark meat w/o skin, roasted	1 cup (5 oz)	286	14	130	0	—
dark meat w/o skin, stewed	1 cup (5 oz)	269	13	104	0	—
dark meat w/o skin, stewed	3 oz	165	8	64	0	—
drumstick w/ skin, batter dipped & fried	1 (2.6 oz)	193	11	194	6	—
drumstick w/ skin, floured & fried	1 (1.7 oz)	120	7	44	1	—
drumstick w/ skin, roasted	1 (1.8 oz)	112	6	47	0	—
drumstick w/ skin, stewed	1 (2 oz)	116	6	43	0	—
drumstick w/o skin, fried	1 (1.5 oz)	82	3	40	0	—
drumstick w/o skin, roasted	1 (1.5 oz)	76	2	42	0	—
drumstick w/o skin, stewed	1 (1.6 oz)	78	3	37	0	—
leg w/ skin, batter dipped & fried	1 (5.5 oz)	431	26	442	14	—
leg w/ skin, floured & fried	1 (3.9 oz)	285	16	99	3	—

FOOD	PORTION	CAL	FAT	SOD	CARB	FIB
leg w/ skin, roasted	1 (4 oz)	265	15	99	0	—
leg w/ skin, stewed	1 (4.4 oz)	275	16	92	0	—
leg w/o skin, fried	1 (3.3 oz)	195	9	90	1	—
leg w/o skin, roasted	1 (3.3 oz)	182	8	87	0	—
leg w/o skin, stewed	1 (3.5 oz)	187	8	78	0	—
light meat w/ skin, batter dipped & fried	4 oz	312	17	324	11	—
light meat w/ skin, floured & fried	2.7 oz	192	9	60	1	—
light meat w/ skin, roasted	2.8 oz	175	9	59	0	—
light meat w/ skin, stewed	3.2 oz	181	9	57	0	—
light meat w/o skin, fried	1 cup (5 oz)	268	8	114	1	—
light meat w/o skin, roasted	1 cup (5 oz)	242	6	108	0	—
light meat w/o skin, stewed	1 cup (5 oz)	223	6	91	0	—
neck w/ skin, stewed	1 (1.3 oz)	94	7	20	0	—
neck w/o skin, stewed	1 (.6 oz)	32	1	12	0	—
skin, batter dipped & fried	4 oz	449	33	663	26	—
skin, batter dipped & fried	from ½ chicken (6.7 oz)	748	55	1105	44	—
skin, floured & fried	1 oz	166	14	18	3	—
skin, floured & fried	from ½ chicken (2 oz)	281	24	30	5	—
skin, roasted	from ½ chicken (2 oz)	254	23	36	0	—
skin, stewed	from ½ chicken (2 oz)	261	24	40	0	—
thigh w/ skin, batter dipped & fried	1 (3 oz)	238	14	248	8	—
thigh w/ skin, floured & fried	1 (2.2 oz)	162	9	55	2	—
thigh w/ skin, roasted	1 (2.2 oz)	153	10	52	0	—
thigh w/ skin, stewed	1 (2.4 oz)	158	10	49	0	—
thigh w/o skin, fried	1 (1.8 oz)	113	5	49	1	—
thigh w/o skin, roasted	1 (1.8 oz)	109	6	46	0	—

FOOD	PORTION	CAL	FAT	SOD	CARB	FIB
broiler/fryer *(cont.)*						
thigh w/o skin, stewed	1 (1.9 oz)	107	5	41	0	—
w/ skin, floured & fried	½ breast (3.4 oz)	218	9	75	2	—
w/ skin, floured fried	½ chicken (11 oz)	844	47	264	10	—
w/ skin, fried	½ chicken (16.4 oz)	1347	81	1360	44	—
w/ skin, neck & giblets, batter dipped & fried	1 chicken (2.3 lbs)	2987	180	2921	93	—
w/ skin, neck giblets, roasted	1 chicken (1.5 lbs)	1598	90	536	tr	—
w/ skin, neck & giblets, stewed	1 chicken (1.6 lbs)	1625	93	494	tr	—
w/ skin, roasted	½ chicken (10.5 oz)	715	41	244	0	—
w/ skin, stewed	½ chicken (11.07 oz)	730	42	224	0	—
w/o skin, roasted	1 cup (5 oz)	266	10	120	0	—
w/o skin, fried	1 cup	307	13	127	2	—
w/o skin, stewed	1 cup (5 oz)	248	9	98	0	—
w/o skin, stewed	1 oz	54	3	18	0	—
wing w/ skin, batter dipped & fried	1 (1.7 oz)	159	11	157	5	—
wing w/ skin, floured & fried	1 (1.1 oz)	103	7	25	1	—
wing w/ skin, roasted	1 (1.2 oz)	99	7	28	0	—
wing w/ skin, stewed	1 (1.4 oz)	100	7	27	0	—
capon w/ skin, neck & giblets, roasted	1 chicken (3.1 lbs)	3211	165	704	1	—
roaster						
dark meat w/o skin, roasted	1 cup (5 oz)	250	12	133	0	—
light meat w/o skin, roasted	1 cup (5 oz)	214	6	71	0	—
w/ skin, neck & giblets, roasted	1 chicken (2.4 lbs)	2363	140	760	1	—
w/ skin, roasted	½ chicken (1.1 lbs)	1071	64	349	0	—
w/o skin, roasted	1 cup (5 oz)	469	28	105	0	—

FOOD	PORTION	CAL	FAT	SOD	CARB	FIB
stewing						
dark meat w/o skin, stewed	1 cup (5 oz)	361	21	133	0	—
w/ skin neck & giblets, stewed	1 chicken (1.3 lbs)	1636	107	419	tr	—
w/ skin, stewed	½ chicken (9.2 oz)	744	49	190	0	—
w/ skin, stewed	6.2 oz	507	34	130	0	—
FROZEN						
Tyson						
Breast Tenders Skinless	3.5 oz	120	1	55	0	—
Breasts Boneless	3.5 oz	210	12	50	0	—
Breasts Boneless Skinless	3.5 oz	130	2	50	0	—
Drums & Thighs	3.5 oz	270	17	110	0	—
Thighs Boneless Skinless	3.5 oz	200	10	70	0	—
FROZEN PREPARED						
Banquet						
Fried Chicken Breast Portions	5.75 oz	220	11	710	13	—
Fried Chicken Thighs & Drumsticks	6.25 oz	250	14	790	14	—
Hot'n Spicy Chicken Nuggets	2.5 oz	240	18	360	10	—
Hot'n Spicy Fried Chicken	6.4 oz	330	19	1210	29	—
Hot'n Spicy Snack'n Chicken	3.75 oz	140	9	480	8	—
Original Fried Chicken	5.6 oz	290	17	1060	26	—
Southern Fried Chicken	5.6 oz	290	17	1060	26	—
Banquet Boneless						
Breast Tenders	2.25 oz	150	6	280	12	—
Chicken Nuggets	2.5 oz	200	13	530	10	—
Chicken Nuggets w/ Cheddar	2.5 oz	240	17	530	10	—
Chicken Patties	2.5 oz	190	12	440	11	—
Chicken Sticks	2.5 oz	210	14	340	10	—
Drum-Snackers	2.5 oz	210	14	510	12	—
Fried Breast Tenders	2.25 oz	160	7	340	13	—

FOOD	PORTION	CAL	FAT	SOD	CARB	FIB
Banquet Boneless *(cont.)*						
Southern Fried Chicken Nuggets	2.5 oz	210	14	500	12	—
Southern Fried Chicken Patties	2.5 oz	200	12	590	12	—
Country Skillet						
Chicken Chunks	3 oz	260	16	470	17	—
Chicken Nuggets	3 oz	250	15	580	14	—
Chicken Patties	3 oz	230	15	560	14	—
Southern Fried Chicken Chunks	3 oz	270	18	570	15	—
Southern Fried Chicken Patties	3 oz	240	15	540	14	—
Healthy Balance						
Baked Boneless Breast Nuggets	2.25 oz	120	4	310	8	—
Baked Boneless Breast Patties	2.25 oz	120	4	310	8	—
Baked Boneless Breast Tenders	2.25 oz	120	4	310	8	—
Swanson						
Chicken Nibbles	3.25 oz	300	19	690	19	—
Chicken Nuggets	3 oz	230	14	360	14	—
Fried Chicken Breast Portion	4.5 oz	360	20	800	21	—
Pre-fried Chicken Parts	3.25 oz	270	16	650	16	—
Thighs And Drumsticks	3.25 oz	290	18	610	17	—
Tyson						
BBQ Breast Fillets	3 oz	110	2	200	13	—
Breaded Patties	3 oz	300	20	—	15	—
Breast Chunks	3 oz	240	17	430	10	—
Breast Fillets	3 oz	190	9	400	15	—
Breast Patties	2.6 oz	220	15	640	11	—
Breast Tenders	3 oz	220	12	500	13	—
Chick'n Cheddar	2.6 oz	220	15	310	11	—
Chick'n Chunks	2.6 oz	220	15	500	11	—
Cordon Bleu Mini	1	90	4	210	5	—
Diced	3 oz	130	3	40	1	—
Grilled Sandwich	3.5 oz	200	5	470	25	—
Hors D'Oeuvres	3.5 oz	100	1	600	1	—
Mesquite Chunks						
Hot BBQ Breast Tenders	2.75 oz	110	3	580	4	—

FOOD	PORTION	CAL	FAT	SOD	CARB	FIB
Mesquite Breast Fillets	2.75 oz	100	2	250	3	—
Mesquite Breast Strips	2.75 oz	100	2	240	2	—
Mesquite Breast Tenders	2.75 oz	110	2	290	2	—
Microwave Breast Sandwich	4.25 oz	328	14	520	33	—
Microwave Chunks	3.5 oz	220	15	—	11	—
Microwave Chunks BBQ Sandwich	4 oz	230	6	600	27	—
Microwave Tenders	3.5 oz	230	11	600	19	—
Roasted Breasts	1 oz	50	3	160	—	—
Roasted Breasts Fillets	1 oz	50	2	160	—	—
Roasted Half Chicken	1 oz	60	4	150	—	—
Roasted Thighs	1 oz	70	5	180	—	—
Roasted Whole Chicken	1 oz	60	4	150	—	—
Southern Fried Breast Fillets	3 oz	220	11	630	15	—
Southern Fried Breast Patties	2.6 oz	220	15	460	9	—
Southern Fried Chick'n Chunks	2.6 oz	220	15	540	11	—
Thick & Crispy Patties	2.6 oz	220	14	490	13	—
Weaver						
Batter Dipped Breast	4.4 oz	310	20	220	13	—
Batter Dipped Drums & Thighs	3 oz	210	14	220	11	—
Batter Dipped Wings	4 oz	400	28	520	20	—
Breast Fillets	4.5 oz	270	13	520	18	—
Breast Fillets Strips	3.3 oz	200	10	500	14	—
Breast Patties	3 oz	205	11	640	14	—
Chicken Nuggets	2.6 oz	190	12	450	10	—
Crispy Dutch Frye Assorted	3.6 oz	290	18	550	16	—
Crispy Dutch Frye Breasts	4.5 oz	350	22	520	17	—
Crispy Dutch Frye Drums & Thighs	3.5 oz	290	19	640	14	—
Crispy Dutch Frye Wings	4 oz	400	28	520	20	—

FOOD	PORTION	CAL	FAT	SOD	CARB	FIB
Weaver *(cont.)*						
Crispy Light Skinless	2.9 oz	170	9	320	9	—
Croquettes	2 pieces	280	16	780	22	—
Croquettes With Gravy	2 pieces + ½ cup gravy	282	18	1040	26	—
Honey Batter Tenders	3 oz	220	12	500	14	—
Hot Wings	2.7 oz	170	11	670	1	—
Mini Drums Crispy	3 oz	210	12	480	13	—
Mini Drums Herbs & Spice	3 oz	200	11	320	13	—
Premium Tenders	3 oz	170	9	500	11	—
Roasted Drumsticks	1 oz	50	3	190	—	—
Rondelets Cheese	1 (2.6 oz)	190	11	520	12	—
Rondelets Italian	1 (2.6 oz)	190	11	560	11	—
Rondelets Original	1 (3 oz)	190	10	610	13	—
Weight Watchers						
Chicken Nuggets	5.9 oz	220	7	500	23	
READY-TO-USE						
Carl Buddig	1 oz	50	3	320	1	0
Dutch Family Roll	1 oz	61	15	—	—	—
Falls BBQ	3 oz	150	8	310	—	—
Healthy Choice Breast Skinless	1 oz	25	tr	240	tr	—
Hebrew National Deli Thin Oven Roasted	1.8 oz	45	1	460	—	—
Hillshire						
Deli Select Breast Oven Roasted	1 slice	10	tr	115	tr	—
Deli Select Breast Smoked	1 slice	10	tr	95	tr	—
Flavor Pack 90–99% Fat Free Breast Smoked	1 slice (0.75 oz)	20	tr	220	tr	—
Longacre Roll	1 oz	65	17	—	—	—
Louis Rich						
Deli-Thin Breast Oven Roasted	4 slices (1.8 oz)	60	2	620	1	0
Breast Deluxe Oven Roasted	1 slice (1 oz)	40	1	330	1	0
Breast Hickory Smoked	1 slice (1 oz)	30	1	360	1	0
White Oven Roasted	1 slice (1 oz)	40	3	350	1	0
Mr. Turkey Breast	1 slice (1 oz)	32	1	—	—	—

FOOD	PORTION	CAL	FAT	SOD	CARB	FIB
Oscar Mayer						
Breast Roast Thin Sliced	1 slice (.4 oz)	13	tr	151	tr	—
Smoked Breast	1 slice (1 oz)	25	tr	397	tr	—
Perdue Done It!						
BBQ Breast Half	1 oz	46	2	150	1	—
BBQ Drumsticks	1 oz	53	2	106	2	—
BBQ Half Dark Meat	1 oz	57	4	108	1	—
BBQ Half White Meat	1 oz	40	1	110	1	—
BBQ Thighs	1 oz	59	3	98	1	—
BBQ Wings	1 oz	62	4	169	1	—
Breast Roasted	1 oz	45	2	116	1	—
Cornish Hen Roasted Dark Meat	1 oz	45	3	72	tr	—
Cornish Hen Roasted White Meat	1 oz	39	1	93	tr	—
Cutlets	3.5 oz	250	14	445	17	—
Drumsticks Roasted	1 oz	40	1	115	0	—
Nuggets Cheese	1 (.67 oz)	54	4	108	3	—
Nuggets Fun Shaped	1 (.73 oz)	54	3	92	4	—
Nuggets Original	1 (.67 oz)	48	3	85	3	—
Tenders	1 oz	62	3	116	4	—
Thighs Roasted	1 oz	46	2	114	tr	—
Whole or Half Roasted Dark Meat	1 oz	51	3	73	tr	—
Whole or Half Roasted White Meat	1 oz	37	1	85	0	—
Wings Garlic & Herb	1 oz	61	4	172	tr	—
Wings Hot & Spicy	1 oz	60	4	190	1	—
Tyson						
Bologna	1 slice	44	1	185	4	—
Breast Hickory Smoked	1 slice	25	1	195	1	—
Breast Honey Flavored	1 slice	25	1	—	1	—
Breast Oven Roasted	1 slice	25	1	185	1	—
Breast Oven Roasted Mesquite	1 slice	25	1	—	1	—
Roll	1 slice	26	1	153	1	—
Wings Barbecue	6–7 (3.5 oz)	218	14	400	0	—
Wings Hot & Spicy	6–7 (3.5 oz)	218	14	400	0	—
Wings Roasted	6–7 (3.5 oz)	218	14	400	0	—
Wings Teriyaki	6–7 (3.5 oz)	218	14	400	0	—

FOOD	PORTION	CAL	FAT	SOD	CARB	FIB
Wampler Longacre						
Breast Stuffed w/ Breading; not prep	8 oz	472	94	—	—	—
Breast Stuffed w/ Cordon Bleu; not prep	6.5 oz	429	39	—	—	—
Breast Deli Sliced Browned Roasted	1 oz	49	11	—	—	—
Breast Meat	1 oz	38	2	—	—	—
Diced Breast	1 oz	38	2	—	—	—
Roll Diced Breast	1 oz	49	11	—	—	—
Roll Sliced	1 oz	63	16	—	—	—
Weaver						
Roasted Wings	1 oz	70	5	180	—	—
Weight Watchers						
Roasted and Smoked Breast	2 slices (0.75 oz)	25	1	220	tr	—
Roasted Ham	2 slices (0.75 oz)	25	1	210	tr	—
chicken roll light meat	1 pkg (6 oz)	271	13	992	4	—
chicken roll light meat	2 oz	90	4	331	1	—
poultry salad sandwich spread	1 oz	238	4	107	2	—
poultry salad sandwich spread	1 tbsp (13 g)	109	2	49	1	—
TAKE-OUT						
boneless breaded & fried						
w/ barbecue sauce	6 pieces (4.6 oz)	330	18	830	25	—
w/ honey	6 pieces (4 oz)	339	18	537	27	—
w/ mustard sauce	6 pieces (4.6 oz)	323	17	791	21	—
w/ sweet & sour sauce	6 pieces (4.6 oz)	346	18	791	29	—
breast & wing breaded & fried	2 pieces (5.7 oz)	494	30	975	20	—
drumstick breaded & fried	2 pieces (5.2 oz)	430	27	756	16	—
thigh breaded & fried	2 pieces (5.2 oz)	430	27	756	16	—

CHICKEN DISHES
see also CHICKEN SUBSTITUTES, DINNER

FOOD	PORTION	CAL	FAT	SOD	CARB	FIB
CANNED						
Chicken & Dumplings (Swanson)	7.5 oz	220	11	980	19	—
Chicken Ala King (Swanson)	5.25 oz	190	12	690	9	—
Chicken Stew (Swanson)	7.63 oz	160	7	990	15	—

FOOD	PORTION	CAL	FAT	SOD	CARB	FIB
FROZEN						
Kibun Chicken Pasta Salad w/ dressing	½ pkg	220	9	—	—	—
Kibun Chicken Pasta Salad w/o dressing	½ pkg	150	2	—	—	—
MicroMagic Chicken Sandwich	1 pkg (4.5 oz)	390	16	650	42	—
Ovenstuffs Chicken Turnover	1 (4.75 oz)	350	16	690	36	—
Weight Watchers Chicken & Broccoli Pita	1 (5.4 oz)	190	5	420	19	—
Weight Watchers Grilled Chicken Sandwich	1 (4 oz)	210	6	420	22	—
HOME RECIPE						
chicken & noodles	1 cup	365	18	600	26	—
chicken a la king	1 cup	470	34	760	12	—
MIX						
Lipton Microeasy Barbeque Chicken	¼ pkg	108	1	981	24	—
Lipton Microeasy Country Chicken	¼ pkg	78	1	844	15	—
Skillet Chicken Helper						
Cheesy Broccoli, as prep	⅕ pkg (7.5 oz)	270	6	790	34	—
Creamy Chicken, as prep	⅕ pkg (8.25 oz)	290	10	800	29	—
Creamy Mushroom, as prep	⅕ pkg (8 oz)	280	8	800	31	—
Fettucine Alfredo, as prep	⅕ pkg (7.5 oz)	270	8	800	29	—
Stir-Fried Chicken, as prep	⅕ pkg (7 oz)	330	11	940	36	—
READY-TO-USE						
Salad (Wampler Longacre)	1 oz	65	16	—	—	—
The Spreadables Chicken Salad	¼ can	100	6	—	—	—
TAKE-OUT						
chicken & dumplings	¾ cup	256	12	1283	12	tr
chicken cacciatore	¾ cup	394	24	671	9	2
chicken paprikash	1½ cups	296	10	—	—	—
chicken pie w/ top crust	1 slice (5.6 oz)	472	31	—	32	1
fillet sandwich, plain	1	515	29	957	39	—

FOOD	PORTION	CAL	FAT	SOD	CARB	FIB
fillet sandwich, w/ cheese, lettuce, mayonnaise & tomato	1	632	39	1238	42	—

CHICKEN SUBSTITUTES

FOOD	PORTION	CAL	FAT	SOD	CARB	FIB
Harvest Direct TVP Poultry Chunks	3.5 oz	280	1	15	32	18
Harvest Direct TVP Poultry Ground	3.5 oz	280	1	15	32	18
Jaclyn's Salsa Chicken Style Dinner	11.5 oz	325	9	290	35	—
Jaclyn's Sesame Chicken Style Dinner	11.5 oz	345	8	635	40	—
LaLoma Chicken Supreme, not prep	¼ cup (16 g)	50	0	450	4	—
LaLoma Chik Nuggets	5 nuggets (85 g)	270	20	530	8	—
LaLoma Fried Chicken	1 piece (57 g)	180	14	570	2	—
LaLoma Fried Chicken w/ Gravy	2 pieces (85 g)	140	10	340	4	—
Worthington						
Chick-ketts	½ cup (84 g)	160	7	640	6	—
ChickStiks	1 (47 g)	110	7	380	4	—
Chicken Sliced	2 slices (57 g)	130	9	460	3	—
CrispyChik	1 patty (71 g)	220	15	620	13	—
CrispyChik	6 nuggets (85 g)	280	19	500	17	—
Cutlets	1.5 slices (92 g)	100	2	270	4	—
Diced Chik	¼ cup (60 g)	90	8	330	2	—
FriChik	2 pieces (90 g)	180	13	610	13	—
Golden Croquettes	5 pieces (106 g)	280	14	890	20	—
Savory Slices	2 slices (60 g)	90	8	330	2	—
Vegetarian Chicken Pie	1 (227 g)	380	20	1200	43	—

CHICKPEAS
CANNED

FOOD	PORTION	CAL	FAT	SOD	CARB	FIB
Goya Spanish Style	7.5 oz	150	2	890	32	9
Green Giant Garbanzo	½ cup	90	2	320	18	5
Hanover	½ cup	100	1	—	—	—
Old El Paso Garbanzo	½ cup	190	tr	250	16	—
Progresso	½ cup	110	1	200	22	6
S&W Garbanzo Lite 50% Less Salt	½ cup	110	0	295	21	—
S&W Garbanzo Premium Large	½ cup	110	1	470	20	—

FOOD	PORTION	CAL	FAT	SOD	CARB	FIB
S&W Garbanzo Water Pack	½ cup	105	1	5	19	—
Chickpeas	1 cup	285	3	718	54	—
DRIED						
Bean Cuisine Garbanzo	½ cup	115	1	5	—	5
Hurst Brand Garbanzo	1 cup	288	4	—	—	—
cooked	1 cup	269	4	11	45	—

CHICORY
FRESH

FOOD	PORTION	CAL	FAT	SOD	CARB	FIB
greens, raw, chopped	½ cup	21	tr	41	4	—
root, raw	1 (2.1 oz)	44	tr	30	11	—
roots, raw, cut up	½ cup (1.6 oz)	33	tr	23	8	—
witloof, head, raw	1 (1.9 oz)	9	tr	1	2	—
witloof, raw	½ cup (1.6 oz)	8	tr	1	2	—

CHILI
CANNED
Dennison's

FOOD	PORTION	CAL	FAT	SOD	CARB	FIB
Chili Beans In Chili Gravy	7.5 oz	180	1	—	—	—
Chili Con Carne w/ Beans	7.5 oz	310	15	—	—	—
Chili Con Carne w/o Beans	7.5 oz	300	19	—	—	—
Chunky Chili w/ Beans	7.5 oz	310	14	—	—	—
Cook-off Chili w/ Beans	7.5 oz	340	19	—	—	—
Hot Chili Con Carne w/ Beans	7.5 oz	310	16	—	—	—
Gebhardt						
Hot With Beans	1 cup	470	27	1000	47	6
Plain	1 cup	530	43	990	20	1
With Beans	1 cup	495	28	1010	47	6
Hain						
Spicy Tempeh	7.5 oz	160	4	1350	24	—
Spicy Vegetarian	7.5 oz	160	1	1060	29	—
Spicy Vegetarian Reduced Sodium	7.5 oz	170	1	200	31	—
Spicy With Chicken	7.5 oz	130	2	1030	19	—
Health Valley						
Mild Vegetarian With Beans	5 oz	160	3	290	21	12

FOOD	PORTION	CAL	FAT	SOD	CARB	FIB
Health Valley *(cont.)*						
Mild Vegetarian With Beans No Salt Added	5 oz	160	3	30	21	12
Mild Vegetarian With Lentils	5 oz	140	4	290	15	7
Mild Vegetarian With Lentils No Salt Added	5 oz	140	4	50	15	7
Spicy Vegetarian With Beans	5 oz	160	4	280	21	12
Healthy Choice Spicy w/ Beans & Ground Turkey	½ can (7.5 oz)	210	5	530	26	—
Healthy Choice Turkey w/ Beans	½ can (7.5 oz)	200	5	560	20	—
Hunt's Chili Beans	4 oz	100	tr	490	18	6
Just Rite						
Hot With Beans	4 oz	195	10	495	16	1
With Beans	4 oz	200	11	500	16	1
Without Beans	4 oz	180	11	515	9	tr
Luck's Hot Chili Beans	7.5 oz	200	2	—	—	—
Manwich Chili Fixin's, as prep	8 oz	290	14	980	20	5
Natural Touch Vegetarian	⅔ cup (190 g)	230	12	890	19	—
Old El Paso Chili Con Carne	1 cup	162	7	510	8	2
Old El Paso Chili With Beans	1 cup	217	10	480	17	6
S&W Chili Beans	½ cup	130	1	520	23	—
S&W Chili Makin's Original	½ cup	100	1	782	20	—
Van Camp's						
Chili Weenee	1 cup	309	16	1057	28	—
Chili With Beans	1 cup	352	23	1215	21	—
Chili Without Beans	1 cup	412	36	1499	12	—
Wolf Brand						
Chili-Mac	7.5 oz	317	20	854	23	—
Extra Spicy With Beans	7.5 oz	324	21	926	21	—
Extra Spicy Without Beans	7.5 oz	363	25	962	15	—
Plain	7.5 oz	330	22	1165	10	—
With Beans	7.5 oz	345	22	1013	22	—
Without Beans	1 cup	387	27	1042	16	—
Worthington	⅔ cup (141 g)	190	10	550	15	—

FOOD	PORTION	CAL	FAT	SOD	CARB	FIB
chili w/ beans	1 cup	286	14	1330	30	—
DRIED						
powder	1 tsp	8	tr	26	1	—
Gebhardt Chili Powder	1 tsp	15	tr	0	3	tr
Gebhardt Chili Quik Seasoning	1 tsp	10	tr	165	2	tr
Hain Hot	¼ pkg	30	1	370	5	—
Hain Medium	¼ pkg	30	1	300	5	—
Hain Mild	¼ pkg	30	1	330	5	—
Old El Paso Seasoning Mix	⅛ pkg	21	1	717	4	1
FROZEN						
Lean Cuisine Three Bean	1 pkg (9 oz)	210	6	460	32	7
Lightlife	4.3 oz	110	3	360	14	—
Stouffer's With Beans	1 pkg (8.75 oz)	270	10	1130	29	8
Swanson Homestyle Chile Con Carne	8¼ oz	270	10	740	26	—
Tyson Chicken Chili	3.5 oz	105	3	420	11	—
TAKE-OUT						
con carne w/ beans	8.9 oz	254	8	1008	22	—

CHINESE CABBAGE
see CABBAGE

CHINESE FOOD
see ORIENTAL FOOD

CHINESE PRESERVING MELON

FOOD	PORTION	CAL	FAT	SOD	CARB	FIB
cooked	½ cup	11	tr	93	3	—

CHIPS
see also POPCORN, PRETZELS, SNACKS

FOOD	PORTION	CAL	FAT	SOD	CARB	FIB
CORN						
Fritos	34 pieces (1 oz)	150	10	220	16	1
Chili Cheese	34 pieces (1 oz)	160	10	300	15	1
Crisp 'N Thin	18 pieces (1 oz)	160	10	240	16	1
Dip Size	13 pieces (1 oz)	150	10	240	16	1
Non-Stop Nacho Cheese	34 pieces (1 oz)	150	9	220	16	1
Rowdy Rustlers Bar-B-Q	34 pieces (1 oz)	150	9	300	17	1
Wild 'N Mild	32 pieces (1 oz)	160	9	240	16	1
Health Valley	1 oz	160	11	90	13	1
Health Valley No Salt Added	1 oz	160	11	1	13	1

FOOD	PORTION	CAL	FAT	SOD	CARB	FIB
Health Valley With Cheddar Cheese	1 oz	160	10	120	15	1
Lance	1 pkg (50 g)	270	17	350	26	—
Lance BBQ	1 pkg (50 g)	260	16	360	25	—
Snyder's	1 oz	160	11	150	14	2
Snyder's BBQ	1 oz	160	11	200	14	2
Weight Watchers Corn Snacker	0.5 oz	60	2	230	10	—
Weight Watchers Corn Snackers Nacho Cheese	0.5 oz	60	2	270	10	—
Wise	1 oz	160	10	180	15	—
Corn Crunchies	1 oz	160	10	180	15	—
Crispy Corn	1 oz	160	10	125	15	—
Crispy Corn Nacho Cheese	1 oz	160	10	190	16	—
MULTIGRAIN						
Sunchips	12 pieces (1 oz)	150	8	100	18	—
Sunchips French Onion	12 pieces (1 oz)	140	7	120	18	—
POTATO						
Cape Cod	19 chips (1 oz)	150	8	110	17	1
Cottage Fries No Salt Added	1 oz	160	11	5	14	—
Eagle						
BBQ Thins	1 oz	150	10	220	15	—
Ranch Ridged	1 oz	160	10	220	15	—
Ridged	1 oz	150	10	220	15	—
Sour Cream & Onion	1 oz	150	10	240	15	—
Thins	1 oz	150	10	220	15	—
Eagle Kettle Fry						
BBQ Crunchy	1 oz	150	8	140	16	—
Cape Cod	1 oz	150	8	120	16	—
Cape Cod No Salt	1 oz	150	8	0	16	—
Cape Cod Waves	1 oz	150	8	120	16	—
Cape Cod Waves No Salt	1 oz	150	8	0	16	—
Dill & Sour Cream	1 oz	150	8	160	16	—
Dill & Sour Cream No Salt	1 oz	150	8	15	16	—
Extra Crunchy	1 oz	150	8	180	16	—
Idaho Russet	1 oz	150	8	180	16	—
Louisiana BBQ	1 oz	150	8	140	16	—
Health Valley						
Country Ripple	1 oz	160	10	60	15	1
Country Ripple No Salt Added	1 oz	160	10	1	15	1

FOOD	PORTION	CAL	FAT	SOD	CARB	FIB
Dip Chips	1 oz	160	10	60	15	1
Dip Chips No Salt Added	1 oz	160	10	1	15	1
Natural	1 oz	160	10	60	15	1
Natural No Salt Added	1 oz	160	10	1	15	1
Kelly's	1 oz	150	9	160	14	2
Bar-B-Q	1 oz	150	9	230	15	1
Crunchy	1 oz	150	9	140	17	2
Rippled	1 oz	150	9	160	14	2
Sour Cream n' Onion	1 oz	150	9	170	15	1
Unsalted	1 oz	150	10	5	14	—
Lance	1 pkg (32 g)	190	15	220	12	—
BBQ	1 pkg (32 g)	190	12	270	18	—
Cajun Style	1 pkg (32 g)	160	11	250	16	—
Hot Fries	1 pkg (28 g)	160	10	220	14	—
Ripple	1 pkg (32 g)	190	15	220	12	—
Sour Cream & Onion	1 pkg (32 g)	190	12	390	18	—
Lay's	17 pieces (1 oz)	150	10	170	15	1
Bar-B-Q	17 pieces (1 oz)	150	9	270	15	1
Cheddar Cheese	17 pieces (1 oz)	150	10	300	14	1
Crunch Tators	16 pieces (1 oz)	150	8	120	17	1
Crunch Tators Amazin' Cajun	16 pieces (1 oz)	150	8	150	17	—
Crunch Tators Hoppin' Jalapeno	16 pieces (1 oz)	140	7	200	18	1
Crunch Tators Mighty Mesquite	16 pieces (1 oz)	150	8	135	17	—
Crunch Tators Supreme Sour Cream	16 pieces (1 oz)	150	8	180	16	—
Flamin' Hot	17 pieces (1 oz)	150	9	190	15	1
Kansas City Style Bar-B-Q	17 pieces (1 oz)	150	9	270	15	1
Salt & Vinegar	17 Pieces (1 oz)	150	10	390	14	1
Sour Cream & Onion	17 pieces (1 oz)	160	10	220	15	1
Tangy Ranch	17 pieces (1 oz)	160	10	210	15	1
Unsalted	17 pieces (1 oz)	150	10	10	15	1
Louise's Fat-Free	1 oz	100	tr	160	23	—
Mr. Phipps Tater Crisps						
Bar-B-Que	11 (0.5 oz)	60	2	160	10	—
Original	11 (0.5 oz)	60	2	130	10	—
Sour Cream 'n Onion	11 (0.5 oz)	60	2	150	10	—
New York Deli	1oz	160	11	120	14	—
Old Dutch Foods	1 oz	150	9	160	16	—

FOOD	PORTION	CAL	FAT	SOD	CARB	FIB
Old Dutch Foods *(cont.)*						
Augratin	1 oz	150	8	220	15	—
BBQ	1 oz	140	8	360	16	—
Dill Flavored	1 oz	150	8	340	16	—
Onion & Garlic	1 oz	150	9	420	15	—
Ripple	1 oz	150	9	150	16	—
Sour Cream & Onion	1 oz	150	10	220	15	—
Pringle's	1 oz	170	13	—	—	—
Butter 'n Herbs	1 oz	170	13	—	—	—
Cheez-ums	1 oz	170	13	—	—	—
Idaho Rippled	1 oz	170	12	—	—	—
Idaho Rippled French Onion	1 oz	170	12	—	—	—
Idaho Rippled Taco 'n Cheddar	1 oz	170	12	—	—	—
Light	1 oz	150	8	—	—	—
Light B-B-Q	1 oz	150	8	—	—	—
Rippled	1 oz	170	12	—	—	—
Sour Cream & Onion	1 oz	170	12	—	—	—
Ruffles	18 chips (1 oz)	150	10	135	15	1
Cheddar Cheese & Sour Cream	18 chips (1 oz)	160	10	250	15	1
Light	18 chips (1 oz)	130	6	140	19	1
Mesquite Grille B-B-Q	18 chips (1 oz)	160	10	270	15	1
Monterey Jack Cheese Flavor Cheese Attack	18 chips (1 oz)	160	10	200	15	1
Ranch	18 chips (1 oz)	160	10	220	15	1
Sour Cream & Onion	18 chips (1 oz)	160	10	220	15	1
Sour Cream & Onion Light	18 chips (1 oz)	130	6	190	18	1
Snyder's	1 oz	150	10	130	13	1
BBQ	1 oz	150	10	370	13	1
Cheddar Bacon	1 oz	150	10	260	13	1
Coney Island	1 oz	150	10	280	13	1
Grilled Steak & Onion	1 oz	150	10	260	13	1
Hot Buffalo Wings	1 oz	150	10	200	13	1
Kosher Dill	1 oz	150	10	400	13	1
No Salt	1 oz	150	10	0	13	1
Salt & Vinegar	1 oz	150	10	200	13	1
Sausage Pizza	1 oz	150	10	230	13	1
Sour Cream & Onion	1 oz	150	10	190	13	1
Sour Cream & Onion Unsalted	1 oz	150	10	10	13	1

FOOD	PORTION	CAL	FAT	SOD	CARB	FIB
Suprimos Cheddar & Jack	1 oz	140	6	180	17	—
Suprimos Cool Onion	1 oz	140	6	170	17	—
Weight Watchers Great Snackers						
Barbecue	0.5 oz	70	3	100	10	—
Cheddar Cheese	0.5 oz	70	3	130	10	—
Sour Cream & Onion	½ oz	70	3	140	10	—
Wise Natural	1 oz	160	11	190	14	—
Wise Ridgles Barbecue	1 oz	150	10	240	14	—
potato	1 oz	152	10	168	15	1
potato	1 pkg (8 oz)	1217	79	1347	120	8
sticks	1 pkg (1 oz)	148	10	71	15	—
sticks	½ cup	94	6	45	10	—
TORTILLA						
Doritos Lightly Salted	16 (1 oz)	150	7	135	18	2
Doritos Salsa 'N Cheese	16 (1 oz)	150	8	180	17	2
Eagle	1 oz	150	8	140	18	—
Nacho	1 oz	150	8	200	17	—
Ranch	1 oz	150	8	150	17	—
Restaurant Style	1 oz	150	7	100	18	—
Strips	1 oz	150	8	140	18	—
Guiltless Gourmet Baked	22–26 chips (1 oz)	110	1	119	21	1
Hain						
Sesame	1 oz	140	7	190	19	—
Sesame No Salt Added	1 oz	140	7	<5	19	—
Sesame Cheese	1 oz	160	8	270	20	—
Taco Style	1 oz	160	11	320	15	—
La FAMOUS	1 oz	140	7	180	18	—
La FAMOUS No Salt Added	1 oz	140	7	5	18	—
Lance Jalapeno Cheese	1 pkg (1.13 oz)	160	8	—	—	—
Lance Nacho	1 pkg (32 g)	160	8	240	19	—
Old El Paso Crispy Corn	16 chips (1 oz)	150	8	106	17	1
Old El Paso NACHIPS	9 chips (1 oz)	150	7	80	18	2
Santitas	1 oz	140	7	50	19	2
Cantina Style	1 oz	140	6	75	19	2
Cantina Style Fajita Flavored	1 oz	140	7	95	19	2
Strips	1 oz	140	7	65	19	2
Snyder's	1 oz	140	7	130	18	2
Enchilada	1 oz	140	7	220	18	2

FOOD	PORTION	CAL	FAT	SOD	CARB	FIB
Snyder's *(cont.)*						
Nacho Cheese	1 oz	140	7	130	18	2
No Salt	1 oz	140	7	0	18	2
Ranch	1 oz	140	7	150	18	2
Tostitos	11 pieces (1 oz)	140	8	160	18	2
Bite Size	16 pieces (1 oz)	150	8	110	18	2
Restaurant Style Lime 'N Chili	7 pieces (1 oz)	150	7	190	18	2
Restaurant Style White Corn	7 pieces (1 oz)	150	6	75	20	2
Tostitos Baked	1 oz	110	1	140	24	2
Cool Ranch	1 oz	130	3	170	21	2
Unsalted	1 oz	110	1	0	24	2
Tyson						
Nacho Cheese	1 oz	140	7	145	17	—
Ranch Flavor	1 oz	140	2	—	17	—
Traditional	1 oz	140	7	95	17	—
Unsalted	1 oz	140	7	7	17	—
Wise BRAVOS	1 oz	150	8	180	18	—

CHITTERLINGS

pork, simmered	3 oz	258	24	33	0	—

CHIVES

freeze-dried	1 tbsp	1	tr	—	tr	—
fresh chopped	1 tbsp	1	tr	0	tr	—
fresh chopped	1 tsp	0	tr	0	tr	—

CHOCOLATE

see also CANDY, CAROB, ICE CREAM TOPPINGS, MILK DRINKS

BAKING

Baker's Semi-Sweet	1 oz	135	9	1	17	—
Baker's Unsweetened	1 oz	141	15	1	9	—
Baker's German Sweet	1 oz	143	10	1	17	—
Baker's German Sweet	¼ cup	200	12	1	27	—
Hershey Premium Semi-Sweet	1 oz	140	8	—	16	—
Hershey Premium Unsweetened	1 oz	190	16	5	7	—
Nestle Choco Bake	½ oz	80	8	0	5	3
Nestle Semi-Sweet	½ oz	70	4	0	9	2
Nestle Unsweetened	½ oz	80	7	0	5	3
Nestle Premier White	½ oz	80	5	15	8	—
baking	1 oz	145	15	1	8	—

FOOD	PORTION	CAL	FAT	SOD	CARB	FIB
CHIPS						
Baker's	1 oz	143	8	25	18	—
Baker's Semi-Sweet	¼ cup	197	9	29	30	—
Baker's Big Milk Chocolate	¼ cup	239	14	42	30	—
Baker's Big Semi-Sweet	¼ cup	220	13	1	31	—
Baker's Real Semi-Sweet	¼ cup	198	12	1	28	—
Hershey						
Chunks Milk Chocolate	1 oz	160	9	25	16	—
Chunks Semi-Sweet	1 oz	140	8	—	15	—
Milk Chocolate	1 oz	150	12	55	27	—
Miniature Semi-Sweet	¼ cup (1.5 oz)	220	12	5	26	—
Mint Chocolate	¼ cup	230	12	—	28	—
Semi-Sweet	¼ cup (1.5 oz)	220	12	5	26	—
Nestle Morsels Milk Chocolate (Nestle)	1 tbsp	70	4	0	10	—
Nestle Morsels Mint Chocolate (Nestle)	1 tbsp	70	4	0	9	2
Nestle Morsels Rainbow (Nestle)	1 tbsp	70	3	0	10	1
Nestle Morsels Semi-Sweet (Nestle)	1 tbsp	40	4	0	9	2
Nestle Morsels Semi-Sweet Mini (Nestle)	1 tbsp	70	4	0	9	2
MIX						
Hershey Chocolate Milk Mix	3 tbsp	90	4	40	22	—
powder	2–3 heaping tsp	75	1	45	20	—
powder, as prep w/ whole milk	9 oz	226	9	165	31	—
SYRUP						
Estee	1 tbsp	20	tr	5	5	—
Hershey's	2 tbsp	80	1	20	17	—
chocolate	1 cup	653	3	287	177	—
chocolate	2 tbsp	82	tr	36	22	—
chocolate, as prep w/ whole milk	9 oz	232	9	156	34	—

CHOCOLATE MILK

see CHOCOLATE, COCOA, MILK DRINKS

CHUTNEY

apple	1.2 oz	68	0	—	18	1
apple cranberry	1 tbsp	16	0	1	4	—

FOOD	PORTION	CAL	FAT	SOD	CARB	FIB
tomato	1.2 oz	54	0	—	14	1
CILANTRO						
fresh	¼ cup	1	tr	1	tr	—
CINNAMON						
ground	1 tsp	6	tr	1	2	—
CISCO						
raw	3 oz	84	2	47	0	—
smoked	1 oz	50	3	135	0	—
smoked	3 oz	151	10	409	0	—
CLAMS						
CANNED						
American Original Foods Quahogs	4 oz	66	tr	—	2	—
Doxsee Chopped	6.5 oz	90	tr	1020	6	—
Doxsee Clam Juice	3 fl oz	4	0	110	0	—
Empress Whole Baby	4 oz	60	1	540	2	—
Gorton's Minced & Chopped	½ can	70	1	640	4	—
Progresso	½ cup	70	tr	140	2	—
Progresso Red Clam Sauce	½ cup	70	3	560	7	—
Progresso White Clam Sauce	½ cup	110	8	280	1	—
S&W Fancy Chopped	2 oz	28	0	280	2	—
S&W Fancy Minced	2 oz	28	0	280	2	—
S&W Whole Baby Chowder Clams	2 oz	33	0	—	1	—
Snow's Minced	6.5 oz	90	tr	1020	6	—
liquid only	1 cup	6	tr	516	tr	—
liquid only	3 oz	2	tr	183	tr	—
meat only	1 cup	236	3	179	8	—
meat only	3 oz	126	2	95	4	—
FRESH						
cooked	20 sm	133	2	100	5	—
cooked	3 oz	126	2	95	4	—
raw	20 sm (180 g)	133	2	100	5	—
raw	3 oz	63	1	47	2	—
raw	9 lg (180 g)	133	2	100	5	—
FROZEN						
Fried (Mrs. Paul's)	2.5 oz	200	9	450	21	—
Microwave Crunchy Clam Strips (Gorton's)	3.5 oz	330	22	430	24	—

FOOD	PORTION	CAL	FAT	SOD	CARB	FIB
Microwave Fried Clams (Mrs. Paul's)	2.5 oz	260	15	410	23	—
HOME RECIPE						
breaded & fried	20 sm	379	21	684	19	—
breaded & fried	3 oz	171	9	309	9	—
TAKE-OUT						
breaded & fried	¾ cup	451	26	833	39	—

CLOVES
ground	1 tsp	7	tr	5	1	—

COCOA
see also CHOCOLATE

FOOD	PORTION	CAL	FAT	SOD	CARB	FIB
Carnation Hot						
Cocoa 70 calorie	3 tsp (21 g)	70	tr	—	—	—
Cocoa Milk Chocolate	1 pkg or 4 heaping tsp (1 oz)	110	1	—	—	—
Cocoa Natural Mint	1 pkg or 4 heaping tsp (1 oz)	110	1	—	—	—
Cocoa Rich Chocolate	1 pkg or 4 heaping tsp (1 oz)	110	1	—	—	—
Cocoa Rich Chocolate w/ Marshmallows	1 pkg or 4 heaping tsp (1 oz)	110	1	—	—	—
Cocoa Sugar Free Mint	1 pkg or 4 heaping tsp (15 g)	50	tr	—	—	—
Cocoa Sugar Free Rich Chocolate	1 pkg or 4 heaping tsp (15 g)	50	tr	—	—	—
Hershey	⅓ cup (1 oz)	120	4	10	13	—
Hershey European Cocoa	1 oz	90	3	15	8	—
Hills Bros. Hot Cocoa	6 oz	110	2	—	—	—
Hills Bros. Hot Cocoa Sugar Free	6 oz	60	2	—	—	—
Nestle	1 tbsp	15	1	0	3	2
Nestle						
Mix	1 oz	110	1	100	23	—
Mix, as prep w/ 2% milk	6 oz	210	5	190	32	—
Mix, as prep w/ skim milk	6 oz	180	1	200	32	—

FOOD	PORTION	CAL	FAT	SOD	CARB	FIB
Nestle *(cont.)*						
Mix, as prep w/ whole milk	6 oz	230	8	240	32	—
Mix With Marshmallows	1 oz	120	1	115	23	—
Mix With Marshmallows, as prep w/ 2% milk	6 oz	220	5	190	32	—
Mix With Marshmallows, as prep w/ skim milk	6 oz	190	1	200	32	—
Mix With Marshmallows, as prep w/ whole milk	6 oz	240	8	240	32	—
Swiss Miss Cocoa						
Diet	6 oz	20	tr	180	3	0
Lite, as prep	6 oz	70	tr	160	17	0
Sugar Free, as prep	6 oz	60	tr	125	10	0
Sugar Free With Sugar Free Marshmallows, as prep	6 oz	50	tr	120	9	0
Swiss Miss Hot						
Cocoa Bavarian Chocolate	6 oz	110	3	170	20	0
Cocoa Double Rich	6 oz	110	1	150	22	0
Cocoa Milk Chocolate	6 oz	110	1	125	24	0
Cocoa With Mini Marshmallows	6 oz	110	1	170	23	0
Ultra Slim-Fast Hot Cocoa, as prep w/ water	8 oz	190	tr	140	35	5
Weight Watchers	1 pkg	60	0	160	10	—
hot cocoa	1 cup	218	9	123	26	—
mix w/ Nutrasweet, as prep w/ water	7 oz	48	tr	173	9	—
mix, as prep w/ water	7 oz	103	1	149	23	—
powder	1 oz	102	1	143	23	—

COCONUT

FOOD	PORTION	CAL	FAT	SOD	CARB	FIB
Angel Flake Toasted (Baker's)	⅓ cup	212	17	83	17	—
Cream of Coconut (Coco Lopez)	2 tbsp	120	5	10	20	—
Premium Shred (Baker's)	⅓ cup	135	9	84	12	—

FOOD	PORTION	CAL	FAT	SOD	CARB	FIB
coconut water	1 cup	46	tr	252	9	—
coconut water	1 tbsp	3	tr	16	1	—
cream, canned	1 cup	568	52	149	25	—
cream, canned	1 tbsp	36	3	10	2	—
dried, sweetened, flaked	1 cup	351	24	189	35	—
dried, sweetened, flaked	7 oz pkg	944	64	509	95	—
dried, sweetened, flaked, canned	1 cup	341	24	15	32	—
dried, sweetened, shredded	1 cup	466	33	244	44	—
dried, sweetened, shredded	7 oz pkg	997	71	522	95	—
dried, toasted	1 oz	168	13	11	13	—
dried, unsweetened	1 oz	187	18	11	7	—
fresh	1 piece (1.5 oz)	159	15	9	7	4
fresh, shredded	1 cup	283	27	16	12	7
milk, canned	1 cup	445	48	29	6	—
milk, canned	1 tbsp	30	3	2	tr	—
milk, frozen	1 cup	486	50	29	13	—
milk, frozen	1 tbsp	30	3	2	1	—

COD
CANNED
atlantic	1 can (11 oz)	327	3	680	0	—
atlantic	3 oz	89	1	185	0	—
roe	3.5 oz	118	3	—	tr	—

DRIED
atlantic	3 oz	246	2	5973	0	—

FRESH
atlantic, raw	3 oz	70	1	46	0	—
atlantic, cooked	1 fillet (6.3 oz)	189	2	141	0	—
atlantic, cooked	3 oz	89	1	66	0	—
pacific, baked	3 oz	95	1	82	0	—
roe, baked w/ butter & lemon juice	3.5 oz	126	3	73	2	—
roe, raw	3.5 oz	130	2	—	2	—

FROZEN
Fishmarket Fresh (Gorton's)	5 oz	110	1	90	0	—
Light Fillets (Mrs. Paul's)	1 fillet	240	11	430	22	—
Light Fillets (Van De Kamp's)	1 piece	250	11	510	20	—

FOOD	PORTION	CAL	FAT	SOD	CARB	FIB
Natural Fillets (Van De Kamp's)	4 oz	90	1	90	0	—

COFFEE
see also COFFEE, BEVERAGES, COFFEE SUBSTITUTES

INSTANT

cappuccino mix, as prep	7 oz	62	2	104	11	—
decaffeinated	1 rounded tsp (1.8 g)	4	0	0	1	—
decaffeinated, as prep	6 oz	4	0	6	1	—
french mix, as prep	7 oz	57	3	—	7	—
kava	1 tsp	2	0	<5	1	—
mocha mix, as prep	7 oz	51	2	36	8	—
regular	1 rounded tsp	4	0	1	1	—
regular, as prep	6 oz	4	0	6	1	—
regular w/ chicory	1 rounded tsp	6	0	5	1	—
regular w/ chicory, as prep	6 oz	6	0	10	1	—

REGULAR

brewed	6 oz	4	0	4	1	—

TAKE-OUT

cafe au lai	1 cup (8 fl oz)	77	4	62	6	—
cafe brulot	1 cup (4.8 fl oz)	48	0	2	3	—
cafe con leche	1 cup (8 fl oz)	77	4	62	6	—
espresso	1 cup (3 fl oz)	2	0	2	tr	—
irish coffee	1 serving (9 fl oz)	107	3	25	3	—
mocha	1 mug (9.6 fl oz)	202	15	28	17	—

COFFEE BEVERAGES
see also COFFEE SUBSTITUTES

Chock o'ccino (Chock Full o' Nuts)						
Cinnamon	8 oz	120	2	55	25	—
Coffee	8 oz	120	2	55	25	—
Mocha	8 oz	120	2	55	25	—
International Coffee						
Cafe Amaretto (General Foods)	6 oz	51	3	—	—	—
Cafe Francais	6 oz	55	3	—	—	—
Cafe Irish Creme	6 oz	55	3	—	—	—
Cafe Vienna	6 oz	59	2	—	—	—
Irish Mocha Mint	6 oz	51	2	—	—	—
Orange Cappuccino	6 oz	59	10	—	—	—
Sugar Free Cafe Francais	6 oz	35	2	—	—	—

FOOD	PORTION	CAL	FAT	SOD	CARB	FIB
Sugar Free Irish Creme	6 oz	31	3	—	—	—
Sugar Free Cafe Vienna	6 oz	29	3	—	—	—
Sugar Free Irish Mocha Mint	6 oz	28	2	—	—	—
Sugar Free Orange Cappuccino	6 oz	29	2	—	—	—
Sugar Free Suisse Mocha	6 oz	29	2	—	—	—
Suisse Mocha	6 oz	53	3	—	—	—

COFFEE SUBSTITUTES

FOOD	PORTION	CAL	FAT	SOD	CARB	FIB
Kaffree Roma Natural Touch	1 tsp	6	0	—	1	—
Postum Instant	6 oz	11	0	3	3	—
Postum Instant Coffee Flavored	6 oz	11	0	3	3	—
powder	1 tsp	9	tr	2	2	—
powder, as prep	6 oz	9	tr	7	2	—
powder, as prep w/ milk	6 oz	121	6	91	10	—

COFFEE WHITENERS
see also MILK SUBSTITUTES

LIQUID

FOOD	PORTION	CAL	FAT	SOD	CARB	FIB
Coffee-Mate	1 oz	31	2	—	—	—
Coffee-Rich	1 tbsp	20	2	—	—	—
Grand Union	1 tbsp	24	2	—	—	—
International Delight (Naturally Yours)						
Amaretto	1 tbsp (0.6 fl oz)	45	2	5	7	0
Cinnamon Hazelnut	1 tbsp (0.6 fl oz)	45	2	5	7	0
Irish Creme	1 tbsp (0.6 fl oz)	45	2	5	7	0
No Fat Amaretto	1 tbsp (0.5 fl oz)	30	0	5	7	0
No Fat French Vanilla	1 tbsp (0.5 fl oz)	30	0	5	7	0
No Fat Hawaiian Macadamia	1 tbsp (0.5 fl oz)	30	0	5	7	0
No Fat Irish Creme	1 tbsp (0.5 fl oz)	30	0	5	7	0
Suisse Chocolate Mocha	1 tbsp (0.6 fl oz)	45	2	10	7	0
nondairy, frzn	1 tbsp	20	2	12	2	—

POWDER

FOOD	PORTION	CAL	FAT	SOD	CARB	FIB
Coffee-Mate	1 pkg (3 g)	16	tr	—	—	—

FOOD	PORTION	CAL	FAT	SOD	CARB	FIB
Coffee-Mate	1 tsp	10	tr	—	—	—
Cremora	1 tsp	12	1	5	1	—
N-Rich Creamer	1 tsp	10	tr	0	1	0
Weight Watchers Dairy Creamer Instant Non-fat Dry Milk	1 pkg	10	0	15	1	—
nondairy	1 tsp	11	tr	4	1	—

COLLARDS

FRESH
cooked	½ cup	17	tr	10	4	—
raw, chopped	½ cup	6	tr	4	1	—

FROZEN
chopped, cooked	½ cup	31	tr	42	6	—

COOKIES
see also BROWNIE, CAKE, DOUGHNUTS, PIE

HOME RECIPE
chocolate chip, as prep w/ butter	1 (0.42 oz)	78	5	55	9	—
chocolate chip, as prep w/ margarine	1 (0.56 oz)	78	5	58	9	—
macaroons	1 (0.8 oz)	97	3	59	17	—
oatmeal	1 (0.5 oz)	67	3	90	10	—
oatmeal w/ raisins	1 (0.52 oz)	65	2	81	10	—
peanut butter	1 (0.7 oz)	95	5	104	12	—
shortbread, as prep w/ butter	1 (0.38 oz)	60	4	51	6	—
shortbread, as prep w/ margarine	1 (0.38 oz)	60	4	56	6	—
sugar, as prep w/ butter	1 (0.49 oz)	66	3	64	8	—
sugar, as prep w/ margarine	1 (0.49 oz)	66	3	69	8	—

MIX
Chocolate Chip (Duncan Hines)	2	130	5	—	—	—
Chocolate Chip Big Batch (Betty Crocker)	2	120	6	100	16	—
Chocolate Chip Cookie Mix (Estee)	1 (2 in)	50	3	40	6	—
Date Bar Classic Dessert (Betty Crocker)	1	60	2	35	9	—
Golden Sugar (Duncan Hines)	2	130	6	—	—	—

FOOD	PORTION	CAL	FAT	SOD	CARB	FIB
Oatmeal Raisin (Duncan Hines)	2	130	6	—	—	—
Peanut Butter (Duncan Hines)	2	140	7	—	—	—
chocolate chip	1 (0.56 oz)	79	4	47	10	—
oatmeal	1 (0.6 oz)	74	3	75	10	tr
READY-TO-EAT						
7-Grain Oatmeal Frookie	1	45	2	35	7	—
Almond Crecents (Sunshine)	2	70	3	55	10	—
Almond Crescents (Archway)	2 (0.8 oz)	100	4	75	17	tr
Almond Toast Mandel (Stella D'Oro)	1	60	1	43	10	—
Aloha (LU)	1	75	5	—	—	—
Amaranth Cookies (Health Valley)	1	70	3	30	12	2
Angel Bars (Stella D'Oro)	1	80	5	15	7	—
Angel Wings (Stella D'Oro)	1	70	5	40	7	—
Angelica Goodies (Stella D'Oro)	1	110	4	45	16	—
Anginetti (Stella D'Oro)	1	30	1	3	5	—
Animal (Little Debbie)	1 pkg (1.5 oz)	190	5	110	33	0
Animal Cookies Candied (Grandma's)	5 (1 oz)	140	6	80	20	—
Animal Crackers (FFV)	9	110	3	—	—	—
Animal Crackers (Sunshine)	7	70	2	60	12	—
Animal Crackers Barnum's (Nabisco)	5 (0.5 oz)	60	2	70	11	—
Animal Frackers (Frookie)	6	60	2	25	9	—
Anisette Sponge (Stella D'Oro)	1	50	1	40	10	—
Anisette Toast (Stella D'Oro)	1	50	1	50	9	—
Anisette Toast Jumbo (Stella D'Oro)	1	110	1	65	23	—
Apple Cinnamon Oat Bran (Frookie)	1	45	2	35	7	—
Apple Cinnamon Oat Bran (Frookie)	1 lg	120	4	100	18	—
Apple Fruitins (Frookie)	1	60	1	25	12	—

FOOD	PORTION	CAL	FAT	SOD	CARB	FIB
Apple N'Raisin (Archway)	1 (1.1 oz)	130	52	105	20	1
Apple Newtons (Nabisco)	1 (0.75 oz)	70	2	70	15	—
Apple Newtons Fat Free (Nabisco)	1 (0.75 oz)	70	0	45	16	—
Apple Pastry Low Sodium (Stella D'Oro)	1	80	3	5	14	—
Apple Raisin Bar (Weight Watchers)	1	100	3	115	18	—
Apricot Filled (Archway)	1 (1 oz)	110	4	90	18	tr
Arrowroot Biscuit (Nabisco)	1 (0.25 oz)	20	1	15	3	—
Bakers Bonus Oatmeal (Nabisco)	1 (0.5 oz)	80	3	65	12	—
Barre Chocolat (LU)	1	65	3	—	—	—
Bavarian Fingers (Sunshine)	1	70	3	55	10	—
Beacon Hill Chocolate Chocolate Walnut (Pepperidge Farm)	1	120	7	65	14	1
Bells And Stars (Archway)	3 (1 oz)	150	7	100	19	tr
Biscos Sugar Wafers (Nabisco)	4 (0.5 oz)	70	3	20	10	—
Biscos Waffle Cremes (Nabisco)	1 (0.25 oz)	40	2	10	6	—
Biscottini Cashews (Stella D'Oro)	1	110	6	50	14	—
Blueberry Filled (Archway)	1 (1 oz)	110	4	115	19	tr
Bordeaux (Pepperidge Farm)	2	70	3	40	11	0
Breakfast Treats (Stella D'Oro)	1	100	4	80	15	—
Brown Edge Wafers (Nabisco)	2½ (0.5 oz)	70	2	45	10	—
Brownie Chocolate Nut (Pepperidge Farm)	2	110	7	45	11	—
Brownie Nut Large (Pepperidge Farm)	1	140	8	65	15	—
Brussels (Pepperidge Farm)	2	110	5	65	13	0

FOOD	PORTION	CAL	FAT	SOD	CARB	FIB
Brussels Mint (Pepperidge Farm)	2	130	7	40	17	—
Bugs Bunny Graham Cookies (Nabisco)	5 (0.5 oz)	60	2	70	11	—
Butter (Pally)	4 (0.88 oz)	100	3	95	17	—
Butter Chessman (Pepperidge Farm)	2	90	4	60	12	—
Butter Flavored Cookies (Sunshine)	2	60	2	55	9	—
Buttercup (Keebler)	3	70	3	110	11	—
Cameo (Nabisco)	1 (0.5 oz)	70	3	50	10	—
Cappucino (Pepperidge Farm)	1	50	3	20	6	—
Capri (Pepperidge Farm)	1	80	5	45	10	—
Caramel Cookie Bars (Little Debbie)	1 pkg (1.2 oz)	160	8	90	23	1
Caramel Patties (FFV)	2	150	7	—	—	—
Carrot Cake (Archway)	1 (1 oz)	120	5	180	18	0
Castelets Chocolate (Stella D'Oro)	1	60	3	33	9	—
Champagne (Pepperidge Farm)	2	110	6	—	—	—
Chantilly (Pepperidge Farm)	1	80	2	35	14	—
Chesapeake Chocolate Chunk Pecan (Pepperidge Farm)	1	120	7	60	14	1
Cherry Filled (Archway)	1 (1 oz)	110	4	100	19	tr
Cherry Nougat (Archway)	3 (1 oz)	150	9	40	18	0
Cheyenne Peanut Butter Milk Chocolate Chunk (Pepperidge Farm)	1	110	6	80	13	1
Chinese Dessert Cookies (Stella D'Oro)	1	170	9	90	19	—
Chip-A-Roos (Sunshine)	1	60	3	45	7	—
Chips Ahoy!						
Bite Size Chocolate Chip (Nabisco)	6 (0.5 oz)	70	3	50	9	—
Chewy Chocolate Chip	1 (0.5 oz)	60	3	40	8	—
Chocolate Chunk Pecan	1 (0.5 oz)	100	6	65	10	—

FOOD	PORTION	CAL	FAT	SOD	CARB	FIB
Chips Ahoy! *(cont.)*						
Chunky Chocolate Chip	1 (0.5 oz)	90	5	90	11	—
Heath Toffee Chunk	1 (0.5 oz)	90	5	90	10	—
Oatmeal Chocolate Chip	1	90	5	50	10	—
Real Chocolate Chip	1 (0.5 oz)	50	2	40	7	—
Rockers Chocolate Chip	1 (0.5 oz)	60	3	40	8	—
Sprinkled Real Chocolate Chip	1 (0.5 oz)	60	3	40	8	—
Striped Chocolate Chip	1 (0.5 oz)	90	5	45	10	—
White Fudge Chunk	1 (0.5 oz)	90	5	75	10	—
Chips Chocolat (LU)	1	85	5	—	—	—
Choc-O-Lunch (Lance)	1 pkg (37 g)	180	7	150	26	—
Choc-O-Mint (Lance)	1 pkg (35 g)	180	10	90	22	—
Chocolate (Weight Watchers)	3	80	3	135	13	—
Chocolate Chip						
(Archway)	1 (1 oz)	130	6	150	19	0
(Drake's)	2 (1 oz)	140	6	110	18	—
(Duncan Hines)	2	110	5	—	—	—
(Dutch Mill)	3 (1.1 oz)	160	10	85	18	1
(Entenmann's)	3 (0.9 oz)	140	7	85	19	—
(Famous Amos)	3 (1 oz)	140	6	100	20	—
(Frookie)	1	45	2	35	7	—
(Frookie)	1 lg	120	4	100	18	—
(Grandma's)	2 (2.75 oz)	370	17	270	50	—
(Nutra/Balance)	1 (2 oz)	260	14	81	34	8
(Pepperidge Farm)	2	100	5	45	12	0
(Weight Watchers)	2	90	2	65	18	—
Chocolate Chip Bag (Archway)	3 (0.9 oz)	130	7	70	17	0
Chocolate Chip Bar (Tastykake)	1 (43 g)	190	8	95	28	1
Chocolate Chip Chewy (Little Debbie)	1 pkg (2 oz)	370	19	280	47	1
Chocolate Chip Crisp (Little Debbie)	1 pkg (1.5 oz)	210	12	150	26	1
Chocolate Chip Drop (Archway)	1 (1 oz)	140	10	105	11	tr
Chocolate Chip Fudge (Lance)	1 (28 g)	130	5	130	20	—

FOOD	PORTION	CAL	FAT	SOD	CARB	FIB
Chocolate Chip Ice Box (Archway)	1 (1 oz)	140	7	80	19	9
Chocolate Chip Large (Pepperidge Farm)	1	130	6	60	16	—
Chocolate Chip Mini (Archway)	12 (1.1 oz)	150	7	95	20	0
Chocolate Chip Mint (Frookie)	1	45	2	35	7	—
Chocolate Chip Pecan (Famous Amos)	3 (1 oz)	150	8	98	18	—
Chocolate Chip Rich'N Chewy (Grandma's)	3 (1 oz)	140	6	80	20	—
Chocolate Chip Snaps (Nabisco)	3 (0.5 oz)	70	2	50	11	—
Chocolate Chip Soft (Lance)	1 (28 g)	130	5	100	19	—
Chocolate Chip & Toffee (Archway)	1 (1 oz)	140	7	120	19	tr
Chocolate-Chocolate Chip (Drake's)	2 (1 oz)	130	5	85	19	—
Chocolate Cookiesaurus (Sunshine)	7	120	5	140	19	—
Chocolate Chunk Macadamia Nut (Tastykake)	1 pkg (56 g)	310	14	180	42	2
Chocolate Chunk Pecan (Pepperidge Farm)	1	70	4	25	8	—
Chocolate Fudge Sandwich (Keebler)	1	80	4	70	12	—
Chocolate Sandwich (Weight Watchers)	2	90	3	90	15	—
Chocolate Snaps (Nabisco)	4 (0.5 oz)	70	2	75	11	—
Chocolu (LU)	1	55	3	—	—	—
Cinnamon Snaps (Archway)	12 (1.1 oz)	150	7	115	19	0
Coated Graham (Lance)	1 pkg	200	10	60	24	—
Coconut (Drake's)	2 (1 oz)	130	5	95	20	—
Coconut Macaroon (Archway)	1 (0.8 oz)	90	5	55	14	2
Coconut Macaroon (Drake's)	1 (1 oz)	135	7	80	17	—
Coconut Macaroons (Dutch Mill)	3 (1 oz)	120	7	115	14	0
Commodore (Keebler)	1	60	2	65	10	—

FOOD	PORTION	CAL	FAT	SOD	CARB	FIB
Como Delight (Stella D'Oro)	1	150	7	60	18	—
Cookie Jar Hermits (Archway)	1 (1 oz)	110	3	160	19	tr
Cookie Wreaths (Little Debbie)	1 pkg (0.6 oz)	90	5	45	11	0
Cookies 'N Fudge Party Grahams (Nabisco)	1 (0.25 oz)	45	2	35	6	—
Cookies 'N Fudge Striped (Nabisco)	1 (0.5 oz)	60	3	60	7	—
Cookies 'N Fudge Striped Wafers (Nabisco)	1 (0.5 oz)	70	4	25	8	—
Cookies Mates (Keebler)	2	50	2	55	8	—
Craquelin (LU)	1	55	3	—	—	—
Creme Filled Chocolate (Little Debbie)	1 pkg (1.8 oz)	260	11	230	36	1
Creme Filled Chocolate (Little Debbie)	1 pkg (1.2 oz)	180	8	115	24	1
Creme Filled Wafers Assorted (Estee)	1	30	2	5	4	—
Creme Filled Wafers Chocolate (Estee)	1	20	1	5	3	—
Creme Filled Wafers Vanilla (Estee)	1	20	1	5	3	—
Crokine (LU)	2	19	0	—	—	—
Dakota Milk Chocolate Oatmeal (Pepperidge Farm)	1	110	6	70	15	1
Danish Imported (Nabisco)	2 (0.5 oz)	70	4	15	9	—
Dark Chocolate (Archway)	1 (1 oz)	110	4	150	20	tr
Date Pecan (Pepperidge Farm)	2	110	5	40	15	—
Deep Night Fudge (Stella D'Oro)	1	65	4	33	8	—
Devil's Food Cakes (Nabisco)	1 (0.75 oz)	70	1	40	15	—
Dinosaur Grrrahams (Mother's)	1	70	2	50	12	—
Dinosaur Grrrahams Chocolate (Salerno)	1 pkg (1.25 oz)	167	5	139	25	1

FOOD	PORTION	CAL	FAT	SOD	CARB	FIB
Dinosaur Grrrahams Cinnamon (Salerno)	1 pkg (1.25 oz)	165	5	144	26	1
Dinosaur Grrrahams Original (Salerno)	1 pkg (1.25 oz)	156	3	114	26	1
Dixi Vanilla (Sunshine)	2	130	5	110	19	—
Dunkaroos (General Mills)	1 pkg (1 oz)	130	5	70	19	—
Dutch Apple Bars (Stella D'Oro)	1	110	3	35	19	—
Dutch Chocolate (Archway)	1 (1 oz)	120	4	110	19	0
Easter Puffs (Little Debbie)	1 pkg (1.2 oz)	140	5	65	25	0
Egg Biscuits Low Sodium (Stella D'Oro)	3	120	3	15	20	—
Egg Biscuits Sugared (Stella D'Oro)	1	80	1	45	14	—
Egg Jumbo (Stella D'Oro)	1	50	1	30	9	—
Euphrates (LU)	2	40	2	—	—	—
Famous Chocolate Wafers (Nabisco)	2½ (0.5 oz)	70	2	100	11	—
Fancy Fruit Chunks (Health Valley)						
Apricot Almond	2	90	4	45	12	2
Date Pecan	2	90	4	45	13	2
Raisin Oat Bran	2	70	2	95	13	2
Tropical Fruit	2	90	3	45	15	2
Fancy Peanut Chunks (Health Valley)	2	90	3	55	12	2
Fat Free (Health Valley)						
Apple Spice	3	75	tr	40	17	3
Apricot Delight	3	75	tr	40	16	3
Date Delight	3	75	tr	40	17	3
Hawaiian Fruit	3	75	tr	40	16	3
Raisin Oatmeal	3	75	tr	40	17	3
Fat Free Jumbos (Health Valley)						
Apple Raisin	1	70	tr	35	16	3
Raisin	1	70	tr	35	16	3
Raspberry	1	70	tr	35	16	3
Fiber Jumbos (Health Valley)						
Blueberry Nut	1	100	3	45	14	3

FOOD	PORTION	CAL	FAT	SOD	CARB	FIB
Fiber Jumbos *(cont.)*						
Chunky Pecan	1	100	3	45	14	3
Raisin Nut	1	100	3	45	14	3
Fig Bar (Lance)	1 pkg (42 g)	150	2	85	30	—
Fig Bar (Mother's)	1 oz	100	2	75	20	—
Fig Bars (Sunshine)	1	50	1	35	10	—
Fig Bars Low Fat (Archway)	2 (1.1 oz)	100	1	105	23	1
Fig Bars Vanilla (FFV)	1	60	1	—	—	—
Fig Bars Whole Wheat (FFV)	1	60	1	—	—	—
Fig Fruitins (Frookie)	1	60	1	25	12	—
Fig Newtons (Nabisco)	1 (0.5 oz)	60	1	60	11	—
Fig Newtons Fat Free (Nabisco)	1 (0.75 oz)	70	0	80	15	—
Figaroos (Little Debbie)	1 pkg (1.5 oz)	160	4	115	31	3
Figaroos (Little Debbie)	1 pkg (2 oz)	200	5	160	40	2
Fortune (La Choy)	1	15	tr	1	4	tr
French Vanilla Creme (Keebler)	1	80	4	80	12	—
Frosty Lemon (Archway)	1 (1 oz)	120	5	110	19	0
Frosty Orange (Archway)	1 (1 oz)	120	4	140	19	1
Fruit & Fitness (Health Valley)	5	200	6	115	34	6
Fruit And Honey Bar (Archway)	1 (1 oz)	110	4	120	18	tr
Fruit Bar No Fat (Archway)	1 (1 oz)	90	0	95	21	0
Fruit Cake (Archway)	1 (1.1 oz)	140	7	100	20	2
Fruit Delight Apple Cinnamon Fat Free (Stella D'Oro)	1	70	0	50	17	—
Fruit Delight Peach Apricot Fat Free (Stella D'Oro)	1	70	0	35	17	—
Fruit Delight Raspberry Fat Free (Stella D'Oro)	1	70	0	40	17	—
Fruit Filled Apricot-Raspberry (Pepperidge Farm)	2	100	4	50	15	—
Fruit Filled Strawberry (Pepperidge Farm)	2	100	5	50	15	—

FOOD	PORTION	CAL	FAT	SOD	CARB	FIB
Fruit Filled Bar Apple (Weight Watchers)	1	80	tr	35	21	—
Fruit Filled Bar Raspberry (Weight Watchers)	1	80	tr	45	22	—
Fruit Jumbos (Health Valley)						
Almond Date	1	70	3	30	10	1
Oat Bran	1	70	2	35	12	2
Raisin Nut	1	70	3	35	10	1
Tropical Fruit	1	70	3	35	10	2
Fruit Slices (Stella D'Oro)	1	60	2	45	9	—
Fruit Slices Fat Free (Stella D'Oro)	1	50	0	60	12	—
Fudge (Estee)	1	30	1	0	4	—
Fudge Bar (Tastykake)	1 (50 g)	200	7	160	35	1
Fudge Chips Chocolate (LU)	1	75	4	—	—	—
Fudge Chocolate Chip (Grandma's)	2 (2.75 oz)	350	13	380	54	—
Fudge Dipped Grahams (Sunshine)	2	80	4	40	11	—
Fudge Family Bears Chocolate With Vanilla Filling (Sunshine)	1	70	3	60	9	—
Fudge Family Bears Peanut Butter (Sunshine)	1	70	3	65	9	—
Fudge Family Bears Vanilla With Fudge Filling (Sunshine)	1	60	3	50	9	—
Fudge Macaroons (Little Debbie)	1 pkg (1 oz)	140	8	65	18	1
Fudge Nut Bar (Archway)	1 (1 oz)	110	5	120	17	tr
Fudge Striped Shortbread (Sunshine)	3	160	8	80	21	—
Fun Chip Mini (Archway)	12 (1.1 oz)	140	6	100	21	0
FundaMiddles Vanilla Creme In Chocolate Graham Shells (General Mills)	1 pkg (0.8 oz)	110	4	120	18	—
Gaufrettes (LU)	2	85	4	—	—	—

FOOD	PORTION	CAL	FAT	SOD	CARB	FIB
Geneva (Pepperidge Farm)	2	130	6	50	14	—
Ginger (Little Debbie)	1 pkg (0.7 oz)	90	3	55	14	1
Ginger Boys Calcium Enriched (FFV)	6	120	3	—	—	—
Ginger Snaps (Bakery Wagon)	4-5 (1 oz)	140	6	105	19	—
Ginger Snaps (Sunshine)	3	60	2	70	9	—
Ginger Snaps Old Fashioned (Nabisco)	2 (0.5 oz)	60	1	80	11	—
Ginger Spice (Frookie)	1	45	2	35	7	—
Gingerman (Pepperidge Farm)	2	70	3	50	10	—
Gingersnaps (Archway)	5 (1.1 oz)	130	5	110	22	0
Golden Bars (Stella D'Oro)	1	110	4	65	16	—
Golden Fruit (Sunshine)	1	70	1	40	14	—
Grab Cookie Bits Chocolate (Grandma's)	8 (1 oz)	140	6	180	19	—
Grab Cookie Bits Peanut Butter (Grandma's)	8 (1 oz)	140	6	125	19	—
Grab Cookie Bits Vanilla (Grandma's)	8 (1 oz)	140	6	75	20	—
Graham (Nabisco)	2 (0.5 oz)	60	1	90	11	—
Graham Amaranth (Health Valley)	7	110	3	110	25	3
Graham Chocolate (Nabisco)	1 (0.5 oz)	50	3	30	7	—
Graham Honey (Health Valley)	7	100	4	125	18	2
Graham Honey Fiber Enriched (Keebler)	2	90	2	110	16	—
Graham Kitchen Rich (Keebler)	2	60	2	55	9	—
Graham Oat Bran (Health Valley)	7	120	3	45	20	5
Grahamy Bears (Sunshine)	4	60	2	55	9	—
Granola No Fat (Archway)	1 (0.5 oz)	50	0	60	11	tr
Hazelnut (Pepperidge Farm)	2	110	6	75	15	—
Hermit (Drakes)	1 (2 oz)	230	7	280	38	—

FOOD	PORTION	CAL	FAT	SOD	CARB	FIB
Heyday Caramel & Peanut (Nabisco)	1 (0.75 oz)	110	6	40	13	—
Heyday Fudge (Nabisco)	1 (0.75 oz)	110	6	40	13	—
Holiday Pak (Archway)	3 (1.1 oz)	150	8	95	19	tr
Holiday Rings & Stars (Stella D'Oro)	1	47	1	12	7	—
Holiday Trinkets (Stella D'Oro)	1	40	2	31	5	—
Homeplate (Keebler)	1	60	2	130	10	—
Honey Jumbos Crisp Cinnamon (Health Valley)	1	70	4	35	9	1
Honey Jumbos Crisp Peanut Butter (Health Valley)	1	70	2	35	11	1
Honey Jumbos Fancy Oat Bran (Health Valley)	2	130	4	50	20	4
Honey Maid Cinnamon (Nabisco)	2 (0.5 oz)	60	1	85	12	—
Honey Maid Grahams (Nabisco)	2 (0.5 oz)	60	1	90	11	—
Hostess Assortment (Stella D'Oro)	1	40	2	20	6	—
Hydrox	1	50	2	45	7	—
Hydrox Doubles (Peanut Butter)	1	60	3	65	8	—
Iced Gingerbread (Archway)	3 (1.1 oz)	140	5	130	23	0
Iced Gingerbread Cookies (Sunshine)	3	70	3	75	10	—
Iced Molasses (Archway)	1 (1 oz)	110	5	170	19	tr
Iced Oatmeal (Archway)	1 (1 oz)	120	5	85	19	1
Ideal Bars Chocolate And Peanut (Nabisco)	1 (0.75 oz)	90	5	80	10	—
Irish Oatmeal (Pepperidge Farm)	2	90	5	80	13	—
Jelly Tarts (FFV)	2	110	4	—	—	—
Jingles (Sunshine)	3	70	3	55	11	—
Keebies (Keebler)	1	80	3	80	12	—
Kichel Low sodium (Stella D'Oro)	21	150	9	25	13	—

FOOD	PORTION	CAL	FAT	SOD	CARB	FIB
Krisp Kreem Wafers (Keebler)	2	50	3	20	7	—
Lady Stella Assortment (Stella D'Oro)	1	40	2	22	6	—
Le Petit-Beurre (LU)	1	40	1	—	—	—
Lem-O-Lunch (Lance)	1 pkg (48 g)	240	11	190	32	—
Lemon Coolers (Sunshine)	2	60	2	45	9	—
Lemon Nekot (Lance)	1 pkg (42 g)	220	11	100	28	—
Lemon Nut Crunch (Pepperidge Farm)	2	110	7	50	13	—
Lemon Snaps (Archway)	12 (1.1 oz)	150	7	120	19	0
Lido (Pepperidge Farm)	1	90	5	30	10	—
Linzer (Pepperidge Farm)	1	120	4	55	20	—
Little Schoolboy (LU)	1	65	3	—	—	—
Lorna Doone (Nabisco)	2 (0.5 oz)	70	4	65	9	—
Mallomars (Nabisco)	1 (0.5 oz)	60	3	20	9	—
Mallopuffs (Sunshine)	1	70	2	35	12	—
Malt (Lance)	1 pkg (35 g)	190	11	125	16	—
Mandarin Chocolate Chip (Frookie)	1	45	2	35	7	—
Margherite Chocolate (Stella D'Oro)	1	70	3	40	10	—
Margherite Vanilla (Stella D'Oro)	1	70	3	45	11	—
Marie LU (LU)	1	50	2	45	8	—
Marshmallow Puffs (Nabisco)	1 (0.75 oz)	90	4	40	14	—
Marshmallow Twirls (Nabisco)	1 (1 oz)	130	5	50	20	—
Milano (Pepperidge Farm)	2	120	6	45	15	—
Milk Chocolate Chip (Duncan Hines)	2	110	5	—	—	—
Milk Chocolate Macadamia (Pepperidge Farm)	2	140	8	—	—	—
Milk Lunch (LU)	1	35	1	—	—	—
Mini Chocolate Chip Cookies (Sunshine)	2	70	4	50	8	—
Mint Milano (Pepperidge Farm)	2	150	7	60	17	—
Mint Sandwich (FFV)	2	160	7	—	—	—

FOOD	PORTION	CAL	FAT	SOD	CARB	FIB
Molasses Crisps (Pepperidge Farm)	2	70	3	50	8	—
Molasses Iced (Bakery Wagon)	1	100	4	120	17	—
Mystic Mint (Nabisco)	1 (0.5 oz)	90	5	65	11	—
Nantucket Chocolate Chunk (Pepperidge Farm)	1	120	6	60	15	1
Nassau (Pepperidge Farm)	1	80	5	45	9	—
New Orleans Cake (Archway)	1 (1 oz)	110	4	105	18	tr
Nilla Wafers (Nabisco)	3½ (0.5 oz)	60	2	45	11	—
Nut-O-Lunch (Lance)	1 oz	140	5	—	—	—
Nutter Butter Bites (Nabisco)	4½ (0.5 oz)	70	3	55	9	—
Nutter Butter Peanut Butter (Nabisco)	1 (0.5 oz)	70	3	50	9	—
Nutter Butter Peanut Creme (Nabisco)	2 (0.5 oz)	80	4	45	8	—
Nutty Nougat (Archway)	3 (1.1 oz)	160	10	60	18	0
Oat Bran Animal Cookies (Health Valley)	7	110	4	50	17	3
Oat Bran Fruit & Nut (Health Valley)	2	110	4	70	17	3
Oat Bran Muffin (Frookie)	1	45	2	35	7	—
Oat Bran Muffin (Frookie)	1 lg	120	4	100	18	—
Oat Bran With Nuts And Raisins (Sunshine)	1	60	3	55	8	—
Oatmeal						
(Archway)	1 (0.9 oz)	110	3	95	19	tr
(Drake's)	2 (1 oz)	120	5	50	19	—
(Lance)	1 (57 G)	130	5	70	20	—
(Mother's)	1	60	3	80	8	—
Oatmeal Apple Spice (Grandma's)	2 (2.75 oz)	330	12	570	51	—
Oatmeal Mini (Archway)	12 (1.1 oz)	150	8	130	19	1
Oatmeal Apple Filled (Archway)	1 (1 oz)	110	3	105	18	0
Oatmeal Calcium Enriched (FFV)	5	130	5	—	—	—

FOOD	PORTION	CAL	FAT	SOD	CARB	FIB
Oatmeal Country Style (Sunshine)	1	70	3	65	10	—
Oatmeal Creme (Drake's)	1 (2 oz)	240	9	250	9	—
Oatmeal Crisp (Little Debbie)	1 pkg (1.5 oz)	210	11	230	27	1
Oatmeal Date Filled (Archway)	1 (1 oz)	110	4	120	18	tr
Oatmeal Date Filled (Bakery Wagon)	1	90	3	100	15	—
Oatmeal Large (Pepperidge Farm)	1	120	6	105	18	—
Oatmeal Lights (Little Debbie)	1 pkg (1.3 oz)	140	4	190	28	1
Oatmeal Pecan (Archway)	1 (1 oz)	120	5	100	18	1
Oatmeal Raisin						
(Archway)	1 (1 oz)	110	4	115	19	tr
(Duncan Hines)	2	110	5	—	—	—
(Dutch Mill)	3 (1 oz)	130	6	75	18	1
(Famous Amos)	3 (1 oz)	134	6	137	19	—
(Frookie)	1	45	2	35	7	—
(Frookie)	1 lg	120	4	100	18	—
(Little Debbie)	1 pkg (2.7 oz)	320	13	330	50	2
Oatmeal Raisin (Nutra/Balance)	1 (2 oz)	240	9	50	36	8
Oatmeal Raisin (Pepperidge Farm)	2	110	5	115	15	—
Oatmeal Raisin (Weight Watchers)	2	90	tr	75	20	—
Oatmeal Raisin Bar (Tastykake)	1 (50 g)	210	8	250	32	1
Oatmeal Raisin Bran (Archway)	1 (1 oz)	110	4	100	19	tr
Oatmeal Soft (Bakery Wagon)	1	100	5	105	15	—
Oatmeal Spice (Weight Watchers)	3	80	2	75	13	—
Old Fashion (Keebler)						
Chocolate Chip	1	80	4	75	11	—
Double Fudge	1	80	4	65	11	—
Oatmeal	1	80	4	110	13	—
Peanut Butter	1	80	4	100	10	—
Sugar	1	80	3	70	13	—

FOOD	PORTION	CAL	FAT	SOD	CARB	FIB
Old Fashioned Chocolate Chip (Pepperidge Farm)	2	100	5	45	12	0
Old Fashioned Molasses (Archway)	1 (1 oz)	120	3	150	20	0
Old Fashioned Windmill (Archway)	1 (0.7 oz)	100	4	95	15	0
Old Time Molasses (Grandma's)	2 (2.75 oz)	320	9	520	58	—
Orange Milano (Pepperidge Farm)	2	150	7	60	17	—
Oreo (Nabisco)	1 (0.5 oz)	50	2	75	8	—
Double Stuf	1 (0.5 oz)	70	4	75	9	—
Fudge Covered	1 (0.75 oz)	110	6	75	13	—
White Fudge Covered	1 (0.75 oz)	110	6	75	14	—
Mini	5 (0.5 oz)	70	3	85	10	—
Orleans (Pepperidge Farm)	3	90	6	30	11	—
Orleans Sandwich (Pepperidge Farm)	2	120	8	40	14	—
Palmito (LU)	1	50	3	—	—	—
Paris (Pepperidge Farm)	2	100	5	—	—	—
Party Treats (Archway)	3 (1.1 oz)	140	7	105	20	0
Peach Apricot Pastry Sodium Free (Stella D'Oro)	1	80	3	0	13	—
Peanut Butter						
(Archway)	1 (1 oz)	140	7	125	16	tr
(Grandma's)	2 (2.75 oz)	410	30	410	43	—
(Little Debbie)	1 pkg (1.5 oz)	210	10	230	27	1
Bar (Frito Lay)	1.75 oz	270	16	65	30	—
Bars (Little Debbie)	1 pkg (1.9 oz)	270	15	190	33	1
Creme Filled Wafer (Lance)	1 pkg (50 g)	240	10	80	34	—
Nougat (Archway)	3 (1.1 oz)	160	9	140	18	1
Sandwich (FFV)	2	170	8	—	—	—
Wafers (Drake's)	1 (2.25 oz)	324	16	135	43	—
Peanut Butter & Chip (Archway)	3 (0.9 oz)	130	7	125	16	0
Peanut Butter & Jelly Sandwiches (Little Debbie)	1 pkg (1.1 oz)	130	5	100	22	1
Peanut Butter n' Chips (Archway)	1 (1 oz)	140	7	115	16	tr
Peanut Cluster (Little Debbie)	1 pkg (1.4 oz)	190	11	125	23	1

FOOD	PORTION	CAL	FAT	SOD	CARB	FIB
Pecan						
Crunch (Archway)	6 (1.1 oz)	150	8	120	18	0
Ice Box (Archway)	1 (1 oz)	140	7	100	18	0
Malted Nougat (Archway)	3 (1.1 oz)	160	10	60	17	2
Shortbread (Little Debbie)	1 pkg (1.5 oz)	220	13	170	26	0
Shortbread (Pepperidge Farm)	1	70	5	15	7	—
Spinwheels (Little Debbie)	1 pkg (1 oz)	110	4	100	16	1
Supremes (Nabisco)	1 (0.5 oz)	80	5	45	9	—
Pfeffernusse (Archway)	2 (1.3 oz)	140	1	100	32	tr
Pfeffernusse Spice Drops (Stella D'Oro)	1	40	1	18	7	—
Pims (LU)	1	50	1	—	—	—
Pineapple Filled (Archway)	1 (0.9 oz)	100	4	75	16	1
Pinwheels (Nabisco)	1 (1 oz)	130	5	35	20	—
Pirouettes Chocolate Laced (Pepperidge Farm)	2	70	4	20	8	—
Pirouettes Original (Pepperidge Farm)	2	70	4	35	9	—
Pitter Patter (Keebler)	1	90	4	115	12	—
Prune Pastry Dietetic (Stella D'Oro)	1	90	3	0	14	—
Pure Chocolate Middles (Nabisco)	1 (0.5 oz)	80	5	35	9	—
Raisin Bran (Pepperidge Farm)	2	110	5	55	13	—
Raisin Oatmeal (Archway)	1 (1 oz)	130	5	40	19	1
Raisin Oatmeal Bag (Archway)	3 (1 oz)	130	6	55	19	1
Raisin Soft (Grandma's)	2 (2.75 oz)	320	10	280	54	—
Raspberry Filled (Archway)	1 (1 oz)	110	4	90	18	tr
Raspberry Newtons (Nabisco)	1 (0.75 oz)	70	2	70	15	—
Regal Grahams (FFV)	2	140	7	—	—	—
Rocky Road (Archway)	1 (1 oz)	130	6	85	18	tr
Roman Egg Biscuits (Stella D'Oro)	1	140	5	125	20	—
Royal Dainty (FFV)	2	120	6	—	—	—

FOOD	PORTION	CAL	FAT	SOD	CARB	FIB
Royal Nuggets (Stella D'Oro)	1	2	tr	—	tr	—
Ruth's Golden Oatmeal (Archway)	1 (1 oz)	120	5	135	19	tr
Sandwich Cookies Chocolate (Estee)	1	50	2	15	7	—
Sandwich Cookies Original (Estee)	1	45	2	5	6	—
Sandwich Cookies Peanut Butter (Estee)	1	50	3	35	5	—
Sante Fe Oatmeal Raisin (Pepperidge Farm)	1	100	4	70	16	1
Sausalito Milk Chocolate Macadamia (Pepperidge Farm)	1	120	7	65	14	0
Schoks-Chocolate (LU)	1	70	4	—	—	—
School House Cookies (Sunshine)	15	120	4	100	20	—
Sea Flappers (Sunshine)	7	140	6	80	20	—
Select Assortment (Archway)	3 (0.9 oz)	130	6	80	18	0
Sesame Regina (Stella D'Oro)	1	50	2	28	6	—
Seville (Pepperidge Farm)	2	100	5	—	—	—
Shortbread (Pepperidge Farm)	2	150	8	85	17	—
Shortbread (Weight Watchers)	3	80	2	95	13	—
Snack Wafer (Estee)						
Chocolate	1	80	4	—	11	—
Chocolate Coated	1	130	7	10	14	—
Strawberry	1	80	4	—	11	—
Vanilla	1	80	4	—	11	—
Snackwell's						
Chocolate Chip	6 (0.5 oz)	60	1	85	11	—
Cinnamon Graham Snacks	9 (0.5 oz)	50	0	50	12	tr
Devil's Food Cakes	1 (0.5 oz)	60	0	30	13	tr
Oatmeal Raisin	1 (0.5 oz)	60	1	65	10	—
Social Tea (Nabisco)	3 (0.5 oz)	70	2	60	11	—
Soft Molasses Drop (Archway)	1 (1 oz)	110	4	160	18	1

FOOD	PORTION	CAL	FAT	SOD	CARB	FIB
Soft Sugar (Archway)	1 (1 oz)	110	4	110	18	0
Soft 'n Chewy Chocolate Chocolate Chip (Tastykake)	1 (32 g)	170	7	110	26	1
Soft 'n Chewy Chocolate Chip (Tastykake)	1 (39 g)	170	7	170	25	1
Soft 'n Chewy Oatmeal Raisin (Tastykake)	1 (39 g)	160	5	160	27	1
Southport (Pepperidge Farm)	2	170	10	—	—	—
Sprinkles Rainbow Topping (Sunshine)	1	70	2	25	13	—
Strawberry Filled (Archway)	1 (1 oz)	110	4	90	18	tr
Strawberry Newtons (Nabisco)	1 (0.75 oz)	70	2	70	15	—
Sugar (Archway)	1 (1 oz)	120	4	190	20	0
Sugar (Pepperidge Farm)	2	100	5	55	13	—
Sugar Wafers (Sunshine)						
Assorted	2	90	4	25	12	—
Chocolate	2	90	4	15	12	—
Peanut Butter	2	80	4	35	10	—
Vanilla	4	90	4	25	12	—
Swiss Fudge (Stella D'Oro)	1	70	3	33	9	—
T. C. Rounds (FFV)	2	160	8	—	—	—
Taffy Creme Sandwich (Mother's)	1-2 (1 oz)	140	8	80	17	—
Tahiti (Pepperidge Farm)	1	90	6	25	9	—
Tango (FFV)	2	160	5	—	—	—
Teddy Grahams (Nabisco)						
Bearwich Chocolate and Vanilla Creme	4 (0.5 oz)	70	3	60	10	—
Bearwich Chocolate Creme With Peanut Butter	4 (0.5 oz)	70	3	65	10	—
Bearwich Cinnamon With Vanilla Creme	4 (0.5 oz)	70	3	60	10	—
Bearwich Vanilla And Chocolate Creme	4 (0.5 oz)	70	3	65	10	—

FOOD	PORTION	CAL	FAT	SOD	CARB	FIB
Chocolate Graham	11 (0.5 oz)	60	2	90	10	—
Cinnamon Graham	11 (0.5 oz)	60	2	80	11	—
Honey Graham	11 (0.5 oz)	60	2	90	11	—
Vanilla And Beach Bears	11 (0.5 oz)	60	2	75	11	—
Vanilla And Holiday Bears	11 (0.5 oz)	60	2	75	11	—
Vanilla And Rockin' Bears	11 (0.5 oz)	60	2	75	11	—
Vanilla Graham	11 (0.5 oz)	60	2	75	10	—
The Great Tofu (Health Valley)	2	90	3	30	14	4
The Great Wheat Free (Health Valley)	2	80	3	35	14	3
Trolley Cakes Devilsfood (FFV)	2	120	2	—	—	—
Tru Blu Chocolate (Sunshine)	2	160	7	140	23	—
Tru Blu Lemon (Sunshine)	1	70	3	65	12	—
Tru Blu Vanilla (Sunshine)	1 (0.5 oz)	80	3	65	12	—
Van-O-Lunch (Lance)	1 pkg (37 g)	180	7	150	26	—
Vanilla Sugar Wafer (Tastykake)	1 (6 g)	36	2	10	4	0
Vanilla Wafer (Archway)	5 (1.1 oz)	130	4	130	22	0
Vanilla Wafers (FFV)	8	120	5	—	—	—
Vanilla Wafers (Keebler)	4	80	4	60	10	—
Vanilla Wafers (Sunshine)	3	70	3	50	9	—
Vienna Fingers (Sunshine)	1 (0.5 oz)	70	3	60	10	—
Wedding Cakes (Archway)	3 (1.1 oz)	160	8	45	20	0
Zurich (Pepperidge Farm)	1	60	2	30	10	—
animal	11 crackers (1 oz)	126	4	112	21	—
animal crackers	1 (2.5 g)	11	tr	10	2	—
animal crackers	1 box (2.4 oz)	299	9	274	51	—
butter	1 (5 g)	23	1	18	3	tr
chocolate chip	1 (0.4 oz)	48	2	32	7	tr
chocolate chip	1 box (1.9 oz)	233	12	188	36	—
chocolate chip low fat	1 (0.25 oz)	45	2	38	7	—
chocolate chip low sugar low sodium	1 (0.24 oz)	31	1	1	5	—

FOOD	PORTION	CAL	FAT	SOD	CARB	FIB
chocolate chip soft-type	1 (0.5 oz)	69	4	49	9	tr
chocolate w/creme filling	1 (0.35 oz)	47	2	36	7	tr
chocolate w/creme filling chocolate coated	1 (0.60 oz)	82	5	55	11	—
chocolate w/creme filling sugar free low sodium	1 (0.35 oz)	46	2	24	7	—
chocolate w/extra creme filling	1 (0.46 oz)	65	3	64	9	—
chocolate wafer	1 (0.2 oz)	26	1	35	4	—
chocolate wafer cookie crumbs	1½ cup (5.9 oz)	728	25	980	120	—
digestive biscuits plain	2	141	7	—	21	1
fig bars	1 (0.56 oz)	56	1	56	11	1
fortune	1 (0.28 oz)	30	tr	22	7	tr
fudge	1 (0.73 oz)	73	1	40	17	tr
gingersnaps	1 (0.24 oz)	29	1	48	5	—
graham	1 squares (0.24 oz)	30	1	42	5	—
graham chocolate covered	1 (0.49 oz)	68	3	41	9	—
graham cracker crumbs	1½ cup (4.4 oz)	540	13	756	97	3
graham honey	1 (0.24 oz)	30	1	42	5	tr
ladyfingers	1 (0.38 oz)	40	1	16	7	—
marshmallow chocolate coated	1 (0.46 oz)	55	2	22	9	—
marshmallow pie chocolate coated	1 (1.4 oz)	165	7	66	26	—
molasses	1 (0.5 oz)	65	2	69	11	—
oatmeal	1 (0.52 oz)	71	4	62	9	tr
oatmeal	1 (0.6 oz)	81	3	69	12	1
oatmeal soft-type	1 (0.5 oz)	61	2	52	10	tr
oatmeal raisin	1 (0.6 oz)	81	3	69	12	1
oatmeal raisin low sugar no sodium	1 (0.24 oz)	31	1	1	5	—
oatmeal raisin soft-type	1 (0.5 oz)	61	2	52	10	tr
peanut butter sandwich	1 (0.5 oz)	67	3	52	9	—
peanut butter sandwich sugar free low sodium	1 (0.35 oz)	54	3	41	5	—
peanut butter soft-type	1 (0.5 oz)	69	4	50	9	tr
raisin soft-type	1 (0.5 oz)	60	2	51	10	—
shortbread	1 (0.28 oz)	40	2	36	5	—
shortbread pecan	1 (0.49 oz)	79	5	39	8	tr

FOOD	PORTION	CAL	FAT	SOD	CARB	FIB
sugar	1 (0.52 oz)	72	3	53	10	—
sugar low sugar sodium free	1 (0.24 oz)	30	1	0	5	—
sugar wafers w/creme filling	1 (0.12 oz)	18	1	5	3	—
sugar wafers w/creme filling sugar free sodium free	1 (0.14 oz)	20	1	0	3	—
vanilla sandwich	1 (0.35 oz)	48	2	35	7	tr
vanilla wafers	1 (0.21 oz)	28	1	18	4	—
REFRIGERATED						
Chocolate Chip (Pillsbury)	1	70	3	55	9	—
Oatmeal Raisin (Pillsbury)	1	60	2	55	10	—
Peanut Butter (Pillsbury)	1	70	3	75	9	—
Sugar (Pillsbury)	1	70	3	70	9	—
chocolate chip	1 (0.42 oz)	59	3	28	8	—
chocolate chip, unbaked	1 oz	126	6	59	17	—
oatmeal	1 (0.4 oz)	56	3	39	8	—
oatmeal raisin	1 (0.4 oz)	56	3	39	8	—
peanut butter	1 (0.4 oz)	60	3	52	7	—
peanut butter dough	1 oz	130	7	112	15	—
sugar	1 (0.42 oz)	58	3	56	8	—
sugar dough	1 oz	124	6	120	17	—

CORIANDER

FOOD	PORTION	CAL	FAT	SOD	CARB	FIB
leaf, dried	1 tsp	2	tr	1	tr	—
leaf, fresh	¼ cup	1	tr	1	tr	—
seed	1 tsp	5	tr	1	1	—

CORN

See also BRAN, CEREAL, CORNMEAL, FLOUR

CANNED

FOOD	PORTION	CAL	FAT	SOD	CARB	FIB
50% Less Salt No Sugar Added (Green Giant)	½ cup	50	1	140	11	2
Corn (Green Giant)	½ cup	70	0	350	10	2
Cream Style (Green Giant)	½ cup	100	tr	390	24	2
Cream Style (Libby)	½ cup	80	0	—	—	—
Cream Style (Owatonna)	½ cup	100	1	—	—	—
Cream Style Diet (S&W)	½ cup	100	1	0	21	—
Cream Style Premium Homestyle (S&W)	½ cup	105	1	435	25	—
Deli Corn (Green Giant)	½ cup	80	tr	350	19	2

FOOD	PORTION	CAL	FAT	SOD	CARB	FIB
Golden Kernel 50% Less Salt (Green Giant)	½ cup	70	tr	175	16	2
Golden Vacuum Packed (Green Giant)	½ cup	80	0	330	20	2
Mexi Corn (Green Giant)	½ cup	80	tr	450	19	2
No Salt No Sugar (Green Giant)	½ cup	80	tr	0	18	2
Sweet 'N Natural (S&W)	½ cup	90	1	180	20	—
Sweet Select (Green Giant)	½ cup	60	1	280	12	2
White Vacuum Packed (Green Giant)	½ cup	80	0	290	20	2
Whole Kernel						
(Seneca)	½ cup	80	1	—	—	—
Natural Pack (Libby)	½ cup	80	1	—	—	—
Natural Pack (Seneca)	½ cup	80	1	—	—	—
Tender Young (S&W)	½ cup	90	1	295	20	—
Vacuum Pack (Owatonna)	½ cup	100	1	—	—	—
Water Pack (S&W)	½ cup	80	1	0	15	—
Whole Kernel In Brine (Owatonna)	½ cup	90	1	—	—	—
cream style	½ cup	93	1	365	23	—
w/red & green peppers	½ cup	86	1	396	21	—
white	½ cup	66	1	—	15	—
yellow	½ cup	66	1	—	15	1
FRESH						
on-the-cob w/butter, cooked	1 ear	155	3	30	32	—
white, cooked	½ cup	89	1	14	21	—
white, raw	½ cup	66	1	12	15	—
yellow, cooked	1 ear (2.7 oz)	83	1	13	19	—
yellow, cooked	½ cup	89	1	14	21	—
yellow, raw	1 ear (3 oz)	77	1	14	17	—
yellow, raw	½ cup	66	1	12	15	—
FROZEN						
Big Ears (Birds Eye)	1 ear	160	1	0	37	—
Cob Corn (Ore-Ida)	1 ear (5.3 oz)	190	tr	10	40	—
Cob Corn Mini-Gold (Ore-Ida)	1 (2.65 oz)	90	tr	5	20	—
Cream Style (Green Giant)	½ cup	110	1	370	25	3
Cut (Big Valley)	3.5 oz	80	1	5	20	—
Fritters (Mrs. Paul's)	2	240	9	560	35	—

FOOD	PORTION	CAL	FAT	SOD	CARB	FIB
Harvest Fresh Niblets (Green Giant)	½ cup	80	1	40	17	2
Harvest Fresh White Shoepeg (Green Giant)	½ cup	90	1	60	19	2
In Butter Sauce (Birds Eye)	½ cup	90	2	170	19	2
In Butter Sauce (Green Giant)	½ cup	100	2	310	19	—
Little Ears (Birds Eye)	2 ears	130	1	0	30	—
Nibblers Corn On The Cob (Green Giant)	1 ear	120	1	10	27	2
Niblet Ears (Green Giant)	1 ear	120	1	10	27	2
Niblets (Green Giant)	½ cup	90	tr	5	19	2
On The Cob (Birds Eye)	1 ear	120	1	0	29	—
One Serve Niblets In Butter Sauce (Green Giant)	1 pkg	120	2	350	24	3
One Serve On the Cob (Green Giant)	1 pkg	120	1	10	26	2
Polybag Cut (Birds Eye)	½ cup	80	1	0	19	2
Polybag Deluxe Tender Sweet (Birds Eye)	½ cup	80	1	0	20	2
Souffle (Stouffer's)	½ cup (2.4 oz)	170	7	490	21	1
Super Sweet Nibblers Corn On The Cob (Green Giant)	2 ears	90	2	10	19	2
Super Sweet Niblet Ears (Green Giant)	1 ear	90	2	10	19	2
Super Sweet Niblet Select (Green Giant)	½ cup	60	1	5	13	2
Sweet (Birds Eye)	½ cup	80	1	0	20	2
White In Butter Sauce (Green Giant)	½ cup	100	2	280	20	2
White Select (Green Giant)	½ cup	90	1	5	19	2
White Shoepeg (Hanover)	½ cup	80	0	—	—	—
White Sweet (Hanover)	½ cup	80	0	—	—	—
Yellow Sweet (Hanover)	½ cup	80	0	—	—	—
cooked	½ cup	67	tr	4	17	—
on-the-cob, cooked	1 ear (2.2 oz)	59	tr	3	14	—
SHELF STABLE						
Golden Whole Kernel (Pantry Express)	½ cup	60	tr	210	18	1

FOOD	PORTION	CAL	FAT	SOD	CARB	FIB
TAKE-OUT						
fritters	1 (1 oz)	62	2	126	9	1
scalloped	½ cup	258	7	246	43	—

CORN CHIPS
see CHIPS

CORNISH HENS
see CHICKEN

CORNMEAL

FOOD	PORTION	CAL	FAT	SOD	CARB	FIB
Albers White	3 tbsp	110	0	0	34	tr
Albers Yellow	3 tbsp	110	0	0	34	tr
Arrowhead Yellow	¼ cup (1.2 oz)	120	1	0	27	3
Aunt Jemima White	3 tbsp	102	1	1	22	1
Aunt Jemima Yellow	3 tbsp	102	1.	1	22	1
Quaker White	3 tbsp	102	1	1	22	1
Quaker Yellow	3 tbsp	102	1	1	22	1
corn grits, cooked	1 cup	146	tr	0	31	—
corn grits, uncooked	1 cup	579	2	1	124	—
degermed	1 cup	506	2	5	107	7
self-rising, degermed	1 cup	489	2	1860	103	—
whole grain	1 cup	442	4	43	94	13
HOME RECIPE						
hush puppies	1 (0.75 oz)	74	3	147	10	1
hush puppies	5 (2.7 oz)	256	12	965	35	4
MIX						
Arrowhead Corn Bread	¼ cup (1.2 oz)	120	1	270	24	4
Aunt Jemima Bolted White Mix	3 tbsp	99	1	337	21	—
Aunt Jemima Buttermilk Self-Rising White Mix	3 tbsp	101	1	439	21	—
Aunt Jemima Self-Rising White Mix	3 tbsp	98	1	381	21	1
Aunt Jemima Self-Rising Yellow Mix	3 tbsp	100	1	490	21	—
Golden Dipt Corny Dog Batter Mix	1 oz	100	0	490	22	—
Golden Dipt Hush Puppy Deluxe Mix	1.25 oz	120	0	520	26	—
Golden Dipt Hush Puppy Jalapeno Mix	1.25 oz	120	0	570	27	—
Golden Dipt Hush Puppy With Onion	1.25 oz	120	0	520	27	—

FOOD	PORTION	CAL	FAT	SOD	CARB	FIB
Hodgson Mill Yellow	¼ cup (1 oz)	100	1	0	22	3
Hodgson Mill Yellow Self Rising	¼ cup (1 oz)	90	1	260	21	3
Kentucky Kernel White corn Meal Mix	¼ cup (1 oz)	100	1	210	22	2
Miracle Maize Complete, as prep	1 piece (1.5 oz)	193	3	193	34	2
Miracle Maize Country Style, as prep	1 piece 2 in × 2 in (1.8 oz)	230	5	406	38	2
Miracle Maize Sweet, as prep	1 piece 2 in × 2 in (1.8 oz)	236	5	260	41	1

CORNSALAD

raw	1 cup	12	tr	—	2	—

CORNSTARCH

Argo	1 cup (128 g)	460	tr	tr	115	—
Argo	1 tbsp (8 g)	30	0	0	7	—
Hodgson Mill	2 tsp (0.4 oz)	35	0	0	9	—
Kingsford's	1 cup (128 g)	460	tr	tr	115	—
Kingsford's	1 tbsp (8 g)	30	tr	0	7	—
cornstarch	⅓ cup	164	tr	4	39	tr

COTTAGE CHEESE

Axelrod Nonfat	½ cup (4.4 oz)	90	0	500	7	0
Borden 4%	½ cup	120	5	400	4	—
Borden Dry Curd 0.5%	½ cup	80	1	20	3	—
Borden Unsalted 4%	½ cup	120	5	40	4	—
Breakstone						
2%	4 oz	100	2	510	4	—
4% Small Curd	4 oz	110	5	370	3	—
4% With Pineapple	4 oz	140	5	260	14	—
Dry Curd No Salt Added	4 oz	90	0	65	6	—
Cabot	4 oz	120	5	455	3	—
Cabot Light	4 oz	90	1	360	3	—
Formagg	1 oz	80	2	—	—	—
Friendship						
California Style	½ cup (4 oz)	115	5	380	4	0
Lowfat No Salt Added	½ cup (4 oz)	90	1	40	4	0
Lowfat Pineapple	½ cup (4 oz)	120	1	300	17	0
Lowfat 1%	½ cup (4 oz)	90	1	360	4	0
Nonfat	½ cup (4 oz)	80	0	380	5	0

FOOD	PORTION	CAL	FAT	SOD	CARB	FIB
Friendship *(cont.)*						
Nonfat Plus Peach	½ cup (4 oz)	110	0	300	15	0
Pot Style	½ cup (4 oz)	90	3	430	3	0
With Pineapple	½ cup (4 oz)	140	4	310	15	0
Knudsen						
2%	4 oz	100	2	370	4	—
2% With Fruit Cocktail	4 oz	130	2	330	16	—
2% With Mandarin Orange	4 oz	110	2	320	11	—
2% With Peach	6 oz	170	2	270	19	—
2% With Pear	4 oz	110	2	320	12	—
2% With Pineapple	6 oz	170	2	300	18	—
2% With Spiced Apple	6 oz	180	2	280	20	—
2% With Strawberry	4 oz	170	2	320	19	—
4% Large Curd	4 oz	120	5	340	4	—
4% Small Curd	4 oz	120	5	370	4	—
Nonfat	4 oz	90	0	420	3	—
Lactaid 1%	4 oz	72	1	406	3	—
Land O'Lakes	4 oz	120	5	—	—	—
Land O'Lakes 2%	4 oz	100	2	—	—	—
Light n' Lively	4 oz	80	2	370	4	—
Light n' Lively 1% Garden Salad	4 oz	80	2	350	5	—
Light n'Lively 1% Peach And Pineapple	4 oz	100	1	320	12	—
Lite-Line Lowfat 1½%	½ cup	90	2	400	4	—
Sargento Pot Cheese	1 oz	26	tr	1	1	—
Sealtest 2%	4 oz	100	2	340	4	—
Viva Nonfat	½ cup	70	0	430	5	—
Weight Watchers 1%	½ cup	90	1	460	4	—
Weight Watchers 2%	½ cup	100	2	460	4	—
creamed	1 cup	217	9	850	6	—
creamed	4 oz	117	5	457	3	—
creamed, w/fruit	4 oz	140	4	457	15	—
dry curd	1 cup	123	1	19	3	—
dry curd	4 oz	96	tr	14	2	—
lowfat 1%	1 cup	164	2	918	6	—
lowfat 1%	4 oz	82	1	459	3	—
lowfat 2%	1 cup	203	4	918	8	—
lowfat 2%	4 oz	101	2	459	4	—

COTTONSEED

FOOD	PORTION	CAL	FAT	SOD	CARB	FIB
kernels, roasted	1 tbsp	51	4	3	2	—

FOOD	PORTION	CAL	FAT	SOD	CARB	FIB
COUGH DROPS						
Halls	1 (3.8 g)	15	0	—	4	—
Halls Plus (Halls)	1 (4.7 g)	18	0	—	5	—
Halls With Vitamin C (Halls)	1 (3.8 g)	14	0	—	4	—
COUSCOUS						
Couscous Lemon Thyme Salad Mix, as prep (Nile Spice)	½ cup	103	5	146	13	—
Golden Couscous Lentil Curry Soup Mix, as prep (Nile Spice)	10 oz	220	tr	590	44	—
Golden Couscous Tomato Minestrone Soup, as prep (Nile Spice)	10 oz	200	0	590	41	—
Golden Couscous Vegetable Chicken Soup, as prep (Nile Spice)	10 oz	220	5	400	34	—
Golden Couscous Vegetable Parmesan Soup, as prep (Nile Spice)	10 oz	200	3	550	35	—
Whole Wheat Lentil & Onion Couscous Pilaf, as prep (Nile Spice)	½ cup	153	4	188	25	—
cooked	½ cup	101	tr	4	21	—
dry	½ cup	346	tr	9	71	—
COWPEAS						
CANNED						
common	1 cup	184	1	718	33	—
DRIED						
catjang, cooked	1 cup	200	1	32	35	—
FRESH						
leafy tips, chopped, cooked	1 cup	12	tr	3	1	—
leafy tips, raw, chopped	1 cup	10	tr	2	2	—
FROZEN						
cooked	½ cup	112	tr	5	20	—

FOOD	PORTION	CAL	FAT	SOD	CARB	FIB
CRAB						
CANNED						
Dungeness Crab (S&W)	3.25 oz	81	2	920	1	—
blue	1 cup	133	2	5	0	—
blue	3 oz	84	1	283	0	—
FRESH						
alaska king, cooked	1 leg (4.7 oz)	129	2	1436	0	—
alaska king, cooked	3 oz	82	1	911	0	—
alaska king, raw	1 leg (6 oz)	144	1	1438	0	—
alaska king, raw	3 oz	71	1	711	0	—
blue, cooked	1 cup	138	2	376	0	—
blue, cooked	3 oz	87	2	237	0	—
blue, raw	1 crab (.7 oz)	18	tr	62	tr	—
blue, raw	3 oz	74	1	249	tr	—
dungeness, raw	1 crab (5.7 oz)	140	2	481	1	—
dungeness, raw	3 oz	73	1	251	1	—
queen, steamed	3 oz	98	1	587	0	—
FROZEN						
Crab Crisp (King & Prince)	4 oz	310	19	—	—	—
Crab Del Rey (King & Prince)	3 oz	153	9	—	—	—
Deviled Crab (Mrs. Paul's)	1 cake	180	9	480	18	—
Deviled Crab Miniatures (Mrs. Paul's)	3½ oz	240	12	540	25	—
READY-TO-USE						
crab cakes	1 cake (2.1 oz)	93	5	198	tr	—
TAKE-OUT						
baked	1 (3.8 oz)	160	2	550	4	—
cake	1 (2 oz)	160	10	492	5	—
soft-shell, fried	1 (4.4 oz)	334	18	1118	31	—
CRACKER CRUMBS						
Corn Flake Crumbs (Kellogg's)	1/4 cup (1 oz)	100	0	290	24	1
Cracker Meal (Golden Dipt)	1 oz	100	0	0	22	
Cracker Meal (Keebler)	1 cup	100	3	5	23	—
Cracker Meal (Lance)	1 oz	100	1	1	21	—
Cracker Meal (Nabisco)	1/4 cup	100	tr	10	23	—
Graham (Sunshine)	1 cup	550	14	—	—	—
Graham Crumbs (Keebler)	1 cup	520	14	630	90	—

FOOD	PORTION	CAL	FAT	SOD	CARB	FIB
Premium Fat Free (Nabisco)	2 tbsp	50	0	0	11	—
Zesty Meal (Keebler)	1 cup	85	10	100	61	—
cracker meal	1 cup	440	2	32	93	—

CRACKERS
see also CRACKER CRUMBS

FOOD	PORTION	CAL	FAT	SOD	CARB	FIB
6 Calorie Wafer (Estee)	1	6	tr	0	1	—
American Classic (Nabisco)						
Cracked Wheat	4 (0.5 oz)	70	4	140	8	—
Dairy Butter (Nabisco)	4 (0.5 oz)	70	3	140	9	—
Golden Sesame (Nabisco)	4 (0.5 oz)	70	3	120	9	—
Toasted Poppy (Nabisco)	4 (0.5 oz)	70	3	140	9	—
Armenian Thin Bread (Venus)	2 (0.9 oz)	100	1	165	19	—
Bacon Cheese (Eagle)	1 oz	140	6	330	18	—
Bacon Flavored (Nabisco)	7 (0.5 oz)	70	4	210	9	—
Better Cheddars (Nabisco)	10 (0.5 oz)	70	4	130	8	—
Better Cheddars Low Salt (Nabisco)	10 (0.5 oz)	70	4	65	8	—
Bonnie (Lance)	1 pkg (34 g)	160	7	170	24	—
Bran Wafers Salt Free (Venus)	5 (0.6 oz)	80	1	0	11	2
Breadflats (J. J. Flats)						
Caraway	1	52	1	126	10	1
Caraway And Salt	1	51	1	213	9	1
Cinnamon	1	53	1	126	10	1
Flavorall	1	52	1	139	10	1
Garlic	1	52	1	127	10	1
Sesame	1	55	2	124	9	1
Oat Bran	1	49	1	141	8	2
Onion	1	53	1	140	10	1
Plain	1	53	1	143	10	1
Poppy	1	53	1	126	9	1
Brown Rice (Sesmark)	15 (1 oz)	120	2	85	25	tr
Butter Crackers (Goya)	1	40	1	60	6	—
Butter Thins (Pepperidge Farm)	4	70	3	115	10	0
Captain Wafers (Lance)	2	30	1	60	5	—

FOOD	PORTION	CAL	FAT	SOD	CARB	FIB
Captain Wafers Very Low Sodium (Lance)	2	30	1	25	5	—
Captain Wafers w/ Cream Cheese & Chives (Lance)	1 pkg (37 g)	170	9	260	23	—
Cheddar Thins (FFV)	7	70	2	—	—	—
Cheddar Wedges (Nabisco)	31 (0.5 oz)	70	3	150	9	—
Cheese (Eagle)	1 oz	130	6	330	18	—
Cheese (Hain)	1 oz	130	6	180	17	—
Cheese Crackers With Peanut Butter (Little Debbie)	1 pkg (0.9 oz)	140	7	290	16	1
Cheese Crackers With Peanut Butter (Little Debbie)	1 pkg (1.4 oz)	210	10	430	23	1
Cheese Filled (Frito-Lay)	6 (1.5 oz)	210	10	470	24	—
Cheese-On-Wheat	1 pkg (37 g)	180	9	260	22	—
Cheese Thins (Sesmark)	15 (1 oz)	130	3	110	26	tr
Cheez 'n Crackers (Handi-Snacks)	1 pkg	120	8	360	9	—
Cheez 'n Crackers Bacon (Handi-Snacks)	1 pkg	130	9	410	8	—
Cheez-It	12	70	4	135	7	—
Cheez-It Low Salt	12	70	4	65	7	—
Chicken In A Biskit (Nabisco)	7 (0.5 oz)	80	5	130	8	—
Club (Keebler)	2	30	2	75	4	—
Corn Crackers Salt Free (Venus)	5 (0.5 oz)	60	1	0	10	2
Cracked Wheat (Pepperidge Farm)	3	100	4	180	14	0
Cracked Wheat Wafers Salt Free (Venus)	5 (0.5 oz)	60	1	0	11	—
Cracker Bread (Venus)	5 (0.5 oz)	60	1	90	11	—
Cracker Crisp Country Butter (McCrackens)	1 oz	140	8	170	18	—
Cracker Crisp Sour Cream & Chives (McCrackens)	1 oz	140	8	170	18	—
Cracker Crisp Tangy Cheddar (McCrackens)	1 oz	140	8	170	18	—
Cracker Crisp Toasted Wheat (McCrackens)	1 oz	140	8	170	18	—

FOOD	PORTION	CAL	FAT	SOD	CARB	FIB
Cracker Snacks Cheddar (Frito-Lay)	13-16 (1 oz)	70	4	150	8	—
Cracker Snacks Zesty Italian (Frito-Lay)	13-16 (1 oz)	70	3	115	9	—
Crackups (Nabisco)	15 (0.5 oz)	70	3	100	10	—
Crisp Bread (Ryvita)						
Dark Finn Crisp	2	38	tr	—	—	—
Dark Rye	1	26	tr	—	—	—
Dark w/Caraway Seeds Finn Crisp	2	38	tr	—	—	—
High Fiber	1	23	tr	—	—	—
Light Rye	1	26	tr	—	—	—
Toasted Sesame Rye	1	31	tr	—	—	—
Crispbread Garlic (Weight Watchers)	2	30	0	55	7	—
Crispy Graham (Pepperidge Farm)	4	70	2	115	13	—
Crown Pilot (Nabisco)	1 (0.5 oz)	70	2	70	11	—
Double Cheddar (FFV)	7	70	2	—	—	—
English Water Biscuits (Pepperidge Farm)	4	70	1	100	13	0
Escort (Nabisco)	3 (0.5 oz)	70	4	115	9	—
Flutters Garden Herb (Pepperidge Farm)	0.75 oz	100	4	190	14	—
Flutters Golden Sesame (Pepperidge Farm)	0.75 oz	110	5	150	13	—
Flutters Original Butter (Pepperidge Farm)	0.75 oz	100	4	150	15	—
Flutters Toasted Wheat (Pepperidge Farm)	0.75 oz	110	5	170	13	—
Garden Vegetable (Pepperidge Farm)	5	60	2	125	10	—
Goldfish (Pepperidge Farm)						
Cheddar Cheese	1 oz	120	4	230	19	1
Cheddar Cheese	1 pkg (1.5 oz)	190	6	340	28	1
Cheese Thins	4	50	2	160	—	0
Original	1 oz	130	5	190	18	1
Parmesan Cheese	1 oz	120	4	330	19	1
Pizza Flavored	1 oz	130	5	220	19	1
Pretzel	1 oz	110	3	160	20	1
Gourmet Flatbread Caraway & Rye (Adrienne's)	2	20	tr	45	4	—

FOOD	PORTION	CAL	FAT	SOD	CARB	FIB
Gourmet Flatbread Classic Island (Adrienne's)	2	20	tr	45	3	—
Gourmet Flatbread Slightly Onion (Adrienne's)	2	20	tr	45	3	—
Gourmet Flatbread Ten Grain (Adrienne's)	2	20	tr	45	3	1
Goya Crackers	1	30	0	45	5	—
Ham & Cheese Crispy Wafers (FFV)	7	70	2	—	—	—
Harvest Crisps 5 Grain (Nabisco)	6 (0.5 oz)	60	2	135	10	—
Harvest Crisps Oat (Nabisco)	6 (0.5 oz)	60	2	135	10	—
Hearty Wheat (Pepperidge Farm)	4	100	5	140	13	1
Herb Stoned Wheat (Health Valley)	13	55	2	80	9	2
Herb Stoned Wheat No Salt (Health Valley)	13	55	2	30	9	2
Hi Ho	4	80	5	—	—	—
Hors D'oeuvre (Venus)	3 (0.5 oz)	60	2	20	11	—
Ideal Crispbread (Extra Thin)	3	48	0	86	9	1
Ideal Crispbread (Fiber Thins)	2	41	1	81	8	2
Ideal Crispbread (Oatbran Thins)	2	50	0	80	8	2
Kavli	1 piece	40	tr	40	10	2
Krispy Saltine (Sunshine)	5	60	1	210	11	—
Krispy Unsalted Tops (Sunshine)	5	60	1	120	11	—
Lanchee (Lance)	1 pkg (35 g)	180	11	110	19	—
Lavash Wafer Bread Crisp Original (Venus)	2 (0.5 oz)	60	1	90	11	—
Lavash Wafer Bread Crisp Sesame (Venus)	2 (0.5 oz)	60	1	70	10	—
Melba Rounds (Devonsheer)						
Garlic	0.5 oz	56	1	132	9	1
Honey Bran	0.5 oz	52	1	98	9	1
Onion	0.5 oz	51	1	120	10	1
Plain	0.5 oz	53	1	111	10	1

FOOD	PORTION	CAL	FAT	SOD	CARB	FIB
Plain Unsalted	0.5 oz	52	1	<5	10	1
Rye	0.5 oz	53	1	130	10	1
Sesame	0.5 oz	57	2	131	8	1
Melba Toast						
Garlic (Keebler)	2	25	54	35	4	—
Long (Keebler)	2	30	tr	10	7	—
Oblong (Lance)	2	30	0	50	7	—
Onion (Keebler)	2	25	tr	35	4	—
Plain (Keebler)	2	25	tr	35	4	—
Plain (Lance)	2	20	0	30	4	—
Pumpernickel (Old London)	0.5 oz	54	1	156	10	1
Round Garlic (Lance)	2	20	0	35	4	—
Round Onion (Lance)	2	20	0	30	4	—
Rye (Old London)	0.5 oz	52	1	132	10	—
Sesame (Keebler)	2	25	tr	35	4	—
Sesame (Lance)	2	25	0	35	4	—
Sesame (Old London)	0.5 oz	55	2	148	8	1
Sesame Unsalted (Old London)	0.5 oz	55	2	5	8	1
Wheat (Old London)	0.5 oz	51	1	121	10	1
White (Old London)	0.5 oz	51	1	111	10	1
White Unsalted (Old London)	0.5 oz	51	1	4	10	1
Whole Grain (Old London)	0.5 oz	52	1	116	9	1
Whole Grain Unsalted (Old London)	0.5 oz	53	1	4	10	1
Multi Grain (Pepperidge Farm)	4	70	2	115	12	—
NAB Cheese Peanut Butter Sandwich (Nabisco)	4 (1 oz)	130	7	320	15	—
NAB Peanut Butter Toast Sandwich (Nabisco)	4 (1 oz)	130	7	300	15	—
Nekot (Lance)	1 pkg (42 g)	210	10	95	24	—
Nip-Chee (Lance)	1 pkg (37 g)	180	8	320	21	—
Nips Cheese (Nabisco)	13 (0.5 oz)	70	3	130	9	—
Oat Bran Krisp (Ralston)	2	60	3	140	6	3
Oat Bran Wafers (Venus)	5 (0.5 oz)	60	1	105	11	2
Oat Bran Wafers Salt Free (Venus)	5 (0.5 oz)	60	1	0	11	1

FOOD	PORTION	CAL	FAT	SOD	CARB	FIB
Oat Thins (Nabisco)	8 (0.5 oz)	70	3	90	10	—
Ocean Crisp (FFV)	1	60	1	—	—	—
Old Brussels Cheddar Waferettes (Venus)	5 (0.5 oz)	80	5	160	7	—
Old Brussels Jalapeno Waferettes (Venus)	5 (0.5 oz)	80	5	160	7	1
Onion (Hain)	1 oz	130	6	160	17	—
Onion No Salt Added (Hain)	1 oz	130	6	5	17	—
Oyster Crackers (Lance)	1 pkg (14 g)	70	2	170	10	—
Oyster Crackers Large (Keebler)	26	80	2	175	13	—
Oyster Crackers Small (Keebler)	50	80	2	175	13	—
Oysterettes (Nabisco)	18 (0.5 oz)	60	1	140	10	—
Peanut Butter Filled (Frito Lay)	6 (1.5 oz)	210	10	450	24	—
Peanut Butter Wheat (Lance)	1 pkg (37 g)	190	11	210	18	—
Peanut Butter & Cheese (Eagle)	1 oz	280	16	450	26	—
Peanut Butter 'n Cheez Crackers (Handi-Snacks)	1 pkg	190	14	180	11	—
Pita Crisps (Tuscany)	1 oz	90	1	—	—	—
Pita Crisps Sesame (Tuscany)	1 oz	96	2	—	—	—
Premium Bits (Nabisco)	16 (0.5 oz)	70	3	160	9	—
Premium Saltine (Nabisco)	5 (0.5 oz)	60	2	180	10	—
Premium Saltine Fat Free (Nabisco)	5 (0.5 oz)	50	0	115	12	—
Premium Saltine Low Salt (Nabisco)	5 (0.5 oz)	60	2	115	10	—
Premium Saltine Unsalted Tops (Nabisco)	5 (0.5 oz)	60	2	135	10	—
Premium Soup And Oyster (Nabisco)	20 (0.5 oz)	60	1	210	10	—
Premium With Multi-Grain (Nabisco)	5 (0.5 oz)	60	2	170	10	—
Rice Bran (Health Valley)	7	130	4	65	19	2
Rice Thins Original (Sesmark)	15 (1 oz)	130	3	150	24	tr

FOOD	PORTION	CAL	FAT	SOD	CARB	FIB
Rice Thins Teriyaki Flavored (Sesmark)	13 (1 oz)	130	3	170	24	tr
Rich (Hain)	1 oz	130	5	160	18	—
Rich No Salt Added (Hain)	1 oz	130	5	15	18	—
Ritz (Nabisco)	4 (0.5 oz)	70	4	120	9	—
Ritz Bits (Nabisco)	22 (0.5 oz)	70	4	120	9	—
Cheese	22 (0.5 oz)	70	4	130	8	—
Cheese Pizza	5 (0.5 oz)	80	5	140	8	—
Cheese Sandwiches	6 (0.5 oz)	80	5	135	7	—
Low Salt	22 (0.5 oz)	70	4	60	9	—
Nacho Cheese	6 (0.5 oz)	80	5	140	8	—
Peanut Butter Sandwiches	6 (0.5 oz)	80	4	110	8	—
Ritz Low Salt (Nabisco)	4 (0.5 oz)	70	4	60	9	—
Ritz Whole Wheat (Nabisco)	5 (0.5 oz)	70	3	110	9	—
Rounds (Old London)						
Bacon	0.5 oz	53	1	126	9	1
Garlic	0.5 oz	56	1	132	9	1
Onion	0.5 oz	52	1	121	10	1
Rye	0.5 oz	52	1	132	10	—
Sesame	0.5 oz	56	2	149	8	1
White	0.5 oz	48	1	111	9	1
Whole Grain	0.5 oz	54	1	102	9	1
Royal Lunch (Nabisco)	1 (0.5 oz)	60	2	80	10	—
Rye (Hain)	1 oz	120	4	200	19	—
Rye No Salt Added (Hain)	1 oz	120	4	10	19	—
Rye Twins (Lance)	2	30	1	65	5	—
Rye Wafers Low Salt (Venus)	5 (0.5 oz)	60	1	110	11	—
Rye-Cheese (Lance)	1 pkg (41 g)	190	9	320	22	—
Rykrisp Natural	2	40	0	75	7	4
Rykrisp Seasoned	2	45	1	105	8	3
Rykrisp Seasoned Twindividuals	2	45	1	105	8	3
Rykrisp Sesame	2	50	2	105	7	3
Saltines (Lance)	2	25	1	65	4	—
Saltines Slug Pack (Lance)	4 crackers	50	1	130	8	—
Savory Thins Original (Sesmark)	15 (1 oz)	125	2	125	25	1
Sesame (Hain)	1 oz	140	7	210	16	—

FOOD	PORTION	CAL	FAT	SOD	CARB	FIB
Sesame (Pepperidge Farm)	4	80	4	140	12	2
Sesame Crisp (FFV)	2	120	3	—	—	—
Sesame No Salt Added (Hain)	1 oz	140	7	5	16	—
Sesame Stoned Wheat (Health Valley)	13	55	2	80	9	2
Sesame Stoned Wheat No Salt Added (Health Valley)	13	55	2	30	9	2
Sesame Thins Cheddar (Sesmark)	9 (1 oz)	150	8	400	15	3
Sesame Thins Garlic (Sesmark)	9 (1 oz)	150	8	340	16	3
Sesame Thins Original (Sesmark)	9 (1 oz)	150	8	380	16	2
Sesame Thins Unsalted (Sesmark)	1 (1 oz)	150	8	1	17	3
Sesame Twins (Lance)	2	40	1	65	6	—
Seven Grain Vegetable Stoned Wheat (Health Valley)	13	55	2	80	9	2
Seven Grain Vegetable Stoned Wheat No Salt Added (Health Valley)	13	55	2	30	9	2
Snack Crackers Toasted Rye (Keebler)	2	30	2	70	4	—
Snack Crackers Toasted Sesame (Keebler)	2	30	2	65	4	—
Snack Crackers Toasted Wheat (Keebler)	2	30	2	60	4	—
Snack Mix Classic (Pepperidge Farm)	1 oz	140	8	360	14	1
Snack Mix Lightly Smoked (Pepperidge Farm)	1 oz	150	9	350	13	1
Snack Sticks Cheese (Pepperidge Farm)	8	130	5	400	19	1
Snack Sticks Pretzel (Pepperidge Farm)	8	120	3	430	23	1

FOOD	PORTION	CAL	FAT	SOD	CARB	FIB
Snack Sticks Pumpernickel (Pepperidge Farm)	8	140	6	330	20	1
Snack Sticks Sesame (Pepperidge Farm)	8	140	5	280	19	1
Snackbread Original Wheat (Ryvita)	1	20	tr	—	—	—
Snackbread High Fiber (Ryvita)	1	14	tr	—	—	—
Snackwell's Cheese	18 (0.5 oz)	60	1	160	11	tr
Snackwell's Wheat	5 (0.5 oz)	50	0	160	12	tr
Snorkles Fun Cheddar (Nabisco)	27 (0.5 oz)	60	2	130	9	—
Snorkles Fun Pizza (Nabisco)	27 (0.5 oz)	60	2	110	10	—
Snorkles Fun Ranch (Nabisco)	27 (0.5 oz)	60	2	110	10	—
Sociables (Nabisco)	6 (0.5 oz)	70	3	135	9	—
Sour Cream & Chive (Hain)	1 oz	130	6	150	15	—
Sour Cream & Chive No Salt Added (Hain)	1 oz	130	6	25	15	—
Sourdough (Hain)	0.5 oz	65	3	100	9	—
Sourdough Low Salt (Hain)	1 oz	130	5	10	18	—
Spicy Lightly Smoked (Pepperidge Farm)	1 oz	140	8	340	14	1
Stoned Wheat (FFV)	4	60	1	—	—	—
Stoned Wheat (Health Valley)	13	55	2	80	9	2
Stone Wheat No Salt Added (Health Valley)	13	55	2	30	9	2
Stoned Wheat Wafers Bite Size (Venus)	7 (0.5 oz)	60	1	180	11	—
Swiss Cheese (Nabisco)	7 (0.5 oz)	70	3	170	11	—
Tam Tams (Manischewitz)	10	147	8	171	17	—
Tam Tams No Salt (Manischewitz)	10	138	7	—	18	—
Tams Garlic (Manischewitz)	10	153	8	165	19	—
Tams Onion (Manischewitz)	10	150	8	157	18	—
Tams Wheat (Manischewitz)	10	150	8	180	18	—

FOOD	PORTION	CAL	FAT	SOD	CARB	FIB
Tid Bits Cheese (Nabisco)	15 (0.5 oz)	70	4	200	8	—
Toastchee (Lance)	1 pkg (39 g)	190	11	310	19	—
Toasted Rice (Pepperidge Farm)	4	60	2	140	10	—
Toasted Snack Bacon (Keebler)	2	30	2	65	4	—
Toasted Snack Onion (Keebler)	2	30	2	70	4	—
Toasted Snack Pumpernickel (Keebler)	2	30	2	55	4	—
Toasted Wheat With Onion (Pepperidge Farm)	4	80	3	140	12	0
Toasty (Lance)	1 pkg (35 g)	180	10	160	17	—
Toasty Crackers With Peanut Butter (Little Debbie)	1 pkg (0.9 oz)	140	7	290	16	1
Toasty Crackers With Peanut Butter (Little Debbie)	1 pkg (1.4 oz)	200	10	350	20	1
Town House (Keebler)	2	35	2	60	4	—
Triscuit (Nabisco)	3 (0.5 oz)	60	2	75	10	—
Triscuit Deli-Style Rye (Nabisco)	3 (0.5 oz)	60	2	80	10	—
Triscuit Low Salt (Nabisco)	3 (0.5 oz)	60	2	35	10	—
Triscuit Wheat 'n Bran (Nabisco)	3 (0.5 oz)	60	2	75	10	—
Tuscany Toast	1 oz	95	2	—	—	—
Tuscany Toast (Pepato)	1 oz	93	2	—	—	—
Tuscany Toast (Pesto)	1 oz	96	2	—	—	—
Tuscany Toast (Tomato)	1 oz	95	2	—	—	—
Twigs Sesame & Cheese Sticks (Nabisco)	7 (0.5 oz)	70	4	140	8	—
Uneeda Biscuit Unsalted Tops (Nabisco)	2 (0.5 oz)	60	2	100	10	—
Unsalted (Estee)	4	60	2	0	9	—
Vegetable (Hain)	1 oz	130	5	180	10	—
Vegetable No Salt Added (Hain)	1 oz	130	5	50	10	—
Vegetable Thins (Nabisco)	6 (0.5 oz)	70	4	140	8	—

FOOD	PORTION	CAL	FAT	SOD	CARB	FIB
Waldorf Sodium Free (Keebler)	2	30	1	0	5	—
Wasa Crispbread						
Breakfast	1	50	1	70	9	1
Extra Crisp	1	25	0	40	5	—
Falu Rye	1	30	0	60	6	2
Fiber Plus	1	35	1	60	5	3
Golden Rye	1	30	0	50	7	3
Hearty Rye	1	50	0	75	10	1
Light Rye	1	25	0	40	5	1
Royal	½	26	0	54	6	1
Savory Sesame	1	30	1	45	4	2
Sesame Rye	1	30	1	45	4	2
Sesame Wheat	1	60	2	65	9	1
Toasted Wheat	1	50	1	70	9	1
Water Crackers Fat Free (Venus)	5 (0.5 oz)	55	0	70	11	—
Waverly (Nabisco)	4 (0.5 oz)	70	3	160	10	—
Waverly Low Salt (Nabisco)	4 (0.5 oz)	70	3	80	10	—
Wheat Crackers With Cheddar Cheese (Little Debbie)	1 pkg (0.9 oz)	140	7	270	16	0
Wheat Crispy Wafers (FFV)	6	70	3	—	—	—
Wheat Twins (Lance)	2	30	1	70	5	—
Wheat Thins (Nabisco)	8 (0.5 oz)	70	3	120	9	—
Wheat Thins Low Salt (Nabisco)	8 (0.5 oz)	70	3	60	9	—
Wheat Thins Multi-Grain (Nabisco)	8 (0.5 oz)	60	2	135	10	—
Wheat Thins Nutty (Nabisco)	7 (0.5 oz)	70	4	170	9	—
Wheat Wafers Low Salt (Venus)	5 (0.5 oz)	60	2	110	10	1
Wheatswafer (Lance)	2	30	1	50	4	—
Wheatsworth Stone Ground (Nabisco)	4 (0.5 oz)	70	3	135	9	—
Wholegrain Wheat (Keebler)	2	30	1	70	5	—
Zesta Saltine (Keebler)	2	25	1	75	4	—
Zesta Saltine Unsalted Top (Keebler)	2	25	1	35	4	—
Zings! Cheddar (Nabisco)	15 (0.5 oz)	70	3	130	9	—

FOOD	PORTION	CAL	FAT	SOD	CARB	FIB
Zings! Original (Nabisco)	15 (0.5 oz)	70	3	115	10	—
Zings! Ranch (Nabisco)	15 (0.5 oz)	70	3	135	9	—
Zwieback (Nabisco)	2 (0.5 oz)	60	1	20	10	—
cheese	1 (1 in sq, 1 g)	5	tr	10	1	—
cheese	14 (0.5 oz)	71	4	141	8	—
cheese, low sodium	1 (1 in sq, 1 g)	5	tr	5	1	—
cheese, low sodium	14 (0.5 oz)	71	4	68	8	—
cheese w/ peanut butter filling	1 (0.24 oz)	34	2	69	4	tr
crispbread	3	61	2	—	9	1
crispbread, rye	1 (0.35 oz)	37	tr	26	8	2
crispbread, rye	3	77	1	—	17	3
melba toast, plain	1 (5 g)	19	tr	41	4	tr
melba toast, pumpernickel	1 (5 g)	19	tr	45	4	tr
melba toast, rye	1 (5 g)	19	tr	45	4	tr
melba toast, wheat	1 (5 g)	19	tr	42	4	tr
milk	1 (0.42 oz)	55	2	71	8	—
oyster cracker	1 (1 g)	4	tr	13	1	tr
peanut butter sandwich	1 (7 g)	34	2	66	4	—
rusk toast	1 (0.35 oz)	41	1	25	7	—
rye w/ cheese filling	1 (0.24 oz)	34	2	73	4	—
rye wafers, plain	1 (0.9 oz)	84	tr	199	20	—
rye wafers, seasoned	1 (0.8 oz)	84	2	195	16	—
saltines	1 (3 g)	13	tr	38	2	tr
saltines, low salt	1 (3 g)	13	tr	19	2	tr
snack cracker	1 (3 g)	15	1	25	2	tr
snack cracker, low salt	1 (3 g)	15	1	11	2	tr
soup cracker	1 (1 g)	4	tr	13	1	tr
water biscuits	3	92	3	—	16	1
wheat w/ cheese filling	1 (0.24 oz)	35	2	64	4	—
wheat w/ peanut butter filling	1 (0.24 oz)	35	2	57	4	—
wheat thins	1 (2 g)	9	tr	16	1	—
wheat thins	7 (0.5 oz)	67	3	113	9	1
wheat thins, low salt	7 (0.5 oz)	67	3	40	9	1
whole wheat	1 (4 g)	18	1	26	3	—
whole wheat, low salt	1 (4 g)	18	1	10	3	--
zwieback	3.5 oz	374	4	263	73	4

CRANBERRIES

CANNED

FOOD	PORTION	CAL	FAT	SOD	CARB	FIB
CranFruit Cranberry Raspberry Sauce (Ocean Spray)	2 oz	100	0	10	23	—

FOOD	PORTION	CAL	FAT	SOD	CARB	FIB
CranFruit Cranberry Strawberry Sauce (Ocean Spray)	2 oz	100	0	10	23	—
CranFruit Cranberry Orange Sauce (Ocean Spray)	2 oz	100	0	10	23	—
Cranberry Sauce Jellied (Ocean Spray)	2 oz	90	0	10	22	—
Cranberry Sauce Jellied Old Fashioned (S&W)	½ cup	90	0	20	22	—
Cranberry Sauce Whole Berry Old Fashioned (S&W)	½ cup	90	0	20	22	—
Whole Berry Sauce (Ocean Spray)	2 oz	90	0	10	23	—
cranberry sauce, sweetened	½ cup	209	tr	40	54	—
FRESH						
Ocean Spray	½ cup	25	0	0	6	—
chopped	1 cup	54	tr	1	14	—
JUICE						
Ocean Spray Cocktail	8 fl oz	140	0	35	34	0
Ocean Spray Cocktail Reduced Calorie	8 fl oz	50	0	35	13	0
Ocean Spray Lightstyle Cranberry Juice Cocktail Low Calorie	8 fl oz	40	0	35	10	0
Seneca Cranberry Juice Cocktail	6 oz	110	0	—	—	—
Seneca Cranberry Juice Cocktail frzn, as prep	6 oz	110	0	—	—	—
Smucker's Juice Sparkler	10 oz	140	tr	5	34	—
Veryfine	8 oz	160	0	<10	40	—
cranberry juice cocktail	1 cup	147	tr	10	38	—
cranberry juice cocktail	6 oz	108	tr	4	27	—
cranberry juice cocktail, low calorie	6 oz	33	0	6	9	—
cranberry juice cocktail frzn	12 oz can	821	0	13	210	—
cranberry juice cocktail frzn, as prep	6 oz	102	0	6	26	—

FOOD	PORTION	CAL	FAT	SOD	CARB	FIB

CRANBERRY BEANS
CANNED
cranberry beans	1 cup	216	1	863	39	—

DRIED
Bean Cuisine	½ cup	115	1	5	—	5
cooked	1 cup	240	1	1	43	—

CRAYFISH
cooked	3 oz	97	1	58	0	—
raw	3 oz	76	1	45	0	—
raw	8	24	tr	14	0	—

CREAM
see also SOUR DREAM, SOUR CREAM SUBSTITUTES, WHIPPED TOPPINGS
LIQUID
Half & Half (Farmland)	2 tbsp	40	3	15	2	0
Half & Half (Land O'Lakes)	1 tbsp	20	2	—	—	—
Light Cream (Farmland)	2 tbsp	30	3	10	1	0
Whipping Cream (Land O'Lakes)	1 tbsp	45	5	—	—	—
Whipping Cream Gourmet Heavy (Land O'Lakes)	1 tbsp	60	6	—	—	—
half & half	1 cup	315	28	98	10	—
half & half	1 tbsp	20	2	6	1	—
heavy whipping	1 tbsp	52	6	6	tr	—
light coffee	1 cup	496	46	95	9	—
light coffee	1 tbsp	29	3	6	1	—
light whipping	1 tbsp	44	5	5	tr	—

WHIPPED
heavy whipping	1 cup	411	44	89	7	—
light whipping	1 cup	345	37	82	7	—

CREAM CHEESE
NEUFCHATEL
Philadelphia Brand Light	1 oz	80	7	115	1	—
Spreadery With Classic Ranch	1 oz	70	7	190	1	—
Spreadery With French Onion	1 oz	70	6	135	2	—
Spreadery With Garden Vegetable	1 oz	70	6	220	2	—
Spreadery With Garlic & Herb	1 oz	70	6	140	1	—

FOOD	PORTION	CAL	FAT	SOD	CARB	FIB
Spreadery With Strawberries	1 oz	70	5	270	tr	—
WisPride Garden Vegetable Cup	2 tbsp (1.1 oz)	60	5	180	2	0
WisPride Garlic & Herb Cup	2 tbsp (1.1 oz)	60	5	180	2	0
neufchatel	1 oz	74	7	113	1	—
neufchatel	1 pkg (3 oz)	221	20	339	3	—
REDUCED CALORIE						
Alpine Lace Fat Free With Chives	2 tbsp (1 oz)	30	0	165	1	0
Alpine Lace Fat Free With Garlic & Herbs	2 tbsp (1 oz)	30	0	165	1	0
Alpine Lace Free N'Lean	1 oz	30	0	—	2	—
Fleur De Lait						
Alouette C'est Light Herbs & Garlic	1 oz	70	6	120	2	—
Alouette C'est Light Spinach	1 oz	65	6	90	2	—
Alouette C'est Light Strawberry	1 oz	75	5	30	5	—
Alouette C'est Light Vegetables Julienne	1 oz	60	5	110	2	—
Chavrie	1 oz	50	4	150	1	—
Ultra Light Chives & Onions	1 oz	60	5	130	2	—
Ultra Light Fresh Vegetables	1 oz	60	5	130	2	—
Ultra Light Garlic & Spices	1 oz	60	5	120	1	—
Ultra Light Mixed Berry	1 oz	80	4	65	8	—
Ultra Light Nacho	1 oz	70	5	175	2	—
Ultra Light Strawberry	1 oz	70	6	70	6	—
Ultra Plain Light	1 oz	60	5	110	1	—
Formagg	1 oz	80	7	—	—	—
Friendship NY Style Reduced Fat	2 tbsp (1 oz)	50	3	120	0	0
Philadelphia Brand Light	1 oz	60	5	160	2	—
Weight Watchers	2 tbsp	35	2	40	1	—
REGULAR						
Fleur De Lait	1 oz	100	9	40	2	—
Philadelphia Brand	1 oz	100	10	90	1	—

FOOD	PORTION	CAL	FAT	SOD	CARB	FIB
Philadelphia Brand With Chives	1 oz	90	9	125	1	—
Philadelphia Brand With Pimentos	1 oz	90	9	150	1	—
cream cheese	1 oz	99	10	84	1	—
cream cheese	1 pkg (3 oz)	297	30	251	2	—
SOFT						
Heluva Good Cheese	1 tbsp (1 oz)	100	10	85	1	0
Philadelphia Brand	1 oz	100	10	100	2	—
With Chives & Onions	1 oz	100	9	100	2	—
With Herb & Garlic	1 oz	100	9	160	2	—
With Olives & Pimento	1 oz	90	8	160	2	—
With Pineapple	1 oz	90	8	90	4	—
With Smoked Salmon	1 oz	90	8	180	1	—
With Strawberries	1 oz	90	8	75	4	—
WHIPPED						
Philadelphia Brand	1 oz	100	10	85	1	—
With Chives	1 oz	90	8	150	1	—
With Onions	1 oz	90	8	170	2	—
With Smoked Salmon	1 oz	90	8	170	2	—

CREAM CHEESE SUBSTITUTES

FOOD	PORTION	CAL	FAT	SOD	CARB	FIB
Better Than Cream Cheese French Onion (Tofutti)	1 oz	80	8	135	1	—
Better Than Cream Cheese Herb & Chive (Tofutti)	1 oz	80	8	135	1	—
Better Than Cream Cheese Plain (Tofutti)	1 oz	80	8	135	1	—

CREAM OF TARTAR

FOOD	PORTION	CAL	FAT	SOD	CARB	FIB
cream of tartar	1 tsp	8	0	2	2	—

CREPES

FOOD	PORTION	CAL	FAT	SOD	CARB	FIB
basic crepe, unfilled	1	75	2	—	—	—

CRESS

see also WATERCRESS

FOOD	PORTION	CAL	FAT	SOD	CARB	FIB
garden, cooked	½ cup	16	tr	5	3	—
garden, raw	½ cup	8	tr	4	1	—

FOOD	PORTION	CAL	FAT	SOD	CARB	FIB
CROAKER						
FRESH						
atlantic, breaded & fried	3 oz	188	11	296	6	—
atlantic, raw	3 oz	89	3	47	0	—
CROISSANT						
All Butter (Sara Lee)	1	170	9	240	19	—
All Butter Petite Size (Sara Lee)	1	120	6	160	13	—
Colonial Wheat Croissants (Rainbo)	1	300	19	—	—	—
Croissant Sandwich Quartet (Pepperidge Farm)	1	170	7	250	22	tr
Petite All Butter (Pepperidge Farm)	1	120	6	170	13	—
apple	1 (2 oz)	145	5	156	21	1
cheese	1 (2 oz)	236	12	316	27	2
croissant	1 (2 oz)	232	12	424	26	2
plain	1 mini (1 oz)	115	6	211	13	1
TAKE-OUT						
w/ egg & cheese	1	369	25	551	24	—
w/ egg, cheese & bacon	1	413	28	889	24	—
w/ egg, cheese & ham	1	475	34	1080	24	—
w/ egg, cheese & sausage	1	524	38	1115	25	—
CROUTONS						
Arnold Crispy						
Cheddar Romano	0.5 oz	64	3	154	8	tr
Cheese Garlic	0.5 oz	60	2	130	9	tr
Fine Herbs	0.5 oz	50	1	150	10	1
Italian	0.5 oz	60	3	150	8	tr
Onion & Garlic	0.5 oz	60	2	190	9	—
Seasoned	0.5 oz	60	3	160	8	—
Brownberry						
Ceasar Salad	0.5 oz	62	3	165	8	1
Cheddar Cheese	0.5 oz	63	3	155	8	tr
Onion And Garlic	0.5 oz	60	2	190	9	tr
Seasoned	0.5 oz	59	2	155	8	1
Toasted	0.5 oz	56	1	145	10	tr
Kellogg's Croutettes	1 cup (1 oz)	100	0	370	20	0
Pepperidge Farm						
Cheddar & Romano Cheese	0.5 oz	60	2	200	10	—

FOOD	PORTION	CAL	FAT	SOD	CARB	FIB
Pepperidge Farm *(cont.)*						
Cheese & Garlic	0.5 oz	70	3	180	9	—
Onion & Garlic	0.5 oz	70	3	160	9	—
Seasoned	0.5 oz	70	3	180	9	—
Sour Cream & Chive	0.5 oz	70	3	170	9	—
plain	1 cup (1 oz)	122	2	209	22	2
seasoned	1 cup (1.4 oz)	186	7	495	25	2
CUCUMBER						
FRESH						
raw	1 (11 oz)	38	tr	6	8	3
raw, sliced	½ (1.8 oz)	7	tr	1	1	1
JARRED						
Rosoff's Salad	3 slices (1 oz)	12	0	220	3	—
Schorr's Cucumber Garden Salad	3 slices (1 oz)	12	0	220	3	—
TAKE-OUT						
cucumber salad	3.5 oz	50	tr	480	11	—
CUMIN						
seed	1 tsp	8	tr	4	1	—
CURRANTS						
DRIED						
zante	½ cup	204	tr	6	53	—
FRESH						
black	½ cup	36	tr	1	9	—
JUICE						
black currant nectar	3.5 oz	55	0	5	13	—
red currant nectar	3.5 oz	54	tr	tr	13	—
CUSK						
FRESH						
fillet, baked	3 oz	106	1	38	0	—
CUSTARD						
Custard (Royal)	mix for 1 serving	60	0	75	16	—
Flan (Jell-O)	½ cup	151	4	65	26	—
Flan Caramel Custard (Royal)	mix for 1 serving	60	0	55	15	—
Golden Egg Americana (Jell-O)	½ cup	160	6	198	23	—
baked	1 cup	305	17	209	29	—
custard, as prep from mix	½ cup	161	5	—	—	—

FOOD	PORTION	CAL	FAT	SOD	CARB	FIB
zabaglione, home recipe	½ cup (57.2 g)	135	5	9	13	0

CUTTLEFISH
steamed	3 oz	134	1	632	1	—

DANDELION GREENS
fresh, cooked	½ cup	17	tr	23	3	—
raw, chopped	½ cup	13	tr	21	3	—

DANISH PASTRY
FROZEN
Apple (Pepperidge Farm)	1	220	8	130	35	—
Apple (Sara Lee)	1	120	6	120	15	—
Apple Danish Twist (Sara Lee)	1 slice (1.9 oz)	190	10	200	22	—
Apple Free & Light (Sara Lee)	1 slice (2 oz)	130	0	120	30	—
Cheese (Pepperidge Farm)	1	240	14	230	25	—
Cheese (Sara Lee)	1	130	8	130	13	—
Cheese Danish Twist (Sara Lee)	1 slice (1.9 oz)	200	12	270	21	—
Cinnamon Raisin (Pepperidge Farm)	1	250	11	170	35	—
Cinnamon Raisin (Sara Lee)	1	150	8	140	17	—
Raspberry (Pepperidge Farm)	1	220	9	140	31	—
Raspberry Danish Twist (Sara Lee)	1 slice (1.9 oz)	200	9	220	25	—

READY-TO-EAT
Coffee Cake Raspberry (Hostess)	1 (1.2 oz)	110	3	110	21	tr
Apple (Hostess)	1 (3.8 oz)	400	22	340	47	2
Apple Fruit Roll (Hostess)	1 (2 oz)	180	4	170	33	1
almond	1 (4¼ in diam, 2.3 oz)	280	16	236	30	2
apple	1 (4¼ in diam, 2.5 oz)	264	13	251	34	1
cheese	1 (3 oz)	353	25	320	29	—
cheese	1 (3 oz)	266	16	319	26	—
cinnamon	1 (3 oz)	349	17	326	47	—

FOOD	PORTION	CAL	FAT	SOD	CARB	FIB
cinnamon	1 (4¼ in diam, 2.3 oz)	262	15	241	29	1
cinnamon nut	1 (4¼ in diam, 2.3 oz)	280	16	236	30	2
fruit	1 (3.3 oz)	335	16	333	45	—
lemon	1 (4¼ in diam, 2.5 oz)	264	13	251	34	1
plain ring	1 (12 oz)	1305	71	1302	152	—
raisin	1 (4¼ in diam, 2.5 oz)	264	13	251	34	1
raisin nut	1 (4¼ in diam, 2.3 oz)	280	16	236	30	2
raspberry	1 (4¼ in diam, 2.5 oz)	264	13	251	34	1
strawberry	1 (4¼ in diam, 2.5 oz)	264	13	251	34	1
REFRIGERATED						
Caramel Danish w/ Nuts (Pillsbury)	1	160	8	240	19	—
Cinnamon Raisin Danish w/ Icing (Pillsbury)	1	150	7	230	20	—
Orange Danish w/ Icing (Pillsbury)	1	150	7	250	19	—

DATES
DRIED

FOOD	PORTION	CAL	FAT	SOD	CARB	FIB
Bordo Diced	2 oz	203	1	5	48	—
California Deglet Noor	10	240	0	—	—	—
Dole Chopped	½ cup	280	0	3	68	—
Dole Pitted	½ cup	280	0	0	62	—
Dromedary Chopped	¼ cup	130	0	0	31	—
Dromedary Pitted	5	100	0	0	23	—
chopped	1 cup	489	1	5	131	—
whole	10	228	tr	2	61	—

DEER
See VENISON

DIETING AIDS
See NUTRITIONAL SUPPLEMENTS

DILL

FOOD	PORTION	CAL	FAT	SOD	CARB	FIB
seed	1 tsp	6	tr	tr	1	—
sprigs, fresh	1 cup	4	tr	5	1	—

FOOD	PORTION	CAL	FAT	SOD	CARB	FIB
sprigs, fresh	5	0	tr	1	tr	—
weed, dry	1 tsp	3	tr	2	1	—

DINNER

See also ORIENTAL FOOD, PASTA DINNERS, POT PIE, SPANISH FOOD

FROZEN

FOOD	PORTION	CAL	FAT	SOD	CARB	FIB
Armour Ham Steak	11 oz	350	13	—	—	—
Armour Classics						
Chicken Fettucini	11 oz	260	9	660	28	—
Chicken & Noodles	11 oz	230	73	660	23	—
Chicken Mesquite	9.5 oz	370	16	660	42	—
Chicken Parmigiana	11.5 oz	370	19	1060	27	—
Chicken w/ Wine & Mushroom Sauce	10.75 oz	280	11	900	24	—
Glazed Chicken	10.75 oz	300	16	960	24	—
Meat Loaf	11.25 oz	360	17	1170	32	—
Salisbury Parmigiana	11.5 oz	410	21	1120	32	—
Salisbury Steak	11.25 oz	350	17	1430	26	—
Swedish Meatballs	11.25 oz	330	18	1140	23	—
Turkey w/ Dressing & Gravy	11.5 oz	320	12	1280	34	—
Veal Parmigiana	11.25 oz	400	22	1320	34	—
Armour Lite						
Beef Pepper Steak	11.25 oz	220	4	970	29	—
Beef Stroganoff	11.25 oz	250	6	510	33	—
Chicken Marsala	10.5 oz	250	7	930	27	—
Chicken Ala King	11.25 oz	290	7	630	38	—
Chicken Burgundy	10 oz	210	2	780	25	—
Chicken Oriental	10 oz	180	1	660	24	—
Salisbury Steak	11.5 oz	300	11	980	29	—
Shrimp Creole	11.25 oz	260	2	900	53	—
Sweet & Sour Chicken	11 oz	240	2	820	39	—
Banquet						
Beans & Frankfurters Dinner	10 oz	350	14	1310	43	—
Beef Platter	9 oz	230	63	770	22	—
Boneless Chicken Drumsnacker Platter	7 oz	290	12	1580	33	—
Boneless Chicken Nugget Platter	6 oz	340	16	790	34	—
Boneless Chicken Pattie Platter	6.75 oz	310	15	820	31	—
Chicken & Dumplings	10 oz	270	10	1080	32	—

FOOD	PORTION	CAL	FAT	SOD	CARB	FIB
Banquet *(cont.)*						
Extra Helping Beef Dinner	15.5 oz	430	13	1220	42	—
Extra Helping Chicken Nuggets w/ Barbecue Sauce	10 oz	540	19	2330	68	—
Extra Helping Chicken Nuggets w/ Sweet & Sour Sauce	10 oz	540	19	2330	68	—
Extra Helping Fried Chicken All White Meat	14.25 oz	760	38	1770	69	—
Extra Helping Fried Chicken Dinner	14.25 oz	790	43	1490	68	—
Extra Helping Meat Loaf	16.25 oz	640	34	3320	60	—
Extra Helping Mexican Style Dinner	19 oz	680	25	3930	102	—
Extra Helping Salisbury Steak Dinner	16.25 oz	590	28	2760	57	—
Extra Helping Southern Fried Chicken Dinner	13.25 oz	790	39	2390	75	—
Extra Helping Turkey Dinner	17 oz	460	12	2030	64	—
Family Entrees Dumplings & Chicken	7 oz	280	14	—	28	—
Fish Platter	8 oz	270	7	650	38	—
Fried Chicken Dinner	9 oz	520	29	1130	41	—
Ham Platter	8.25 oz	200	5	1050	27	—
Italian Style Dinner	9 oz	180	2	790	35	—
Meat Loaf Dinner	9.5 oz	340	19	1220	32	—
Mexican Style Combination Dinner	11 oz	360	12	1290	52	—
Mexican Style Dinner	11 oz	410	17	1330	53	—
Noodles & Chicken	10 oz	170	4	740	26	—
Salisbury Steak Dinner	9 oz	280	13	1050	30	—
Southern Fried Chicken Platter	8.75 oz	400	16	3640	33	—
Veal Parmagian	9.25 oz	330	16	1140	35	—
Western Style Dinner	9 oz	300	16	1280	28	—
White Meat Fried Chicken Platter	8.75 oz	390	13	1620	37	—
White Meat Hot'n Spicy Fried Chicken Platter	9 oz	440	15	2280	43	—

FOOD	PORTION	CAL	FAT	SOD	CARB	FIB
Banquet Cookin' Bag						
Chicken Ala King	4 oz	110	5	—	—	—
Creamed Chipped Beef	4 oz	100	4	—	9	—
Gravy & Salisbury Steak	5 oz	190	14	—	8	—
Gravy & Sliced Beef	4 oz	100	5	—	5	—
Gravy & Sliced Turkey	5 oz	100	6	—	5	—
Turkey Chili	4 oz	80	2	15	11	—
Banquet Entree						
Chicken and Noodles	8.5 oz	240	10	1120	23	—
Gravy and Turkey w/ Dressing	7 oz	220	8	1410	26	—
Birds Eye Easy Recipe Beef Burgundy, not prep	½ pkg	120	5	670	17	4
Birds Eye Easy Recipe Beef Fajitas, not prep	½ pkg	80	3	390	14	3
Budget Gourmet						
Beef Cantonese	1 pkg (9.1 oz)	270	9	880	31	—
Beef Pot Roast	1 pkg (10.5 oz)	230	7	510	19	—
Beef Stroganoff	1 pkg (8.75 oz)	260	10	840	27	—
Chicken And Egg Noodles	1 pkg (10 oz)	440	26	880	28	—
Chicken Au Gratin	1 pkg (9.1 oz)	230	8	820	23	—
Chicken Breast Parmigiana	1 pkg (11 oz)	270	9	530	30	—
Chicken Marsala	1 pkg (9 oz)	260	8	730	31	—
Chicken With Fettucini	1 pkg (10 oz)	400	21	700	29	—
Chinese Style Vegetables And Chicken	1 pkg (10 oz)	280	7	590	47	—
French Recipe Chicken	1 pkg (10 oz)	220	9	870	21	—
Glazed Turkey	1 pkg (9 oz)	260	5	710	38	—
Ham And Asparagus Au Gratin	1 pkg (8.75 oz)	300	14	860	26	—
Herbed Chicken Breast With Fettucini	1 pkg (11 oz)	240	6	430	30	—
Italian Style Vegetables And Chicken	1 pkg (10.25 oz)	310	8	690	50	—
Mandarin Chicken	1 pkg (10 oz)	240	5	710	38	—
Mesquite Chicken Breast	1 pkg (11 oz)	250	6	550	33	—
Orange Glazed Chicken	1 pkg (9 oz)	270	3	870	46	—

FOOD	PORTION	CAL	FAT	SOD	CARB	FIB
Budget Gourmet *(cont.)*						
Oriental Beef	1 pkg (10 oz)	290	8	840	36	—
Oriental Chicken With Vegetables	1 pkg (9 oz)	280	6	690	44	—
Pepper Steak With Rice	1 pkg (10 oz)	300	8	720	40	—
Roast Chicken With Homestyle Gravy	1 pkg (11 oz)	280	8	560	36	—
Roast Sirloin Supreme	1 pkg (9 oz)	320	15	630	28	—
Sirloin Cheddar Melt	1 pkg (9.4 oz)	380	21	950	29	—
Sirloin Of Beef In Herb Sauce	1 pkg (9.5 oz)	250	9	860	21	—
Sirloin Of Beef In Wine Sauce	1 pkg (11 oz)	280	8	560	36	—
Sirloin Salisbury Steak	1 pkg (11 oz)	280	9	530	30	—
Sirloin Salisbury Steak	1 pkg (9 oz)	220	8	730	24	—
Sirloin Tips and Country Vegetables	1 pkg (10 oz)	290	17	810	19	—
Special Recipe Sirloin Of Beef	1 pkg (11 oz)	250	9	560	29	—
Stuffed Turkey Breast	1 pkg (11 oz)	250	6	570	31	—
Swedish Meatballs With Noodles	1 pkg (10 oz)	590	38	920	37	—
Sweet And Sour Chicken	1 pkg (10 oz)	340	5	620	55	—
Teriyaki Beef	1 pkg (10.75 oz)	260	7	530	37	—
Teriyaki Chicken Breast	1 pkg (11 oz)	300	8	480	41	—
Dining Light						
Chicken Ala King	9 oz	240	7	780	30	—
Chicken w/ Noodles	9 oz	240	7	570	28	—
Salisbury Steak	9 oz	200	8	1000	14	—
Sauce & Swedish Meatballs	9 oz	280	10	660	34	—
Healthy Choice						
Barbecue Beef Ribs	11 oz	330	6	530	40	—
Beef Pepper Steak	11 oz	290	6	530	34	—
Breast of Turkey	10.5 oz	290	5	420	39	—
Cacciatore Chicken	12.5 oz	310	3	430	47	—
Chicken A'L' Orange	9 oz	240	2	220	36	—
Chicken And Vegetables	11.5 oz	210	1	490	31	—
Chicken Dijon	11 oz	260	3	420	38	—
Chicken Oriental	11.25 oz	230	1	460	36	—

FOOD	PORTION	CAL	FAT	SOD	CARB	FIB
Chicken Parmigiana	11.5 oz	270	3	240	38	—
Chicken & Pasta Divan	11.5 oz	310	4	510	45	—
Glazed Chicken	8.5 oz	220	3	390	27	—
Herb Roasted Chicken	12.3 oz	290	4	430	39	—
Lemon Pepper Fish	10.7 oz	300	5	370	52	—
Mandarin Chicken	11 oz	260	2	400	39	—
Mesquite Chicken	10.5 oz	340	1	290	58	—
Roasted Turkey & Mushroom Gravy	8.5 oz	200	3	380	26	—
Salisbury Steak	11.5 oz	300	7	480	41	—
Salisbury Steak w/ Mushroom Gravy	11 oz	280	6	500	35	—
Salsa Chicken	11.25 oz	240	2	450	36	—
Seafood Newburg	8 oz	200	3	440	30	—
Shrimp Creole	11.25 oz	230	2	430	45	—
Shrimp Marinara	10.25 oz	260	1	320	51	—
Sirloin Beef w/ Barbecue Sauce	11 oz	300	6	320	40	—
Sirloin Tips	11.75 oz	280	8	370	30	—
Sliced Turkey w/ Gravy And Dressing	10 oz	270	4	530	30	—
Sole Au Gratin	11 oz	270	5	470	40	—
Sole w/ Lemon Butter	8.25 oz	230	4	430	33	—
Sweet & Sour Chicken	11.5 oz	280	2	260	44	—
Turkey Tetrazzini	12.6 oz	340	6	490	49	—
Yankee Pot Roast	11 oz	250	4	360	34	—
Kid Cuisine						
Chicken Nuggets	6.8 oz	360	17	660	39	—
Chicken Sandwiches	8.2 oz	470	17	830	61	—
Fish Sticks	7 oz	360	14	1050	46	—
Fried Chicken	7.5 oz	430	22	890	42	—
Hot Dogs w/ Buns	6.7 oz	450	19	880	57	—
Mexican Style	5.7 oz	290	85	610	45	—
Kid Cuisine Mega Meal						
Chicken Nuggets	8.4 oz	470	20	1010	51	—
Fried Chicken	10.8 oz	720	41	1400	53	—
Hot Dog w/ Bun	8.25 oz	500	25	1260	32	—
Le Menu						
Beef Sirloin Tips	11.5 oz	400	18	760	29	—
Beef Stroganoff	10 oz	430	24	980	28	—
Chicken A La King	10.25	330	13	830	29	—
Chicken Cordon Bleu	11 oz	460	20	850	47	—
Chicken In Wine Sauce	10 oz	280	7	680	27	—

FOOD	PORTION	CAL	FAT	SOD	CARB	FIB
Le Menu *(cont.)*						
Chicken Parmigiana	11.75	410	20	1030	31	—
Chopped Sirloin Beef	12.25 oz	430	24	1010	28	—
Ham Steak	10 oz	300	11	1500	31	—
LightStyle Glazed Chicken Breast	10 oz	230	3	480	25	—
LightStyle Herb Roasted Chicken	10 oz	240	7	400	18	—
LightStyle Salisbury Steak	10 oz	280	9	400	31	—
LightStyle Sliced Turkey	10 oz	210	5	540	21	—
LightStyle Sweet And Sour Chicken	10 oz	250	7	530	29	—
LightStyle Turkey Divan	10 oz	260	7	420	23	—
LightStyle Veal Marsala	10 oz	230	3	700	28	—
Pepper Steak	11.5 oz	370	13	1020	36	—
Salisbury Steak	10.5 oz	370	20	880	28	—
Sliced Breast of Turkey w/ Mushroom Gravy	10.5 oz	300	7	1020	38	—
Sweet & Sour Chicken	11.25 oz	400	18	1020	41	—
Veal Parmigiana	11.25 oz	390	17	840	36	—
Yankee Pot Roast	10 oz	330	13	700	27	—
Le Menu Entree LightStyle						
Chicken A La King	8.25 oz	240	5	670	29	—
Chicken Dijon	8 oz	240	7	500	21	—
Empress Chicken	8.25 oz	210	5	690	26	—
Glazed Turkey	8.25 oz	260	6	720	34	—
Herb Roast Chicken	7.75 oz	260	6	500	29	—
Swedish Meatballs	8 oz	260	8	700	30	—
Traditional Turkey	8 oz	200	5	610	19	—
Lean Cuisine						
Baked Chicken	1 pkg (8 oz)	240	5	480	31	3
Beef Pot Roast	1 pkg (9 oz)	210	7	570	21	3
Chicken a l'Orange	1 pkg (8 oz)	260	3	260	40	1
Chicken And Vegetables	1 pkg (10.5 oz)	240	5	520	30	5
Chicken In Honey Barbecue Sauce	1 pkg (8.75 oz)	250	5	560	35	6

FOOD	PORTION	CAL	FAT	SOD	CARB	FIB
Chicken In Peanut Sauce	1 pkg (9 oz)	280	6	590	33	3
Chicken Italiano	1 pkg (9 oz)	270	6	560	31	3
Chicken Marsala	1 pkg (8.1 oz)	180	4	470	13	5
Chicken Parmesan	1 pkg (10.9 oz)	220	5	530	22	5
Chicken Pie	1 pkg (9.5 oz)	320	10	590	39	3
Fiesta Chicken	1 pkg (8.5 oz)	240	5	590	31	3
Fish Divan	1 pkg (10.4 oz)	210	6	490	15	3
Glazed Chicken	1 pkg (8.5 oz)	240	6	460	24	2
Homestyle Turkey	1 pkg (9.4 oz)	230	5	590	26	3
Honey Mustard Chicken	1 pkg (7.5 oz)	250	5	460	32	4
Meatloaf	1 pkg (9.4 oz)	270	10	530	24	4
Oriental Beef	1 pkg (9 oz)	250	8	480	30	4
Roasted Turkey Breast	1 pkg (9.75 oz)	290	40	530	48	3
Salisbury Steak With Macaroni & Cheese	1 pkg (9.5 oz)	200	10	590	22	2
Stuffed Cabbage	1 pkg (9.5 oz)	220	7	460	27	5
Swedish Meatballs	1 pkg (9.1 oz)	290	8	590	32	3
Sweet And Sour Chicken	1 pkg (10.4 oz)	260	3	440	43	3
Turkey Pie	1 pkg (9.5 oz)	300	9	590	34	3
Morton						
Beans & Franks w/ Sauce	8.5 oz	300	11	1270	39	—
Fish w/ Mashed Potatoes And Carrots	9.25 oz	350	12	860	44	—
Glazed Ham	8 oz	230	3	1120	40	—
Gravy & Charbroiled Beef Patty	9 oz	270	12	1310	26	—
Gravy & Salisbury Steak	9 oz	270	16	1270	21	—
Tomato Sauce & Meatloaf	9 oz	280	16	1360	24	—
Veal Parmagian	8.75 oz	230	7	1330	31	—
Stouffer's						
Chicken A La King	1 pkg (9.5 oz)	320	10	750	43	3
Chicken Divan	1 pkg (8 oz)	210	10	570	10	1
Creamed Chicken	1 pkg (6.5 oz)	280	20	720	8	1
Creamed Chipped Beef	½ cup (4.5 oz)	150	11	690	6	1
Creamed Chipped Beef Over Country Biscuit	1 pkg (9 oz)	460	28	1650	40	3

FOOD	PORTION	CAL	FAT	SOD	CARB	FIB
Stouffer's *(cont.)*						
Escalloped Chicken & Noodles	1 pkg (10 oz)	440	29	880	28	2
Green Pepper Steak	1 pkg (10.5 oz)	330	9	650	45	3
Ham And Asparagus Bake	1 pkg (9.5 oz)	520	36	1040	32	2
Homestyle Baked Chicken	1 pkg (8.9 oz)	270	12	750	19	2
Homestyle Beef Pot Pie	1 pkg (8.9 oz)	270	10	640	25	4
Homestyle Breaded Chicken Tenders	1 pkg (6.6 oz)	380	18	1060	33	4
Homestyle Chicken Parmigiana	1 pkg (10.9 oz)	320	10	890	30	4
Homestyle Chicken & Noodles	1 pkg (10 oz)	310	14	1030	23	2
Homestyle Chicken Monterey	1 pkg (9.4 oz)	410	20	700	35	4
Homestyle Fish Filet With Macaroni & Cheese	1 pkg (9 oz)	430	21	930	37	2
Homestyle Fried Chicken	1 pkg (7.1 oz)	330	16	780	29	3
Homestyle Meatloaf	1 pkg (9.9 oz)	380	24	910	24	3
Homestyle Roast Turkey	1 pkg (7.9 oz)	280	11	950	25	1
Homestyle Salisbury Steak	1 pkg (9.6 oz)	370	19	1220	26	—
Homestyle Sliced Beef And Potatoes	1 pkg (8.1 oz)	270	10	900	25	2
Homestyle Veal Parmigiana	1 pkg (11.9 oz)	420	19	1200	43	6
Lunch Express Chicken With Garden Vegetables	1 pkg (9.9 oz)	340	11	750	45	2
Lunch Express Mandarin Chicken	1 pkg (9.75 oz)	270	6	520	41	2
Lunch Express Mexican Style Rice With Chicken	1 pkg (9 oz)	270	8	390	39	3
Lunch Express Oriental Beef	1 pkg (6.2 oz)	260	8	1220	34	4
Lunch Express Rice And Chicken Stir-Fry	1 pkg (9 oz)	280	9	590	39	3
Stuffed Pepper	1 pkg (10 oz)	200	8	900	24	1
Swedish Meatballs	1 pkg (9.25 oz)	440	23	840	36	3

FOOD	PORTION	CAL	FAT	SOD	CARB	FIB
Swanson						
Beans & Franks	10.5 oz	440	19	900	53	—
Beef	11.25 oz	310	6	770	38	—
Beef In Barbecue Sauce	11 oz	460	17	860	51	—
Chicken Duet Gourmet Nuggets Pizza Style	3 oz	210	12	—	—	—
Chopped Sirloin Beef	10.75 oz	340	16	790	28	—
Fish 'n Chips	10 oz	500	21	960	60	—
Fried Chicken Dark Meat	9.75 oz	560	28	1130	55	—
Fried Chicken White Meat	10.25 oz	550	25	1460	60	—
Homestyle Chicken Cacciatore	10.95 oz	260	8	1030	33	—
Homestyle Chicken Nibbles	4.25 oz	340	20	730	29	—
Homestyle Fish & Fries	6.5 oz	340	16	670	37	—
Homestyle Fried Chicken	7 oz	390	21	1100	33	—
Homestyle Salisbury Steak	10 oz	320	16	980	22	—
Homestyle Scalloped Potatoes And Ham	9 oz	300	13	1080	26	—
Homestyle Seafood Creole With Rice	9 oz	240	6	810	40	—
Homestyle Sirloin Tips In Burgundy Sauce	7 oz	160	5	550	16	—
Homestyle Turkey With Dressing & Potatoes	9 oz	290	11	1010	30	—
Homestyle Veal Parmigiana	10 oz	330	13	960	33	—
Hungry-Man Boneless Chicken	17.75	700	28	1530	65	—
Hungry-Man Chopped Beef Steak	16.75 oz	640	37	1600	41	—
Hungry-Man Fried Chicken Dark Meat	14.25 oz	860	45	1660	77	—
Hungry-Man Fried Chicken White Meat	14.25 oz	870	46	2150	80	—
Hungry-Man Salisbury Steak	16.5 oz	680	41	1730	37	—

FOOD	PORTION	CAL	FAT	SOD	CARB	FIB
Swanson *(cont.)*						
Hungry-Man Sliced Beef	15.25 oz	450	12	1060	49	—
Hungry-Man Turkey	17 oz	550	18	1810	61	—
Hungry-Man Veal Parmigiana	18.25 oz	590	26	1840	57	—
Loin Of Pork	10.75 oz	280	12	790	27	—
Macaroni & Beef	12 oz	370	15	930	48	—
Meatloaf	10.75 oz	360	15	960	41	—
Noodles & Chicken	10.5 oz	280	8	740	45	—
Salisbury Steak	10.75 oz	400	17	880	43	—
Swedish Meatballs	8.5 oz	360	20	790	26	—
Swiss Steak	10 oz	350	11	700	37	—
Turkey	11.5 oz	350	11	1090	42	—
Turkey	8.75 oz	270	11	—	—	—
Veal Parmigiana	12.25 oz	430	20	1010	42	—
Western Style	11.5	430	19	1060	43	—
Tyson						
Beef Champignon	1 pkg (10.5 oz)	370	15	830	31	—
Chicken Picante	1 pkg (9 oz)	250	4	390	26	—
Chicken Supreme	1 pkg (oz)	230	6	480	23	—
Francais	1 pkg (9.5 oz)	280	14	1130	20	—
Glazed Chicken With Sauce	1 pkg (9.25 oz)	240	4	930	29	—
Grilled Chicken	1 pkg (7.75 oz)	220	3	520	22	—
Grilled Italian Chicken	1 pkg (9 oz)	210	3	420	19	—
Healthy Portions BBQ Chicken	1 pkg (12.5 oz)	400	8	600	56	—
Healthy Portions Chicken Marinara	1 pkg (13.75 oz)	340	7	590	37	—
Healthy Portions Herb Chicken	1 pkg (13.75 oz)	340	4	550	43	—
Healthy Portions Honey Mustard Chicken	1 pkg (13.75 oz)	390	6	520	52	—
Healthy Portions Italian Style Chicken	1 pkg (13.75 oz)	310	4	600	38	—
Healthy Portions Mesquite Chicken	1 pkg (13.25 oz)	330	5	600	38	—
Healthy Portions Salsa Chicken	1 pkg (13.75 oz)	370	6	470	52	—
Healthy Portions Sesame Chicken	1 pkg (13.5 oz)	400	6	400	59	—

FOOD	PORTION	CAL	FAT	SOD	CARB	FIB
Honey Roasted Chicken	1 pkg (9 oz)	220	4	500	23	—
Kiev	1 pkg (9.25 oz)	450	25	950	39	—
Marsala	1 pkg (9 oz)	200	4	670	19	—
Mesquite	1 pkg (9 oz)	320	8	660	39	—
Picatta	1 pkg (9 oz)	200	4	550	18	—
Roasted Chicken	1 pkg (9 oz)	200	2	430	21	—
Sweet & Sour	1 pkg (11 oz)	420	15	850	50	—
Turkey With Gravy	1 pkg (9.5 oz)	320	12	900	34	—
Ultra Slim-Fast						
Beef Pepper Steak	12 oz	270	4	590	36	0
Chicken Fettucini	12 oz	380	12	980	38	1
Chicken & Vegetable	12 oz	290	3	850	45	4
Country Style Vegetable & Beef Tips	12 oz	230	5	960	26	4
Mesquite Chicken	12 oz	360	1	300	61	5
Roasted Chicken In Mushroom Sauce	12 oz	280	6	830	30	0
Shrimp Creole	12 oz	240	4	730	45	5
Shrimp Marinara	12 oz	290	3	880	53	0
Sweet & Sour Chicken	12 oz	330	2	340	57	0
Turkey Medallions In Herb Sauce	12 oz	280	6	950	33	0
Weight Watchers						
Barbecue Glazed Chicken	7 oz	200	6	450	22	—
Beef Sirloin Tips	7.5 oz	210	6	560	20	—
Beef Stroganoff	8.5 oz	280	9	590	29	—
Chicken Ala King	9 oz	230	4	460	30	—
Chicken Cordon Bleu	7.7 oz	170	5	560	15	—
Chicken Kiev	7 oz	190	5	470	22	—
Homestyle Chicken And Noodles	9 oz	240	7	450	25	—
Imperial Chicken	8.5 oz	210	4	420	26	—
London Broil	7.5 oz	110	3	320	4	—
Oven Baked Fish	7 oz	150	4	260	6	—
Southern Baked Chicken	6.3 oz	170	7	520	10	—
Stuffed Turkey Breast	8.5 oz	270	8	520	31	—
Veal Patty Parmigiana	8.2 oz	150	4	550	5	—

DIP

FOOD	PORTION	CAL	FAT	SOD	CARB	FIB
Avocado Guacamole (Kraft)	2 tbsp	50	4	210	3	—

FOOD	PORTION	CAL	FAT	SOD	CARB	FIB
Bacon & Horseradish (Kraft)	2 tbsp	60	5	200	3	—
Bacon & Horseradish Premium (Kraft)	2 tbsp	50	5	270	2	—
Bacon & Onion Premium (Kraft)	2 tbsp	60	5	170	2	—
Bacon And Horseradish (Breakstone)	2 tbsp	70	6	270	2	—
Bacon And Horseradish (Sealtest)	2 tbsp	70	6	270	2	—.
Bacon And Onion Gourmet (Breakstone)	2 tbsp	70	6	210	2	—
Bean (Eagle)	1 oz	35	2	140	4	—
Black Bean Mild (Guiltless Gourmet)	1 oz	25	0	80	5	1
Black Bean Spicy (Guiltless Gourmet)	1 oz	25	0	80	5	1
Blue Cheese Premium (Kraft)	2 tbsp	50	4	210	2	—
Chesapeake Clam Gourmet (Breakstone)	2 tbsp	50	4	200	2	—
Clam (Breakstone)	2 tbsp	50	4	220	2	—
Clam (Kraft)	2 tbsp	60	4	240	3	—
Clam (Sealtest)	2 tbsp	50	4	220	2	—
Clam Premium (Kraft)	2 tbsp	45	4	210	2	—
Creamy Cucumber Premium (Kraft)	2 tbsp	50	4	130	2	—
Creamy Onion Premium (Kraft)	2 tbsp	45	4	160	2	—
Cucumber And Onion (Breakstone)	2 tbsp	50	4	160	2	—
Cucumber And Onion (Sealtest)	2 tbsp	50	4	160	2	—
Fiesta Bean (Chi-Chi's)	1 oz	32	1	156	4	—
Fiesta Cheese (Chi-Chi's)	1 oz	37	2	258	4	—
French Onion (Breakstone)	2 tbsp	50	5	140	2	—
French Onion (Kraft)	2 tbsp	60	4	240	3	—
French Onion (Sealtest)	2 tbsp	50	4	140	2	—
French Onion Premium (Kraft)	2 tbsp	45	4	150	2	—
Frito-Lay Cheddar Cheese	1 oz	45	3	180	3	—
Frito-Lay French Onion	1 oz	50	4	180	3	—
Frito-Lay Jalapeno Bean	1 oz	30	1	115	4	—

FOOD	PORTION	CAL	FAT	SOD	CARB	FIB
Frito-Lay Picante Sauce	1 oz	10	0	160	3	—
Green Onion (Kraft)	2 tbsp	60	4	170	3	—
Hain Hot Bean	4 tbsp	70	1	250	10	—
Hain Mexican Bean	4 tbsp	60	1	260	9	—
Hain Onion Bean	4 tbsp	70	1	270	10	—
Hain Taco Dip & Sauce	4 tbsp	25	1	350	1	—
Heluva Good Cheese Bacon Horseradish	2 tbsp (1.1 oz)	60	5	200	2	0
Heluva Good Cheese Clam	2 tbsp (1.1 oz)	50	5	130	2	0
Heluva Good Cheese French Onion	2 tbsp (1.1 oz)	50	5	160	2	0
Heluva Good Cheese French Onion Light	2 tbsp (1.1 oz)	35	2	180	3	0
Heluva Good Cheese Homestyle Onion	2 tbsp (1.1 oz)	60	5	290	3	0
Heluva Good Cheese Jalapeno Cheddar Light	2 tbsp (1.1 oz)	40	2	160	3	0
Heluva Good Cheese Ranch	2 tbsp (1.1 oz)	60	5	180	2	0
Jalapeno Cheddar Gourmet (Breakstonc)	2 tbsp	70	6	90	2	—
Jalapeno Cheese Premium (Kraft)	1 tbsp	50	4	160	3	—
Jalapeno Pepper (Kraft)	2 tbsp	50	4	160	3	—
Mushroom And Herb Gourmet (Breakstone)	2 tbsp	50	4	150	2	—
Nacho Cheese Premium (Kraft)	2 tbsp	55	4	200	2	—
Pinto Bean (Guiltless Gourmet)	1 oz	25	0	80	5	1
Synder's Mustard Pretzel	2 tbsp (1.2 oz)	90	4	20	13	1
Toasted Onion Gourmet (Breakstone)	2 tbsp	50	5	170	2	—
Wise Jalapeno Flavored Bean	2 tbsp	25	0	100	5	—
Wise Taco	2 tbsp	12	0	115	3	—
DOCK						
fresh, cooked	3.5 oz	20	1	3	3	—
raw, chopped	½ cup	15	tr	3	2	—
DOGFISH						
raw	3.5 oz	193	15	14	0	—

FOOD	PORTION	CAL	FAT	SOD	CARB	FIB

DOLPHINFISH
FRESH

FOOD	PORTION	CAL	FAT	SOD	CARB	FIB
baked	3 oz	93	1	96	0	—
fillet, baked	5.6 oz	174	1	179	0	—

DOUGHNUTS
see also DUNKIN' DONUTS, WINCHELL'S

FOOD	PORTION	CAL	FAT	SOD	CARB	FIB
Assorted Regular (Hostess)	1 (1.6 oz)	200	11	230	23	tr
Cider (Dutch Mill)	1 (2.1 oz)	240	10	220	35	1
Cinnamon (Dutch Mill)	1 (1.8 oz)	210	11	250	26	1
Cinnamon (Tastykake)	1 (47 g)	180	8	210	26	1
Cinnamon Family Pack (Hostess)	1 (1 oz)	110	5	140	15	tr
Cinnamon Apple (Earth Grains)	1	310	17	—	—	—
Cinnamon Swirl (Hostess)	1 (1.6 oz)	180	7	220	28	tr
Crumb Regular (Hostess)	1 (1 oz)	130	8	115	14	tr
Crumb Topped (Entenmann's)	1 (2.1 oz)	260	12	220	34	—
Devil's Food (Earth Grains)	1	330	21	—	—	—
Devil's Food Crumb (Entenmann's)	1 (2.1 oz)	250	12	200	34	—
Donut Holes Double-Dipped Chocolate (Dutch Mill)	3 (1.4 oz)	220	16	140	19	0
Donut Holes Shootin' Stars (Dutch Mill)	3 (1.4 oz)	190	10	110	23	0
Donut Sticks (Little Debbie)	1 pkg (1.6 oz)	210	13	210	25	1
Donut Sticks (Little Debbie)	1 pkg (2 oz)	250	15	250	30	1
Donut Sticks (Little Debbie)	1 pkg (2.5 oz)	320	19	310	37	1
Donut Sticks (Little Debbie)	1 pkg (3 oz)	390	23	370	45	1
Double-Dipped Chocolate (Dutch Mill)	1 (2.1 oz)	280	17	360	31	1
Frosted Regular (Hostess)	1 (1.4 oz)	180	11	170	20	1
Frosted Rich (Tastykake)	1 (57 g)	260	16	200	28	3

FOOD	PORTION	CAL	FAT	SOD	CARB	FIB
Frosted Rich Mini (Tastykake)	1 (14 g)	44	3	60	8	1
Gem Donettes Cinnamon (Hostess)	6 (3 oz)	320	11	390	53	1
Gem Donettes Frosted (Hostess)	6 (3 oz)	390	23	360	42	2
Gem Donettes Frosted Strawberry Filled (Hostess)	3 (3 oz)	240	13	210	29	1
Gem Donettes Powdered (Hostess)	6 (3 oz)	350	16	380	47	1
Gem Donettes Powdered Strawberry Filled (Hostess)	3 (3 oz)	210	9	210	31	tr
Glazed (Dutch Hill)	1 (2.1 oz)	250	12	220	34	1
Glazed Chocolate (Dutch Hill)	1 (2.4 oz)	270	11	380	40	1
Glazed Old Fashioned (Earth Grains)	1	310	18	—	—	—
Glazed Party (Hostess)	1 (2.3 oz)	260	10	310	39	1
Honey Wheat (Tastykake)	1 (57 g)	210	8	200	32	1
Honey Wheat Mini (Tastykake)	1 (12 g)	40	1	50	7	0
Hostess O's Raspberry Filled Powdered (Hostess)	1 (2.2 oz)	230	10	230	35	tr
Jumbo Frosted (Hostess)	1 (2 oz)	260	16	240	28	1
Jumbo Plain (Hostess)	1 (1.1 oz)	140	7	190	16	tr
Jumbo Powdered (Hostess)	1 (1.3 oz)	160	9	170	19	tr
Mini Chocolate (Hostess)	5 (2 oz)	220	9	220	33	1
Old Fashion Donuts (Drake's)	1 (1.7 oz)	182	8	238	25	—
Old Fashioned Glazed (Hostess)	1 (2.1 oz)	250	12	230	33	tr
Old Fashioned Glazed Honey Wheat (Hostess)	1 (2.1 oz)	250	12	270	33	1
Old Fashioned Plain (Hostess)	1 (1.5 oz)	170	9	230	21	tr
Orange Glazed (Tastykake)	1 (57 g)	210	9	180	32	1
Plain (Dutch Hill)	1 (1.8 oz)	210	12	270	25	1

FOOD	PORTION	CAL	FAT	SOD	CARB	FIB
Plain (Tastykake)	1 (47 g)	190	10	170	22	1
Plain Regular (Hostess)	1 (1 oz)	120	6	160	13	tr
Powdered Family Pack (Hostess)	1 (1 oz)	110	6	135	15	1
Powdered Old Fashioned (Earth Grains)	1	290	19	—	—	—
Powdered Sugar (Tastykake)	1 (46 g)	180	9	220	24	1
Powdered Sugar Donut Delites (Drake's)	7 (2.5 oz)	300	15	316	38	—
Powdered Sugar Mini (Tastykake)	1 (12 g)	40	1	70	7	0
Rich Frosted (Entenmann's)	1 (2 oz)	280	18	210	27	—
Sugared (Dutch Mill)	1 (1.8 oz)	220	11	260	27	1
cake type, unsugared	1 (1.6 oz)	198	11	257	23	1
chocolate, glazed	1 (1.5 oz)	175	8	143	24	1
chocolate, coated	1 (1.5 oz)	204	13	185	21	1
creme, filled	1 (3 oz)	307	21	262	26	—
french cruller, glazed	1 (1.4 oz)	169	8	142	24	—
frosted	1 (1.5 oz)	204	13	185	21	1
honey bun	1 (2.1 oz)	242	14	205	27	1
jelly	1 (3 oz)	289	16	249	33	—
old fashioned	1 (1.6 oz)	198	11	257	23	1
sugared	1 (1.6 oz)	192	10	181	23	1
wheat, glazed	1 (1.6 oz)	162	9	160	19	—
wheat, sugared	1 (1.6 oz)	162	9	160	19	—
yeast, glazed	1 (2.1 oz)	242	14	205	27	1

DRESSING
see STUFFING/DRESSING

DRINK MIXER
see also SODA, MINERAL WATER/BOTTLED WATER

FOOD	PORTION	CAL	FAT	SOD	CARB	FIB
Bloody Mary Mix (Libby)	6 oz	40	0	1120	8	—
Bloody Mary Mix Extra Spicy (Tabasco)	8 fl oz	58	tr	1645	11	2
Margarita Mix w/ rum (Bacardi)	8 fl oz	160	0	0	24	—
Margarita Mix w/o liquor (Bacardi)	8 fl oz	100	0	0	25	—
Pina Colada (Bacardi)	8 fl oz	140	0	10	34	—
Rum Runner (Bacardi)	8 fl oz	140	0	10	35	—
Schweppes Collins Mixer	6 oz	70	0	—	—	—

FOOD	PORTION	CAL	FAT	SOD	CARB	FIB
Schweppes Lemon Sour	6 oz	75	0	—	—	—
Strawberry Daiquiri w/o liquor (Bacardi)	8 fl oz	140	0	0	35	—
Tabasco Bloody Mary Mix (McIlhenny)	8 fl oz	56	tr	1548	11	1
whiskey sour mix	2 oz	55	0	66	14	—

DRUM
FRESH
freshwater, fillet, baked	5.4 oz	236	10	148	0	—
freshwater, baked	3 oz	130	5	82	0	—

DUCK
w/ skin, roasted	½ duck (13.4 oz)	1287	108	227	0	—
w/ skin, roasted	6 oz	583	49	103	0	—
w/o skin, roasted	½ duck (7.8 oz)	445	25	143	0	—
w/o skin, roasted	3.5 oz	201	11	65	0	—
wild breast w/o skin, raw	½ breast (2.0 oz)	102	4	47	0	—
wild w/ skin, raw	½ duck (9.5 oz)	571	41	152	0	—

DUMPLING
FROZEN
Apple Dumpling (Pepperidge Farm)	1 (3 oz)	260	13	230	33	—

DURIAN
fresh	3.5 oz	141	2	1	29	—

EEL
FRESH
cooked	1 fillet (5.6 oz)	375	24	104	0	—
cooked	3 oz	200	13	55	0	—
raw	3 oz	156	10	43	0	—

EGG
see also EGG DISHES, EGG SUBSTITUTES
CHICKEN
fried w/ margarine	1	91	7	162	1	—
frozen	1	75	5	63	1	—
frozen	1 cup	363	24	307	3	—
hard cooked	1	77	5	62	1	—
hard cooked, chopped	1 cup	210	14	169	2	—
poached	1	74	4	140	1	—
raw	1	75	5	63	1	—
scrambled, plain	2	200	15	211	2	—

FOOD	PORTION	CAL	FAT	SOD	CARB	FIB
scrambled, w/ whole milk & margarine	1	101	7	171	1	—
scrambled, w/ whole milk & margarine	1 cup	365	27	616	5	—
white only	1	17	0	5	tr	—
white only	1 cup	121	0	399	2	—
OTHER POULTRY						
duck, raw	1	130	10	102	1	—
goose, raw	1	267	19	—	2	—
quail, raw	1	14	1	—	tr	—
turkey, raw	1	135	9	—	1	—

EGG DISHES
FROZEN

FOOD	PORTION	CAL	FAT	SOD	CARB	FIB
Chefwich Cheese Omelet	5 oz	380	17	—	—	—
Chefwich Ham & Cheese Omelet	5 oz	340	14	—	—	—
Chefwich Sausage & Cheese Omelet	5 oz	400	19	—	—	—
Chefwich Western Style Omelet	5 oz	350	13	—	—	—
Downyflake Scrambled Eggs With Ham And Hash Browns	1 pkg (6.25 oz)	360	26	730	17	—
Downyflake Scrambled Eggs With Ham And Pecan Twirl	1 pkg (6.25 oz)	470	28	670	40	—
Downyflake Scrambled Eggs With Hash Browns And Sausage	1 pkg (6.25 oz)	420	34	790	17	—
Downyflake Scrambled Eggs With Sausage And Pecan Twirl	1 pkg (6.25 oz)	510	33	710	39	—
Great Starts Egg, Sausage & Cheese	5.5 oz	460	28	1310	35	—
Great Starts						
Omelet With Cheese And Ham	7 oz	390	29	1220	15	—
Reduced Cholesterol Eggs With Mini Oatbran Muffins	4.75 oz	250	12	400	27	—
Scrambled Eggs With Cheese & Cinnamon Pancakes	3.4 oz	290	23	380	14	—

FOOD	PORTION	CAL	FAT	SOD	CARB	FIB
Scrambled Eggs & Bacon With Home Fries	5.6 oz	340	26	690	16	—
Scrambled Eggs & Home Fries	4.6 oz	260	19	380	14	—
Scrambled Eggs & Sausage With Hash Browns	6.5 oz	430	34	760	19	—
Kid Cuisine Egg Patties w/ Cheese	4.8 oz	200	10	650	15	—
Kid Cuisine Scrambled Eggs	4.1 oz	270	17	520	21	—
Quaker Scrambled Eggs Cheddar Cheese & Fried Potatoes	1 pkg (5.9 oz)	250	13	910	22	—
Quaker Scrambled Eggs & Sausage With Hash Browns	1 pkg (5.7 oz)	290	20	810	14	—
Quaker Scrambled Eggs & Sausage With Pancakes	1 pkg (5.2 oz)	270	14	880	21	—
Weight Watchers Garden Vegetable Omelet Sandwich	1 (3.6 oz)	210	6	—	28	—
Weight Watchers Ham And Cheese Handy Omelet	4 oz	180	5	—	18	—
HOME RECIPE						
deviled	2 halves	145	13	180	1	—
TAKE-OUT						
salad	½ cup	307	28	565	2	—
sandwich w/ cheese	1	340	19	804	26	—
sandwich w/ cheese & ham	1	348	16	1005	31	—
scotch egg	1 (4.2 oz)	301	21	—	16	2

EGG SUBSTITUTES

FOOD	PORTION	CAL	FAT	SOD	CARB	FIB
Egg Beaters	¼ cup	25	0	80	1	0
Egg Beaters Cheese Omelette	½ cup	110	5	480	2	—
Egg Beaters Vegetable Omelette	½ cup	50	0	170	5	—
Egg Watchers	2 oz	50	2	100	2	—
Healthy Choice Cholesterol Free	¼ cup	30	tr	90	1	—

FOOD	PORTION	CAL	FAT	SOD	CARB	FIB
Morningstar Farms						
Better'n Eggs	¼ cup (57 g)	30	0	100	1	—
Scramblers Links Muffins	1 pkg (4 oz)	220	10	400	22	—
Scramblers Cheese Home Fries	1 pkg (5 oz)	210	9	310	20	—
Scramblers Sandwich w/ Cheese	1 (3.5 oz)	220	7	420	29	—
Scramblers Sandwich w/ Pattie	1 (4.5 oz)	300	12	590	29	—
Scramblers Sandwich w/ Pattie, Cheese	1 (5 oz)	350	15	780	33	—
Scramblers Links Hash Browns	1 pkg (5 oz)	240	13	580	20	—
Scramblers	¼ cup (57 g)	60	3	125	3	—
Second Nature No Cholesterol	2 fl oz	60	2	90	3	—
Second Nature No Fat	2 fl oz	40	0	100	3	—
Second Nature No Fat With Garden Vegetables	2.5 fl oz	40	0	100	4	—
Simple Eggs	1.75 fl oz	35	1	130	1	1
frozen	1 cup	384	27	479	8	—
frozen	¼ cup	96	7	120	2	—
liquid	1.5 oz	40	2	83	tr	—
liquid	1 cup	211	8	444	2	—
powder	0.35 oz	44	1	79	2	—
powder	0.70 oz	88	3	158	4	—

EGGNOG

FOOD	PORTION	CAL	FAT	SOD	CARB	FIB
Borden	4 fl oz	160	9	80	16	—
Borden Light	½ cup	130	2	80	23	—
Land O'Lakes	8 oz	300	15	—	—	—
eggnog	1 cup	342	19	138	34	—
eggnog	1 qt	1368	76	553	138	—
eggnog flavor mix, as prep w/ milk	9 oz	260	8	163	39	—

EGGPLANT

FOOD	PORTION	CAL	FAT	SOD	CARB	FIB
CANNED						
Caponata (Progresso)	½ can	70	4	260	4	—
FRESH						
cubed, cooked	½ cup	13	tr	2	3	—
raw, cut up	½ cup (1.4 oz)	11	tr	1	2	—
whole, peeled, raw	1 (1 lb)	117	1	14	28	—

FOOD	PORTION	CAL	FAT	SOD	CARB	FIB
FROZEN						
Parmigiana (Mrs. Paul's)	5 oz	240	16	600	18	—
TAKE-OUT						
baba ghannouj	¼ cup	55	4	95	5	—
ELDERBERRIES						
FRESH						
elderberries	1 cup	105	1	—	27	—
JUICE						
elderberry	3.5 oz	38	0	1	8	—
ELK						
roasted	3 oz	124	2	52	0	—
ENDIVE						
fresh	3.5 oz	9	tr	53	tr	2
raw, chopped	½ cup	4	tr	6	1	—
ENGLISH MUFFIN						
FROZEN						
Great Starts Egg, Beefsteak & Cheese	5.9 oz	360	20	730	27	—
Great Starts Egg, Canadian Bacon & Cheese	4.1 oz	290	15	770	25	—
Healthy Choice English Muffin Sandwich	1 (4.5 oz)	200	3	510	30	—
Healthy Choice Turkey Sausage Omelet On English Muffin	1 (4.75 oz)	210	4	470	30	—
Healthy Choice Western Style Omelet On English Muffin	1 (4.75 oz)	200	3	480	29	—
Weight Watchers Sandwich With Egg, Ham And Cheese	1 (4 oz)	230	8	590	25	—
HOME RECIPE						
cinnamon raisin	1	186	3	123	38	—
english muffin	1	158	2	122	30	—
honey bran	1	153	3	154	30	—
whole wheat	1	167	tr	135	34	—
READY-TO-USE						
Matthew's Cinnamon Raisin	1	160	2	290	33	4

FOOD	PORTION	CAL	FAT	SOD	CARB	FIB
Matthew's Golden White	1	140	4	340	23	1
Matthew's Whole Wheat	1	150	2	340	31	4
Pepperidge Farm Cinnamon Apple	1	140	1	210	27	—
Pepperidge Farm Cinnamon Chip	1	160	3	180	28	—
Pepperidge Farm Cinnamon Raisin	1	150	2	200	29	—
Pepperidge Farm Plain	1	140	220	27	—	—
Pepperidge Farm Sourdough	1	135	1	260	27	—
Roman Meal	1 (2.2 oz)	135	1	332	25	3
Shop 'n Save	1	130	1	—	—	—
Tastykake	1 (57 g)	130	1	240	26	—
Tastykake Cinnamon Raisin	1 (64 g)	150	1	150	31	—
Tastykake Sourdough	1 (57 g)	130	1	210	25	—
Thomas'	1	130	1	206	25	—
Thomas' Honey Wheat	1	128	1	199	24	—
Thomas' Oat Bran	1	116	1	192	26	3
Thomas' Raisin Cinnamon	1	151	1	183	31	—
Thomas' Sandwich Size	1 (92 g)	210	2	330	42	2
Thomas' Sour Dough	1	131	1	210	25	—
apple cinnamon	1	138	2	255	28	—
granola	1	155	1	275	31	—
mixed grain	1	155	1	275	31	—
plain	1	134	1	265	26	—
plain, toasted	1	133	1	262	26	—
raisin cinnamon	1	138	2	255	28	—
sourdough	1	134	1	265	26	—
wheat	1	127	1	218	26	—
whole wheat	1	134	1	420	27	4
REFRIGERATED						
Roman Meal	½ muffin (1.1 oz)	66	tr	95	14	1
Roman Meal Honey Nut Oat Bran	½ muffin (1.1 oz)	81	1	114	16	1
TAKE-OUT						
w/ butter	1	189	6	386	30	—
w/ cheese & sausage	1	394	24	1036	29	—
w/ egg, cheese & bacon	1	487	31	1135	31	—
w/ egg, cheese & canadian bacon	1	383	20	785	31	—

FOOD	PORTION	CAL	FAT	SOD	CARB	FIB
EPPAW						
raw	½ cup	75	1	6	16	—
FALAFEL						
mix						
Near East, as prep	3 patties (3.7 oz)	310	2	740	22	7
TAKE-OUT						
falafel	1 (1.2 oz)	57	3	50	5	—
falafel	3 (1.8 oz)	170	9	150	16	—

FAST FOODS
see INDIVIDUAL NAMES

FAT
   see also BUTTER, BUTTER BLENDS, BUTTER SUBSTITUTES, MARGARINE, OIL

FOOD	PORTION	CAL	FAT	SOD	CARB	FIB
Crisco	1 tbsp	110	12	—	—	—
Crisco Butter Flavor	1 tbsp	110	12	—	—	—
Wesson Shortening	1 tbsp	100	12	0	0	0
beef suet	1 oz	242	27	—	0	—
beef tallow	1 tbsp (13 g)	115	13	0	0	—
beef, cooked	1 oz	193	20	12	0	—
chicken	1 cup	1846	205	—	0	—
chicken	1 tbsp	115	13	—	0	—
cocoa butter	1 tbsp	120	14	—	0	—
duck	1 tbsp	115	13	—	0	—
goose	1 tbsp	115	13	—	0	—
lamb new zealand, raw	1 oz	182	19	6	0	—
lard	1 cup (205 g)	1849	205	tr	0	—
lard	1 tbsp (13 g)	115	13	0	0	—
nutmeg butter	1 tbsp	120	14	—	0	—
pork backfat	1 oz	230	25	—	—	—
pork, cured	1 oz	164	17	—	—	—
pork, cured, roasted	1 oz	167	18	—	—	—
pork, cooked	1 oz	200	21	9	0	—
salt pork	1 oz	212	23	404	0	—
shortening	1 cup	1812	205	—	0	—
shortening	1 tbsp	113	13	—	0	—
turkey	1 tbsp	115	13	—	0	00
ucuhuba butter	1 tbsp	120	14	—	0	—

FAVA BEANS
CANNED

FOOD	PORTION	CAL	FAT	SOD	CARB	FIB
Progresso	½ cup	90	tr	420	15	12

FOOD	PORTION	CAL	FAT	SOD	CARB	FIB
FEIJOA						
fresh	1 (1.75 oz)	25	tr	2	5	—
puree	1 cup	119	2	7	26	—
FENNEL						
fresh bulb	1 (8.2 oz)	72	tr	122	17	—
fresh, sliced	1 cup	27	tr	45	6	—
seed	1 tsp	7	tr	2	1	—
FENUGREEK						
seed	1 tsp	12	tr	2	2	—
FIBER						
Natural Delta Fiber (Delta)	½ cup (1 oz)	20	tr	20	2	20
FIGS						
CANNED						
Kadota Figs Whole Fancy (S&W)	½ cup	100	0	—	28	—
in heavy syrup	3	75	tr	1	19	—
in light syrup	3	58	tr	1	15	—
water pack	3	42	tr	1	11	—
DRIED						
California	½ cup (3.5 oz)	200	1	11	58	17
cooked	½ cup	140	1	6	16	—
whole	10	477	2	20	122	17
FRESH						
fig	1 med	50	tr	1	10	—
FILBERTS						
dried, blanched	1 oz	191	19	1	5	—
dried, unblanched	1 oz	179	18	1	4	—
dry roasted, unblanched	1 oz	188	19	1	5	—
oil roasted, unblanched	1 oz	187	18	1	5	2
FISH						
see also FISH SUBSTITUTES, INDIVIDUAL NAMES						
CANNED						
Progresso Mixed Seafood Sauce	½ cup	110	6	445	12	—
Progresso Seafood	½ cup	190	15	570	5	tr
FRESH						
roe	3.5 oz	39	2	—	tr	—
FROZEN						
Cajun Cookin' Seafood Gumbo	17 oz	330	7	1330	51	—

FOOD	PORTION	CAL	FAT	SOD	CARB	FIB
Gorton's						
Crispy Batter Dipped Fillets	2	290	19	550	18	—
Crispy Batter Sticks	4	260	18	480	16	—
Crunch Fillets	2	230	13	420	16	—
Crunchy Sticks	4	210	13	240	15	—
Light Recipe Lightly Breaded Fish Fillets	1 fillet	180	8	380	16	—
Light Recipe Tempura Fillets	1 fillet	200	14	400	8	—
Microwave Crispy Batter Large Cut Fillets	1	320	21	680	20	—
Microwave Entree Fillets In Herb Butter	1 pkg	190	8	450	3	—
Microwave Fillets	2	340	26	400	17	—
Microwave Larger Cut Fillets	1	320	22	500	20	—
Microwave Larger Cut Ranch Fillet	1	330	21	520	24	—
Microwave Sticks	6	340	22	420	24	—
Potato Crisp Fillets	2	300	20	360	18	—
Potato Crisp Sticks	4	260	16	390	21	—
Value Pack Portions	1 portion	180	11	490	13	—
Value Pack Sticks	4	190	9	420	17	—
Mrs. Paul's						
40 Crunchy Fish Sticks	4 (2.75 oz)	200	10	340	18	—
Batter Dipped Fish Fillets	2 fillets	330	17	650	28	—
Battered Fish Portions	2 portions	300	19	540	21	—
Battered Fish Sticks	4 sticks	210	12	590	15	—
Combination Seafood Platter	9 oz	600	33	408	55	—
Crispy Crunchy Breaded Fish Portions	2 portions	230	15	300	14	—
Crispy Crunchy Breaded Fish Sticks	4 sticks	140	6	340	14	—
Crispy Crunchy Fish Fillets	2 fillets	220	9	380	23	—
Crispy Crunchy Fish Sticks	4 sticks	190	8	560	18	—
Crunchy Batter Fish Fillets	2 fillets	280	14	730	26	—
Fish Cakes	2	190	7	690	24	—
Light Fillets In Butter Sauce	1 fillet	140	6	520	1	—

FOOD	PORTION	CAL	FAT	SOD	CARB	FIB
Mrs. Paul's *(cont.)*						
Light Seafood Entrees Fish Dijon	8.75 oz	200	5	650	17	—
Light Seafood Entrees Fish Florentine	8 oz	220	8	820	10	—
Light Seafood Entrees Fish Mornay	9 oz	230	10	670	12	—
Microwave Buttered Fillet	1 fillet	80	4	130	10	—
Microwave Fillet Sandwich	1	280	15	460	27	—
Microwave Fillets	1 fillet	280	19	390	16	—
Microwave Fish Sticks	5	290	20	330	18	—
Van De Kamp's						
Battered Fish Fillets	1	170	10	350	13	—
Battered Fish Sticks	4	160	9	350	12	—
Breaded Fish Fillets	2	280	18	280	18	—
Breaded Fish Sticks	4	200	12	290	15	—
Fish Sticks Value Pack	4	170	10	270	13	—
Crispy Microwave Fillets	1 piece	140	9	210	9	—
Crispy Microwave Fishsticks	3 pieces	130	7	280	11	—
Crispy Microwave Large Fillets	1 piece	290	17	640	21	—
breaded fillet	1 (2 oz)	155	7	332	14	—
sticks	1 stick (1 oz)	76	3	163	7	—
MIX						
Beer Batter Fry (Golden Dipt)	1 oz	100	0	650	22	—
Cajun Style Fish Fry (Golden Dipt)	0.66 oz	60	0	470	14	—
Fish & Chips Batter Mix (Golden Dipt)	1.25 oz	120	0	910	27	—
Fish Fry (Golden Dipt)	0.66 oz	60	0	430	14	—
Seafood Frying Mix (Golden Dipt)	0.66 oz	60	0	600	14	—
Tempura Batter Mix (Golden Dipt)	1 oz	100	0	130	22	—
TAKE-OUT						
kedgeree	5.6 oz	242	11	—	15	1

FOOD	PORTION	CAL	FAT	SOD	CARB	FIB
sandwich w/ tartar sauce	1	431	55	615	41	—
sandwich w/ tartar sauce & cheese	1	524	29	939	48	—
taramasalata	3.5 oz	446	46	—	4	—

FISH PASTE
fish paste	2 tsp	15	1	—	tr	0

FISH SUBSTITUTES
LaLoma Ocean Platter, mix not prep	½ cup (16 g)	50	0	260	5	—
Worthington Fillets	2 (85 g)	180	9	910	9	—
Worthington Tuno	2 oz (57 g)	100	7	310	3	—

FLATFISH
FRESH
cooked	1 fillet (4.5 oz)	148	2	133	0	—
cooked	3 oz	99	1	89	0	—

TAKE-OUT
battered & fried	3.2 oz	211	11	484	15	—
breaded & fried	3.2 oz	211	11	484	15	—

FLAX
Seeds (Arrowhead)	3 tbsp (1 oz)	140	10	0	11	6

FLOUNDER
FROZEN
Crunchy Batter Fillets (Mrs. Paul's)	2 fillets	220	9	560	23	—
Fishmarket Fresh (Gorton's)	5 oz	110	1	170	1	—
Flounder Primavera (King & Prince)	6 oz	180	9	—	—	—
Flounder Del Rey (King & Prince)	4.5 oz	163	8	—	—	—
Light Fillets (Mrs. Paul's)	1 fillet	240	10	450	20	—
Light Fillets (Van De Kamp's)	1 piece	260	12	480	21	—
Microwave Entree Stuffed (Gorton's)	1 pkg	350	18	850	21	—
Natural Fillets (Van De Kamp's)	4 oz	100	2	100	0	—

FOOD	PORTION	CAL	FAT	SOD	CARB	FIB
FLOUR						
50/50 Flour (Hodgson Mill)	¼ cup (1 oz)	100	1	0	21	2
All Purpose						
(Ballard)	1 cup	400	1	0	87	—
(Ceresota)	1 cup	390	1	0	83	—
(Gold Medal)	1 cup	400	1	0	87	—
(Heckers)	1 cup	390	1	0	83	—
(Robin Hood)	1 cup	400	1	0	85	—
Best (Pillsbury)	1 cup	400	1	0	87	—
(Red Band)	1 cup	390	1	—	—	—
(White Deer)	1 cup	400	1	—	—	—
Best For Bread (Hodgson Mill)	¼ cup (1 oz)	100	0	0	22	1
Bohemian Style Rye and Wheat Best (Pillsbury)	1 cup	400	1	0	86	—
Bread Best (Pillsbury)	1 cup	400	2	0	83	—
Buckwheat (Hodgson Mill)	⅓ cup (1.6 oz)	160	1	10	33	2
Drifted Snow (General Mills)	1 cup	400	1	—	—	—
Kamut (Arrowhead)	¼ cup (1.2 oz)	110	1	0	25	4
La Pina (Gold Medal)	1 cup	390	1	—	—	—
Oat Blend (Gold Medal)	1 cup	390	3	0	81	—
Oat Bran Blend (Hodgson Mill)	¼ cup (1 oz)	110	1	120	24	3
Oat Bran Flour (Hodgson Mill)	¼ cup (1 oz)	110	2	4	23	3
Pastry (Arrowhead)	⅓ cup (1.1 oz)	100	1	0	22	3
Rye (Hodgson Mill)	¼ cup (1 oz)	90	1	0	22	5
Rye Medium Best (Pillsbury)	1 cup	400	2	0	83	—
Rye Stone Ground (Robin Hood)	1 cup	360	2	10	86	13
Rye Whole Grain (Arrowhead)	¼ cup (1.6 oz)	160	1	0	34	6
Seasoned Flour (Hodgson Mill)	¼ cup (1 oz)	90	0	1360	20	0
Self-Rising						
(Aunt Jemima)	¼ cup	109	tr	794	24	1
(Ballard)	1 cup	380	1	1290	84	—
Best (Pillsbury)	1 cup	380	1	1290	84	—
(Gold Medal)	1 cup	380	1	1520	83	—

FOOD	PORTION	CAL	FAT	SOD	CARB	FIB
(Red Band)	1 cup	380	1	—	—	—
(Robin Hood)	1 cup	380	1	1520	83	—
Shake & Blend Best (Pillsbury)	2 tbsp	50	0	0	11	—
Softasilk (General Mills)	¼ cup	100	0	—	—	—
Spelt (Arrowhead)	¼ cup (1.2 oz)	100	1	0	24	5
Teff (Arrowhead)	¼ cup (1.4 oz)	140	1	5	29	5
Unbleached (Gold Medal)	1 cup	400	1	0	87	—
Unbleached (Robin Hood)	1 cup	400	1	0	85	—
Unbleached Best (Pillsbury)	1 cup	400	1	0	86	—
Unbleached White (Arrowhead)	⅓ cup (1.6 oz)	160	1	0	33	0
White (Hodgson Mill)	¼ cup (1 oz)	100	0	0	23	3
Whole Grain Wheat (Arrowhead)	¼ cup (1.6 oz)	160	1	0	34	7
Whole Wheat (Arrowhead)	¼ cup (1.2 oz)	130	1	0	25	4
(Ceresota)	1 cup	400	2	0	80	—
(Gold Medal)	1 cup	350	2	0	78	10
(Heckers)	1 cup	400	2	0	80	—
(Hodgson Mill)	¼ cup (1 oz)	100	1	0	22	3
Whole Wheat Best (Pillsbury)	1 cup	400	2	10	80	—
Whole Wheat Blend (Gold Medal)	1 cup	380	2	0	84	8
Wondra	1 cup	400	1	—	—	—
corn masa	1 cup	416	4	6	87	—
corn whole grain	1 cup	422	5	6	90	8
cottonseed, lowfat	1 oz	94	tr	10	10	—
peanut, defatted	1 cup	196	tr	108	21	—
peanut, defatted	1 oz	92	tr	50	10	—
peanut, lowfat	1 cup	257	13	0	19	—
potato	1 cup (6.3 oz)	628	1	61	143	—
rice, brown	1 cup	574	4	12	121	4
rice, white	1 cup	578	2	1	127	2
rye, dark	1 cup	415	3	2	88	—
rye, light	1 cup	374	1	2	82	7
rye, medium	1 cup	361	2	3	79	7
sesame, lowfat	1 oz	95	tr	11	10	—
triticale, whole grain	1 cup	440	2	3	95	9
white, all-purpose	1 cup	455	1	2	95	2
white, bread	1 cup	495	2	2	99	—

FOOD	PORTION	CAL	FAT	SOD	CARB	FIB
white, cake	1 cup	395	tr	2	85	—
white, self-rising	1 cup	442	1	1587	93	—
whole wheat	1 cup	407	2	6	87	8

FRANKFURTER
see HOTDOG

FRENCH BEANS
DRIED

cooked	1 cup	228	1	11	43	—

FRENCH FRIES
see POTATO

FRENCH TOAST
FROZEN

Aunt Jemima	3 oz	166	4	554	27	1
Aunt Jemima Cinnamon Swirl	3 oz	171	4	516	28	1
Downyflake	2	270	12	380	34	—
Downyflake Extra Thick	1	150	9	340	11	—
Downflake Texas Style & Sausage	1 pkg (4.25 oz)	400	24	550	37	—
Great Starts Cinnamon Swirl With Sausage	5.5 oz	390	21	530	37	—
Great Starts French Toast With Sausage	5.5 oz	380	21	550	35	—
Great Starts Mini French Toast With Sausage	2.5 oz	190	9	320	22	—
Great Starts Oatmeal French Toast With Lite Links	4.65 oz	310	13	500	35	—
Healthy Starts French Toast With LeanLinks	6.5 oz	400	13	595	51	—
Kid Cuisine	4.11 oz	260	12	320	28	—
Quaker French Toast Sticks & Syrup	1 pkg (5.2 oz)	400	20	640	48	—
Quaker French Toast Wedges & Sausage	1 pkg (5.3 oz)	360	17	780	40	—
Weight Watchers French Toast With Cinnamon	2 slices (3 oz)	160	5	280	24	—
Weight Watchers French Toast With Links	4.5 oz	270	11	—	24	—
french toast	1 slice (2 oz)	126	4	292	19	2

FOOD	PORTION	CAL	FAT	SOD	CARB	FIB
HOME RECIPE						
as prep w/ 2% milk	1 slice	149	7	311	16	—
as prep w/ whole milk	1 slice	151	7	311	16	—
TAKE-OUT						
w/ butter	2 slices	356	19	513	36	—

FROG'S LEGS

frog leg, as prep w/ seasoned flour & fried	1 (0.8)	70	5	—	15	—

FROSTING
see CAKE

FRUCTOSE

Fructose Estee	1 tsp	12	0	0	3	—

FRUIT DRINKS
see also LEMONADE

FROZEN						
Five Alive Berry Citrus	8 fl oz	120	0	0	30	—
Five Alive Citrus	8 fl oz	120	0	0	30	—
Five Alive Tropical Citrus	8 fl oz	120	0	25	29	—
Minute Maid						
Berry Punch	8 fl oz	130	0	5	31	—
Citrus Punch	8 fl oz	120	0	5	31	—
Fruit Punch	8 fl oz	120	0	5	31	—
Limeade	8 fl oz	100	0	0	26	—
Pineapple Orange	8 fl oz	120	0	0	31	—
Tropical Punch	8 fl oz	120	0	5	31	—
Seneca Cranberry Apple Cocktail, as prep	6 oz	110	0	—	—	—
Seneca Grape Cranberry Cocktail, as prep	6 oz	110	0	—	—	—
Seneca Raspberry Cranberry Cocktail, as prep	6 oz	110	0	—	—	—
Tree Top						
Apple Citrus, as prep	6 oz	90	0	10	22	—
Apple Cranberry, as prep	6 oz	100	0	10	25	—
Apple Grape, as prep	6 oz	100	0	10	25	—
Apple Pear, as prep	6 oz	90	0	10	22	—
Apple Raspberry, as prep	6 oz	80	0	10	21	—

FOOD	PORTION	CAL	FAT	SOD	CARB	FIB
citrus juice drink, as prep	1 cup	114	0	7	28	—
citrus juice drink, not prep	1 can (12 fl oz)	684	tr	12	171	—
fruit punch, not prep	1 can (12 fl oz)	678	tr	34	173	—
fruit punch, as prep w/ water	1 cup	113	tr	11	29	—
limeade	1 can (6 oz)	408	tr	—	108	—
limeade, as prep w/ water	1 cup	102	tr	6	27	—
MIX						
Crystal Light Berry Blend Sugar Free	8 oz	3	0	—	0	—
Crystal Light Fruit Punch Sugar Free	8 oz	3	0	—	0	—
Crystal Light Lemon-Lime	8 oz	4	0	—	0	—
Crystal Light Tropic Quencher	8 oz	5	0	—	0	—
Kool-Aid						
Lemon-Lime	8 oz	98	0	—	25	—
Purplesaurus Rex	8 oz	98	0	6	25	—
Rainbow Punch	8 oz	98	0	—	25	—
Raspberry	8 oz	98	0	27	25	—
Sharkleberry Fin	8 oz	98	0	—	25	—
Strawberry	8 oz	98	0	27	25	—
Sugar Free Berry Blue	8 oz	3	0	6	0	—
Sugar Free Berry Punch	8 oz	3	0	33	0	—
Sugar Free Purplesaurus Rex	8 oz	3	0	6	0	—
Sugar Free Rainbow Punch	8 oz	4	0	—	0	—
Sugar Free Sharkleberry Fin	8 oz	3	0	—	0	—
Sugar Free Tropical Punch	8 oz	3	0	8	0	—
Sugar Sweetened Mountain Berry Punch	8 oz	98	0	15	25	—
Sugar Sweetened Purplesaurus Rex	8 oz	84	0	6	21	—
Sugar Sweetened Rainbow Punch	8 oz	84	0	20	21	—

FOOD	PORTION	CAL	FAT	SOD	CARB	FIB
Sugar Sweetened Sharkleberry Fin	8 oz	84	0	—	21	—
Sugar Sweetened Sunshine Punch	8 oz	83	0	—	21	—
Sugar Sweetened Surfin' Berry Punch	8 oz	79	0	27	20	—
Sugar Sweetened Tropical Punch	8 oz	84	0	—	21	—
Tropical Punch	8 oz	98	0	—	25	—
Unsweetened Berry Blue	8 oz	98	0	6	25	—
Wylers Drink Mix Unsweetened Bunch O' Berries	8 oz	2	0	28	1	—
Wylers Drink Mix Unsweetened Pink Wyler's	8 fl oz	3	0	19	1	—
Wylers Drink Mix Unsweetened Tropical Punch	8 oz	2	0	tr	1	—
fruit punch, as prep w/ water	9 oz	97	0	38	25	—
READY-TO-DRINK						
Bright & Early Fruit Punch Frozen	8 fl oz	130	0	5	31	—
Chiquita Orange Banana	6 fl oz	90	0	—	—	—
Crystal Geyser Juice Squeeze Citrus Grape	1 bottle (12 fl oz)	145	0	20	35	—
Crystal Geyser Juice Squeeze Orange & Passion Fruit	1 bottle (12 fl oz)	125	0	20	31	—
Crystal Geyser Juice Squeeze Passion Fruit & Mango	1 bottle (12 fl oz)	130	0	20	31	—
Dole						
New Breakfast Juice Pineapple Orange	6 fl oz	90	tr	20	23	—
New Breakfast Juice Pineapple Orange Banana	6 fl oz	90	tr	10	21	—
New Breakfast Juice Pineapple Orange Guava	6 fl oz	100	tr	10	21	—
New Breakfast Juice Pineapple Passion Banana	6 fl oz	100	tr	10	21	—

FOOD	PORTION	CAL	FAT	SOD	CARB	FIB
Dole *(cont.)*						
Pineapple Grapefruit	6 fl oz	90	tr	25	23	—
Pineapple Orange	6 fl oz	90	tr	20	23	—
Pineapple Orange Banana	6 fl oz	90	tr	10	21	—
Pineapple Pink Grapefruit	6 fl oz	100	tr	5	25	—
Five Alive Citrus	6 fl oz	90	0	20	22	—
Five Alive Citrus	1 bottle (16 fl oz)	120	0	25	31	—
Five Alive Citrus	1 can (11.5 fl oz)	170	0	35	43	—
Five Alive Citrus Chilled	8 fl oz	120	0	25	30	—
Hawaiian Punch						
Fruit Juicy Red	6 fl oz	90	0	—	—	—
Island Fruit Cocktail	6 fl oz	90	0	—	—	—
Lite Fruit Juicy Red	6 fl oz	60	0	—	—	—
Tropical Fruits	6 fl oz	90	0	—	—	—
Very Berry	6 fl oz	90	0	—	—	—
Wild Fruit	6 fl oz	90	0	—	—	—
Hi-C						
Boppin' Berry	8 fl oz	130	0	30	32	—
Boppin' Berry Box	8.45 fl oz	140	0	30	33	—
Double Fruit Box	8.45 fl oz	130	0	35	32	—
Double Fruit Cooler	8 fl oz	130	0	30	31	—
Ecto Cooler	1 can (11.5 fl oz)	180	0	40	45	—
Ecto Cooler	8 fl oz	130	0	25	32	—
Ecto Cooler Box	8.45 fl oz	130	0	35	32	—
Fruit Punch	1 can (11.5 fl oz)	190	0	40	46	—
Fruit Punch	8 fl oz	130	0	30	32	—
Fruit Punch Box	8.45 fl oz	140	0	30	32	—
Fruity Bubble Gum	8 fl oz	120	0	25	30	—
Fruit Bubble Gum Box	8.45 fl oz	130	0	30	32	—
Hula Punch	1 can (11.5 fl oz)	170	0	40	42	—
Hula Punch	8 fl oz	120	0	30	29	—
Hula Punch	8.45 fl oz	120	0	30	30	—
Jammin' Apple Box	8.45 fl oz	130	0	30	33	—
Stompin' Banana Berry	8 fl oz	130	0	30	31	—
Stompin' Banana Berry Box	8.45 fl oz	130	0	30	32	—
Wild Berry	8 fl oz	120	0	30	30	—
Wild Berry Box	8.45 fl oz	130	0	30	32	—
Juice Works Appleberry	6 fl oz	100	0	—	—	—
Juicy Juice						
Apple Grape	6 fl oz	90	0	10	22	—

FOOD	PORTION	CAL	FAT	SOD	CARB	FIB
Berry	6 fl oz	90	0	10	22	—
Berry	8.45 fl oz	130	0	15	30	—
Punch	6 fl oz	100	0	10	23	—
Punch	8.45 fl oz	140	0	10	33	—
Tropical	6 fl oz	110	0	10	26	—
Tropical	8.45 fl oz	150	0	10	36	—
Kern's						
Appricot Orange Nectar	6 fl oz	112	0	<10	28	—
Apricot Pineapple Nectar	6 fl oz	110	0	10	25	—
Banana Pineapple Nectar	6 fl oz	120	0	10	29	—
Coconut Pineapple Nectar	6 fl oz	120	0	40	26	—
Passionfruit Orange Nectar	6 fl oz	110	0	10	28	—
Strawberry Banana Nectar	6 fl oz	100	0	10	25	—
Tropical Nectar	6 fl oz	112	0	10	29	—
Kool-Aid Koolers						
Mountainberry Punch	1 pkg (8.45 fl oz)	142	0	3	37	—
Rainbow Punch	1 pkg (8.45 fl oz)	135	0	3	36	—
Sharkleberry Fin	1 pkg (8.45 fl oz)	140	0	3	37	—
Tropical Punch	1 pkg (8.45 fl oz)	132	0	3	35	—
Libby's Passion Fruit Orange Nectar	8 fl oz	150	0	10	36	—
Libby's Strawberry Banana Nectar	8 fl oz	150	0	5	35	—
Mauna La'i Island Guava Hawaiian Guava Fruit Juice Drink	8 fl oz	130	0	35	32	0
Mauna La'i Mango & Hawaiian Guava Fruit Juice Drink	8 fl oz	130	0	35	33	0
Mauna La'i Paradise Guava Hawaiian Guava & Passion Fruit Juice Drink	8 fl oz	130	0	35	32	0
Minute Maid						
Berry Punch Box	8.45 fl oz	130	0	25	31	—
Berry Punch Chilled	8 fl oz	130	0	25	31	—
Citrus Punch Chilled	8 fl oz	130	0	25	31	—
Fruit Punch Box	8.45 fl oz	120	0	25	31	—

FOOD	PORTION	CAL	FAT	SOD	CARB	FIB
Minute Maid *(cont.)*						
Fruit Punch Chilled	8 fl oz	120	0	25	31	—
Grape Punch Chilled	8 fl oz	130	0	25	32	—
Juices To Go Citrus Punch	1 bottle (10 fl oz)	160	0	35	39	—
Juices To Go Citrus Punch	1 can (11.5 fl oz)	180	0	40	45	—
Juices To Go Concord Punch	1 bottle (10 fl oz)	160	0	35	40	—
Juices To Go Concord Punch	1 bottle (16 fl oz)	130	0	25	32	—
Juices To Go Concord Punch	1 can (11.5 fl oz)	180	0	40	46	—
Juices To Go Fruit Punch	1 bottle (10 fl oz)	160	0	35	39	—
Juices To Go Fruit Punch	1 bottle (16 fl oz)	120	0	25	31	—
Juices To Go Fruit Punch	1 can (11.5 fl oz)	180	0	40	44	—
Juices To Go Orange Blend	1 bottle (10 fl oz)	150	0	35	37	—
Juices To Go Orange Blend	1 can (11.5 fl oz)	170	0	40	43	—
Naturals Apple Cranberry	8 fl oz	170	0	25	42	—
Naturals Concord Medley	8 fl oz	130	0	25	32	—
Naturals Fruit Medley	8 fl oz	120	0	25	31	—
Naturals Orange Grape Medley	8 fl oz	120	0	25	30	—
Naturals Tropical Medley	8 fl oz	120	0	25	31	—
Tropical Punch Box	8.45 fl oz	130	0	25	32	—
Tropical Punch Chilled	8 fl oz	120	0	25	31	—
Mott's						
Apple Cranberry	6 fl oz	83	0	—	—	—
Apple Cranberry	8.45 fl oz	136	0	—	—	—
Apple Cranberry	9.5 fl oz	167	0	—	—	—
Apple Grape	9.5 fl oz	139	0	—	—	—
Fruit Punch	9.5 fl oz	150	0	—	—	—
Grape Apple	9.5 fl oz	158	0	—	—	—
Ocean Spray						
Cran.Blueberry	8 fl oz	160	0	35	41	0

FOOD	PORTION	CAL	FAT	SOD	CARB	FIB
Cran.Cherry	6 fl oz	160	0	35	39	0
Cran.Grape	8 fl oz	170	0	35	41	0
Cran.Raspberry	8 fl oz	140	0	35	36	0
Cran.Raspberry Reduced Calorie	8 fl oz	50	0	35	13	0
Cran. Strawberry	8 fl oz	140	0	35	36	tr
Cranapple	8 fl oz	160	0	35	41	tr
Cranapple Reduced Calorie	8 fl oz	50	0	35	13	0
Cranicot	8 fl oz	160	0	35	40	0
Crantastic	8 fl oz	150	0	35	37	0
Fruit Punch	8 fl oz	130	0	35	32	0
Lightstyle Cran.Grape Low Calorie	8 fl oz	40	0	35	9	0
Lightstyle Cran.Raspberry Low Calorie	8 fl oz	40	0	35	10	0
Refreshers Citrus Cranberry Juice Drink	8 fl oz	140	0	35	35	0
Refreshers Citrus Peach Juice Drink	8 fl oz	120	0	35	30	0
Refreshers Orange Cranberry Juice Drink	8 fl oz	130	0	35	33	0
Ruby Red & Tangerine Grapefruit Juice Cocktail	8 fl oz	130	0	35	32	0
S&W Apricot Pineapple Nectar	6 fl oz	120	0	10	29	—
S&W Apricot Pineapple Nectar Diet	6 fl oz	80	0	10	20	—
Seneca Cranberry Apple Cocktail	6 fl oz	110	0	—	—	—
Seneca Raspberry Cranberry Cocktail	6 fl oz	110	0	—	—	—
Sipps Fruit Punch	8.45 oz	130	0	—	—	—
Sipps Lemon Lime Cooler	8.45 oz	130	0	—	—	—
Sipps Mixed Berry	8.45 oz	130	0	—	—	—
Sipps Sunshine Punch	8.45 oz	130	0	—	—	—
Smucker's Apple Cranberry Juice	8	120	0	10	32	—
Smucker's Orange Banana Juice	8 oz	120	0	10	30	—
Sunny Delight	6 fl oz	90	0	—	—	—

FOOD	PORTION	CAL	FAT	SOD	CARB	FIB
Tang Mixed Fruit	8.45 fl oz	137	0	2	36	—
Tang Strawberry	8.45 fl oz	121	0	1	32	—
Tang Tropical Orange	8.45 fl oz	146	0	3	37	—
Tree Top Apple						
Citrus	6 fl oz	90	0	10	22	—
Cranberry	6 fl oz	100	0	10	25	—
Grape	6 fl oz	100	0	10	25	—
Pear	6 fl oz	90	0	10	22	—
Raspberry	6 fl oz	80	0	10	21	—
Veryfine						
Apple Cherryberry	8 fl oz	130	0	<25	33	—
Apple Cranberry	8 fl oz	130	0	<10	33	—
Apple Raspberry	8 fl oz	110	0	<15	27	—
Fruit Punch	8 fl oz	130	0	<35	33	—
Guava Strawberry	8 fl oz	120	0	<25	30	—
Lemon & Lime	8 fl oz	120	0	<10	30	—
Papaya Punch	8 fl oz	120	0	<10	30	—
Passionfruit Orange	8 fl oz	110	0	<25	26	—
Pineapple Orange	8 fl oz	130	0	<10	32	—
White House Apple Cherry	6 fl oz	90	0	10	22	0
cranberry apple drink	6 fl oz	123	0	4	32	—
cranberry apricot drink	6 fl oz	118	0	4	30	—
fruit punch	6 fl oz	87	tr	41	22	—
orange & apricot	8 fl oz	128	tr	—	32	—
orange grapefruit juice	8 fl oz	107	tr	8	25	—
pineapple & grapefruit	8 fl oz	117	tr	14	29	—
pineapple & orange drink	8 fl oz	125	0	9	29	—

FRUIT MIXED

see also INDIVIDUAL NAMES

CANNED

FOOD	PORTION	CAL	FAT	SOD	CARB	FIB
Chunky Mixed Diet (S&W)	½ cup	40	0	5	10	—
Chunky Mixed Natural Style (S&W)	½ cup	90	0	5	21	—
Chunky Mixed Unsweetened (S&W)	½ cup	40	0	5	10	—
Fruit Cocktail						
Hunt's	4 oz	90	tr	7	23	tr
Diet (S&W)	½ cup	40	0	5	10	—
Heavy Syrup (S&W)	½ cup	90	0	15	24	—
Natural Lite (S&W)	½ cup	60	0	5	15	—

FOOD	PORTION	CAL	FAT	SOD	CARB	FIB
Natural Style (S&W)	½ cup	90	0	5	21	—
Unsweetened (S&W)	½ cup	40	0	5	10	—
Tropical Fruit Salad Dole	½ cup	70	tr	10	17	—
fruit cocktail, in heavy syrup	½ cup	93	tr	7	24	—
fruit cocktail, juice pack	½ cup	56	tr	4	15	—
fruit cocktail, water pack	½ cup	40	tr	5	10	—
fruit salad, in heavy syrup	½ cup	94	tr	7	24	—
fruit salad, in light syrup	½ cup	73	tr	7	19	—
fruit salad, juice pack	½ cup	62	tr	7	16	—
fruit salad, water pack	½ cup	37	tr	4	10	—
mixed fruit, in heavy syrup	½ cup	92	tr	5	24	—
tropical fruit salad, in heavy syrup	½ cup	110	tr	3	29	—
DRIED						
Fruit 'n Nut Mix (Planters)	1 oz	150	9	90	13	—
mixed	11 oz pkg	712	1	52	188	—
FROZEN						
Mixed (Big Valley)	3.5 oz	45	tr	0	10	—
Mixed Fruit (Birds Eye)	½ cup	120	0	5	31	1
mixed fruit sweetened	1 cup	245	tr	8	61	—

FRUIT SNACKS
Brock

Beauty And The Beast	1 pkg (0.9 oz)	90	0	25	21	—
Cinderella	1 pkg (0.9 oz)	90	0	25	21	—
Dinosaurs	1 pkg (0.9 oz)	90	0	25	21	—
Ninja Trolls	1 pkg (0.9 oz)	90	0	25	21	—
Sharks	1 pkg (0.9 oz)	90	0	25	21	—
Fruit Bites Jungle Pals	1 pkg (0.9 oz)	90	1	15	21	—
Fruit By The Foot Cherry	1	80	2	45	18	—
Fruit By The Foot Grape	1	80	2	45	18	—
Fruit By The Foot Strawberry	1	80	2	45	18	—
Fruit Roll-Ups						
Cherry	1 (0.5 oz)	50	tr	40	12	—
Crazy Colors	1 (0.5 oz)	50	tr	40	12	—
Fruit Punch	1 (0.5 oz)	50	tr	40	12	—
Grape	1 (0. oz)	50	tr	40	12	—
Raspberry	1 (0.5 oz)	50	tr	40	12	—
Strawberry	1 (0.5 oz)	50	tr	40	12	—
Garfield And Friends						
1-2 Punch	1 pkg	100	1	60	22	—

FOOD	PORTION	CAL	FAT	SOD	CARB	FIB
Garfield And Friends *(cont.)*						
Cat Cooler	1 pkg	100	1	60	22	—
Fat Cat Funnies	1 (0.5 oz)	50	tr	20	12	—
Fruit Party	1 (0.5 oz)	50	tr	40	12	—
Very Strawberry	1 pkg	100	1	60	22	—
Hanna Barbera Flintstones	1 pkg (1 oz)	100	0	15	22	—
Hanna Barbera Jetsons	1 pkg (1 oz)	100	0	15	22	—
Hanna Barbera Yo Yogi!	1 pkg (1 oz)	100	0	15	22	—
Health Valley						
Bakes Apple	1 bar	100	3	25	16	3
Bakes Date	1 bar	100	3	25	16	3
Bakes Raisin	1 bar	100	3	20	16	3
Fat Free Fruit Bars 100% Organic Apple	1 bar	140	tr	10	33	4
Fat Free Fruit Bars 100% Organic Apricot	1 bar	140	tr	10	33	4
Fat Free Fruit Bars 100% Organic Date	1 bar	140	tr	10	33	4
Fat Free Fruit Bars 100% Organic Raisin	1 bar	140	tr	10	33	4
Fruit & Fitness Bars	2 bars	200	5	75	35	5
Oat Bran Bakes Apricot	1 bar	100	3	15	16	2
Oat Bran Bakes Fig & Nut	1 bar	100	3	10	16	2
Oat Bran Jumbo Fruit Bars Almond	1 bar	170	5	10	28	7
Oat Bran Jumbo Fruit Bars Raisin & Cinnamon	1 bar	160	2	10	32	6
Rice Bran Jumbo Fruit Bars Almond & Date	1 bar	160	5	5	27	4
Shark Bites & Berry Bears Assorted Fruit	1 pkg	100	tr	20	22	—
Shark Bites & Berry Bears Fruit Punch	1 pkg	100	tr	20	22	—
Squeezit						
Berry B. Wild	1 (6.75 oz)	90	0	0	22	—
Chucklin' Cherry	1 (6.75 oz)	90	0	5	23	—
Grumpy Grape	1 (6.75 oz)	90	0	0	23	—
Mean Green Puncher	1 (6.75 oz)	90	0	0	23	—

FOOD	PORTION	CAL	FAT	SOD	CARB	FIB
Silly Billy Strawberry	1 (6.75 oz)	90	0	0	23	—
Smarty Arty Orange	1 (6.75 oz)	90	0	50	23	—
Sunbelt						
Fruit Boosters Apple	1 (1.3 oz)	130	2	60	27	0
Fruit Boosters Blueberry	1 (1.3 oz)	130	2	60	27	1
Fruit Jammers	1 (1 oz)	100	1	20	23	0
Sunkist						
Fruit Flippits Cherry	0.8 oz	107	4	18	18	—
Fruit Flippits Strawberry	0.8 oz	107	4	18	18	—
Fruit Roll Apricot	1	76	1	17	18	0
Fruit Roll Cherry	1	75	tr	18	18	0
Fruit Roll Grape	1	76	tr	13	19	0
Fruit Roll Raspberry	1	75	tr	20	18	0
Fruit Roll Strawberry	1	74	tr	11	18	0
Fun Fruit Animals	0.9 oz	100	1	10	22	0
Fun Fruit Dinosaurs Strawberry	0.9 oz	100	1	10	22	0
Fun Fruit Galactic Gems	0.9 oz	100	1	10	22	—
Fun Fruit Mario Nintendo	0.9 oz	100	tr	10	22	—
Fun Fruit Meteorites	0.9 oz	100	1	10	22	—
Fun Fruit Spooky Fruit	1 pkg	100	1	10	22	0
Fun Fruit Strawberry	0.9 oz	100	1	10	22	—
Fun Fruit Wacky Players	0.9 oz	100	1	10	22	—
Surf's Up! Sun Splash	1 pkg	100	1	30	22	—
Surf's Up! Tutti Frutti	1 pkg	100	1	20	22	—
Thunder Jets Associated Fruit Squadron	1 pkg	100	1	30	24	—
Thunder Jets Mach 1 Fruit Mix	1 pkg	100	1	30	24	—
Tiny Toons Bunch Of Berries	1 pkg (0.9 oz)	100	1	10	22	—
Tiny Toons Fruit Assortment	1 pkg (0.9 oz)	100	1	10	22	—
Tiny Toons Paaaarrrty Punch	1 pkg (0.9 oz)	100	1	10	22	—
Weight Watchers						
Apple	0.5 oz	50	tr	140	13	—
Cinnamon	0.5 oz	50	tr	140	13	—

FOOD	PORTION	CAL	FAT	SOD	CARB	FIB
Weight Watchers *(cont.)*						
Peach	0.5 oz	50	tr	140	13	—
Strawberry	0.5 oz	50	tr	140	13	—

GARBANZO
see CHICKPEAS

GARLIC

clove	1	4	tr	1	1	—
powder	1 tsp	9	tr	1	2	—

GEFILTE FISH
READY-TO-USE

Manischewitz	1 piece	107	4	—	4	—
Manischewitz Gefiltefish & Pike	1 piece	99	4	—	5	—
Manischewitz Gefiltefish & Pike Sweet	1 piece	129	4	—	9	—
Manischewitz Homestyle	1 piece	111	4	—	6	—
Manischweitz Sweet	1 piece	132	4	—	9	—
sweet	1 piece (1.5 oz)	35	1	220	3	—

GELATIN
DRINKS

Orange Flavored Drinking Gelatin w/ NutraSweet (Knox)	1 pkg	39	tr	17	4	0

MIX

Apple (Royal)	½ cup	80	0	95	19	—
Apricot (Jell-O)	½ cup	82	tr	51	19	0
Black Cherry (Jell-O)	¼ cup	82	tr	51	19	tr
Black Raspberry (Jell-O)	½ cup	82	tr	37	19	tr
Blackberry (Jell-O)	½ cup	82	tr	51	19	tr
Blackberry (Royal)	½ cup	80	0	95	19	—
Cherry (D-Zerta)	½ cup	8	0	4	0	—
Cherry (Royal)	½ cup	80	0	95	19	—
Cherry Sugar free (Diamond Crystal)	½ cup	8	tr	—	—	—
Cherry Sugar Free (Jell-O)	½ cup	9	0	81	0	—
Cherry Sugar Free (Royal)	½ cup	8	0	90	1	—
Concord Grape (Jell-O)	½ cup	82	tr	37	19	0
Concord Grape (Royal)	½ cup	80	0	130	19	—

FOOD	PORTION	CAL	FAT	SOD	CARB	FIB
Fruit Punch (Royal)	½ cup	80	0	90	19	—
Gelatin Desserts (Estee)	½ cup	8	0	0	tr	—
Hawaiian Pineapple Sugar Free (Jell-O)	½ cup	8	tr	50	0	—
Kosher-Jel (Emes)	½ cup (4 fl oz)	60	0	7	15	—
Kosher-Jel Plain (Emes)	1 tbsp (7 g)	21	0	tr	5	1
Lemon (D-Zerta)	½ cup	8	0	4	0	—
Lemon (Jell-O)	½ cup	82	tr	75	19	0
Lemon (Royal)	½ cup	80	0	250	19	—
Lemon Sugar Free (Diamond Crystal)	½ cup	8	tr	—	—	—
Lemon Sugar Free (Jell-O)	½ cup	8	0	60	0	—
Lemon-Lime (Royal)	½ cup	80	0	95	19	—
Lime (D-Zerta)	½ cup	9	0	4	0	—
Lime (Jell-O)	½ cup	82	tr	58	19	tr
Lime (Royal)	½ cup	80	0	125	19	—
Lime Sugar Free (Diamond Crystal)	½ cup	8	tr	—	—	—
Lime Sugar Free (Jell-O)	½ cup	9	0	63	0	—
Lime Sugar Free (Royal)	½ cup	8	0	100	1	—
Mixed Berry (Royal)	½ cup	80	0	90	19	—
Mixed Fruit (Jell-O)	½ cup	82	tr	51	19	tr
Mixed Fruit Sugar Free (Jell-O)	½ cup	8	0	50	0	—
Orange (D-Zerta)	½ cup	8	0	4	0	—
Orange (Jell-O)	½ cup	82	tr	51	19	tr
Orange (Royal)	½ cup	80	0	95	19	—
Orange Sugar Free (Diamond Crystal)	½ cup	8	tr	—	—	—
Orange Sugar Free (Jell-O)	½ cup	8	0	53	0	—
Orange Sugar Free (Royal)	½ cup	10	0	90	1	—
Peach (Royal)	½ cup	80	0	95	19	—
Peach Sugar Free (Jell-O)	½ cup	8	tr	49	0	—
Pineapple (Royal)	½ cup	80	0	95	19	—
Raspberry (D-Zerta)	½ cup	8	0	4	0	—
Raspberry (Royal)	½ cup	80	0	125	19	—
Raspberry Sugar Free (Diamond Crystal)	½ cup	8	tr	—	—	—
Raspberry Sugar Free (Jell-O)	½ cup	8	0	57	0	—
Raspberry Sugar Free (Royal)	½ cup	8	0	90	1	—

FOOD	PORTION	CAL	FAT	SOD	CARB	FIB
Strawberry (D-Zerta)	½ cup	8	0	4	0	—
Strawberry (Royal)	½ cup	80	0	105	19	—
Strawberry Banana Sugar Free (Royal)	½ cup	8	0	85	1	—
Strawberry Banana Sugar Free (Jell-O)	½ cup	9	0	55	0	—
Strawberry Orange (Royal)	½ cup	80	0	110	19	—
Strawberry Sugar Free (Diamond Crystal)	½ cup	8	tr	—	—	—
Strawberry Sugar Free (Jell-O)	½ cup	9	0	64	0	—
Strawberry Sugar Free (Royal)	½ cup	8	0	90	1	—
Triple Berry Sugar Free (Jell-O)	½ cup	8	tr	50	0	—
Tropical Fruit (Royal)	½ cup	80	0	110	19	—
Wild Strawberry (Jell-O)	½ cup	81	tr	75	19	tr
fruit flavored	½ cup	70	0	55	17	—
low calorie	½ cup	8	0	9	0	0

GIBLETS

FOOD	PORTION	CAL	FAT	SOD	CARB	FIB
capon, simmered	1 cup (5 oz)	238	8	80	0	—
chicken, floured & fried	1 cup (5 oz)	402	19	164	6	—
chicken, simmered	1 cup (5 oz)	228	7	85	1	—
turkey, simmered	1 cup (5 oz)	243	7	85	3	—

GINGER

FOOD	PORTION	CAL	FAT	SOD	CARB	FIB
ground	1 tsp	6	tr	1	1	—
root, fresh	¼ cup	17	tr	3	4	—
root, fresh	5 slices	8	tr	1	2	—
root, fresh, sliced	¼ cup	17	tr	3	4	—

GINKGO NUTS

FOOD	PORTION	CAL	FAT	SOD	CARB	FIB
canned	1 oz	32	tr	87	6	—
dried	1 oz	99	tr	4	21	—
raw	1 oz	52	tr	1	11	—

GIZZARDS

FOOD	PORTION	CAL	FAT	SOD	CARB	FIB
chicken, simmered	1 cup (5 oz)	222	5	97	2	—
turkey, simmered	1 cup (5 oz)	236	6	79	1	—

GOAT

FOOD	PORTION	CAL	FAT	SOD	CARB	FIB
roasted	3 oz	122	3	73	0	—

FOOD	PORTION	CAL	FAT	SOD	CARB	FIB
GOOSE						
FRESH						
w/ skin, roasted	½ goose (1.7 lbs)	2362	170	543	0	—
w/ skin, roasted	6.6 oz	574	41	132	0	—
w/o skin, roasted	½ goose (1.3 lbs)	1406	75	447	0	—
w/o skin, roasted	5 oz	340	18	108	0	—
GOOSEBERRIES						
fresh	1 cup	67	1	1	15	—
canned, in light syrup	½ cup	93	tr	3	24	—
GRANOLA						
BARS						
Fi-Bar Coconut	1	120	4	30	20	6
Fi-Bar Peanut Butter	1	130	4	30	20	6
Grist Mill						
Chewy Apple Cinnamon	1 (1 oz)	120	4	35	21	1
Chewy Chocolate Chip	1 (1 oz)	130	4	30	21	1
Chewy Chunky Nut And Raisin	1 (1 oz)	130	6	35	18	1
Chewy Peanut Butter	1 (1 oz)	130	5	45	20	1
Chewy Peanut Butter Chocolate	1 (1 oz)	130	4	40	20	2
Chocolate Snack Chocolate Chip	1 (1.2 oz)	180	10	60	21	1
Chocolate Snack Nutty Fudge	1 (1.3 oz)	190	11	90	19	2
Crunchy Cinnamon	1 (0.8 oz)	110	5	60	16	1
Crunchy Oats 'N Honey	1 (0.8 oz)	110	5	60	15	1
Hershey						
Chocolate Covered Chocolate Chip	1 (1.2 oz)	170	8	50	22	—
Chocolate Covered Cocoa Creme	1 (1.2 oz)	180	9	50	22	—
Chocolate Covered Cookies & Creme	1 (1.2 oz)	170	8	50	22	—
Chocolate Covered Peanut Butter	1 (1.2 oz)	180	10	65	19	—
Kudos						
Chocolate Chip	1 (1 oz)	130	5	75	18	1
Milk and Cookies	1 (1 oz)	130	5	65	19	1
Nutty Fudge	1 (1 oz)	130	5	60	18	1
Peanut Butter	1 (1 oz)	130	5	90	18	1

FOOD	PORTION	CAL	FAT	SOD	CARB	FIB
Nature Valley						
Cinnamon	1	120	5	70	17	1
Oat Bran Honey Graham	1	110	4	90	16	1
Oats N'Honey	1	120	5	65	17	1
Peanut Butter	1	120	6	70	15	1
Rice Bran Cinnamon Graham	1	90	4	75	13	1
New Trail Chocolate Covered Cookies and Creme	1	200	11	85	23	—
Quaker						
Chewy Chocolate Chip	1	128	5	90	19	1
Chewy Chunky Nut & Raisin	1	131	6	86	17	2
Chewy Cinnamon Raisin	1	128	5	92	19	1
Chewy Honey & Oats	1	125	4	95	19	1
Chewy Peanut Butter	1	128	5	116	18	1
Chewy Peanut Butter Chocolate Chip	1	131	6	112	17	1
Dipps Caramel Nut	1	148	6	81	21	1
Dipps Chocolate Chip	1	139	6	78	19	1
Dipps Chocolate Fudge	1	160	8	74	20	—
Dipps Peanut Butter	1	170	9	74	9	1
Dipps Peanut Butter Chocolate Chip	1	174	10	102	10	—
Dipps Rocky Road	1	140	7	—	—	—
Sunbelt						
Chewy Chocolate Chip	1 (1.8 oz)	220	10	95	32	2
Chewy Chocolate Chip	1 (1.25 oz)	160	7	65	23	2
Chewy Oats & Honey	1 (1.7 oz)	210	9	105	32	2
Chewy With Almonds	1 (1.5 oz)	190	10	95	25	2
Chewy With Almonds	1 (1 oz)	130	7	60	17	2
Chewy With Raisins	1 (1.2 oz)	150	6	65	25	2
Fudge Dipped Chewy Chocolate Chip	1 (1.5 oz)	190	8	80	28	2
Fudge Dipped Chewy Macaroon	1 (1.4 oz)	200	13	60	22	2
Fudge Dipped Chewy Macaroon	1 (2 oz)	280	17	90	32	3
Fudge Dipped Chewy With Peanuts	1 (2 oz)	270	15	95	32	2
Fudge Dipped Chewy With Peanuts	1 (1.5 oz)	210	12	65	24	2

FOOD	PORTION	CAL	FAT	SOD	CARB	FIB
CEREAL						
Erewhon						
Date Nut	1 oz	130	6	45	17	—
Honey Almond	1 oz	130	6	65	17	—
Maple	1 oz	130	5	55	17	—
Spiced Apple	1 oz	130	6	55	17	—
Sunflower Crunch	1 oz	130	4	60	18	—
With Bran	1 oz	130	6	10	17	4
Good Shepherd						
Crunchy	1 oz	130	5	15	19	2
Honey Almond	1 oz	120	4	10	20	2
Organic 5 Grain Muesli	1 oz	160	3	55	27	3
Organic Brown Rice	1 oz	130	4	35	16	4
Organic Wheat Free	1 oz	90	3	3	39	2
Organic Wheat Free Apple Cinnamon	1 oz	125	4	35	20	3
Organic Wheat Free Blueberry Amaranth	1 oz	110	1	10	22	2
Organic Wheat Free Strawberry Amaranth	1 oz	110	1	12	22	2
Grist Mill Low-Fat With Raisins	⅔ cup (1.9 oz)	220	3	100	42	3
Kellogg's Low Fat	⅓ cup (1 oz)	110	2	35	22	2
Kellogg's Low Fat With Raisins	⅓ cup (1.1 oz)	120	2	35	25	2
Nature Valley Cinnamon & Raisin	⅓ cup (1 oz)	120	4	90	20	1
Nature Valley Fruit & Nut	⅓ cup (1 oz)	130	5	75	19	1
Nature Valley Toasted Oat	⅓ cup (1 oz)	130	5	90	20	1
Post Hearty	¼ cup (1 oz)	128	4	78	21	1
Quaker Sun Country 100% Natural With Almonds	¼ cup	130	5	11	19	1
Quaker Sun Country 100% Natural With Raisins & Dates	¼ cup	123	5	9	20	2
Quaker Sun Country With Raisins	¼ cup	125	5	10	19	2
Sunbelt Banana Nut	1.9 oz	250	9	60	37	4
Sunbelt Fruit & Nut	1.9 oz	230	7	100	38	4
Sunbelt Low Fat	1.9 oz	200	3	80	42	4
granola	¼ cup	138	8	3	16	—

FOOD	PORTION	CAL	FAT	SOD	CARB	FIB

GRAPEFRUIT

CANNED

FOOD	PORTION	CAL	FAT	SOD	CARB	FIB
Sections Unsweetened (S&W)	½ cup	40	0	0	9	—
Sections In Light Syrup (S&W)	½ cup	80	0	0	14	—
Sections Natural Style (S&W)	½ cup	40	0	—	9	—
juice pack	½ cup	46	tr	9	11	—
unsweetened	1 cup	93	tr	3	22	—
water pack	½ cup	44	tr	2	11	—

FRESH

FOOD	PORTION	CAL	FAT	SOD	CARB	FIB
Chiquita Ruby	½ fruit	40	0	—	—	—
Dole	½	50	0	0	14	6
Ocean Spray White	½ med	45	0	0	12	—
Ocean Spray Pink	½ med	50	0	0	13	—
pink	½	37	tr	0	9	1
pink sections	1 cup	69	tr	1	18	1
red	½	37	tr	0	9	—
red sections	1 cup	69	tr	1	18	—
white	½	39	tr	0	10	1
white sections	1 cup	76	tr	0	19	1

JUICE

FOOD	PORTION	CAL	FAT	SOD	CARB	FIB
Crystal Geyser Juice Squeeze	1 bottle (12 fl oz)	150	0	20	36	—
Libby's	6 oz	70	0	0	17	—
Minute Maid						
Frozen	8 fl oz	100	0	25	23	—
Juices To Go	1 bottle (10 fl oz)	120	0	35	29	—
Juices To Go	1 bottle (16 fl oz)	100	0	25	23	—
Juices To Go	1 can (11.5 fl oz)	140	0	40	33	—
Juices To Go Pink Cocktail	1 bottle (10 fl oz)	140	0	35	34	—
Juices To Go Pink Cocktail	1 bottle (16 fl oz)	110	0	25	27	—
Juices To Go Pink Juice Cocktail	8 fl oz	160	0	40	39	—
Mott's	10 oz	124	0	—	—	—
Mott's Grapefruit	9.5 oz	118	0	—	—	—
Ocean Spray 100%	8 oz	100	0	35	24	tr
Ocean Spray Lightstyle Pink Grapefruit Juice Cocktail Low Calorie	8 fl oz	40	0	35	9	0

FOOD	PORTION	CAL	FAT	SOD	CARB	FIB
Ocean Spray Pink Grapefruit Juice Cocktail	8 oz	110	0	35	28	0
Ocean Spray Ruby Red Grapefruit Drink	8 oz	130	0	35	33	0
S&W Unsweetened	6 oz	80	0	—	18	—
Tree Top	6 oz	80	0	0	19	—
Veryfine 100%	8 oz	101	0	<10	23	—
Veryfine Pink Grapefruit	8 oz	120	0	<20	29	—
fresh	1 cup	96	tr	2	23	—
frzn, as prep	1 cup	102	tr	2	24	—
frzn, not prep	6 oz	302	1	6	72	—
sweetened	1 cup	116	tr	4	28	—

GRAPES
CANNED

FOOD	PORTION	CAL	FAT	SOD	CARB	FIB
Thompson Seedless Premium (S&W)	½ cup	100	0	5	25	—
Thompson seedless in heavy syrup	½ cup	94	tr	7	25	—
Thompson seedless water pack	½ cup	48	tr	7	13	—

FRESH

FOOD	PORTION	CAL	FAT	SOD	CARB	FIB
Dole	1½ cup	85	0	3	24	2
grapes	10	36	tr	1	9	tr

JUICE

FOOD	PORTION	CAL	FAT	SOD	CARB	FIB
BAMA	8.45 fl oz	120	0	25	29	—
Bright & Early Frozen	8 fl oz	140	0	5	34	—
Hawaiian Punch	6 oz	90	0	—	—	—
Hi-C	1 can (11.5 fl oz)	180	0	45	46	—
Hi-C	8 fl oz	130	0	30	32	—
Hi-C Box	8.45 fl oz	130	0	30	33	—
Juice Works	6 oz	100	0	—	—	—
Juicy Juice	6 oz	90	0	5	22	—
Juicy Juice	8.45 oz	130	0	10	31	—
Kool-Aid	8 oz	98	0	—	25	—
Kool-Aid Sugar Free	8 oz	3	0	—	0	—
Kool-Aid Sugar Sweetened	8 oz	80	0	24	21	—
Minute Maid Chilled	8 fl oz	130	0	5	33	—
Minute Maid Grape Punch Frozen	8 fl oz	130	0	5	32	—
S&W Concord Unsweetened	6 oz	100	0	9	25	—
Seneca	6 oz	115	0	—	—	—

FOOD	PORTION	CAL	FAT	SOD	CARB	FIB
Seneca Grape frzn, as prep	6 oz	100	0	—	—	—
Seneca Natural frzn, as prep	6 oz	115	0	—	—	—
Seneca White Grape Juice frzn, as prep	6 oz	110	0	—	—	—
Sippin' Pak 100% Pure	8.45 fl	130	0	25	32	—
Sipps Grape	8.45 oz	130	0	—	—	—
Tang Fruit Box	8.45 oz	131	0	2	34	—
Tree Top	6 oz	120	0	10	30	—
Tree Top Sparkling Juice	6 oz	120	0	—	29	—
Veryfine 100%	8 oz	153	0	<20	37	—
Veryfine Grape Drink	8 oz	130	0	<10	34	—
Wylers Drink Mix Unsweetened	8 oz	2	0	12	1	—
bottled	1 cup	155	tr	7	38	—
frzn sweetened, as prep	1 cup	128	tr	5	32	—
frzn sweetened, not prep	6 oz	386	1	15	96	—
grape drink	6 oz	84	0	12	22	—

GRAVY
see also SAUCE

FOOD	PORTION	CAL	FAT	SOD	CARB	FIB
Au Jus (Franco-American)	2 oz	10	0	330	2	—
Beef (Franco-American)	2 oz	25	1	340	4	—
Chicken (Franco-American)	2 oz	45	4	240	3	—
Chicken Giblet (Franco-American)	2 oz	30	2	310	3	—
Cream (Franco-American)	2 oz	35	2	220	4	—
Gravymaster	¼ tsp	3	0	14	1	—
Mushroom (Franco-American)	2 oz	25	1	290	3	—
Pork (Franco-American)	2 oz	40	3	330	3	—
Turkey (Franco-American)	2 oz	30	2	290	3	—
au jus	1 cup	38	tr	—	6	—
beef	1 can (10 oz)	155	7	1630	14	—
beef	1 cup	124	6	1305	11	—
chicken	1 cup	189	14	1375	13	—
mushroom	1 cup	120	6	1259	13	—
turkey	1 cup	122	5	—	12	—
DRY						
Bournvita	2 heaping tsp	34	1	—	7	—
Bovril	1 heaping tsp	9	0	—	tr	0
Brown (Hain)	¼ pkg	16	0	600	3	—
Brown (Pillsbury)	¼ cup	15	0	300	3	—

FOOD	PORTION	CAL	FAT	SOD	CARB	FIB
Brown Gravy Quik, as prep (LaLoma)	2 tsp	45	4	150	2	—
Chicken (Diamond Crystal)	2 oz	30	1	—	—	—
Chicken (Pillsbury)	¼ cup	25	1	230	4	—
Chicken Gravy Quik, as prep (LaLoma)	2 tsp	45	4	180	2	—
Country Quik Gravy, as prep (LaLoma)	2 tsp	10	tr	200	2	—
Home Style (Pillsbury)	¼ cup	15	0	300	3	—
Marmite	1 heaping tsp	9	0	—	tr	—
Mushroom Quik Gravy, as prep (LaLoma)	2 tsp	10	tr	160	2	—
Oil-Less Roux And Gravy Mix (Cajun King)	3.5 oz	394	4	348	78	—
Onion Quik Gravy, as prep (LaLoma)	2 tsp	10	tr	120	2	—
au jus, as prep w/ water	1 cup	32	1	964	4	—
brown, as prep w/ water	1 cup	75	2	1076	13	—
chicken, as prep	1 cup	83	2	1133	14	—
mushroom, as prep	1 cup	70	1	1402	14	—
onion, as prep w/ water	1 cup	77	1	1013	16	—
pork, as prep	1 cup	76	2	1235	13	—
turkey, as prep	1 cup	87	2	1498	15	—

GREAT NORTHERN BEANS
CANNED

FOOD	PORTION	CAL	FAT	SOD	CARB	FIB
Green Giant	½ cup	80	1	290	18	5
Hanover	½ cup	110	0	—	—	—
Trappey's	½ cup	80	1	410	16	—
Great Northern	1 cup	300	1	11	55	14

DRIED

FOOD	PORTION	CAL	FAT	SOD	CARB	FIB
Bean Cuisine	½ cup	115	1	5	—	5
Hurst Brand	1 cup	277	1	—	—	—
cooked	1 cup	210	1	4	37	—

GREEN BEANS
CANNED

FOOD	PORTION	CAL	FAT	SOD	CARB	FIB
Almondine (Green Giant)	½ cup	45	3	300	5	2
Cut						
Green Giant	½ cup	16	0	300	4	1
Hanover	½ cup	20	0	—	—	—
Libby	½ cup	20	0	—	—	—
Owatonna	½ cup	20	0	—	—	—
Seneca	½ cup	20	0	—	—	—

FOOD	PORTION	CAL	FAT	SOD	CARB	FIB
Cut Natural Pack (Libby)	½ cup	20	1	—	—	—
Cut Premium Blue Lake (S&W)	½ cup	20	0	385	4	—
Cut Water Pack (S&W)	½ cup	20	0	5	4	—
Cuts Natural Pack (Seneca)	½ cup	20	0	—	—	—
Dilled (S&W)	½ cup	60	0	385	15	—
French						
(Green Giant)	½ cup	16	0	330	4	1
(Libby)	½ cup	20	0	—	—	—
(Owatonna)	½ cup	20	0	—	—	—
(Seneca)	½ cup	20	0	—	—	—
French Natural (Libby)	½ cup	20	1	—	—	—
French Natural Pack (Seneca)	½ cup	20	0	—	—	—
French Style Premium Blue (S&W)	½ cup	20	0	385	4	—
Green Beans & Wax Beans (S&W)	½ cup	20	0	385	5	—
Kitchen Sliced (Green Giant)	½ cup	16	0	280	4	1
Whole (Libby)	½ cup	20	0	—	—	—
Whole (Seneca)	½ cup	20	0	—	—	—
Whole Fancy Stringless (S&W)	½ cup	20	0	385	4	—
Whole Vertical Pack (S&W)	½ cup	20	0	385	4	—
FROZEN						
Cut (Birds Eye)	½ cup	25	0	0	6	2
Cut (Hanover)	½ cup	20	0	—	—	—
Cut Beans (Southland)	3 oz	25	0	—	—	—
Cut In Butter Sauce (Green Giant)	½ cup	30	1	230	4	2
Farm Fresh Whole (Birds Eye)	¾ cup	30	0	0	7	2
French (Southland)	3 oz	25	0	—	—	—
French Cut (Birds Eye)	½ cup	25	0	0	6	2
French Style Blue Lake (Hanover)	½ cup	25	0	—	—	—
Green Bean Mushroom Casserole (Stouffer's)	½ cup (1.9 oz)	130	8	530	13	2
Green Giant	½ cup	14	0	10	4	2
Harvest Fresh Cut (Green Giant)	½ cup	16	0	95	4	1

FOOD	PORTION	CAL	FAT	SOD	CARB	FIB
In Sauce French Green Beans With Toasted Almonds (Birds Eye)	½ cup	50	2	340	8	2
Italian (Birds Eye)	½ cup	30	0	0	7	3
Italian Cut (Hanover)	½ cup	35	0	—	—	—
One Serve In Butter Sauce (Green Giant)	1 pkg	60	2	370	8	3
Polybag Cut (Birds Eye)	½ cup	25	0	0	6	2
Polybag Deluxe Whole (Birds Eye)	½ cup	20	0	0	4	2
Polybag French Cut (Birds Eye)	½ cup	25	0	0	6	2
Whole Blue Lake (Hanover)	½ cup	30	0	—	—	—
Whole Deluxe (Birds Eye)	½ cup	45	0	0	5	2
SHELF STABLE						
Cut (Pantry Express)	½ cup	12	0	20	3	1

GROUNDCHERRIES
fresh	½ cup	37	tr	—	8	—

GROUPER
FRESH

cooked	1 fillet (7.1 oz)	238	3	107	0	—
cooked	3 oz	100	1	45	0	—
raw	3 oz	78	1	45	0	—

GUAVA
fresh	1	45	1	2	11	—
guava sauce	½ cup	43	tr	4	11	—
JUICE						
Kern's Nectar	6 oz	110	0	10	28	—
Libby's Nectar	6 oz	110	0	15	26	—
Libby's Ripe Nectar	8 oz	140	0	20	35	—

GUINEA HEN
w/ skin, raw	½ hen (12.1 oz)	545	22	—	0	—
w/o skin, raw	½ hen (9.3 oz)	292	7	—	0	—

HADDOCK
cooked	1 fillet (5.3 oz)	168	1	131	0	—
cooked	3 oz	95	1	74	0	—
raw	3 oz	74	1	58	0	—
roe, raw	3.5 oz	130	2	—	2	—
FROZEN						
Battered (Van De Kamp's)	2 pieces	250	15	580	19	—

FOOD	PORTION	CAL	FAT	SOD	CARB	FIB
Breaded Fillets (Van De Kamp's)	2 pieces	270	16	290	19	—
Crunchy Batter Fillets (Mrs. Paul's)	2 fillets	190	5	580	22	—
Fishmarket Fresh (Gorton's)	5 oz	110	1	120	0	—
Light Fillets (Mrs. Paul's)	1 fillet	220	9	350	15	—
Light Fillets (Van De Kamp's)	1 piece	240	11	590	21	—
Microwave Entree Haddock In Lemon Butter (Gorton's)	1 pkg	360	21	730	19	—
Natural Fillets (Van De Kamp's)	4 oz	90	1	125	0	—
SMOKED						
smoked	1 oz	33	tr	214	0	—
smoked	3 oz	99	1	649	0	—

HAKE
raw	3.5 oz	84	1	101	0	—

HALIBUT
FRESH

atlantic & pacific, cooked	½ fillet (5.6 oz)	223	5	110	0	—
atlantic & pacific, cooked	3 oz	119	2	59	0	—
atlantic & pacific, raw	3 oz	93	2	46	0	—
greenland, baked	3 oz	203	15	87	0	—
greenland, baked	5.6 oz	380	28	163	0	—
FROZEN						
Battered (Van De Kamp's)	2 pieces	150	6	400	16	—

see also HAM DISHES, PORK, TURKEY

HAM
Armour

Golden Star Boneless	1 oz	33	1	—	—	—
Golden Star Canned	1 oz	32	tr	—	—	—
Lower Salt 93% Fat Free	1 oz	35	1	221	—	—
Lower Salt Boneless	1 oz	34	1	—	—	—
Star Boneless	1 oz	41	2	—	—	—
Star Canned	1 oz	34	1	—	—	—
Star Speedy Cut	1 oz	44	3	—	—	—
1877 Boneless	1 oz	42	2	—	—	—
Carl Buddig	1 oz	50	3	400	1	0
Carl Buddig Honey Ham	1 oz	50	3	400	1	—

FOOD	PORTION	CAL	FAT	SOD	CARB	FIB
Hansel 'n Gretel						
Baked Virginia	1 oz	34	1	245	2	—
Black Forest	1 oz	32	1	—	tr	—
Cappy	1 oz	31	1	—	1	—
Cooked Fresh	1 oz	33	1	120	tr	—
Deluxe	1 oz	31	1	245	1	—
Honey Valley	1 oz	31	1	260	1	—
Jalapeno	1 oz	25	1	260	1	—
Lessalt	1 oz	30	1	200	1	—
Lessalt Virginia	1 oz	32	1	190	1	—
Light AM	1 oz	27	1	200	1	—
Travane	1 oz	31	1	210	tr	—
Healthy Choice						
Cooked	1 oz	30	1	240	tr	—
Honey	1 oz	30	1	300	1	—
Smoked	1 oz	30	1	210	tr	—
Virginia	1 oz	30	1	250	1	—
Hillshire						
Brown Sugar	1 oz	40	2	440	2	—
Cooked Ham	1 oz	30	1	470	tr	—
Deli Select Baked Ham	1 slice	10	tr	95	tr	—
Deli Select Brown Sugar Baked	1 slice	10	tr	90	tr	—
Deli Select Cajun Ham	1 slice	10	tr	120	tr	—
Deli Select Honey Ham	1 slice	10	tr	100	tr	—
Deli Select Lower Salt	1 slice	10	tr	80	tr	—
Deli Select Smoked Ham	1 slice	10	tr	95	tr	—
Flavor Pack 90-99% Fat Free Brown Sugar Baked	1 slice (0.6 oz)	20	tr	170	1	—
Flavor Pack 90-99% Fat Free Honey Ham	1 slice (0.6 oz)	20	tr	180	1	—
Flavor Pack 90-99% Fat Free Smoked	1 slice (0.6 oz)	20	tr	170	tr	—
Genuine Baked	1 oz	35	1	290	1	—
Honey Ham	1 oz	35	1	470	1	—
Lower Salt	1 oz	30	1	300	1	—
Jones Family Ham	1 slice	40	2	290	tr	—
Jones Ham Slices	1 slice	30	1	200	tr	—
Krakus	1 oz	25	1	355	1	—
Louis Rich						
Carving Board Baked With Natural Juices	2 slices (1.6 oz)	45	1	510	1	0

FOOD	PORTION	CAL	FAT	SOD	CARB	FIB
Louis Rich *(cont.)*						
Carving Board Honey With Natural Juices	2 slices (1.6 oz)	50	2	530	1	0
Carving Board Honey With Natural Juices Carved Thin	6 slices (2.1 oz)	70	2	760	2	0
Carving Board Smoked Cooked With Natural Juices	1 slice (1.6 oz)	50	2	560	0	0
Dinner Slices Baked	1 slice (3.3 oz)	80	2	1150	1	0
Oscar Mayer						
Baked Cooked	1 slice (0.75 oz)	21	1	238	tr	—
Boiled	1 slice (0.75 oz)	23	1	275	tr	—
Boiled Thin Sliced	1 (0.4 oz)	13	tr	157	tr	—
Breakfast Ham	1 slice (1.5 oz)	47	2	582	1	—
Chopped	1 slice (1 oz)	41	2	303	1	—
Cracked Black Pepper	1 slice (0.75 oz)	22	1	284	tr	—
Ham And Cheese Loaf	1 slice (1 oz)	66	5	358	1	—
Honey Ham	1 slice (0.75 oz)	23	1	268	1	—
Honey Ham Thin Sliced	1 slice (0.4 oz)	13	tr	153	tr	—
Jubilee Boneless	1 oz	43	2	365	tr	—
Jubilee Canned	1 oz	29	1	287	tr	—
Jubilee Slice	1 oz	29	1	335	1	—
Jubilee Steak	2 oz	57	2	754	tr	—
Lower Salt	1 slice (0.75 oz)	23	1	174	1	—
Peppered Chopped	1 slice (1 oz)	55	4	312	1	—
Smoked Cooked	1 slice (21 g)	22	1	266	tr	—
Russer Lil' Salt Cooked	1 oz	30	1	220	1	—
Russer Lil' Salt Smoked	1 oz	30	1	220	1	—
The Spreadables Ham Salad	¼ can	100	6	—	—	—
Underwood Deviled	2.08 oz	220	19	430	tr	—
Underwood Deviled Light	2.08 oz	120	8	250	1	—
Underwood Deviled Smoked	2.08 oz	190	18	260	tr	—
Weight Watchers						
Deli Thin Oven Roasted	5 slices (0.33 oz)	12	tr	95	tr	—
Deli Thin Oven Roasted Honey Ham	5 slices (0.33 oz)	12	tr	95	tr	—

FOOD	PORTION	CAL	FAT	SOD	CARB	FIB
Deli Thin Premium Smoked	5 slices (0.33 oz)	12	tr	85	tr	—
Oven Roasted Honey Ham	2 slices (0.75 oz)	25	1	220	tr	—
Oven Roasted Smoked	2 slices (0.75 oz)	25	1	220	tr	—
Premium Cooked	2 slices (0.75 oz)	25	1	220	tr	—
boneless, 11% fat	3 oz	151	8	—	—	—
boneless extra lean, roasted	3 oz	140	7	—	—	—
canned, 13% fat	1 oz	54	4	—	—	—
canned, 13% fat	3 oz	192	13	800	tr	—
canned, extra lean	1 oz	41	2	—	—	—
canned, extra lean	3 oz	142	7	—	—	—
canned, extra lean, 4% fat	3 oz	116	4	965	tr	—
center slice, lean & fat	4 oz	229	15	1566	tr	—
center slice, lean only	4 oz	220	9	—	—	—
chopped	1 oz	65	5	389	0	—
chopped, canned	1 oz	68	5	387	tr	—
ham & cheese loaf	1 oz	73	6	762	1	—
ham & cheese spread	1 oz	69	5	339	1	—
ham & cheese spread	1 tbsp	37	3	179	tr	—
ham salad spread	1 oz	61	4	259	3	—
ham salad spread	1 tbsp	32	2	137	2	—
minced	1 oz	75	6	353	1	—
patties, uncooked	1 (2.3 oz)	206	18	—	—	—
patties, grilled	1 patty (2 oz)	203	18	—	—	—
sliced, extra lean, 5% fat	1 oz	37	1	405	tr	—
sliced, regular, 11% fat	1 oz	52	3	373	1	—
steak, boneless, extra lean	1 oz	35	1	360	0	—
whole, lean & fat, roasted	3 oz	207	14	—	—	—
whole, lean only, roasted	3 oz	133	5	—	—	—

HAM DISHES
FROZEN

FOOD	PORTION	CAL	FAT	SOD	CARB	FIB
Handy Pocket Cheese Sauce & Ham (Weight Watchers)	1 (4 oz)	200	6	490	24	—

FOOD	PORTION	CAL	FAT	SOD	CARB	FIB
Ovenstuffs Ham/Turkey (Deli Melt)	1 (4.75 oz)	360	15	1050	35	—
HOME RECIPE						
croquettes	1 (3.1 oz)	217	14	475	11	tr
salad	½ cup	287	23	671	5	tr
TAKE-OUT						
sandwich w/ cheese	1	353	15	772	33	—

HAMBURGER
see also BEEF

FOOD	PORTION	CAL	FAT	SOD	CARB	FIB
FROZEN						
Kid Cuisine Beef Patty Sandwich/ Cheese	6.25 oz	430	22	550	45	—
Kid Cuisine Mega Meal Double Beef Patty Sandwich w/ Cheese	9.1 oz	480	20	1040	55	—
MicroMagic Cheeseburger	1 pkg (4.75 oz)	450	25	790	29	—
MicroMagic Hamburger	1 pkg (4 oz)	350	18	500	26	—
White Castle Cheeseburger	1 (2.3 oz)	200	11	360	16	—
White Castle Hamburger	1 (2.1 oz)	160	8	270	15	—
TAKE-OUT						
double patty w/ bun	1 reg	544	28	554	43	—
double patty w/ catsup, cheese, mayonnaise, mustard, pickle, tomato & bun	1 lg	706	44	1149	40	—
double patty w/ catsup, mayonnaise, onion, pickle tomato & bun	1 reg	649	35	920	53	—
double patty w/ catsup, mustard, mayonnaise, onion, pickle, tomato & bun	1 lg	540	27	791	40	—
double patty w/ catsup, mustard, onion, pickle & bun	1 reg	576	32	742	39	—
double patty w/ cheese & bun	1 reg	457	28	635	22	—
double patty w/ cheese & double bun	1 reg	461	22	892	44	—
double patty w/ cheese, catsup, mayonnaise,	1 reg	416	21	1051	35	—

FOOD	PORTION	CAL	FAT	SOD	CARB	FIB
onion, pickle, tomato & bun						
single patty w/ bacon, catsup, cheese, mustard, onion, pickle & bun	1 lg	609	37	1044	37	—
single patty w/ bun	1 lg	400	23	474	25	—
single patty w/ bun	1 reg	275	12	387	31	—
single patty w/ catsup, cheese, ham, mayonnaise, pickle, tomato & bun	1 lg	745	48	1713	38	—
single patty w/ catsup, mustard, mayonnaise, onion, pickle, tomato & bun	1 reg	279	13	504	27	—
single patty w/ cheese & bun	1 lg	608	33	1589	47	—
single patty w/ cheese & bun	1 reg	320	15	500	32	—
triple patty w/ catsup, mustard, pickle & bun	1 lg	693	41	713	29	—
triple patty w/ cheese & bun	1 lg	769	51	1211	27	—

HEART

FOOD	PORTION	CAL	FAT	SOD	CARB	FIB
beef, simmered	3 oz	148	5	54	tr	—
chicken, simmered	1 cup (5 oz)	268	11	69	tr	—
lamb, braised	3 oz	158	7	54	2	—
pork, braised	1 heart (4.3 oz)	191	7	—	—	—
turkey, simmered	1 cup (5 oz)	257	9	79	3	—
veal, braised	3 oz	158	6	50	tr	—

HERBAL TEA
see TEA/HERBAL TEA

HERBS/SPICES
see also INDIVIDUAL NAMES

FOOD	PORTION	CAL	FAT	SOD	CARB	FIB
Ac'cent Flavor Enhancer	½ tsp	5	0	300	0	0
Ac'cent Herbal All Purpose Seasoning	½ tsp	0	0	0	0	0
All Purpose Seafood (Golden Dipt)	¼ tsp	2	0	85	0	—

FOOD	PORTION	CAL	FAT	SOD	CARB	FIB
Bar-B-Q Shaker (Diamond Crystal)	½ tsp	4	0	—	—	—
Blackened Red Fish (Golden Dipt)	¼ tsp	2	0	140	0	—
Broiled Fish (Golden Dipt)	¼ tsp	2	0	125	0	—
Cajun Style Shrimp & Crab (Golden Dipt)	¼ tsp	2	0	200	0	—
Chef Seasoning (Diamond Crystal)	1 pkg (0.45 oz)	2	0	—	—	—
Chef Shaker (Diamond Crystal)	½ tsp	4	0	—	—	—
Cleopatra's Secret (Nile Spice)	⅛ tsp	0	0	20	0	—
Desert Spice (Nile Spice)	⅛ tsp	0	0	5	0	—
French Shaker (Diamond Crystal)	½ tsp	4	0	—	—	—
Ginger Curry (Nile Spice)	⅛ tsp	0	0	5	0	—
Italian Shaker (Diamond Crystal)	½ tsp	4	0	—	—	—
Lemon Pepper Seafood (Golden Dipt)	¼ tsp	8	0	115	1	—
Maya Maize Popcorn Seasoning (Nile Spice)	½ tsp	0	tr	25	0	—
Mexican Shaker (Diamond Crystal)	½ tsp	4	0	—	—	—
Mrs. Dash						
Extra Spicy	1 tsp (3.4 g)	12	tr	4	3	—
Garlic & Herb	1 tsp (3.4 g)	12	tr	2	2	—
Lemon & Herb	1 tsp (3.4 g)	12	tr	4	3	—
Low Pepper Blend	1 tsp (3.4 g)	12	tr	4	3	—
Original	1 tsp (3.4 g)	12	tr	4	2	—
Table Blend	1 tsp (3.4 g)	12	tr	4	2	—
Nile Spice	⅛ tsp	0	0	20	0	—
Seasoning Blend Sloppy Joe (Lawry's)	1 pkg	126	tr	3442	28	1
curry powder	1 tsp	6	tr	1	1	—
poultry seasoning	1 tsp	5	tr	tr	1	—
pumpkin pie spice	1 tsp	6	tr	1	1	—
JARRED						
Crab Boil (McIlhenny)	3 oz	378	17	95	40	32

FOOD	PORTION	CAL	FAT	SOD	CARB	FIB
HERRING						
CANNED						
roe	3.5 oz	118	3	—	tr	—
FRESH						
atlantic, cooked	1 fillet (5 oz)	290	17	165	0	—
atlantic, cooked	3 oz	172	10	98	0	—
atlantic, raw	3 oz	134	8	76	0	—
pacific fillet, baked	5.1 oz	360	26	137	0	—
pacific, baked	3 oz	213	15	81	0	—
roe, raw	3.5 oz	130	2	—	2	—
READY-TO-USE						
atlantic, kippered	1 fillet (1.4 oz)	87	5	367	0	—
atlantic, pickled	0.5 oz	39	3	131	1	—
HICKORY NUTS						
dried	1 oz	187	18	0	5	—
HOMINY						
canned, canned	½ cup	57	tr	168	11	—
HONEY						
Burleson's						
Clover	1 tbsp	60	0	1	16	0
Creamed	1 tbsp	60	0	1	16	0
Natural	1 tbsp	60	0	1	16	0
Pure	1 tbsp	60	0	1	16	0
Raw	1 tbsp	60	0	1	16	0
Rocky Mountain Clover	1 tbsp	60	0	1	16	0
Golden Blossom	1 tsp	20	0	tr	5	—
Smucker's Single Serving	0.5 oz	45	0	—	11	—
honey	1 cup	1030	0	17	279	—
honey	1 tbsp	65	0	1	17	—
HONEYDEW						
Chiquita	1 cup	70	0	—	—	—
Dole	1⁄10	50	0	50	12	1
cubed	1 cup	60	tr	17	16	—
fresh	1⁄10	46	tr	13	12	—
HORSE						
roasted	3 oz	149	5	47	0	—
HORSERADISH						
Gold's Hot	1 tsp	4	tr	60	tr	—

FOOD	PORTION	CAL	FAT	SOD	CARB	FIB
Gold's Red	1 tsp	4	0	75	tr	—
Gold's White	1 tsp	4	tr	55	tr	—
Hebrew National White	1 tbsp	7	0	160	1	—
Heluva Good Cheese	1 tsp (5 g)	0	0	6	0	—
Kraft Cream Style	1 tbsp	12	1	85	1	—
Kraft Horseradish Mustard	1 tbsp	14	1	135	1	—
Kraft Prepared	1 tbsp	10	0	140	1	—
Rosoff's Red	1 tbsp (0.5 oz)	8	0	160	2	—
Rosoff's White	1 tbsp (0.5 oz)	7	0	160	1	—
Sauceworks Horseradish	1 tbsp	50	5	105	2	—
Schorr's Red	1 tbsp (0.5 oz)	8	0	160	2	—
Schorr's White	1 tbsp (0.5 oz)	7	0	160	1	—

HOT CAKES
see PANCAKES

HOT DOG
see also MEAT SUBSTITUTES, SAUSAGE, SAUSAGE SUBSTITUTES

CHICKEN

FOOD	PORTION	CAL	FAT	SOD	CARB	FIB
Health Valley Wieners	1	96	8	90	1	0
Tyson	1	115	10	700	1	—
Tyson Cheese	1	145	11	680	1	—
Wampler Longacre	1 (1.6 oz)	115	35	—	—	—
Wampler Longacre	1 (2 oz)	144	44	—	—	—
chicken	1 (1.5 oz)	116	9	617	3	—

MEAT

Armour

FOOD	PORTION	CAL	FAT	SOD	CARB	FIB
Lower Salt Jumbo	1	170	15	450	—	—
Lower Salt Jumbo Beef	1	170	15	460	—	—
Star Jumbo	1	190	18	590	—	—
Star Jumbo Beef	1	190	18	590	—	—
Chefwich Chili Dog	5 oz	380	15	—	—	—
Hebrew National						
Beef	1 (1.7 oz)	150	14	370	—	—
Cocktail Beef	6 (1.8 oz)	160	15	410	—	—
Dinner Beef	1 (4 oz)	350	34	890	—	—
Reduced Fat Beef	1 (1.7 oz)	120	10	350	—	—
Hillshire						
Franks Bun Size Beef	2 oz	180	16	560	2	—
Franks Jumbo Light & Mild	1 link	110	8	570	2	—

FOOD	PORTION	CAL	FAT	SOD	CARB	FIB
Lit'l Franks Beef	2 oz	180	16	580	1	—
Lit'l Wieners	2 oz	180	16	560	2	—
Wieners Bun Size	2 oz	180	16	550	2	—
Wieners Light & Mild	1 link	90	7	580	2	—
Wieners Natural Casing	2 oz	180	17	470	2	—
Nathan's Famous Natural Casing Franks	1	158	14	422	1	—
Nathan's Famous Skinless Franks	1	176	16	463	1	—
Oscar Mayer						
Bacon & Cheddar Cheese	1 (1.5 oz)	137	12	501	1	—
Beef Franks	1 (1.5 oz)	144	13	460	1	—
Beef Franks With Cheddar	1 (1.5 oz)	136	12	492	1	—
Bun-Length Beef	1 (2 oz)	182	17	568	1	—
Bun-Length Wieners	1 (2 oz)	184	17	571	1	—
Cheese Hot Dogs	1 (1.5 oz)	143	13	480	1	—
Light Beef Franks	1 (2 oz)	131	11	594	1	—
Wieners Light	1 (2 oz)	127	11	623	tr	—
Wieners	1 (1.5 oz)	144	13	455	1	—
Wieners Little	1 (0.33 oz)	28	3	94	tr	—
Shofar Kosher Beef	1 (1.8 oz)	150	14	370	0	0
Shofar Kosher Beef Reduced Fat Reduced Sodium	1 (1.8 oz)	120	10	360	0	0
beef	1 (1.5)	142	13	462	1	—
beef	1 (2 oz)	180	16	585	1	—
beef & pork	1 (1.5 oz)	144	13	504	1	—
beef & pork	1 (2 oz)	183	17	639	1	—
pork cheesefurter smokie	1 (1.5 oz)	141	12	465	1	—
TAKE-OUT						
corndog	1	460	19	972	56	—
w/ bun chili	1	297	13	480	31	—
w/ bun plain	1	242	15	671	18	—
TURKEY						
Bil Mar Foods Cheese Franks	1 (1.6 oz)	109	9	—	—	—
Health Valley Wieners	1	96	8	112	1	0
Louis Rich	1 (1.5 oz)	80	6	480	1	0

FOOD	PORTION	CAL	FAT	SOD	CARB	FIB
Louis Rich	1 (1.6 oz)	90	7	500	1	0
Louis Rich Bun Length	1 (2 oz)	110	8	630	2	0
Louis Rich Turkey Cheese Franks	1 (1.6 oz)	90	7	490	2	0
Mr. Turkey Franks	1 (1.6 oz)	106	9	—	—	—
Mr. Turkey Franks	1 (0.5 oz)	79	7	—	—	—
Mr. Turkey Franks	1 (2 oz)	132	11	—	—	—
Wampler Longacre	1 (1.6 oz)	102	31	—	—	—
turkey	1 (1.5 oz)	102	8	642	1	—

HUMMUS

hummus	1 cup	420	21	599	50	—
hummus	⅓ cup	140	7	200	17	—

HYACINTH BEANS

DRIED

cooked	1 cup	228	1	13	40	—

ICE CREAM AND FROZEN DESSERTS

see also ICES AND ICE POPS, PUDDING POPS, SHERBET, YOGURT FROZEN

All Flavors Avari Creme Glace	1 oz	10	0	35	3	—
All Flavors Ice Cream (Bresler's)	3.5 oz	230	12	—	23	—
All Flavors Royale Cremes (Bresler's)	4 oz	260	16	—	24	—
All Flavors Royale Lites (Bresler's)	4 oz	217	0	—	49	—
Almond Praline Light (Edy's)	4 oz	140	5	50	18	—
American Glory (Sealtest)	½ cup (2.4 oz)	130	6	45	17	0
Banana Bob (Good Humor)	1 (3 fl oz)	155	7	55	22	0
Banana Cream (Fi-Bar)	1 bar	93	tr	—	21	—
Banana-Politan Light (Edy's)	4 oz	110	4	50	15	—
Berry Berry Berry (Mocha Mix)	3.5 oz	209	9	99	30	tr
Berry Swirl Bar, Raspberry (Carnation)	1 bar	70	3	—	—	—
Berry Swirl Bar, Strawberry (Carnation)	1 bar	70	3	—	—	—

FOOD	PORTION	CAL	FAT	SOD	CARB	FIB
Black Cherry Free (Sealtest)	½ cup	100	0	45	25	—
Black Cherry Fat Free (Borden)	½ cup	90	tr	40	21	—
Bordeaux Cherry (Healthy Choice)	4 oz	120	1	50	23	—
Bounty Cherry/Dark (M&M's)	1 (0.84 fl oz)	70	5	20	8	0
Bounty Coconut/Dark (M&M's)	1 (0.84 fl oz)	70	5	20	7	0
Bounty Coconut/Milk (M&M's)	1 (0.84 fl oz)	70	5	20	7	0
Brownie Marble Fudge Light (Breyers)	½ cup (2.6 oz)	150	5	55	23	tr
Bubble O'Bill (Good Humor)	1 (3.6 fl oz)	170	10	45	20	1
Bubble Play (Good Humor)	1	110	1	5	25	—
Butter Almond (Breyers)	½ cup	170	11	120	15	0
Butter Pecan (Breyers)	½ cup (2.6 oz)	180	12	125	15	0
Butter Pecan (Frusen Gladje)	½ cup	280	21	160	16	—
Butter Pecan (Haagen-Dazs)	4 oz	390	24	100	29	—
Butter Pecan (Sealtest)	½ cup (2.4 oz)	160	9	115	16	0
Butter Pecan Light (Edy's)	4 oz	140	5	50	18	—
Butter Pecan (Borden)	½ cup	180	12	65	16	—
Cafe Au Lait Light (Edy's)	4 oz	110	4	50	13	—
Candy Bar Light (Edy's)	4 oz	140	5	50	20	—
Candy Cane Crunch (Sealtest)	½ cup (2.4 oz)	150	6	50	21	0
Candy Center Crunch Classic (Good Humor)	1 (3.1 fl oz)	260	19	60	21	1
Cappuccino (Rice Dream)	½ cup	130	5	80	17	—
Caramel Almond Crunch Bar (Haagen-Dazs)	1	240	18	65	17	—
Caramel Nut Sundae (Haagen-Dazs)	4 oz	310	21	100	26	—

FOOD	PORTION	CAL	FAT	SOD	CARB	FIB
Carob (Rice Dream)	½ cup	130	5	80	20	—
Carob (Tofu Ice Creme)	4 fl oz	190	8	55	28	—
Carob Almond (Rice Dream)	½ cup	140	6	80	20	—
Carob Chip (Rice Dream)	½ cup	140	6	80	20	—
Carob Chip Mint (Rice Dream)	½ cup	140	6	80	20	—
Cheesecake Bar Original (Carnation)	1 bar	120	6	—	—	—
Cheesecake Bar Strawberry (Carnation)	1 bar	125	6	—	—	—
Cherry & Ice Cream Swirl (Chiquita)	1 bar	80	3	—	—	—
Cherry Garcia (Ben & Jerry's)	1 pop (3.7 fl oz)	250	18	100	25	2
Cherry Garcia (Ben & Jerry's)	½ cup (4 fl oz)	230	16	35	23	0
Cherry Vanilla (Breyers)	½ cup	150	7	40	17	0
Chip Burrrger (Good Humor)	1 (4.7 oz)	320	15	190	44	1
Chip Sandwich (Good Humor)	1 (4.7 fl oz)	320	15	190	44	1
Choco Taco (Good Humor)	1 (4.4 fl oz)	320	17	100	38	1
Chocolate						
(Ben & Jerry's)	½ cup (4 fl oz)	230	14	25	24	0
(Breyers)	½ cup (2.6 oz)	160	8	30	19	1
(Cyrk)	3 oz	209	16	32	18	0
(Frusen Gladje)	½ cup	240	17	65	17	—
(Haagen-Dazs)	4 oz	270	17	50	24	—
(Healthy Choice)	4 oz	130	2	70	24	—
(Sealtest)	½ cup (2.4 oz)	140	7	50	19	tr
(Simple Pleasures)	4 oz	140	tr	—	25	—
(Ultra Slim-Fast)	4 oz	100	tr	45	19	2
Chocolate American Dream (Edy's)	3 oz	90	11	45	20	—
Chocolate Bar (Rice Dream)	1	270	16	115	33	—
Chocolate Butter Pecan (Sealtest)	½ cup (2.4 oz)	150	8	85	17	0
Chocolate Caramel Sundae Light (Simple Pleasures)	4 oz	90	tr	—	20	—

FOOD	PORTION	CAL	FAT	SOD	CARB	FIB
Chocolate Chip (Breyers)	½ cup (2.5 oz)	170	10	40	18	0
Chocolate Chip (Sealtest)	½ cup (2.4 oz)	150	8	50	18	0
Chocolate Chip (Simple Pleasures)	4 oz	150	3	—	25	—
Chocolate Chip American Dream (Edy's)	3 oz	100	1	45	22	—
Chocolate Chip Cookie Dough (Ben & Jerry's)	1 pop (2.5 fl oz)	240	16	110	26	1
Chocolate Chip Cookie Dough (Ben & Jerry's)	½ cup (4 fl oz)	260	17	65	29	0
Chocolate Chip Cookie Dough (Breyers)	½ cup (2.5 oz)	190	10	45	20	0
Chocolate Chip Ice Milk (Weight Watchers)	½ cup	120	4	80	18	—
Chocolate Chip Light (Edy's)	4 oz	120	4	50	16	—
Chocolate Chip Light (Light n' Lively)	½ cup (2.4 oz)	130	4	45	20	0
Chocolate Chocolate Chip Light (Light n' Lively)	½ cup (2.4 oz)	130	4	40	20	tr
Chocolate Chocolate Chip (Breyers)	½ cup (2.5 oz)	180	10	30	21	1
Chocolate Chip (Frusen Gladje)	½ cup	270	18	60	21	—
Chocolate Chocolate Chip (Haagen-Dazs)	4 oz	290	20	40	28	—
Chocolate Chocolate Chip Reduced Fat (Breyers)	½ cup (2.4 oz)	150	5	50	21	tr
Chocolate Chocolate Mint (Haagen-Dazs)	4 oz	300	20	50	26	—
Chocolate Free (Sealtest)	½ cup	100	0	50	23	—
Chocolate Light (Breyers)	½ cup (2.4 oz)	130	4	55	19	tr
Chocolate Light (Simple Pleasures)	4 oz	80	tr	—	16	—

FOOD	PORTION	CAL	FAT	SOD	CARB	FIB
Chocolate Peanut Butter Twirl (Breyers)	½ cup (2.6 oz)	220	13	75	20	1
Chocolate Dark Chocolate Bar (Haagen-Dazs)	1	390	27	60	32	—
Chocolate Dip Bar (Weight Watches)	1 (2 oz)	110	7	45	10	—
Chocolate Eclair Classic (Good Humor)	1 (3.1 fl oz)	170	9	60	21	1
Chocolate Fat Free (Borden)	½ cup	100	tr	50	21	—
Chocolate Fat Free Frozen Dessert (Weight Watchers)	½ cup	80	0	75	19	—
Chocolate Fudge (Ultra Slim-Fast)	4 oz	120	tr	65	24	2
Chocolate Fudge Brownie (Ben & Jerry's)	½ cup (4 fl oz)	250	14	85	29	1
Chocolate Fudge Mousse Light (Edy's)	4 oz	130	5	50	18	—
Chocolate Fudge Swirl Dessert Bar Free (Sealtest)	1	90	0	30	19	—
Chocolate Fudge Twirl Light (Breyers)	½ cup (2.6 oz)	140	4	55	22	1
Chocolate Ice Milk (Borden)	½ cup	100	2	80	18	—
Chocolate Malted Bars (Carnation)	1 bar	70	3	—	—	—
Chocolate Mousse Bar Sugar Free (Weight Watchers)	1 (1.75 oz)	35	tr	30	9	—
Chocolate Nutty Bar (Rice Dream)	1	330	23	110	29	—
Chocolate Peanut Butter Chocolate Chip Cookie Dough (Ben & Jerry's)	½ cup (4 fl oz)	280	18	60	28	0
Chocolate Swirl (Borden)	½ cup	130	6	65	18	—

FOOD	PORTION	CAL	FAT	SOD	CARB	FIB
Chocolate Swirl Fat Free Frozen Dessert (Weight Watchers)	½ cup	90	0	75	22	—
Chocolate Treat Bar Sugar Free (Weight Watchers)	1 (2.75 oz)	90	0	75	18	—
Chunky Monkey (Ben & Jerry's)	½ cup (4 fl oz)	270	19	25	27	0
Classic Almond Bar (Good Humor)	1 (3.1 fl oz)	210	12	50	21	1
Classic Candy Center Crunch Vanilla (Good Humor)	1	280	21	75	21	0
Classic Chip Cookie Sandwich (Good Humor)	1 (4.1 fl oz)	300	13	215	43	1
Classic Toasted Almond Bar (Good Humor)	1 (3.1 fl oz)	170	9	40	22	1
Classic Vanilla Bar (Good Humor)	1 (3.1 fl oz)	190	10	35	22	0
Cocoa Marble Fudge (Rice Dream)	½ cup	140	6	80	19	—
Cocoa-Fudge 'N Cream (Fi-Bar)	1 bar	93	tr	—	21	—
Coconut Chocolate (Sealtest)	½ cup (2.4 oz)	160	8	55	18	tr
Coffee (Breyers)	½ cup (2.6 oz)	150	8	45	15	0
Coffee (Haagen-Dazs)	4 oz	270	17	55	23	—
Coffee (Sealtest)	½ cup (2.4 oz)	140	7	55	16	0
Coffee (Simple Pleasures)	4 oz	120	tr	—	22	—
Coffee Heath Bar Crunch (Ben & Jerry's)	½ cup (4 fl oz)	270	19	100	26	0
Coffee Light (Light n' Lively)	½ cup (2.4 oz)	110	3	45	18	0
Colonel Crunch Chocolate (Good Humor)	1 (3.1 oz)	160	7	60	21	1
Colonel Crunch Strawberry (Good Humor)	1 (3.1 oz)	170	8	45	22	0

FOOD	PORTION	CAL	FAT	SOD	CARB	FIB
Combo Cup (Good Humor)	1 (6.2 fl oz)	200	10	65	25	1
Cookies 'N' Cream American Dream (Edy's)	3 oz	100	1	45	22	—
Cookies 'N' Cream Light (Edy's)	4 oz	120	5	50	18	—
Cookies N' Cream (Healthy Choice)	4 oz	130	2	80	24	—
Cookies n' Cream Light (Light n' Lively)	½ cup (2.4 oz)	130	3	70	21	0
Cookies n' Cream (Breyers)	½ cup (2.6 oz)	170	9	55	19	0
Cookies n' Cream (Simple Pleasures)	4 oz	150	2	—	25	—
Cool 'N Creamy Amaretto With Chocolate Swirl	1 bar	62	2	50	10	—
Cool 'N Creamy Chocolate/Vanilla	1 bar	54	2	51	7	—
Cool 'N Creamy Double Chocolate Fudge	1 bar	55	2	57	7	—
Cool 'N Creamy Orange/Vanilla	1 bar	31	1	18	5	—
Creamee Burrrger (Good Humor)	1 (4.7 oz)	310	17	150	40	1
Creamy Lites Bar Chocolate (Carnation)	1 bar	50	2	—	—	—
Creamy Lites Bar Strawberry (Carnation)	1 bar	50	2	—	—	—
Cupid's Scoops (Sealtest)	½ cup (2.5 oz)	140	6	55	20	0
Deep Chocolate (Haagen-Dazs)	4 oz	290	14	70	26	—
Deep Chocolate Fudge (Haagen-Dazs)	4 oz	290	14	90	26	—
Deluxe Rocky Road (Breyers)	½ cup (2.5 oz)	190	9	30	24	1
Dinosaur Bar (Good Humor)	1	110	2	5	25	—
Double Fudge Bar (Weight Watchers)	1 (1.75 oz)	60	1	50	12	—

FOOD	PORTION	CAL	FAT	SOD	CARB	FIB
Dove Bar						
Almond	1 (3.67 fl oz)	335	22	75	30	0
Caramel Pecan	1 (3.67 fl oz)	350	35	85	35	0
Chocolate Milk Chocolate	1 (3.8 fl oz)	340	21	80	35	0
Coffee Cashew	1 (3.67 fl oz)	335	22	55	31	0
Crunchy Cookie	1 (3.8 fl oz)	340	21	65	35	0
Peanut	1 (3.8 fl oz)	380	25	100	35	0
Vanilla Dark Chocolate	1 (3.8 fl oz)	340	22	65	34	0
Vanilla Milk Chocolate	1 (3.8 fl oz)	340	21	60	34	0
Dove Bite Size						
Almond Praline	1 (0.75 fl oz)	80	5	15	8	0
Cherry Royale	1 (0.75 fl oz)	70	5	10	8	0
Classic Vanilla	1 (0.75 fl oz)	70	5	10	7	0
French Vanilla	1 (0.75 fl oz)	70	5	10	7	0
Mint Supreme	1 (0.75 fl oz)	80	5	5	8	0
Dream Pie Chocolate (Rice Dream)	1	380	19	225	47	—
Dream Pie Mint (Rice Dream)	1	380	19	225	47	—
Dream Pie Mocha (Rice Dream)	1	380	19	225	47	—
Dream Pie Vanilla (Rice Dream)	1	380	19	225	47	—
Dreamy Caramel Cream Light (Edy's)	4 oz	140	4	50	16	—
Dutch Chocolate (Mocha Mix)	3.5 oz	210	12	135	25	tr
Dutch Chocolate Olde Fashioned Recipe (Borden)	½ cup	130	6	65	16	—
English Toffee Crunch Bar (Weight Watchers)	1 (2 oz)	120	11	60	11	—
Fat Frog (Good Humor)	1 (3.6 fl oz)	150	8	45	19	1
Fosters Freeze (Vanilla)	1 oz	43	1	—	—	—
French Vanilla (Breyers)	(2.5 oz)	170	10	45	15	0
French Vanilla (Sealtest)	½ cup (2.4 oz)	140	8	50	16	0
Fresh Lites Chocolate Chip (Dole)	1 bar	60	1	30	10	—

FOOD	PORTION	CAL	FAT	SOD	CARB	FIB
Fudge Bar (Ultra Slim-Fast)	1	90	tr	50	17	2
Fudge Pop Bar (Haagen-Dazs)	1	210	14	50	19	—
Fudge Royale (Sealtest)	½ cup (2.5 oz)	150	7	55	19	0
Fun Box Ice Cream Sandwich (Good Humor)	1 (3.1 fl oz)	160	5	140	27	1
Heath Bar Crunch (Ben & Jerry's)	1 pop (2.5 fl oz)	260	18	65	25	0
Heath Bar Crunch (Ben & Jerry's)	1 pop (3.7 fl oz)	340	23	90	35	0
Heath Bar Crunch (Ben & Jerry's)	½ cup (4 fl oz)	270	19	100	26	0
Heaven Bars Vanilla Caramel Nut (Carnation)	1 bar	225	15	—	—	—
Heaven Bars Vanilla Nut Fudge (Carnation)	1 bar	222	15	—	—	—
Heaven Sundae Bars Chocolate Fudge (Carnation)	1 bar	150	9	—	—	—
Heaven Sunday Bars Vanilla Fudge (Carnation)	1 bar	150	9	—	—	—
Heavenly Hash (Mocha Mix)	3.5 oz	244	13	116	29	tr
Heavenly Hash (Sealtest)	½ cup (2.4 oz)	150	7	50	20	tr
Heavenly Hash Light (Breyers)	½ cup (2.4 oz)	150	5	55	22	tr
Heavenly Hash Light (Light n' Lively)	½ cup (2.4 oz)	140	4	45	23	tr
Heavenly Hash Reduced Fat (Breyers)	½ cup (2.4 oz)	150	5	55	22	tr
Honey Vanilla (Haagen-Dazs)	4 oz	250	16	55	22	—
Ice Cream Sandwich (Good Humor)	1	190	8	120	28	1
King Cone (Good Humor)	1 (5.7 fl oz)	300	14	110	38	2

FOOD	PORTION	CAL	FAT	SOD	CARB	FIB
King Cone Classic Vanilla (Good Humor)	1 (4.8 oz)	300	10	110	48	1
King Cone Strawberry (Good Humor)	1 (5.7 oz)	250	10	105	38	1
Klondike (Good Humor)						
Almond Bar	1 (5.2 fl oz)	310	21	90	26	3
Caramel Crunch	1 (5.2 fl oz)	300	18	95	31	tr
Chocolate Chocolate Bar	1 (5.2 fl oz)	280	20	60	22	tr
Coffee Bar	1 (5.2 fl oz)	290	20	65	25	0
Dark Chocolate Bar	1 (5.2 fl oz)	290	20	75	24	tr
Gold Bar	1 (5.2 fl oz)	340	23	60	30	1
Krispy Bar	1 (5.2 fl oz)	300	20	85	28	0
Krunch	1 (3.1 fl oz)	200	13	160	17	1
Lite Bar	1 (2.3 fl oz)	110	6	55	14	1
Lite Bar Caramel	1 (2.4 fl oz)	120	6	65	18	1
Lite Sandwich	1 (2.9 fl oz)	100	2	105	18	1
Movie Bites Chocolate	8 pieces (4.6 fl oz)	340	26	50	22	1
Movie Bites Vanilla	8 pieces (4.6 fl oz)	320	22	60	27	1
Original Bar	1 (5.2 fl oz)	290	20	65	24	0
Sandwich Chocolate	1 (5.2 fl oz)	270	10	200	41	2
Sandwich Vanilla	1 (5.2 fl oz)	250	9	230	37	1
Lemon (Rice Dream)	½ cup	130	5	80	17	—
Macadamia Brittle (Haagen-Dazs)	4 oz	280	18	60	25	—
Magnum Almond (Good Humor)	1 (4.2 fl oz)	270	12	50	35	5
Magnum Chocolate (Good Humor)	1 (4.2 fl oz)	260	12	60	38	2
Malt Ball 'N' Fudge Light (Edy's)	4 oz	140	5	50	20	—
Maple Walnut (Cyrk)	3 oz	299	22	34	25	1
Maple Walnut (Sealtest)	½ cup (2.4 oz)	160	9	50	16	0
Marble Fudge Light (Edy's)	4 oz	120	4	50	15	—
Mars Almond Bar	1 (1.85 fl oz)	210	14	45	20	0
Milk Chocolate Almond (Ben & Jerry's)	1 pop (2.5 fl oz)	250	19	85	16	3
Milk Way Single Chocolate/Milk	1 (2 fl oz)	210	11	60	24	0

FOOD	PORTION	CAL	FAT	SOD	CARB	FIB
Milk Way Single Vanilla/Dark	1 (2 fl oz)	200	12	50	24	0
Milk Way Snack Chocolate/Milk	1 (0.72 fl oz)	70	4	25	9	0
Milk Way Snack Vanilla/Dark	1 (0.72 fl oz)	70	4	25	9	0
Mint Chocolate Chip (Breyers)	½ cup (2.6 oz)	170	10	40	18	0
Mint Chocolate Chip (Cyrk)	3 oz	258	18	40	22	0
Mint Chocolate Chocolate Chip (Simple Pleasures)	4 oz	150	2	—	26	—
Mint Cookie (Ben & Jerry's)	½ cup (4 fl oz)	250	17	100	25	0
Mixed Berry & Ice Cream Swirl (Chiquita)	1 bar	80	3	—	—	—
Mocha Almond Fudge (Breyers)	½ cup (2.7 oz)	190	10	45	20	1
Mocha Almond Fudge (Mocha Mix)	3.5 oz	229	11	113	29	tr
Mocha Almond Fudge Reduced Fat (Breyers)	½ cup (2.5 oz)	160	6	55	20	tr
Mocha Almond Fudge American Dream (Edy's)	3 oz	110	1	45	24	—
Mocha Almond Fudge Light (Edy's)	4 oz	140	5	50	19	—
Neapolitan (Healthy Choice)	4 oz	120	2	60	22	—
Neapolitan (Mocha Mix)	3.5 oz	208	11	120	26	tr
Neapolitan Fat Free Frozen Dessert (Weight Watchers)	½ cup	80	0	75	19	—
New York Super Fudge (Ben & Jerry's)	1 pop (2.5 fl oz)	330	26	125	22	3
New York Super Fudge (Ben & Jerry's)	1 pop (3.7 fl oz)	330	26	135	22	3
New York Super Fudge (Ben & Jerry's)	½ cup (4 fl oz)	290	20	40	26	0
Number One Bar (Good Humor)	1 (4.1 fl oz)	190	11	45	22	1

FOOD	PORTION	CAL	FAT	SOD	CARB	FIB
ONE-ders						
(Weight Watchers)						
Brownies 'n Creme	4 oz	130	4	115	20	—
Chocolate Chip	4 oz	120	4	80	18	—
Heavenly Hash	4 oz	130	3	90	22	—
Pralines 'n Creme	4 oz	130	4	90	19	—
Strawberry	4 oz	110	3	75	17	—
Olde Nut Sundae Cone	1 (3.9 oz)	230	9	100	32	2
(Good Humor)						
Orange & Cream Pop	1	130	6	25	18	—
(Haagen-Dazs)						
Orange & Ice Cream Swirl (Chiquita)	1 bar	80	3	—	—	—
Orange Vanilla Treat Bar Sugar Free Fat Free (Weight Watchers)	1 (1.75 oz)	30	0	40	9	—
Peach (Breyers)	½ cup (2.6 oz)	130	6	30	18	0
Peach (Mocha Mix)	3.5 oz	198	9	96	28	tr
Peach (Ultra Slim-Fast)	4 oz	100	tr	55	22	2
Peach Free (Sealtest)	½ cup	100	0	45	23	—
Peach (Simple Pleasures)	4 oz	120	tr	—	21	—
Peach Fat Free (Borden)	½ cup	90	tr	40	21	—
Peanut Butter Crunch Bar (Haagen-Dazs)	1	270	21	55	16	—
Peanut Butter Fudge (Rice Dream)	½ cup	160	7	100	19	—
Peanut Butter & Chocolate Light (Edy's)	4 oz	130	5	50	19	—
Pecan Praline (Simple Pleasures)	4 oz	140	2	—	25	—
Pecan Pralines 'n Creme Ice Milk (Weight Watchers)	½ cup	130	4	90	20	—
Popsicle Ice Cream Sandwich (Good Humor)	1 (3.6 fl oz)	190	8	120	28	1
Popsicle Ice Cream Bar (Good Humor)	1 (3.1 fl oz)	160	11	35	15	1
Praline Almond Crunch Reduced Fat (Breyers)	½ cup (2.4 oz)	140	5	70	20	tr

FOOD	PORTION	CAL	FAT	SOD	CARB	FIB
Praline Almond Crunch Light (Light n' Lively)	½ cup (2.4 oz)	130	3	65	20	0
Praline & Caramel (Healthy Choice)	4 oz	130	2	70	26	—
Pralines And Caramel (Ultra Slim-Fast)	4 oz	120	tr	95	25	2
Rain Forest Crunch (Ben & Jerry's)	1 pop (3.7 fl oz)	350	27	195	26	2
Rain Forest Crunch (Ben & Jerry's)	½ cup (4 fl oz)	270	21	100	21	0
Raspberries 'N Cream (Fi-Bar)	1 bar	93	tr	—	21	—
Raspberry Truffle Light (Edy's)	4 oz	110	5	50	19	—
Raspberry & Ice Cream Swirl (Chiquita)	1 bar	80	3	—	—	—
Rocky Road (Healthy Choice)	4 oz	140	1	70	29	—
Rocky Road American Dream (Edy's)	3 oz	110	1	45	24	—
Rocky Road Deluxe Light (Breyers)	½ cup (2.4 oz)	150	5	50	22	tr
Rocky Road Light (Edy's)	4 oz	130	5	50	17	—
Rum Raisin (Haagen-Dazs)	4 oz	250	17	45	21	—
Rum Raisin (Simple Pleasures)	4 oz	130	tr	—	35	—
Sandwich Giant Neapolitan (Good Humor)	1 (5.2 fl oz)	260	10	150	39	1
Sandwich Giant Vanilla (Good Humor)	1 (5.2 fl oz)	240	10	160	35	1
Sandwich Vanilla (Breyers)	1 (2.8 oz)	250	11	160	32	1
Sidewalk Sundae Bar (Good Humor)	1	280	20	65	21	2
Sidewalk Sundae Cone (Good Humor)	1 (4.2 oz)	270	14	125	31	1
Sidewalk Sundae Sandwich (Good Humor)	1 (3.1 oz)	160	5	140	27	1

FOOD	PORTION	CAL	FAT	SOD	CARB	FIB
Snickers (Single)	1 (2 fl oz)	220	13	65	22	0
Snickers (Snack)	1 (1 fl oz)	110	7	35	11	0
Sprinkle Sandwich (Good Humor)	1 (3.1 fl oz)	180	6	65	28	1
Strawberries 'N Cream Olde Fashioned Recipe (Borden)	½ cup	130	5	55	19	—
Strawberry						
(Borden)	½ cup	130	6	55	18	—
(Breyers)	½ cup (2.6 oz)	130	6	35	15	0
(Cyrk)	3 oz	208	15	31	17	tr
(Frusen Gladje)	½ cup	230	15	60	20	—
(Haagen-Dazs)	4 oz	250	15	40	23	—
(Healthy Choice)	4 oz	110	1	50	21	—
(Rice Dream)	½ cup	130	5	80	17	—
(Sealtest)	½ cup (2.4 oz)	130	6	45	19	0
(Simple Pleasures)	4 oz	120	tr	—	22	—
Strawberry American Dream (Edy's)	3 oz	70	tr	40	16	—
Strawberry Free (Sealtest)	½ cup	100	0	40	23	—
Strawberry Light (Breyers)	½ cup (2.4 oz)	120	4	45	18	0
Strawberry Shortcake Bar Classic (Good Humor)	1 (3.1 fl oz)	160	8	60	20	1
Strawberry & Ice Cream Swirl (Chiquita)	1 bar	80	3	—	—	—
Strawberry Bar (Rice Dream)	1	260	15	110	31	—
Strawberry Fat Free (Borden)	½ cup	90	tr	40	21	—
Strawberry Ice Milk (Borden)	½ cup	90	2	65	17	—
Strawberry Light (Edy's)	4 oz	110	4	50	15	—
Strawberry Swirl (Mocha Mix)	3.5 oz	209	9	98	30	tr
Sundae Cone (Borden)	1	210	12	110	23	—
Sundae Cone (Meadow Gold)	1	210	12	110	23	—
Sundae Twist Cup (Good Humor)	1	160	3	100	33	0

FOOD	PORTION	CAL	FAT	SOD	CARB	FIB
Swiss Almond Fudge Twirl Reduced Fat (Breyers)	½ cup (2.5 oz)	160	6	55	22	tr
Swiss Chocolate Candy Almond (Frusen Gladje)	½ cup	270	19	60	18	—
Musketeers Single Chocolate	1 (2 fl oz)	160	10	30	16	0
Musketeers Single Vanilla	1 (2 fl oz)	160	10	30	16	0
Musketeers Snack Chocolate	1 (0.72 fl oz)	60	4	10	6	0
Musketeers Snack Vanilla	1 (0.72 fl oz)	60	4	10	6	0
Toasted Almond (Mocha Mix)	3.5 oz	229	13	117	26	tr
Toasted Almond American Dream (Edy's)	3 oz	110	1	45	24	—
Toffee Bar Crunch (Breyers)	½ cup (2.5 oz)	180	11	65	18	0
Toffee Bar Crunch Light (Light n' Lively)	½ cup (2.4 oz)	130	4	55	20	0
Toffee Crunch (Simple Pleasures)	4 oz	130	tr	—	22	—
Toffee Fudge Parfait Light (Breyers)	½ cup (2.6 oz)	150	5	55	23	tr
Toffee Taco (Good Humor)	1 (4.4 fl oz)	300	16	120	35	1
Tofulite	4 oz	150	7	—	—	—
Tofutti Frutti Vanilla Apple Orchard (Tofutti)	4 fl oz	100	0	90	20	—
Triple Chocolate Passion (Sealtest)	½ cup (2.5 oz)	160	7	50	21	tr
Vanilla						
(Ben & Jerry's)	½ cup (4 fl oz)	215	16	30	18	0
(Breyers)	½ cup (2.6 oz)	150	8	45	15	0
(Cyrk)	3 oz	209	16	30	16	0
(Eagle Brand)	½ cup	150	9	55	16	—
(Frusen Gladje)	½ cup	230	17	70	16	—
(Haagen-Dazs)	4 oz	260	17	55	23	—
(Healthy Choice)	4 oz	120	2	60	21	—
(Land O'Lakes)	4 oz	140	7	—	—	—

FOOD	PORTION	CAL	FAT	SOD	CARB	FIB
(Mocha Mix)	3.5 oz	209	11	117	26	tr
(Rice Dream)	½ cup	130	5	80	17	—
(Sealtest)	½ cup (2.4 oz)	140	7	55	16	0
(Simple Pleasures)	4 oz	120	tr	—	22	—
(Tofu Ice Creme)	4 fl oz	190	8	55	28	—
(Ultra Slim-Fast)	4 oz	90	tr	55	19	2
Vanilla American Dream (Edy's)	3 oz	80	tr	45	18	—
Vanilla Bar (Breyers)	1 (2.7 oz)	250	17	45	21	tr
Vanilla Bar (Rice Dream)	1	275	16	120	33	—
Vanilla Bar With Chocolate Coating (Breyers)	1 (2.6 oz)	230	15	45	20	0
Vanilla Brownie (Ben & Jerry's)	1 bar (4 fl oz)	260	14	165	32	0
Vanilla Caramel Praline (Breyers)	½ cup (2.6 oz)	190	10	90	23	0
Vanilla Chocolate (Breyers)	½ cup (2.5 oz)	160	8	35	17	0
Vanilla Chocolate Chunk (Ben & Jerry's)	½ cup (4 fl oz)	250	18	30	24	0
Vanilla Chocolate Sandwich (Ultra Slim-Fast)	1	140	2	220	28	1
Vanilla Chocolate Strawberry (Breyers)	½ cup (2.5 oz)	150	8	35	16	0
Vanilla Chocolate Strawberry (Edy's)	4 oz	110	4	50	14	—
Vanilla Chocolate Strawberry (Sealtest)	½ cup (2.4 oz)	140	6	50	18	0
Vanilla Chocolate Strawberry American Dream (Edy's)	3 oz	80	1	45	18	—
Vanilla Chocolate Strawberry Light (Breyers)	½ cup (2.4 oz)	120	4	50	18	0
Vanilla Chocolate Strawberry Light (Light n' Lively)	½ cup (2.4 oz)	110	3	45	19	0
Vanilla Fat Free (Borden)	½ cup	90	tr	50	20	—

FOOD	PORTION	CAL	FAT	SOD	CARB	FIB
Vanilla Fat Free Frozen Dessert (Weight Watchers)	½ cup	80	0	75	20	—
Vanilla Free (Sealtest)	½ cup	100	0	45	24	—
Vanilla Fudge (Haagen-Dazs)	4 oz	270	17	100	26	—
Vanilla Fudge (Rice Dream)	½ cup	140	6	80	21	—
Vanilla Fudge Cookie (Ultra Slim-Fast)	4 oz	110	tr	90	24	2
Vanilla Fudge Royale Free (Sealtest)	½ cup	100	0	50	24	—
Vanilla Fudge Swirl Dessert Bar Free (Sealtest)	1	80	0	30	18	—
Vanilla Fudge Twirl (Breyers)	½ cup (2.6 oz)	160	8	50	19	tr
Vanilla Fudge Swirl Light (Simple Pleasures)	4 oz	90	tr	—	20	—
Vanilla Ice Milk (Borden)	½ cup	90	2	65	17	—
Vanilla Ice Milk (Land O'Lakes)	4 oz	90	3	—	—	—
Vanilla Light (Breyers)	½ cup (2.4 oz)	130	5	55	18	0
Vanilla Light (Light n' Lively)	½ cup (2.4 oz)	110	3	50	19	0
Vanilla Light (Simple Pleasures)	4 oz	80	tr	—	16	—
Vanilla Peanut Butter Fudge Sundae (Breyers)	½ cup (2.5 oz)	170	9	65	18	0
Vanilla Strawberry Royale Free (Sealtest)	½ cup	100	0	35	25	—
Vanilla Strawberry Swirl Dessert Bar Free (Sealtest)	1	80	0	40	17	—
Vanilla Caramel Swirl Bar With Chocolate Peanut Brittle Coating (Breyers)	1 (2.7 oz)	260	15	65	26	0
Vanilla Cookie Crunch Bar (Ultra Slim-Fast)	1	90	4	70	14	1

FOOD	PORTION	CAL	FAT	SOD	CARB	FIB
Vanilla Crunch Bar (Haagen-Dazs)	1	220	16	55	16	—
Vanilla Light (Edy's)	4 oz	100	4	50	13	—
Vanilla Milk Chocolate Brittle Bar (Haagen-Dazs)	1	370	25	160	32	—
Vanilla Milk Chocolate Almond Bar (Haagen-Dazs)	1	370	27	55	27	—
Vanilla Milk Chocolate Bar (Haagen-Dazs)	1	360	27	55	26	—
Vanilla Nutty Bar (Rice Dream)	1	330	23	100	29	—
Vanilla Oatmeal Sandwich (Ultra Slim-Fast)	1	150	3	160	26	3
Vanilla Old Fashioned (Healthy Choice)	4 oz	120	2	60	21	—
Vanilla Olde Fashioned Recipe (Borden)	½ cup	130	7	55	15	—
Vanilla Peanut Butter Swirl (Haagen-Dazs)	4 oz	280	21	120	19	—
Vanilla Sandwich (Ultra Slim-Fast)	1	140	2	220	28	1
Vanilla Sandwich Bar Fat Free (Weight Watchers)	1 (2.5 oz)	130	0	170	30	—
Vanilla Swiss Almond (Frusen Gladje)	½ cup	270	19	65	18	—
Vanilla Swiss Almond (Haagen-Dazs)	4 oz	290	19	55	24	—
Vanilla Swiss Almond (Rice Dream)	½ cup	140	6	80	20	—
Vanilla With Orange Sherbet (Sealtest)	½ cup (2.7 oz)	130	4	45	22	0
Viennetta Chocolate (Good Humor)	1 (4.2 fl oz)	160	9	60	19	1
Viennetta Vanilla (Good Humor)	1 (4.2 fl oz)	160	10	80	15	0
Vinalla Fudge Royale Light (Light n' Lively)	½ cup (2.6 oz)	120	3	50	21	0
WWF Bar (Good Humor)	1 (3.7 fl oz)	200	10	100	24	1

FOOD	PORTION	CAL	FAT	SOD	CARB	FIB
Wild Berry Swirl (Healthy Choice)	4 oz	120	2	60	23	—
Wildberry (Rice Dream)	½ cup	130	5	80	17	—
Wildberry Cream (Fi-Bar)	1 bar	93	tr	—	21	—
X-Men Bar (Good Humor)	1 (3 fl oz)	150	6	90	23	0
french vanilla soft serve	1 cup	377	23	153	38	—
french vanilla soft serve	½ gal	3014	180	1228	306	—
vanilla 10% fat	1 cup	269	14	116	32	—
vanilla 10% fat	½ gal	2153	115	929	254	—
vanilla 16% fat	1 cup	349	24	108	32	—
vanilla 16% fat	½ gal	2805	190	868	256	—
vanilla ice milk	1 cup	184	6	105	29	—
vanilla ice milk	½ gal	1469	45	836	232	—
vanilla ice milk, soft serve	1 cup	223	5	163	38	—
vanilla ice milk, soft serve	½ gal	1787	37	1303	307	—
TAKE-OUT						
cone, vanilla, ice milk, soft serve	1 (4.6 oz)	164	6	92	24	—
sundae caramel	1 (5.4 oz)	303	9	195	49	—
sundae hot fudge	1 (5.4 oz)	284	9	182	48	—
sundae strawberry	1 (5.4 oz)	269	8	92	45	—

ICE CREAM CONES AND CUPS

FOOD	PORTION	CAL	FAT	SOD	CARB	FIB
Comet Rainbow Cups	1 (4.5 oz)	16	tr	10	4	—
Comet Cups	1 (4.5 g)	18	tr	5	4	—
Comet Sugar Cone	1 (0.5 oz)	50	tr	40	11	—
Comet Waffle Cone	1 (0.5 oz)	70	tr	30	15	—
Dutch Mill Chocolate Covered Wafer Cups	1 (0.5 oz)	80	5	—	8	0
Keebler Sugar Cones	1	45	tr	35	11	—
Keebler Vanilla Cups	1	15	tr	20	4	—
sugar cone	1	40	tr	32	8	tr
wafer cone	1	17	tr	6	3	tr

ICE CREAM TOPPINGS
see also SYRUP

FOOD	PORTION	CAL	FAT	SOD	CARB	FIB
Butterscotch (Kraft)	1 tbsp	60	1	70	13	—

FOOD	PORTION	CAL	FAT	SOD	CARB	FIB
Butterscotch (Smucker's)	2 tbsp	140	1	75	33	—
Butterscotch Special Recipe (Smucker's)	2 tbsp	160	3	40	33	—
Caramel (Kraft)	1 tbsp	60	0	45	13	—
Carmel (Smucker's)	2 tbsp	140	1	110	33	—
Chocolate (Kraft)	1 tbsp	50	0	15	11	—
Chocolate (Smucker's)	2 tbsp	130	0	35	27	—
Chocolate Fudge (Hershey)	2 tbsp	100	4	30	14	—
Chocolate Fudge (Smucker's)	2 tbsp	130	1	50	31	—
Chocolate Fudge Magic Shell (Smucker's)	2 tbsp	190	15	50	16	—
Chocolate Magic Shell (Smucker's)	2 tbsp	190	15	25	16	—
Chocolate Nut Magic Shell (Smucker's)	2 tbsp	200	16	40	25	—
Dark Chocolate Special Recipe (Smucker's)	2 tbsp	130	1	45	31	—
Hot Caramel (Smucker's)	2 tbsp	150	4	75	28	—
Hot Fudge (Kraft)	1 tbsp	70	0	50	11	—
Hot Caramel (Smucker's)	2 tbsp	150	4	75	28	—
Hot Fudge (Kraft)	1 tbsp	70	0	50	11	—
Hot Fudge (Smucker's)	2 tbsp	110	4	55	18	—
Hot Fudge Special Recipe (Smucker's)	2 tbsp	150	5	60	23	—
Hot Fudge Light (Smucker's)	2 tbsp	70	tr	35	19	—
Hot Toffee Fudge (Smucker's)	2 tbsp	110	4	55	18	—
Marshmallow (Smucker's)	2 tbsp	120	0	0	29	—
Marshmallow Creme (Kraft)	1 oz	90	0	20	23	—
Peanut Butter Caramel (Smucker's)	2 tbsp	150	2	120	29	—
Pecans in Syrup (Smucker's)	2 tbsp	130	1	0	28	—
Pineapple (Kraft)	1 tbsp	50	0	0	13	—
Pineapple (Smucker's)	2 tbsp	130	0	0	32	—
Strawberry (Kraft)	1 tbsp	50	0	5	14	—

FOOD	PORTION	CAL	FAT	SOD	CARB	FIB
Strawberry (Smucker's)	2 tbsp	120	0	0	30	—
Swiss Milk Chocolate Fudge (Smucker's)	2 tbsp	140	1	70	31	—
Walnuts in Syrup (Smucker's)	2 tbsp	130	1	0	27	—

ICED TEA
see TEA/HERBAL TEA

ICES AND ICE POPS
see also ICE CREAM AND FROZEN DESSERTS, PUDDING POPS, SHERBET, YOGURT FROZEN

FOOD	PORTION	CAL	FAT	SOD	CARB	FIB
Ben & Jerry's						
Cherry Pop	1	330	24	—	28	—
Lemon Ice	4 oz	105	0	—	—	—
Raspberry	4 oz	105	0	—	—	—
Strawberry Ice	4 oz	77	0	—	—	—
Chiquita Fruit & Cream						
Banana	1 bar	80	2	—	—	—
Blueberry	1 bar	80	1	—	—	—
Peach	1 bar	80	1	—	—	—
Raspberry	1 bar	80	1	—	—	—
Strawberry	1 bar	80	1	—	—	—
Strawberry Banana	1 bar	80	2	—	—	—
Chiquita Fruit & Juice Bar						
Cherry	1 bar (2 oz)	50	0	—	—	—
Raspberry	1 bar (2 oz)	50	0	—	—	—
Strawberry	1 bar (2 oz)	50	0	—	—	—
Strawberry Banana	1 bar (2 oz)	50	0	—	—	—
Crystal Light						
Berry Blend	1 bar	13	0	2	2	—
Cherry	1 bar	13	0	4	2	—
Fruit Punch	1 bar	14	0	2	2	—
Orange	1 bar	13	0	3	2	—
Pina Colada	1 bar	14	0	2	2	—
Pineapple	1 bar	14	0	2	2	—
Pink Lemonade	1 bar	14	0	2	2	—
Raspberry	1 bar	13	0	4	2	—
Strawberry	1 bar	13	0	2	2	—
Strawberry Daiquiri	1 bar	14	0	2	2	—
Cyrk						
Ice, Chocolate	4 oz	85	1	19	21	—
Ice, Vanilla	4 oz	75	tr	14	17	—

FOOD	PORTION	CAL	FAT	SOD	CARB	FIB
Sorbet, Apricot	4 oz	104	tr	2	27	1
Sorbet, Apricot, Sugar Free	4 oz	36	tr	1	9	1
Sorbet, Blueberry	4 oz	77	tr	1	20	2
Sorbet, Cherry	4 oz	98	tr	1	25	1
Sorbet, Mango	4 oz	83	tr	2	22	tr
Sorbet, Mango, Sugar Free	4 oz	48	tr	2	13	2
Sorbet, Pina Colada	4 oz	135	4	29	27	tr
Sorbet, Pina Colada, Sugar Free	4 oz	66	3	3	11	1
Sorbet, Plum	4 oz	90	tr	1	23	1
Sorbet, Raspberry	4 oz	88	tr	1	23	2
Sorbet, Raspberry, Sugar Free	4 oz	35	tr	1	9	3
Sorbet, Strawberry	4 oz	79	tr	2	21	1
Sorbet, White Peach	4 oz	96	tr	1	26	1
Dole						
Fresh Lites, Cherry	1 bar	25	tr	10	6	—
Fresh Lites, Lemon	1 bar	25	tr	20	5	—
Fresh Lites, Pineapple Orange	1 bar	25	tr	33	6	—
Fresh Lites, Raspberry	1 bar	25	tr	5	6	—
Fruit N' Cream Bar, Peach	1 bar	90	1	15	18	—
Fruit N' Cream Bar, Raspberry	1 bar	90	1	20	19	—
Fruit N' Cream Bar, Strawberry	1 bar	90	1	20	18	—
Fruit N' Juice Bar, Pineapple	1 bar	70	tr	5	17	—
Fruit N' Juice Bar, Pineapple Orange Banana	1 bar	70	tr	10	17	—
Fruit N' Juice Bar, Raspberry	1 bar	70	tr	15	15	—
Fruit N' Juice Bar, Strawberry	1 bar	70	tr	10	15	—
Sorbet, Mandarin Orange	4 oz	110	tr	10	28	—
Sorbet, Peach	4 oz	110	tr	10	27	—
Sorbet, Pineapple	4 oz	110	tr	10	26	—
Sorbet, Raspberry	4 oz	110	tr	10	27	—

FOOD	PORTION	CAL	FAT	SOD	CARB	FIB.
Dole *(cont.)*						
Sorbet, Strawberry	4 oz	100	tr	10	25	—
SunTops, Grape	1 bar	40	tr	5	9	—
SunTops, Lemonade	1 bar	40	tr	5	9	—
SunTops, Orange	1 bar	40	tr	5	9	—
Fi-Bar Juice Bar						
Lemoney-Lime	1 bar	63	tr	—	15	—
Strawberry Nectar	1 bar	63	tr	—	15	—
Tropical Delight	1 bar	63	tr	—	15	—
Frozfruit Strawberry	1 (4 oz)	80	0	20	20	1
Fruit N' Juice Bar, Peach Passion Fruit (Dole)	1 bar	70	tr	10	18	—
Frusen Gladje Sorbet, Raspberry	1/2 cup	140	0	10	36	—
Good Humor						
Big Stick Cherry Pineapple	1 (3.6 fl oz)	50	0	—	12	0
Big Stick Popsicle Alpine Lace	1 (3.6 fl oz)	50	0	5	12	—
Calippo Cherry	1 (3.8 fl oz)	100	0	5	23	—
Calippo Grape Lemon	1 (3.9 fl oz)	90	0	0	22	—
Calippo Orange	1 (3.9 fl oz)	90	0	0	23	—
Citrus Bites	1 (1.8 fl oz)	35	0	0	9	—
Creamsicle, Sugar Free	1 (1.8 fl oz)	25	0	10	5	—
Creamsicle Bar, Orange	1 (2.8 fl oz)	110	3	30	20	0
Creamsicle Pop, Orange Raspberry	1 (2.6 fl oz)	100	3	25	19	0
Creamsicle Pop, Orange	1 (1.8 fl oz)	70	2	15	13	0
Flintstones Push-Up Yabba Dabba Doo, Orange	1 (2.75 fl oz)	90	1	20	20	—
Fudgsicle Bar	1 (2.8 fl oz)	90	1	55	17	1
Fudgsicle Pop	1 (1.8 fl oz)	60	1	40	12	0
Fudgsicle, Sugar Free	1 (1.8 fl oz)	40	1	35	8	1
Fun Box Fudge Bar	1 (2.3 fl oz)	80	1	65	16	0
Fun Box Pops	1 (2 fl oz)	35	0	5	10	—
Fun Box Twin Pop, Banana	1 (2.6 fl oz)	50	0	10	14	—
Fun Box Twin Pop, Blue Raspberry	1 (2.6 fl oz)	50	0	10	14	—

FOOD	PORTION	CAL	FAT	SOD	CARB	FIB
Fun Box Twin Pop, Cherry	1 (2.6 fl oz)	50	0	10	14	—
Fun Box Twin Pop, Cherry Lemon	1 (2.6 fl oz)	50	0	10	14	—
Fun Box Twin Pop, Orange, Cherry, Grape	1 (2.6 fl oz)	50	0	10	14	—
Fun Box Twin Pop, Root Beer	1 (2.6 fl oz)	50	0	10	14	—
Garfield Bar	1 (3.9 fl oz)	90	0	0	22	—
Great White	1 (3.1 fl oz)	70	1	0	18	—
Hyperstripe	1 (2.8 fl oz)	80	0	0	21	—
Ice Stripe, Cherry Orange	1 (1.5 fl oz)	35	0	0	9	0
Ice Stripe, Grape Lemon	1 (1.5 fl oz)	35	0	0	9	0
Jumbo Jet Star	1 (4.7 fl oz)	80	0	0	20	—
Laser Blazer	1 (2.6 oz)	70	0	5	16	—
Popsicle, All Natural	1 (1.8 fl oz)	45	0	5	10	—
Popsicle, Orange, Cherry, Grape	1 (1.8 fl oz)	45	0	0	11	—
Popsicle, Rainbow Pops	1 (1.8 fl oz)	45	0	0	11	—
Popsicle, Rootbeer, Banana, Lime	1 (1.8 fl oz)	45	0	0	11	—
Popsicle, Strawberry, Raspberry, Wildberry	1 (1.8 fl oz)	45	0	0	11	—
Popsicle, Supersicle Firecracker	1 (4.7 fl oz)	90	0	0	20	—
Popsicle, Supersicle Traffic Signal	1	80	0	0	20	—
Popsicle Twin Pop, Cherry	1 (2.6 fl oz)	70	0	0	16	—
Popsicle Twin Pop, Orange, Cherry, Grape, Lime	1 (2.6 fl oz)	70	0	5	16	—
Snow Cone	1	60	0	5	14	—
Snowfruit Coconut Bar	1 (3.75 fl oz)	150	4	35	27	1
Snowfruit Orange Bar	1	140	0	10	34	tr
Snowfruit Strawberry Bar	1	120	0	15	31	tr

FOOD	PORTION	CAL	FAT	SOD	CARB	FIB
Good Humor *(cont.)*						
Snowfruit Tropical Fruit Bar	1	110	0	10	28	—
Sunkist Orange Juice Bar	1 (3.4 fl oz)	80	1	5	19	—
Sunkist Wildberry	1 (3.4 fl oz)	120	1	10	27	—
Super Mario Bar	1	120	1	10	27	—
Supersicle, Cherry Banana	1 (4.7 fl oz)	80	0	0	20	—
Supersicle, Cherry Cola	1 (4.7 fl oz)	80	0	0	20	—
Supersicle, Double Fudge	1 (4.7 fl oz)	150	2	95	29	1
Supersicle, Firecracker Jr.	1	72	0	0	10	—
Supersicle, Sour Tower	1	80	0	0	20	—
Swirl, Bubble Gum	1 (2.7 fl oz)	55	0	0	13	—
Swirl, Cherry Banana	1 (2.7 fl oz)	55	0	0	13	—
Torpedo, Cherry	1 (1.8 fl oz)	35	0	5	10	0
Twister, Blue Raspberry, Cherry, Cherry Cola, Cherry	1 (1.8 fl oz)	45	0	0	10	—
Twister, Cherry, Lemon, Orange	1 (1.8 fl oz)	45	0	0	10	—
Vampire's Deadly Secret	1 (2.8 fl oz)	100	0	10	24	—
Watermelon Bar	1 (3.6 fl oz)	80	0	0	20	—
Haagen-Dazs						
Sorbet & Cream Blueberry	4 oz	190	8	35	25	—
Sorbet & Cream Keylime	4 oz	190	7	30	29	—
Sorbet & Cream Orange	4 oz	190	8	35	27	—
Sorbet & Cream Raspberry	4 oz	180	8	35	23	—
Ice All Flavors Bresler's	3.5 oz	120	0	—	30	—
Jell-O						
Berry Punch	1 bar	31	tr	23	7	—
Lemon Lime	1 bar	33	tr	23	8	—
Mixed Berry	1 bar	31	tr	23	7	—
Orange	1 bar	31	tr	23	7	—
Orange Pineapple	1 bar	31	tr	23	7	—

FOOD	PORTION	CAL	FAT	SOD	CARB	FIB
Raspberry	1 bar	29	tr	24	7	—
Raspberry Peach	1 bar	29	tr	24	7	—
Side By Side Apple Cherry	1 bar	36	tr	7	8	—
Side By Side Grape Lemon	1 bar	36	tr	7	8	—
Strawberry	1 bar	31	tr	23	7	—
Strawberry Banana	1 bar	31	tr	23	7	—
Kool-Aid Cherry	1 bar	42	0	2	11	—
Kool-Aid Grape	1 bar	42	0	2	11	—
Kool-Aid Mountain Berry Punch	1 bar	42	0	2	11	—
Lifesavers Ice Pops	1	35	0	0	9	0
Lifesavers Ice Pops, Sugar Free	1	12	0	5	3	0
Tofutti Frutti Apricot Mango	4 fl oz	100	0	90	20	—
Tofutti Frutti Three Berry	4 fl oz	100	0	90	20	—
Vitari Passion-Fruit	4 oz	80	0	—	—	—
Vitari Peach	4 oz	80	0	—	—	—

ICING
see CAKE

INSTANT BREAKFAST
see BREAKFAST DRINKS

JACKFRUIT

fresh	3.5 oz	70	tr	2	4	—

JAM/JELLY/PRESERVES
ALL FRUIT

Apple Butter Simply Fruit (Smucker's)	1 tsp	12	0	0	3	—
Blueberry Fruit Spread (Pritikin)	1 tsp	14	0	—	—	—
Peach Fruit Spread (Pritikin)	1 tsp	14	0	—	—	—
Red Raspberry Fruit Spread (Pritikin)	1 tsp	14	0	—	—	—
Simply Fruit Spread All Flavors (Smucker's)	1 tsp	16	0	0	4	—
Strawberry Fruit Spread (Pritikin)	1 tsp	14	0	—	—	—

FOOD	PORTION	CAL	FAT	SOD	CARB	FIB
REDUCED CALORIE						
All Flavors Jelly (Estee)	1 tsp	2	0	10	0	—
All Flavors Preserves (Louis Sherry)	1 tsp	2	0	10	0	—
All Flavors Slenderella (Fruit Spread)	1 tsp	7	0	0	2	—
Apricot Pineapple Preserves (S&W)	1 tsp	4	0	0	1	—
Blueberry Jam (S&W)	1 tsp	4	0	0	1	—
Concord Grape Jelly (S&W)	1 tsp	4	0	0	1	—
Grape Jelly (Kraft)	1 tsp	6	0	5	2	—
Grape Spread (Weight Watchers)	1 tsp	8	0	0	2	—
Imitation Blackberry Jelly Single Serving (Smucker's)	1 pkg (0.4 oz)	4	0	<10	1	—
Imitation Cherry Jelly Single Serving (Smucker's)	1 pkg (0.4 oz)	4	0	<10	1	—
Imitation Grape Jelly Single Serving (Smucker's)	1 pkg (0.4 oz)	4	0	<10	1	—
Low Sugar Spread All Flavors (Smucker's)	1 tsp	8	0	<10	2	—
Orange Marmalade (S&W)	1 tsp	4	0	0	1	—
Raspberry Spread (Weight Watchers)	1 tsp	8	0	0	2	—
Red Raspberry Jam (S&W)	1 tsp	4	0	0	1	—
Red Tart Cherry Preserves (S&W)	1 tsp	4	0	0	1	—
Strawberry Preserves (Kraft)	1 tsp	6	0	5	2	—
Strawberry Spread (Weight Watchers)	1 tsp	8	0	0	2	—
Strawberry Jam (S&W)	1 tsp	4	0	0	1	—
REGULAR						
All Flavors Jelly (Kraft)	1 tsp	17	0	0	4	—
All Flavors Preserves (Kraft)	1 tsp	17	0	0	4	—
All Flavors Jam (Kraft)	1 tsp	17	0	0	4	—
Apple Butter (BAMA)	2 tsp	25	0	5	6	—

FOOD	PORTION	CAL	FAT	SOD	CARB	FIB
Apple Butter (White House)	1 oz	50	0	5	12	1
Apple Butter Autumn Harvest (Smucker's)	1 tsp	12	0	0	3	—
Apple Butter Natural (Smucker's)	1 tsp	12	0	0	3	—
Apple Cider Butter (Smucker's)	1 tsp	12	0	0	3	—
Apple Jelly (BAMA)	2 tsp	30	0	5	8	—
Blueberry Jam (Whistling Wings)	1 oz	50	tr	2	12	tr
Grape Jelly (BAMA)	2 tsp	30	0	5	8	—
Jam All Flavors (Smucker's)	1 tsp	18	0	0	4	—
Jelly All Flavors (Home Brands)	2 tsp	35	0	—	—	—
Jelly All Flavors (Smucker's)	1 tsp	18	0	tr	4	—
Jelly Single Serving All Flavors (Smucker's)	0.5 oz	38	0	<10	9	—
Orange Marmalade (Smucker's)	1 tsp	18	0	0	4	—
Peach Butter (Smucker's)	1 tsp	15	0	0	4	—
Peach Preserves (BAMA)	2 tbsp	30	0	5	8	—
Preserves All Flavors (Home Brands)	2 tsp	35	0	—	—	—
Preserves All Flavors (Smucker's)	1 tsp	18	0	0	4	—
Preserves Single Serving All Flavors (Smucker's)	0.5 oz	38	0	<10	9	—
Pumpkin Butter Autumn Harvest (Smucker's)	1 tsp	12	0	14	3	—
Raspberry Jam (Whistling Wings)	1 oz	60	tr	1	14	1
Red Plum Jam (BAMA)	2 tsp	30	0	5	8	—
Strawberry Preserves (BAMA)	2 tsp	30	0	5	8	—
apply jelly	3.5 oz	259	0	15	65	—
apricot jam	3.5 oz	250	0	—	62	—
blackberry jam	3.5 oz	237	0	—	59	—

FOOD	PORTION	CAL	FAT	SOD	CARB	FIB
cherry jam	3.5 oz	250	0	—	62	—
orange jam	3.5 oz	243	0	11	60	—
plum jam	3.5 oz	241	0	—	60	—
quince jam	3.5 oz	236	0	—	59	—
raspberry jam	3.5 oz	248	0	—	61	—
raspberry jelly	3.5 oz	259	0	—	65	—
red currant jelly	3.5 oz	265	0	4	66	—
red currant jam	3.5 oz	237	0	—	59	—
rose hip jam	3.5 oz	250	0	5	62	—
strawberry jam	3.5 oz	234	0	—	58	—

JAPANESE FOOD
see ORIENTAL FOOD

JAVA PLUM
fresh	1 cup	82	tr	18	21	—
fresh	3	5	tr	1	1	—

JELLY
see JAM/JELLY/PRESERVES

JERUSALEM ARTICHOKE
see ARTICHOKE

JEW'S EAR
pepeao, dried	½ cup	36	tr	8	10	—
pepeao, raw, sliced	1 cup	25	tr	9	7	—

JUJUBE
fresh	3.5 oz	105	tr	3	24	—

KALE
FRESH
Dole chopped	½ cup	17	1	15	3	—
chopped, cooked	½ cup	21	tr	15	4	—
raw, chopped	½ cup	21	tr	15	3	—
scotch chopped, cooked	½ cup	18	tr	29	4	—

FROZEN
chopped, cooked	½ cup	20	tr	10	4	—

KEFIR
kefir	3.5 oz	66	4	46	5	—

KIDNEY
beef, simmered	3 oz	122	3	114	0	—
lamb, braised	3 oz	117	3	128	1	—
pork, braised	3 oz	128	4	—	—	—

FOOD	PORTION	CAL	FAT	SOD	CARB	FIB
veal, braised	3 oz	139	5	93	0	—

KIDNEY BEANS
CANNED

FOOD	PORTION	CAL	FAT	SOD	CARB	FIB
B&M Red Baked Beans	8 oz	250	7	640	42	11
Friends Red Baked	8 oz	340	4	1060	57	—
Goya Spanish Style	7.5 oz	140	1	760	29	10
Green Giant Dark Red	½ cup	90	0	250	20	5
Green Giant Light Red	½ cup	90	0	250	20	5
Hanover Dark Red	½ cup	110	0	—	—	—
Hanover Light Red In Sauce	½ cup	120	0	—	—	—
Hunt's Red	4 oz	100	tr	400	20	5
Luck's Seasoned w/ Pork	7.5 oz	220	6	—	—	—
Progresso Red	½ cup	100	tr	210	21	7
S&W Dark Red Lite 50% Less Salt	½ cup	120	0	355	22	—
S&W Dark Red Premium	½ cup	120	1	—	22	—
S&W Water Pack	½ cup	90	0	0	16	—
Trappey's Dark Red	½ cup	90	0	—	—	—
Trappey's Jalapeno Light Red	½ cup	90	0	—	—	—
Trappey's Light Red	½ cup	90	0	—	—	—
Trappey's New Orleans Style	½ cup	100	2	410	16	—
Trappey's Red w/Chili Gravy	½ cup	100	1	—	—	—
Van Camp's Dark Red	1 cup	182	1	830	35	—
Van Camp's Light Red	1 cup	184	1	650	36	—
Van Camp's New Orleans Style Red	1 cup	178	1	940	34	—
kidney beans	1 cup	208	1	889	38	—
red	1 cup	216	1	873	40	—

DRIED

FOOD	PORTION	CAL	FAT	SOD	CARB	FIB
Arrowhead Red	¼ cup (1.6 oz)	160	1	0	29	10
Hurst Brand	1 cup	254	1	—	—	—
California red, cooked	1 cup	219	tr	7	40	—
cooked	1 cup	225	1	4	40	—
red, cooked	1 cup	225	1	4	40	—
royal red, cooked	1 cup	218	tr	8	39	—

SPROUTS

FOOD	PORTION	CAL	FAT	SOD	CARB	FIB
cooked	1 lb	152	3	—	21	—
raw	½ cup	27	tr	—	4	—

FOOD	PORTION	CAL	FAT	SOD	CARB	FIB
KIWIS						
California Kiwifruit Commission	2 (4.9 oz)	90	1	0	18	4
Dole	2	90	1	0	18	4
fresh	1 med	46	tr	4	11	3
KOHLRABI						
FRESH						
raw, sliced	½ cup	19	tr	14	4	—
sliced, cooked	½ cup	24	tr	17	5	—
KUMQUATS						
fresh	1	12	tr	1	3	—
LAMB						
see also LAMB DISHES						
FRESH						
cubed lean only, braised	3 oz	190	7	60	0	—
cubed lean only, broiled	3 oz	158	6	65	0	—
ground, broiled	3 oz	240	17	69	0	—
leg lean & fat Choice, roasted	3 oz	219	14	56	14	—
loin chop w/bone lean & fat Choice, broiled	1 chop (2.3 oz)	201	15	49	0	—
loin chop w/bone lean only Choice, broiled	1 chop (1.6 oz)	100	5	39	0	—
rib chop lean & fat Choice, broiled	3 oz	307	25	64	0	—
rib chop lean only Choice, broiled	3 oz	200	11	73	0	—
shank lean & fat Choice, braised	3 oz	206	11	61	0	—
shank lean & fat Choice, roasted	3 oz	191	11	55	0	—
shoulder chop w/bone lean only Choice, braised	1 chop (1.9 oz)	152	8	41	0	—
shoulder chop w/bone lean & fat Choice, braised	1 chop (2.5 oz)	244	17	51	0	—
sirloin lean & fat Choice, roasted	3 oz	248	21	58	0	—

FOOD	PORTION	CAL	FAT	SOD	CARB	FIB
FROZEN						
New Zealand, lean & fat, cooked	3 oz	259	19	39	0	—
New Zealand lean only, cooked	3 oz	175	8	43	0	—
LAMB DISHES						
TAKE-OUT						
curry	¾ cup	345	17	258	22	—
moussaka	5.6 oz	312	21	—	16	1
stew	¾ cup	124	5	140	11	2
LAMB'S QUARTERS						
FRESH						
chopped, cooked	½ cup	29	1	—	5	—
LECITHIN						
see SOY						
LEEKS						
DRIED						
freeze dried	1 tbsp	1	0	0	r	—
FRESH						
chopped, cooked	¼ cup	8	tr	3	2	—
cooked	1 (4.4 oz)	38	tr	13	9	—
raw	1 (4.4 oz)	76	tr	25	18	—
raw, chopped	¼ cup	16	tr	5	4	—
LEMON						
Dole	1	18	0	10	4	0
lemon	1 med	22	tr	3	12	—
peel	1 tbsp	0	tr	0	1	—
wedge	1	5	tr	1	3	—
JUICE						
ReaLemon	1 fl oz	6	0	5	2	—
Seneca	1 tbsp	6	0	—	—	—
bottled	1 tbsp	3	tr	3	1	—
fresh	1 tbsp	4	0	0	1	—
frozen	1 tbsp	3	tr	0	1	—
LEMON CURD						
lemon curd made w/ egg	2 tsp	29	1	—	4	0
lemon curd made w/ starch	2 tsp	28	—	—	6	0

FOOD	PORTION	CAL	FAT	SOD	CARB	FIB

LEMON EXTRACT
Virginia Dare	1 tsp	22	0	—	—	—

LEMONADE
FROZEN
Bright & Early	8 fl oz	120	0	5	30	—
Minute Maid	8 fl oz	110	0	0	29	—
Country Style	8 fl oz	120	0	0	30	—
Cranberry Lemonade	8 fl oz	80	0	0	30	—
Pink	8 fl oz	120	0	0	30	—
Raspberry	8 fl oz	120	0	0	30	—
as prep w/water	1 cup	100	tr	8	26	—
lemonade, not prep	1 can (6 oz)	397	tr	8	103	—

MIX
4C Instant, as prep	8 fl oz	80	0	0	20	—
Country Time	8 fl oz	82	0	21	21	—
Country Time Pink	8 fl oz	82	0	21	21	—
Country Time Pink Sugar Free	8 fl oz	4	0	—	0	—
Country Time Sugar Free	8 fl oz	4	0	—	0	—
Crystal Light	8 fl oz	5	0	—	0	—
Kool-Aid	8 fl oz	99	0	8	25	—
Pink	8 fl oz	99	0	8	25	—
Sugar Free	8 fl oz	4	0	—	0	—
Sugar Sweetened Pink	8 fl oz	82	0	—	21	—
Wylers Drink Mix Unsweetened Wyler's	8 oz	3	0	19	1	—
powder, as prep w/ water	9 fl oz	113	tr	19	29	—
powder w/NutraSweet	1 pitcher (67 oz)	40	0	58	10	—

READY-TO-DRINK
Crystal Geyser Juice Squeeze Pink	1 bottle (12 fl oz)	140	0	20	34	—
Diet Rite Salt/Sodium Free	8 fl oz	2	0	0	1	—
Fruitopia	8 fl oz	120	0	25	29	—
Kool-Aid Koolers Lemonade	1 pkg (8.45 fl oz)	120	0	3	32	—
Minute Maid Chilled	8 fl oz	110	0	25	28	—

FOOD	PORTION	CAL	FAT	SOD	CARB	FIB
Cranberry Chilled	8 fl oz	120	0	25	31	—
Juices To Go	1 bottle (16 fl oz)	110	0	25	28	—
Juices To Go	1 can (11.5 fl oz)	160	0	40	40	—
Juices to Go Cranberry Lemonade	1 bottle (16 fl oz)	110	0	25	29	—
Juices To Go Raspberry Lemonade	1 bottle (16 fl oz)	120	0	25	29	—
Pink Chilled	8 fl oz	110	0	25	28	—
Raspberry Chilled	8 fl oz	120	0	0	30	—
Nehi Royal Crown	8 fl oz	130	0	35	35	—
Newman's Own Roadside Virginia	8 fl oz	100	tr	0	22	—
Ocean Spray	8 fl oz	110	0	35	29	0
Ocean Spray With Cranberry Juice	8 fl oz	110	0	35	26	0
Ocean Spray With Raspberry Juice	8 fl oz	110	0	35	27	0
Royal Mistic Lemonade Limeade	16 fl oz	230	0	19	57	—
Royal Mistic Tropical Pink	16 fl oz	230	0	11	57	—
Shasta	12 fl oz	146	0	—	—	—
Sipps Lemonade	8.45 fl oz	85	0	—	—	—
Veryfine	8 fl oz	120	0	<25	30	—
Wylers	1 can (6 fl oz)	64	0	33	17	—

LENTILS

CANNED

Health Valley Fast Menu Hearty Lentils Garden Vegetables	7.5 oz	150	4	200	16	16
Health Valley Fast Menu Organic Lentils With Tofu Wieners	7.5 oz	170	5	260	15	15

DRIED

Hurst Brand cooked	1 cup	258	tr	—	—	—
cooked	1 cup	231	1	4	40	—

FROZEN

Natural Touch Lentil Rice Loaf	2.5 in slice (113 g)	200	11	420	18	—

FOOD	PORTION	CAL	FAT	SOD	CARB	FIB
SPROUTS						
raw	½ cup	40	tr	4	8	—
LETTUCE						
Dole Butter Lettuce	1 head	21	tr	8	4	2
Dole Iceberg	⅙ med head	20	0	10	4	1
Dole Leaf, shredded	1½ cup	12	0	40	1	1
Dole Romaine, shredded	1½ cups	18	1	40	2	1
bibb	1 head (6 oz)	21	tr	8	4	2
boston	1 head (6 oz)	21	tr	8	4	2
boston	2 leaves	2	tr	1	tr	tr
iceberg	1 head (19 oz)	70	1	48	11	5
iceberg	1 leaf	3	tr	2	tr	tr
looseleaf, shredded	½ cup	5	tr	3	1	—
romaine shredded	½ cup	4	tr	2	1	tr
LIMA BEANS						
CANNED						
Dennison's w/Ham	7.5 oz	250	7	—	—	—
Libby	½ cup	80	0	—	—	—
Luck's Small Seasoned w/Pork	7.5 oz	220	7	—	—	—
Luck's Giant Seasoned w/Pork	7.5 oz	230	7	—	—	—
S&W Small Fancy	½ cup	80	0	390	16	—
Seneca	½ cup	80	0	—	—	—
Trappey's Baby Green	½ cup	90	1	410	16	—
Trappey's Baby White	½ cup	90	1	410	17	—
large	1 cup	191	tr	809	36	—
lima beans	½ cup	93	tr	309	17	—
DRIED						
Hurst Brand Baby	1 cup	262	1	—	—	—
baby, cooked	1 cup	229	1	5	42	17
cooked	½ cup	104	tr	14	20	—
large, cooked	1 cup	217	1	4	39	14
FROZEN						
Birds Eye Baby	½ cup	130	0	115	24	—
Birds Eye Fordhook	½ cup	100	0	10	19	—
Green Giant Harvest Fresh	½ cup	80	0	170	18	4
Green Giant In Butter Sauce	½ cup	100	3	390	17	5
Hanover Baby	½ cup	110	0	—	—	—
Hanover Fordhook	½ cup	100	0	—	—	—

FOOD	PORTION	CAL	FAT	SOD	CARB	FIB
cooked	½ cup	94	tr	26	18	—
fordhook, cooked	½ cup	85	tr	45	16	—

LIME
FRESH
| lime | 1 | 20 | tr | 1 | 7 | — |

JUICE
ReaLime	1 oz	6	0	10	2	—
bottled	1 tbsp	3	tr	2	1	—
fresh	1 tbsp	4	tr	0	1	—

LING
FRESH
baked	3 oz	95	1	147	0	—
blue, raw	3.5 oz	83	1	—	0	—
fillet, baked	5.3 oz	168	1	261	0	—

LING COD
| baked | 3 oz | 93 | 1 | 64 | 0 | — |
| fillet, baked | 5.3 oz | 164 | 2 | 114 | 0 | — |

LIQUOR/LIQUEUR
see also BEER AND ALE, CHAMPAGNE, DRINK MIXERS, MALT, WINE, WINE COOLERS

anisette	0.66 oz	74	0	—	7	0
apricot brandy	0.66 oz	64	0	—	6	0
benedictine	0.66 oz	69	0	—	7	0
bloody mary	5 oz	116	tr	332	5	—
bourbon & soda	4 oz	105	0	16	0	—
coffee liqueur	1.5 oz	174	tr	4	24	—
coffee w/cream liqueur	1.5 oz	154	7	43	10	—
creme de menthe	1.5 oz	186	tr	3	21	—
curacao liqueur	0.66 oz	54	0	—	6	0
daiquiri	2 oz	111	0	1	4	—
gin	1.5 oz	110	0	1	0	—
gin & tonic	7.5 oz	171	0	10	16	—
gin rickey	4 oz	150	0	—	—	—
manhattan	2 oz	128	0	2	2	—
martini	2.5 oz	156	0	2	tr	—
mint julep	10 oz	210	0	—	3	0
old-fashioned	2.5 oz	127	0	—	3	0
pina colada	4.5 oz	262	3	9	40	—
planter's punch	3.5 oz	175	0	—	—	—
rum	1.5 oz	97	0	0	0	—
screwdriver	7 oz	174	tr	2	18	—
sloe gin fizz	2.5 oz	132	0	1	4	0

FOOD	PORTION	CAL	FAT	SOD	CARB	FIB
tequila sunrise	5.5 oz	189	tr	7	15	—
tom collins	7.5 oz	121	0	39	3	—
vodka	1.5 oz	97	0	0	0	—
whiskey	1.5 oz	105	0	0	tr	—
whiskey sour	3 oz	123	tr	10	5	—
whiskey sour mix, as prep	3.6 oz	169	0	48	16	—
whiskey sour mix, not prep	1 pkg (0.6 oz)	64	0	46	16	—

LIVER
see also PATE

FOOD	PORTION	CAL	FAT	SOD	CARB	FIB
Beef, raw (Dakota Lean)	3 oz	100	1	—	8	—
beef, braised	3 oz	137	4	59	3	—
beef, pan-fried	3 oz	184	7	90	7	—
chicken, stewed	1 cup (5 oz)	219	8	71	1	—
duck, raw	1 (1.5 oz)	60	2	—	2	—
goose, raw	1 (3.3 oz)	125	4	132	6	—
lamb, braised	3 oz	187	7	48	2	—
lamb, fried	3 oz	202	11	105	3	—
pork, braised	3 oz	141	4	42	3	—
sheep, raw	3.5 oz	131	4	95	0	—
turkey, simmered	1 cup (5 oz)	237	8	89	5	—
veal, braised	3 oz	140	6	45	2	—
veal, fried	3 oz	208	10	112	3	—

LOBSTER
CANNED

FOOD	PORTION	CAL	FAT	SOD	CARB	FIB
Progresso Rock Lobster Sauce	½ cup	120	8	430	11	2
FRESH						
northern, cooked	1 cup	142	1	551	2	—
northern, cooked	3 oz	83	1	323	1	—
northern, raw	1 lobster (5.3 oz)	136	1	—	1	—
northern, raw	3 oz	77	1	—	tr	—
spiny, steamed	1 (5.7 oz)	233	3	370	5	—
spiny, steamed	3 oz	122	2	193	3	—
FROZEN						
Crawfish Etouffee Cajun Cookin'	12 oz	390	10	1110	51	—
Gulfstream Tails King & Prince	6 oz	170	1	—	—	—

FOOD	PORTION	CAL	FAT	SOD	CARB	FIB
TAKE-OUT						
newburg	1 cup	485	27	127	13	—
LOGANBERRIES						
frozen	1 cup	80	tr	1	19	—
LONGANS						
fresh	1	2	0	0	tr	—
LOQUATS						
fresh	1	5	tr	0	1	—
LOTUS						
root, raw, sliced	10 slices	45	tr	33	14	—
root, sliced, cooked	10 slices	59	tr	40	14	—
seeds, dried	1 oz	94	1	1	18	—
LOX						
see SALMON						

LUNCHEON MEATS/COLD CUTS
see also CHICKEN, HAM, MEAT SUBSTITUTES, TURKEY

FOOD	PORTION	CAL	FAT	SOD	CARB	FIB
Armour Beef Bologna Lower Salt	1 oz	90	8	—	—	—
Armour Bologna Lower Salt	1 oz	90	8	—	—	—
Armour Salami Lower Salt	1 oz	80	7	—	—	—
Carl Buddig Beef	1 oz	40	2	430	1	0
Carl Buddig Corned Beef	1 oz	40	2	380	1	0
Carl Buddig Pastrami	1 oz	40	2	320	1	0
Hansel 'n Gretel						
Healthy Deli Bologna Beef & Pork	1 oz	41	2	200	1	—
Healthy Deli Cooked Corn Beef	1 oz	35	1	210	1	—
Healthy Deli Italian Roast Beef	1 oz	31	1	140	tr	—
Healthy Deli Pastrami Round	1 oz	34	1	195	1	—
Healthy Deli Regular Roast Beef	1 oz	30	tr	130	tr	—
Healthy Deli St. Paddy's Corned Beef	1 oz	24	tr	290	1	—
Healthy Choice Bologna	1 oz	30	1	280	2	—

FOOD	PORTION	CAL	FAT	SOD	CARB	FIB
Hebrew National						
Bologna Beef	2 oz	180	16	440	—	—
Bologna Beef Reduced Fat	2 oz	130	12	320	—	—
Bologna Lean Chub	2 oz	90	6	430	—	—
Bologna Midget	2 oz	180	16	440	—	—
Deli Express Corned Beef	2 oz	80	3	450	—	—
Deli Express Tongue Sliced	2 oz	120	9	330	—	—
Deli Pastrami	2 oz	80	8	510	—	—
Salami Beef	2 oz	170	14	420	—	—
Salami Beef Reduced Fat	2 oz	110	8	380	—	—
Salami Lean Chub	2 oz	90	6	340	—	—
Salami Midget	2 oz	170	14	420	—	—
Hillshire						
Bologna Large	1 oz	90	8	260	tr	—
Bologna Ring	1 oz	90	8	230	tr	—
Braunschweiger	1 oz	95	8	270	2	—
Deli Select Bologna Light	1 slice	12	1	85	tr	—
Deli Select Corned Beef	1 slice	10	tr	100	tr	—
Deli Select Oven Roasted Cured Beef	1 slice	10	tr	95	tr	—
Deli Select Pastrami	1 slice	10	tr	100	tr	—
Deli Select Roast Beef	1 slice	10	tr	135	tr	—
Deli Select Smoked Beef	1 slice	10	tr	100	tr	—
Flavor Pack 90-99% Fat Free Pastrami	1 slice (0.6 oz)	18	tr	180	tr	—
Lunch 'N Munch Bologna/American/ Snickers	1 pkg (4.25 oz)	490	34	1110	31	—
Lunch 'N Munch Bologna/American/ Snickers/Hi-C	1 pkg (4.25 oz + 6 fl oz)	590	34	1130	55	—
Lunch 'N Munch Bologna/American	1 pkg (4.5 oz)	480	37	1390	20	—
Lunch 'N Munch Cooked Ham/Swiss/ Snickers/Hi-C	1 pkg (4.25 oz + 6 fl oz)	470	21	1180	54	—

FOOD	PORTION	CAL	FAT	SOD	CARB	FIB
Lunch 'N Munch Cooked Ham/Swiss/ Oreo	1 pkg (4.125 oz)	370	21	1160	30	—
Lunch 'N Munch Cooked Ham/Swiss	1 pkg (4.5 oz)	360	22	1380	19	—
Lunch 'N Munch Cotto Salami/ Monterey Jack	1 pkg (4.5 oz)	440	32	1270	21	—
Lunch 'N Munch Honey Ham/ Cheddar/Snickers/ Hi-C	1 pkg (4.25 oz + 6 fl oz)	500	23	1030	56	—
Lunch 'N Munch Pepperoni/American	1 pkg (4.5 oz)	570	46	1670	20	—
Lunch 'N Munch Smoked Chicken/ Monterey Jack	1 pkg (4.5 oz)	350	20	1260	19	—
Lunch 'N Munch Smoked Chicken/ Monterey/Snickers	1 pkg (4.25 oz)	400	23	1080	31	—
Lunch 'N Munch Smoked Turkey/ Cheddar	1 pkg (4.5 oz)	350	21	1130	20	—
Lunch 'N Munch Smoked Turkey/ Cheddar/Brownie	1 pkg (4.5 oz)	400	22	1240	34	—
Lunch 'N Munch Turkey/Cheddar/ Brownie/Hi-C	1 pkg (4.5 oz + 6 fl oz)	500	22	1260	58	—
Pepperoni	1 oz	110	10	450	0	—
Salame Hard	1 oz	90	7	470	1	—
Salami Hard	1 oz	100	9	450	0	—
Summer Sausage	2 oz	180	16	670	1	—
Summer Sausage Beef	2 oz	190	17	612	1	—
Summer Sausage Light	2 oz	150	12	630	1	—
Summer Sausage w/ Cheddar Cheese	2 oz	200	18	605	1	—
Jones Liver Sausage	1 slice	80	7	180	tr	—
Jones Liver Sausage Chub	1 slice	80	7	230	tr	—
Oscar Mayer						
Bar-B-Q Loaf	1 slice (1 oz)	46	2	333	2	—

FOOD	PORTION	CAL	FAT	SOD	CARB	FIB
Oscar Mayer *(cont.)*						
Bologna	1 slice (1 oz)	90	8	311	1	—
Bologna Beef	1 slice (1 oz)	90	8	304	1	—
Bologna Beef Lebanon	1 slice	46	3	302	tr	—
Bologna Beef Light	1 slice (1 oz)	64	5	316	1	—
Bologna Garlic Beef	1 slice (1 oz)	90	8	301	1	—
Bologna Light	1 slice (1 oz)	64	5	310	1	—
Bologna With Cheese	1 slice	74	7	232	1	—
Braunschweiger German Brand	1 oz	96	9	329	1	—
Braunschweiger Sliced	1 slice (1 oz)	96	9	327	1	—
Braunschweiger Tube	1 oz	97	9	301	1	—
Corned Beef	1 slice (0.5 oz)	17	tr	204	tr	—
Cotto Salami	1 slice	45	3	296	tr	—
Genoa Salami	1 slice	34	3	162	tr	—
Hard Salami	1 slice	33	3	169	tr	—
Head Cheese	1 slice (1 oz)	54	4	347	tr	—
Honey Loaf	1 slice (1 oz)	34	1	378	1	—
Liver Cheese	1 slice	116	10	418	1	—
Lunchables Bologna/ American	1 pkg (4.5 oz)	480	38	1520	20	—
Lunchables Chicken/ Monterey Jack	1 pkg (4.5 oz)	360	22	1580	17	—
Lunchables Chicken/ Roast Beef	1 pkg (5.1 oz)	400	23	1560	23	—
Lunchables Chicken/ Turkey	1 pkg (5.1 oz)	380	22	1730	24	—
Lunchables Chocolate Pudding/ Honey Ham/ American	1 pkg (6.2 oz)	430	23	1360	30	—
Lunchables Chocolate Fudge Pudding/Chicken/ Monterey Jack	1 pkg (6.2 oz)	380	22	1030	35	—
Lunchables Cookies/ Ham/Swiss	1 pkg (4.2 oz)	380	23	1370	29	—
Lunchables Ham/ Cheddar	1 pkg (4.5 oz)	370	25	1680	18	—
Lunchables Ham/ Roast Beef	1 pkg (5.1 oz)	410	25	1730	24	—

FOOD	PORTION	CAL	FAT	SOD	CARB	FIB
Lunchables Ham/ Swiss	1 pkg (4.5 oz)	340	21	1660	18	—
Lunchables Honey Ham/Chicken	1 pkg (5.1 oz)	380	22	1650	24	—
Lunchables Salami/ Mozzarella	1 pkg (4.5 oz)	410	29	1250	19	—
Lunchables Trail Mix/Honey Turkey/ Cheddar	1 pkg (5 oz)	460	27	1190	44	—
Lunchables Turkey/ Cheddar	1 pkg (4.5 oz)	360	22	1600	19	—
Lunchables Turkey/ Ham	1 pkg (5.1 oz)	370	20	1760	23	—
Lunchables Turkey/ Monterey Jack	1 pkg (4.5 oz)	360	22	1600	18	—
Luncheon Meat	1 slice (1 oz)	94	9	323	1	—
New England Brand Sausage	1 slice	29	1	291	tr	—
Old Fashioned Loaf	1 slice (1 oz)	62	4	337	2	—
Olive Loaf	1 slice (1 oz)	63	4	392	3	—
Pastrami	1 slice (0.5 oz)	16	tr	217	tr	—
Peppered Loaf	1 slice (1 oz)	39	2	367	1	—
Pickle And Pimiento Loaf	1 slice (1 oz)	66	4	370	4	—
Picnic Loaf	1 slice (1 oz)	61	4	337	1	—
Salami For Beer	1 slice	50	4	286	tr	—
Salami For Beer Beef	1 slice	63	6	280	tr	—
Sandwich Spread	1 oz	67	5	273	4	—
Smoked Beef	1 slice (0.5 oz)	14	tr	173	tr	—
Summer Sausage	1 slice	69	6	331	tr	—
Summer Sausage Beef	1 slice	70	6	325	tr	—
Russer Lil' Salt						
Bologna	1 oz	70	5	200	1	—
Bologna Beef	1 oz	80	5	200	1	—
Braunschweiger	1 oz	70	5	200	2	—
Cooked Salami	1 oz	60	4	200	1	—
Old Fashioned Loaf	1 oz	60	4	200	2	—
P&P Loaf	1 oz	60	4	200	3	—
Shofar Salami Beef	2 oz	160	15	410	0	0
Underwood Liverwurst	2.08 oz	180	15	470	4	—
Weight Watchers Bologna	2 slices (¾ oz)	35	2	220	1	—

FOOD	PORTION	CAL	FAT	SOD	CARB	FIB
barbecue loaf, pork & beef	1 oz	49	3	378	2	—
beerwurst, beef	1 slice (2¾ in x ¹⁄₁₆ in)	20	2	62	tr	—
beerwurst, beef	1 slice (4 in x ⅛ in)	75	7	214	tr	—
beerwurst, pork	1 slice (2¾ in x ¹⁄₁₆ in)	14	1	74	tr	—
beerwurst, pork	1 slice (4 in x ⅛ in)	55	4	285	tr	—
berliner, pork & beef	1 oz	65	4	368	1	—
blood sausage	1 oz	95	9	—	tr	—
bologna, beef	1 oz	88	8	278	tr	—
bologna, beef & pork	1 oz	89	8	289	1	—
bologna, pork	1 oz	70	6	336	tr	—
braunschweiger, pork	1 oz	102	9	324	1	—
braunschweiger, pork	1 slice (2½ in x ¼ in)	65	6	206	1	—
corned beef loaf	1 oz	43	2	270	0	—
dried beef	1 oz	47	1	—	tr	—
dried beef	5 slices (21 g)	35	tr	—	tr	—
dutch brand loaf, pork & beef	1 oz	68	5	354	2	—
headcheese, pork	1 oz	60	5	356	tr	—
honey loaf, pork & beef	1 oz	36	1	374	2	—
honey roll, sausage, beef	1 oz	42	2	304	1	—
lebanon bologna, beef	1 oz	60	4	379	1	—
liver cheese, pork	1 oz	86	7	347	1	—
liverwurst, pork	1 oz	92	8	—	1	—
luncheon meat, beef	1 oz	87	7	377	1	—
luncheon meat, pork & beef	1 oz	100	9	367	1	—
luncheon meat, pork, canned	1 oz	95	9	365	1	—
luncheon sausage, pork & beef	1 oz	74	6	335	tr	—
luxury loaf, pork	1 oz	40	1	347	1	—
mortadella, beef & pork	1 oz	88	7	353	1	—
mother's loaf, pork	1 oz	80	6	320	2	—
new england sausage, pork & beef	1 oz	46	2	346	1	—

FOOD	PORTION	CAL	FAT	SOD	CARB	FIB
olive loaf, pork	1 oz	67	5	421	3	—
peppered loaf, pork & beef	1 oz	42	2	432	1	—
pepperoni, pork & beef	1 slice (0.2 oz)	27	2	112	tr	—
pepperoni, pork & beef	1 (9 oz)	1248	110	5120	7	—
pickle & pimiento loaf, pork	1 oz	74	6	394	2	—
picnic loaf, pork & beef	1 oz	66	5	330	1	—
salami, cooked, beef & pork	1 oz	71	6	302	1	—
salami, hard, pork	1 pkg (4 oz)	460	38	2554	2	—
salami, hard, pork	1 slice (0.33 oz)	41	4	226	3	—
salami, hard, pork & beef	1 pkg (4 oz)	472	39	2101	3	—
salami, hard, pork & beef	1 slice (0.33 oz)	42	3	186	tr	—
sandwich spread, pork & beef	1 oz	67	5	287	3	—
sandwich spread, pork & beef	1 tbsp	35	3	152	2	—
summer sausage, thuringer, cervelat	1 oz	98	8	412	1	—
TAKE-OUT						
submarine w/salami, ham, cheese, lettuce, tomato, onion & oil	1	456	19	1650	51	—

LUPINES
DRIED

cooked	1 cup	197	5	7	16	—

LYCHEES

fresh	1	6	tr	0	2	—

MACADAMIA NUTS

Candy Glazed (Mauna Loa)	1 oz	170	14	80	11	—
Chocolate Covered (Mauna Loa)	1 oz	170	13	21	12	—
Honey Roasted (Mauna Loa)	1 oz	200	17	80	8	—
Macadamia Nut Brittle (Mauna Loa)	1 oz	150	8	140	19	—

FOOD	PORTION	CAL	FAT	SOD	CARB	FIB
Roasted & Salted (Mauna Loa)	1 oz	210	21	75	4	—
dried	1 oz	199	21	1	4	—
oil roasted	1 oz	204	22	3	4	—

MACARONI
see PASTA

MACE
ground	1 tsp	8	1	1	1	—

MACKEREL
CANNED

FOOD	PORTION	CAL	FAT	SOD	CARB	FIB
Jack Empress	4 oz	140	8	480	0	—
jack	1 can (12.7 oz)	563	23	1368	0	—
jack	1 cup	296	12	720	0	—
FRESH						
atlantic, cooked	3 oz	223	15	71	0	—
atlantic, raw	3 oz	174	12	76	0	—
jack, baked	3 oz	171	9	94	0	—
jack fillet, baked	6.2 oz	354	18	194	0	—
king, baked	3 oz	114	2	172	0	—
king fillet, baked	5.4 oz	207	4	312	0	—
pacific, baked	3 oz	171	9	94	0	—
pacific fillet, baked	6.2 oz	354	18	194	0	—
spanish, cooked	1 fillet (5.1 oz)	230	9	96	0	—
spanish, cooked	3 oz	134	5	56	0	—
spanish, raw	3 oz	118	5	50	0	—

MALT
Bartles & Jaymes

FOOD	PORTION	CAL	FAT	SOD	CARB	FIB
Malt Cooler Berry	12 fl oz	210	0	5	32	—
Malt Cooler Berry Light	12 fl oz	140	0	0	29	—
Malt Cooler Black Cherry	12 fl oz	190	0	5	30	—
Malt Cooler Mandarin Lemon	12 fl oz	210	0	5	34	—
Malt Cooler Margarita	12 fl oz	250	0	40	44	—
Malt Cooler Original	12 fl oz	180	0	0	27	—
Malt Cooler Peach	12 fl oz	200	0	5	31	—
Malt Cooler Pina Colada	12 fl oz	270	0	5	48	—
Malt Cooler Planter's Punch	12 fl oz	220	0	5	35	—

FOOD	PORTION	CAL	FAT	SOD	CARB	FIB
Malt Cooler Red Sangria	12 fl oz	190	0	5	29	—
Malt Cooler Strawberry	12 fl oz	200	0	5	31	—
Malt Cooler Strawberry Daiquiri	12 fl oz	220	0	5	35	—
Malt Cooler Tropical	12 fl oz	220	0	5	36	—
Olde English	12 oz	163	0	—	10	—
Schaefer	12 oz	165	0	20	12	—
Schlitz	12 oz	177	0	21	15	—
nonalcoholic	12 fl oz	32	0	—	5	—

MALTED MILK

FOOD	PORTION	CAL	FAT	SOD	CARB	FIB
Carnation Chocolate	3 heaping tsp (21 g)	79	tr	—	—	—
Carnation Original	3 heaping tsp (21 g)	90	2	—	—	—
Kraft Instant Chocolate	3 tsp	90	1	45	18	—
Kraft Instant Natural	3 tsp	90	2	100	16	—
chocolate, as prep w/ milk	1 cup	229	9	172	30	—
chocolate flavor powder	3 heaping tsp (0.75 oz)	79	1	53	18	—
natural flavor, as prep w/milk	1 cup	237	10	223	27	—
natural flavor powder	1 heaping tsp (0.75 oz)	87	2	103	19	—

MAMMY-APPLE

FOOD	PORTION	CAL	FAT	SOD	CARB	FIB
fresh	1	431	4	127	106	—

MANGO

FOOD	PORTION	CAL	FAT	SOD	CARB	FIB
fresh	1	135	1	4	35	—
JUICE						
Kern's Nectar	6 oz	110	0	10	27	—
Libby's Nectar	6 oz	110	0	0	26	—

MARGARINE

see also BUTTER BLENDS, BUTTER SUBSTITUTES

REDUCED CALORIE

FOOD	PORTION	CAL	FAT	SOD	CARB	FIB
Fleischmann's Diet	1 tbsp	50	6	50	0	—
Fleischmann's Extra Light Corn Oil Spread	1 tbsp	50	6	55	0	—
Mazola Diet	1 cup (235 g)	815	93	2160	1	—
Mazola Diet	1 tbsp (14 g)	50	6	130	0	—

FOOD	PORTION	CAL	FAT	SOD	CARB	FIB
Mazola Light Corn Oil Spread	1 cup (235 g)	835	94	1690	0	—
Mazola Light Corn Oil Spread	1 tbsp (14 g)	50	6	100	0	—
Parkay Diet Soft	1 tbsp	50	6	110	0	—
Smart Beat	1 tbsp	25	3	110	0	—
Smart Beat Unsalted	1 tbsp	25	3	0	0	—
Weight Watchers Extra Light Sweet Unsalted Tub	1 tbsp	50	6	0	0	—
Weight Watchers Extra Light Tub	1 tbsp	50	6	130	0	—
Weight Watchers Light Stick	1 tbsp	60	7	130	0	—
diet	1 cup	800	90	2226	1	—
diet	1 tsp	17	2	46	0	—
REGULAR						
Blue Bonnet	1 tbsp	100	11	95	0	—
Fleischmann's	1 tbsp	100	11	95	0	—
Fleischmann's Light Corn Oil Stick	1 tbsp	80	8	70	0	—
Fleischmann's Sweet Unsalted	1 tbsp	100	11	0	0	—
Hain Safflower	1 tbsp	100	11	170	0	—
Hain Safflower Unsalted	1 tbsp	100	11	<5	0	—
Hollywood Safflower	1 tbsp	100	11	130	0	—
Hollywood Safflower Unsalted Sweet	1 tbsp	100	11	2	0	—
Krona Lever	1 tbsp	100	11	—	—	—
Land O'Lakes Spread	1 tbsp (0.5 oz)	90	10	95	0	—
Land O'Lakes Spread With Sweet Cream	1 tbsp (0.5 oz)	90	10	95	0	—
Land O'Lakes Spread With Sweet Cream Unsalted	1 tbsp (0.5 oz)	90	10	0	0	—
Mazola	1 cup (229 g)	1650	184	1650	3	—
Mazola	1 tbsp (14 g)	100	11	100	0	—
Mazola Unsalted	1 cup (229 g)	1635	184	8	0	—
Mazola Unsalted	1 tbsp (14 g)	100	11	1	0	—
Mother's	1 tbsp	100	11	—	—	—
Mother's Unsalted	1 tbsp	100	11	—	—	—
Nucanola	1 tbsp	90	10	90	0	—
Nucanola	1 tbsp (14 g)	90	10	90	0	—
Parkay	1 tbsp	100	11	105	0	—

FOOD	PORTION	CAL	FAT	SOD	CARB	FIB
Promise	1 tbsp	90	10	—	—	—
corn	1 stick (4 oz)	815	91	1070	1	—
corn	1 tsp	34	4	44	0	—
salted	1 stick (4 oz)	815	91	1069	1	—
salted	1 tsp	39	4	44	0	—
unsalted	1 stick (4 oz)	809	91	2	1	—
unsalted	1 tsp	34	4	tr	0	—
SOFT						
Blue Bonnet	1 tbsp	100	11	95	0	—
Chiffon	1 tbsp	90	10	95	0	—
Chiffon Stick	1 tbsp	100	11	105	0	—
Chiffon Unsalted	1 tbsp	90	10	0	0	—
Fleischmann's	1 tbsp	100	11	95	0	—
Fleischmann's Light Corn Oil Spread	1 tbsp	80	8	70	0	—
Fleischmann's Sweet Unsalted	1 tbsp	100	11	0	0	—
Hain Safflower	1 tbsp	100	11	170	0	—
Hollywood Soft Spread	1 tbsp	90	10	135	1	0
I Can't Believe It's Not Butter! (Lever)	1 tbsp	90	10	—	—	—
Land O'Lakes Spread Tub	1 tbsp (0.5 oz)	80	8	90	0	—
Land O'Lakes Spread With Sweet Cream Tub	1 tbsp (0.5 oz)	80	8	70	0	—
Mother's Unsalted	1 tbsp	100	11	—	—	—
Mother's Salted	1 tbsp	100	11	—	—	—
Parkay Soft	1 tbsp	100	11	105	0	—
Parkay Spread	1 tbsp	60	7	110	0	—
corn	1 cup	1626	183	2449	1	—
corn	1 tsp	34	4	51	0	—
safflower	1 cup	1626	183	2449	1	—
safflower	1 tsp	34	4	51	0	—
soybean, salted	1 cup	1626	183	2449	1	—
soybean, salted	1 tsp	34	4	51	0	—
soybean, unsalted	1 cup	1626	182	63	2	—
soybean, unsalted	1 tsp	34	4	1	0	—
tub, salted	1 cup	1626	183	2449	1	—
tub, salted	1 tsp	34	4	51	0	—
tub, unsalted	1 cup	1626	182	63	0	—
tub, unsalted	1 tsp	34	4	1	0	—
SQUEEZE						
Parkay Squeeze	1 tbsp	90	10	110	0	—
soybean & cottonseed	1 tsp	34	4	37	0	—

FOOD	PORTION	CAL	FAT	SOD	CARB	FIB
WHIPPED						
Blue Bonnet Whipped Spread	1 tbsp	80	9	100	0	—
Chiffon	1 tbsp	70	8	80	0	—
Fleischmann's Lightly Salted	1 tbsp	70	7	60	0	—
Fleischmann's Unsalted	1 tbsp	70	7	0	0	—
Miracle Brand	1 tbsp	60	7	70	0	—
Miracle Brand Stick	1 tbsp	70	7	65	0	—
Parkay	1 tbsp	70	7	70	0	—
Parkay Stick	1 tbsp	70	7	65	0	—

MARJORAM

FOOD	PORTION	CAL	FAT	SOD	CARB	FIB
dried	1 tsp	2	tr	tr	tr	—

MARSHMALLOW

FOOD	PORTION	CAL	FAT	SOD	CARB	FIB
Campfire	2 lg	40	0	10	10	—
Campfire Miniature	24	40	0	10	10	—
Funmallows Kraft	1	30	0	15	7	—
Funmallows Miniature Kraft	10	18	0	5	5	—
Jet-Puffed Kraft	1	25	0	5	6	—
Marshmallow Fluff	1 heaping tap (18 g)	59	tr	12	14	—
Miniature Kraft	10	18	0	5	5	—
marshmallow	1 oz	90	0	25	23	—

MATZO

FOOD	PORTION	CAL	FAT	SOD	CARB	FIB
American Matzo (Manischewitz)	1	115	2	—	22	—
Daily Thin Tea (Manischewitz)	1	103	tr	1	22	tr
Dietetic Thins (Manischewitz)	1	91	tr	tr	19	tr
Egg Dark Chocolate Coated (Manischewitz)	½ matzo (1 oz)	97	3	7	17	1
Egg Milk Chocolate Coated (Horowitz Margareten)	1 oz	97	4	7	16	1
Egg n' Onion (Manischewitz)	1	112	tr	180	23	—
Lightly Salted (Streit's)	1 (1 oz)	110	1	65	23	1
Matzo Ball Mix 50% Less Salt (Goodman's)	2 tbsp (0.5 oz)	50	0	150	11	0

FOOD	PORTION	CAL	FAT	SOD	CARB	FIB
Matzo Ball Mix, as prep (Goodman's)	2 tbsp (0.5 oz)	60	0	190	12	1
Matzo Cracker Miniatures (Manischewitz)	10	90	tr	—	20	—
Matzo Farfel (Manischewitz)	1 cup	180	1	2	60	—
Matzo Meal (Manischewitz)	1 cup	514	1	3	109	tr
Matzoh Meal (Streit's)	¼ cup (1 oz)	110	1	0	24	1
Passover (Manischewitz)	1	129	tr	—	27	—
Passover (Streit's)	1 (1 oz)	110	1	0	25	1
Passover Egg (Manischewitz)	1	132	2	—	27	—
Passover Egg Matzo Crackers (Manischewitz)	10	108	2	—	20	—
Salted Thin (Manischewitz)	1	100	tr	—	21	tr
Unsalted (Manischewitz)	1	110	tr	1	24	tr
Unsalted (Streit's)	1 (0.9 oz)	100	1	0	22	1
Wheat Matzo Crackers (Manischewitz)	10	90	1	—	18	—
Whole Wheat (Streit's)	1 (1 oz)	110	1	0	24	4
Whole Wheat w/Bran (Manischewitz)	1	110	1	1	21	1
egg	1 (1 oz)	111	1	6	22	1
egg & onion	1 (1 oz)	111	1	81	22	1
plain	1 (1 oz)	112	tr	0	24	1
whole wheat	1 (1 oz)	99	tr	1	22	3

MAYONNAISE

see also MAYONNAISE-TYPE SALAD DRESSING, RELISH

REDUCED CALORIE

Best Foods Cholesterol Free Reduced Calorie	1 cup (233 g)	760	75	1210	17	—
Best Foods Cholesterol Free Reduced Calorie	1 tbsp (15 g)	50	5	80	1	—
Best Foods Light	1 cup (233 g)	760	78	1815	16	—
Best Foods Light	1 tbsp (15 g)	50	5	115	1	—
Diamond Crystal	1 tbsp	50	5	—	—	—

FOOD	PORTION	CAL	FAT	SOD	CARB	FIB
Estee	1 tbsp	50	5	80	1	—
Hain Canola	1 tbsp	60	5	160	2	—
Hain Light Low Sodium	1 tbsp	60	6	95	2	—
Hellman's Cholesterol Free Reduced Calorie	1 cup (233 g)	760	75	1210	17	—
Hellmann's Cholesterol Free Reduced Calorie	1 tbsp (15 g)	50	5	80	1	—
Hellman's Light Reduced Calorie	1 cup (233 g)	760	78	1815	16	—
Hellman's Light Reduced Calorie	1 tbsp (15 g)	50	5	115	1	—
Kraft Free	1 tbsp	12	0	190	3	—
Kraft Light	1 tbsp	50	5	110	1	—
Smart Beat Canola Oil	1 tbsp	40	4	110	1	—
Smart Beat Corn Oil	1 tbsp	40	4	110	1	—
Weight Watchers Fat Free	1 tbsp	12	0	125	4	—
Weight Watchers Light	1 tbsp	50	5	100	1	—
Weight Watchers Low Sodium	1 tbsp	50	1	45	1	—
reduced calorie	1 cup	556	46	1193	38	—
reduced calorie	1 tbsp	34	3	75	2	—
REGULAR						
BAMA	1 tbsp	100	11	65	0	—
Bennett's	1 tbsp	110	12	65	1	—
Best Foods Real	1 cup	1570	175	1255	tr	—
Best Foods Real	1 tbsp	100	11	80	tr	—
Hain Canola	1 tbsp	100	11	100	tr	—
Hain Cold Processed	1 tbsp	110	12	70	0	—
Hain Eggless No Salt Added	1 tbsp	110	12	<5	0	—
Hain Real No Salt Added	1 tbsp	110	12	0	0	—
Hain Safflower	1 tbsp	110	12	70	0	—
Hellman's	1 cup (220 g)	1570	173	1255	1	—
Hellman's	1 tbsp	100	11	80	tr	—
Hollywood	1 tbsp	110	12	80	0	—
Hollywood Canola	1 tbsp	100	11	100	tr	—
Hollywood Safflower	1 tbsp	100	12	75	0	—
Kraft Real	1 tbsp	100	12	70	0	—
Kraft Sandwich Spread	1 tbsp	50	5	95	3	—
McIlhenny Spicy	1 tbsp (0.5 oz)	108	12	94	1	tr

FOOD	PORTION	CAL	FAT	SOD	CARB	FIB
Mother's	1 tbsp	100	11	—	—	—
mayonnaise	1 cup	1577	175	1250	6	—
mayonnaise	1 tbsp	99	11	78	tr	—
sandwich spread	1 tbsp	60	5	—	3	—

MAYONNAISE-TYPE SALAD DRESSING
see also MAYONNAISE, RELISH

REDUCED CALORIE

FOOD	PORTION	CAL	FAT	SOD	CARB	FIB
Miracle Whip Free	1 tbsp	20	0	210	5	—
Miracle Whip Light	1 tbsp	45	4	125	2	—
Smart Beat	1 tbsp (15 g)	12	0	130	3	—
Weight Watchers Fat Free Whipped Dressing	1 tbsp	16	0	115	4	—
reduced calorie w/o cholesterol	1 cup	1084	107	794	36	—
reduced calorie w/o cholesterol	1 tbsp	68	7	49	2	—

REGULAR

FOOD	PORTION	CAL	FAT	SOD	CARB	FIB
BAMA	1 tbsp	50	4	105	3	—
Bright Day Dressing	1 tbsp	60	6	—	—	—
Miracle Whip Coleslaw Dressing	1 tbsp	70	6	105	3	—
Spin Blend	1 tbsp	60	5	110	3	—
Spin Blend Cholesterol-Free	1 tbsp	40	4	110	2	—
home recipe	1 cup	400	24	1872	38	—
home recipe	1 tbsp	25	2	117	2	—
mayonnaise-type salad dressing	1 tbsp	57	5	—	4	—
mayonnaise-type salad dressing	1 cup	916	78	1670	56	—

MEAT STICKS
DRIED

FOOD	PORTION	CAL	FAT	SOD	CARB	FIB
Tombstone Beef Jerky	1	35	0	310	tr	0
Tombstone Beef Sticks	1	110	10	270	0	0
Tombstone Snappy Sticks	1	110	10	260	tr	0

MEAT SUBSTITUTES
see also BACON SUBSTITUTES, CHICKEN SUBSTITUTES, SAUSAGE SUBSTITUTES, TURKEY SUBSTITUTES

FOOD	PORTION	CAL	FAT	SOD	CARB	FIB
Better Than Burger? (Sovex)	½ cup (1.9 oz)	165	2	52	25	9

FOOD	PORTION	CAL	FAT	SOD	CARB	FIB
Harvest Direct						
TVP Beef Chunks	3.5 oz	280	1	15	32	18
TVP Beef Chunks Flavored	3.5 oz	250	1	2000	30	17
TVP Beef Ground	3.5 oz	280	1	15	32	18
TVP Beef Ground Flavored	3.5 oz	250	1	2000	30	17
TVP Beef Strips	3.5 oz	280	1	15	32	18
Jaclyn's Salisbury Steak Style Dinner	11 oz	260	8	320	37	—
Jaclyn's Sirloin Strips Style Dinner	12 oz	290	6	320	37	—
Ken & Robert's Veggie Burger	1 (62 g)	110	2	390	19	—
LaLoma						
Big Franks	1 (51 g)	110	6	190	2	—
Corn Dogs	1 (71 g)	190	8	400	15	—
Dinner Cuts	2 pieces (99 g)	110	1	340	2	—
Griddle Steaks	1 piece (54 g)	140	7	390	4	—
Nuteena	½-in slice (65 g)	160	12	110	6	—
Patty Mix	¼ cup (16 g)	50	0	200	4	—
Redi-Burger	½ in slice (68 g)	130	6	340	5	—
Sandwich Spread	3 tbsp (48 g)	70	4	300	4	—
Savory Dinner Loaf Mix, not prep	¼ cup (16 g)	50	0	380	4	—
Savory Meatballs	7 (70 g)	190	8	420	7	—
Sizzle Burger	1 patty (71 g)	220	12	420	10	—
Sizzle Franks	2 (68 g)	170	13	340	3	—
Swiss Steak	1 piece (92 g)	170	10	360	7	—
Tender Bits	4 pieces (57 g)	80	3	260	5	—
Tender Rounds	6 pieces (73 g)	120	4	310	7	—
Vege-Burger	½ cup (108 g)	110	2	190	3	—
Vita-Burger Chunk	¼ cup (21 g)	70	0	150	6	—
Vita-Burger Granules	3 tbsp (21 g)	70	0	150	6	—
Lightlife						
American Grill	2.75 oz	110	3	325	8	—
Barbecue Grill	2.75 oz	130	6	336	10	—
Smart Deli Slices	2 slices (1.5 oz)	44	0	290	1	—
Smart Dogs	1 (1.5 oz)	40	0	290	1	—
Smart Dogs To Go	1 (5 oz)	115	0	300	19	—
Tofu Pups	1 (1.5 oz)	92	5	—	—	—
Vegetarian Sloppy Joe	4.3 oz	130	6	310	11	—
Midland Harvest						
Burger n' Loaf Chili	0.8 oz	90	3	225	7	2

FOOD	PORTION	CAL	FAT	SOD	CARB	FIB
w/o Beans						
Burger n' Loaf Herbs & Spice	3.2 oz	140	5	250	7	4
Burger n' Loaf Italian	3.2 oz	140	5	375	7	4
Burger n' Loaf Original	3.2 oz	140	5	350	7	4
Burger n' Loaf Sloppy Joe w/o Sauce	0.8 oz	80	2	165	9	1
Burger n' Loaf Taco	2.7 oz	90	2	250	7	1
Morningstar Farms						
Breaded Cutlet	1 patty (71 g)	230	14	390	12	—
Deli Franks	1 (35 g)	90	6	420	2	—
Sandwich Burger Pattie w/Cheese	1 (4.75 oz)	370	17	700	32	—
Sandwich Pattie Biscuit	1 (3.5 oz)	280	11	570	31	—
Natural Touch						
Dinner Entree	1 patty (85 g)	230	14	300	6	—
Garden Pattie	1 (67 g)	120	4	300	8	—
Loaf Mix, as Prep	4 oz	180	7	670	12	—
Okara Pattie	1 (64 g)	160	10	420	7	—
Stroganoff Mix, as prep	4 oz	90	3	700	10	—
Taco Mix, as prep	2 tbsp	90	2	210	6	—
Spring Creek Soysage	1 patty (1.6 oz)	63	tr	237	11	—
Worthington						
Beef Style Meatless	4 slices (70 g)	130	6	750	7	—
Bolono	2 slices (38 g)	60	2	390	2	—
Choplets	2 slices (92 g)	100	2	440	4	—
Corn Beef Sliced	4 slices (57 g)	120	6	740	8	—
Country Stew	9.5 oz (270 g)	220	10	760	23	—
Dinner Roast	2 oz	120	8	440	5	—
FriPats	1 (64 g)	180	12	360	5	—
Granburger, not prep	6 tbsp (33 g)	110	1	730	7	—
Multigrain Cutlet	2 slices (92 g)	90	2	550	5	—
Non-Meat Balls	3 (54 g)	100	6	210	5	—
Numete	½-in slice (68 g)	150	11	410	7	—
Prime Stakes	1 piece (92 g)	160	10	410	7	—
Prosage Patties	2 (76 g)	210	14	780	4	—
Prosage Roll	2⅜-in slice (70 g)	180	12	570	4	—
Protose	½-in slice (76 g)	180	8	470	9	—

FOOD	PORTION	CAL	FAT	SOD	CARB	FIB
Worthington *(cont.)*						
Salami Meatless	2 slices (38 g)	70	4	460	2	—
Savory Slices	2 slices (56 g)	100	6	340	4	—
Smoked Beef Slices	6 slices (56 g)	120	6	790	7	—
Stakelets	1 piece (71 g)	150	8	460	7	—
Veelets	1 patty (71 g)	230	14	390	12	—
Vegetable Skallops	½ cup (85 g)	90	2	430	4	—
Vegetable Skallops No Added Salt	½ cup (85 g)	80	1	80	4	—
Vegetable Steaks	2.5 pieces (90 g)	110	2	400	5	—
Vegetarian Burger	½ cup (113 g)	150	4	780	9	—
Vegetarian Burger No Added Salt	½ cup (113 g)	150	4	170	7	—
Vegetarian Beef Pie	1 (227 g)	360	16	1940	44	—
Wham	3 slices (68 g)	120	7	940	3	—
simulated sausage	1 link (25 g)	64	5	222	2	—
simulated sausage	1 patty (38 g)	97	7	137	4	—
simulated meat product	1 oz	88	1	3	11	—

MELON
see also individual names

FRESH

Chiquita Cantalene	1 cup	60	0	—	—	—
Chiquita Honey Mist	1 cup	80	0	—	—	—
FROZEN						
Mixed Balls (Big Valley)	3/5 oz	35	1	20	8	—
melon balls	1 cup	55	tr	53	14	—

MILK
see also CHOCOLATE, COCOA, MILK DRINKS

CANNED

Carnation Evaporated	2 tbsp	40	3	35	3	—
Carnation Evaporated Lowfat	2 tbsp	25	1	35	3	—
Carnation Sweetened Condensed	2 tbsp	130	3	45	22	—
Carnation Lite Evaporated Skimmed Carnation	½ cup (4 fl oz)	100	tr	150	14	—
Eagle Sweetened Condensed	⅓ cup	320	9	120	52	—

FOOD	PORTION	CAL	FAT	SOD	CARB	FIB
Pet Evaporated Filled	½ cup	150	8	140	12	—
Pet Evaporated Light Skimmed	½ cup	100	tr	150	14	—
Pet Evaporated	½ cup	170	10	140	12	—
condensed, sweetened	1 cup	982	27	389	166	—
condensed, sweetened	1 oz	123	3	49	21	—
evaporated	½ cup	169	10	122	13	—
evaporated skim	½ cup	99	tr	147	14	—
DRIED						
Carnation Nonfat	⅓ cup dry	80	0	125	12	—
Flash Instant	8 oz	80	tr	—	—	—
Lactose Reduced, as prep (Nutra/Balance)	8 oz	80	tr	125	12	—
Sanalac, as prep	8 oz	80	tr	125	12	0
buttermilk	1 tbsp	25	tr	34	3	—
nonfat, instantized	1 pkg (3.2 oz)	244	tr	499	47	—
LIQUID, LOWFAT						
1%	1 cup	102	3	123	12	—
1%	1 qt	409	10	493	47	—
1% protein fortified	1 cup	119	3	143	14	—
1% protein fortified	1 qt	477	12	574	54	—
2%	1 cup	121	5	122	12	—
2%	1 qt	485	19	487	47	—
Borden Acidophilus 1%	8 fl oz	100	2	130	11	—
Borden Golden Churn Lowfat Buttermilk	8 fl oz	120	4	250	11	—
Borden Hi-Protein 2%	8 fl oz	140	5	150	13	—
Buttermilk (Land O'Lakes)	8 oz	100	2	—	—	—
CalciMilk	8 fl oz	102	3	123	12	0
Easylac 1% (Farmland)	8 fl oz	100	2	125	11	—
Farmland 1% (Farmland)	8 fl oz	100	3	130	12	0
Farmland 2% (Farmland)	8 fl oz	130	5	130	12	0
Lactaid 1%	8 fl oz	102	3	123	12	0
Land O'Lakes 1%	8 oz	100	3	—	—	—
Land O'Lakes 2%	8 oz	120	5	—	—	—
Viva 2%	8 fl oz	120	5	125	11	—
buttermilk	1 cup	99	2	257	12	—
buttermilk	1 qt	396	9	1028	47	—
LIQUID, REGULAR						
Borden	8 fl oz	150	8	130	11	—
Borden Hi-Calcium	8 fl oz	150	8	130	11	—

FOOD	PORTION	CAL	FAT	SOD	CARB	FIB
Farmland Cholesterol Reduced	8 oz	150	8	125	11	—
Farmland 2% (Farmland)	8 fl oz	150	8	130	12	0
Land O'Lakes	8 oz	150	8	—	—	—
Friendship Buttermilk	8 fl oz	120	4	125	12	0
Land O'Lakes	8 oz	150	8	—	—	—
buffalo	3.5 oz	112	8	40	5	—
camel	3.5 oz	80	4	30	5	—
donkey	3.5 oz	43	1	—	6	—
goat	1 cup	168	10	122	11	—
goat	1 qt	672	40	486	43	—
human	1 cup	171	11	42	17	—
indian buffalo	1 cup	236	17	127	13	—
low sodium	1 cup	149	8	6	11	—
mare	3.5 oz	49	2	—	6	—
sheep	1 cup	264	17	108	13	—
whole	1 cup	150	8	120	11	—
LIQUID, SKIM						
Borden	8 fl oz	90	1	130	12	—
Borden Skim-line	8 fl oz	100	1	150	13	—
Easylac Nonfat (Farmland)	8 fl oz	90	0	125	12	—
Farmland	8 fl oz	80	0	130	12	0
Farmland Skim Plus	8 fl oz	100	tr	150	13	—
Lactaid Nonfat	8 fl oz	86	tr	126	12	0
Land O'Lakes	8 oz	90	tr	—	—	—
Viva	8 fl oz	100	1	150	13	—
Weight Watchers	1 cup	90	tr	140	13	—
skim	1 cup	86	tr	125	12	—
skim	1 qt	342	2	505	48	—
skim protein fortified	1 cup	100	1	144	14	—
skim protein fortified	1 qt	400	2	578	55	—

MILK DRINKS

see also BREAKFAST DRINKS, CHOCOLATE, COCOA

FOOD	PORTION	CAL	FAT	SOD	CARB	FIB
Chocolate Lowfat Dutch Brand (Borden)	8 fl oz	180	5	180	25	—
Chocolate Milk (Land O'Lakes)	8 oz	210	8	—	—	—
Chocolate Milk (Meadow Gold)	8 fl oz	210	8	240	25	—
Chocolate Milk 1% (Lactaid)	8 fl oz	158	3	152	26	tr

FOOD	PORTION	CAL	FAT	SOD	CARB	FIB
Chocolate Milk 1% (Land O'Lakes)	8 oz	160	3	—	—	—
Chocolate Milk 2% (Hershey)	1 cup	190	5	130	29	—
Chocolate Skim Milk (Land O'Lakes)	8 oz	140	tr	—	—	—
Quik Banana Lowfat Milk (Nestle)	8 oz	190	4	115	30	—
Quik Chocolate (Nestle)	2.5 tsp (0.75 oz)	90	1	25	20	—
Quik Chocolate Lowfat Milk (Nestle)	8 oz	200	5	150	29	—
Quik Chocolate, as prep w/2% milk (Nestle)	8 oz	210	5	150	31	—
Quik Chocolate, as prep w/skim milk (Nestle)	8 oz	170	1	150	31	—
Quik Chocolate, as prep w/whole milk (Nestle)	8 oz	230	9	140	31	—
Quik Lite Ready To Drink Chocolate Lowfat (Nestle)	8 oz	130	5	150	13	—
Quik Ready To Drink Chocolate (Nestle)	8 oz	230	9	120	30	—
Quik Ready To Drink Strawberry (Nestle)	8 oz	230	8	140	32	—
Quik Strawberry (Nestle)	2½ tsp (0.75 oz)	80	0	0	21	—
Quik Strawberry Lowfat Milk (Nestle)	8 oz	200	4	120	33	—
Quik Strawberry, as prep w/2% milk (Nestle)	8 oz	200	5	120	32	—
Quik Strawberry, as prep w/skim milk (Nestle)	8 oz	160	0	125	32	—
Quik Strawberry, as prep w/whole milk (Nestle)	8 oz	220	8	120	32	—
Quik Sugar Free Chocolate (Nestle)	1 heaping tsp (5.8 g)	18	tr	35	3	—
Quik Sugar Free Chocolate, as prep w/2% milk (Nestle)	8 oz	140	5	150	15	—

FOOD	PORTION	CAL	FAT	SOD	CARB	FIB
Quik Syrup Chocolate (Nestle)	1¾ tbsp	100	1	45	22	—
Quik Syrup Chocolate, as prep w/2% milk (Nestle)	8 oz	220	5	160	34	—
Quik Syrup Chocolate, as prep w/skim milk (Nestle)	8 oz	220	9	160	34	—
Quik Syrup Chocolate, as prep w/whole milk (Nestle)	8 oz	240	9	160	33	—
Quik Syrup Strawberry (Nestle)	1¾ tbsp	100	0	0	24	—
Quik Syrup Strawberry, as prep w/ 2% milk (Nestle)	8 oz	220	5	120	36	—
Quik Syrup Strawberry, as prep w/ skim milk (Nestle)	8 oz	180	0	130	36	—
Quik Syrup Strawberry, as prep w/whole milk (Nestle)	8 oz	240	8	120	36	—
Quik Vanilla Lowfat Milk (Nestle)	8 oz	200	4	115	31	—
Whole Chocolate Milk (Hershey)	8 oz	210	9	120	28	—
chocolate milk	1 cup	208	8	149	26	—
chocolate milk	1 qt	833	34	596	103	—
chocolate milk 1%	1 cup	158	3	152	26	—
chocolate milk 1%	1 qt	630	10	607	104	—
chocolate milk 2%	1 cup	179	5	150	26	—
strawberry flavor mix, as prep w/whole milk	9 oz	234	8	128	33	—

MILK SUBSTITUTES
see also COFFEE WHITENERS

FOOD	PORTION	CAL	FAT	SOD	CARB	FIB
Better Than Milk						
Carob	8 fl oz	130	5	175	20	—
Chocolate	8 fl oz	125	5	175	17	—
Light	8 fl oz	80	tr	120	15	—
Natural	8 fl oz	90	5	120	10	—
Edensoy	8.45 fl oz	140	4	120	14	—
Edensoy Extra	8.45 fl oz	140	4	110	14	—
First Alternative	8 fl oz	80	2	210	7	—

FOOD	PORTION	CAL	FAT	SOD	CARB	FIB
Rice Dream						
Carob Lite	8 fl oz	150	3	80	32	—
Chocolate	8 fl oz	190	3	80	44	—
Chocolate	8 fl oz	190	3	80	44	—
Organic Original Lite	8 fl oz	130	2	80	28	—
Vanilla Lite	8 fl oz	130	2	80	30	—
Spring Creek Honey Vanilla	1 oz	23	5	7	3	—
Spring Creek Original	1 oz	21	5	6	3	—
Spring Creek Plain	1 oz	15	5	4	1	—
Vegelicious	8 fl oz	100	2	125	18	—
Vitamite	8 fl oz	100	5	—	—	—
Vitasoy						
Carob Supreme	8 fl oz	150	4	110	22	—
Cocoa Light	8 fl oz	140	2	80	25	—
Cocoa Rich	8 fl oz	160	4	130	24	—
Original Creamy	8 fl oz	100	5	130	10	—
Original Light	8 fl oz	90	2	90	15	—
Vanilla Delite	8 fl oz	150	4	100	23	—
Vanilla Light	8 fl oz	110	2	100	20	—
Westoy Cocoa Lite	8 fl oz	140	2	95	25	—
Westoy Plain Lite	8 fl oz	100	2	100	16	—
Westoy Vanilla Lite	8 fl oz	110	2	80	20	—
imitation milk	1 cup	150	8	191	15	—
imitation milk	1 qt	600	33	764	60	—

MILKFISH

FOOD	PORTION	CAL	FAT	SOD	CARB	FIB
baked	3 oz	162	7	—	0	—

MILK SHAKE

FOOD	PORTION	CAL	FAT	SOD	CARB	FIB
Chocolate (Frostee)	8 fl oz	200	8	160	30	—
Chocolate (MicroMagic)	1 (10.5 oz)	290	8	90	46	—
Chocolate Fudge (Weight Watchers)	1 pkg	70	tr	150	11	—
Milk Way Shake	1 (10 fl oz)	390	16	235	54	0
Orange Sherbet (Weight Watchers)	1 pkg	70	tr	210	12	—
Strawberry (Frostee)	8 fl oz	180	7	150	27	—
chocolate	10 oz	360	11	273	58	—
strawberry	10 oz	319	8	234	53	—
thick shake chocolate	10.6 oz	356	8	333	63	—
thick shake vanilla	11 oz	350	10	299	56	—
vanilla	10 oz	314	8	232	51	—

FOOD	PORTION	CAL	FAT	SOD	CARB	FIB

MILLET
cooked	½ cup	143	1	2	28	—

MINERAL/BOTTLED WATER
Artesia

FOOD	PORTION	CAL	FAT	SOD	CARB	FIB
Almund	7 oz	0	0	—	—	—
Cranberi	7 oz	0	0	—	—	—
Lemin	7 oz	0	0	—	—	—
Orange	7 oz	0	0	—	—	—
Crystal Geyser						
Sparkling Lemon	1 bottle (12 fl oz)	0	0	70	0	—
Sparkling Mineral	1 bottle (12 fl oz)	0	0	70	0	—
Sparkling Natural Cola Berry	1 bottle (12 fl oz)	0	0	70	0	—
Sparkling Natural Wild Cherry	1 bottle (12 fl oz)	0	0	70	0	—
Sparkling Orange	1 bottle (12 fl oz)	0	0	70	0	—
Diamond Spring	1 qt	0	0	—	—	—
Evian	1 liter	0	0	5	0	0
Glenpatrick Spring Pure Irish	8 oz	0	0	—	—	—
LaCroix						
Sparkling Berry	12 fl oz	0	0	—	—	—
Sparkling Lemon	12 fl oz	0	0	—	—	—
Sparkling Lime	12 fl oz	0	0	—	—	—
Sparkling Orange	12 fl oz	0	0	—	—	—
Sparkling Regular	12 fl oz	0	0	—	—	—
Mountain Valley	1 qt	0	0	—	—	—
San Pellegrino	1 liter (33.8 oz)	0	0	41	0	—
Saratoga Sparkling	1 liter	0	0	19	0	—
Schweppes Vichy	6 oz	0	0	—	—	—

MISO
miso	½ cup	284	8	5036	39	7

MOCHA
FOOD	PORTION	CAL	FAT	SOD	CARB	FIB
Bavarian Mint Mocha (Hills Bros.)	6 oz	50	1	—	—	—
Bavarian Mint Mocha Sugar Free (Hills Bros.)	6 oz	35	1	—	—	—

FOOD	PORTION	CAL	FAT	SOD	CARB	FIB
Cafe Mocha (Hills Bros.)	6 oz	50	1	—	—	—
Cafe Mocha (MJB Co.)	6 oz	50	1	—	—	—
Cherry Mocha (MJB Co.)	6 oz	50	1	—	—	—
Fudge Mocha Sugar Free (MJB Co.)	6 oz	40	2	—	—	—
Mint Mocha (MJB Co.)	6 oz	50	1	—	—	—
Mint Mocha Sugar Free (MJB Co.)	6 oz	35	1	—	—	—
Swiss Mocha (Hills Bros.)	6 oz	40	2	—	—	—
Vanilla Mocha Sugar Free (MJB Co.)	6 oz	40	2	—	—	—

MOLASSES

FOOD	PORTION	CAL	FAT	SOD	CARB	FIB
Brer Rabbit Dark	2 tbsp	110	0	20	28	—
Brer Rabbit Light	2 tbsp	110	0	15	29	—
Grandma's Gold Label	1 tbsp	70	0	—	—	—
Grandma's Green Label	1 tbsp	70	0	—	—	—
McIlhenny	1 tbsp (0.7 oz)	66	tr	9	16	tr
blackstrap	2 tbsp	85	0	38	22	—
molasses	2 tbsp	85	0	38	22	—

MONKFISH

FOOD	PORTION	CAL	FAT	SOD	CARB	FIB
baked	3 oz	82	2	20	0	—

MOOSE

FOOD	PORTION	CAL	FAT	SOD	CARB	FIB
roasted	3 oz	114	1	58	0	—

MOTH BEANS
DRIED

FOOD	PORTION	CAL	FAT	SOD	CARB	FIB
cooked	1 cup	207	1	17	37	—

MOUSSE
FROZEN

FOOD	PORTION	CAL	FAT	SOD	CARB	FIB
Chocolate (Sara Lee)	1 slice (2.7 oz)	260	17	100	23	—
Chocolate (Weight Watchers)	1 (2.5 oz)	160	3	160	27	—
Chocolate Light (Sara Lee)	1 (3 oz)	170	8	60	20	—
Light Classics Strawberry (Sara Lee)	1 slice (53.8 g)	180	11	—	—	—
Praline Pecan (Weight Watchers)	1 (2.71 oz)	180	4	180	30	—

FOOD	PORTION	CAL	FAT	SOD	CARB	FIB
San Francisco Chocolate Mousse (Pepperidge Farm)	1	490	34	75	41	—
HOME RECIPE						
crab	¼ cup	364	20	—	—	—
orange	½ cup	87	5	24	19	—
MIX						
Amaretto (Estee)	½ cup	70	3	50	10	—
Black Forest Mousse Tiarra Dessert (Duncan Hines)	½ cake	260	13	—	—	—
Cherries & Cream Mousse Tiarra Dessert (Duncan Hines)	½ cake	250	11	—	—	—
Chocolate (Weight Watchers)	½ cup	70	3	—	7	—
Chocolate Amaretto Mousse Tiarra Dessert (Duncan Hines)	½ cake	270	16	—	—	—
Chocolate Fudge Rich And Luscious (Jell-O)	½ cup	143	6	74	20	—
Chocolate Mousse No-Bake (Royal)	⅛ pie	130	4	190	21	—
Chocolate Mousse Tiarra Dessert (Duncan Hines)	½ cake	270	16	—	—	—
Chocolate Rich And Luscious (Jell-O)	½ cup	145	6	73	21	—
Dark Chocolate, as prep (Knorr)	½ cup	90	5	50	10	—
Milk Chocolate, as prep (Knorr)	½ cup	90	5	50	11	—
Orange Chocolate (Estee)	½ cup	70	3	50	9	—
Unflavored, as prep (Knorr)	½ cup	80	5	45	8	—
White Chocolate Almond Mousse (Weight Watchers)	½ cup	70	3	105	7	—
White Chocolate, as prep (Knorr)	½ cup	80	4	50	10	—

FOOD	PORTION	CAL	FAT	SOD	CARB	FIB
MUFFIN						
FROZEN						
Almond & Date Oat Bran Fancy Fruit (Health Valley)	1	180	4	80	31	8
Apple Oat Bran (Sara Lee)	1	190	6	300	36	—
Apple Spice (Healthy Choice)	1 (2.5 oz)	190	4	90	40	—
Apple Spice (Sara Lee)	1	220	8	280	36	—
Apple Spice Fat Free (Health Valley)	1	140	tr	110	30	5
Banana Fat Free (Healthy Valley)	1	130	tr	110	29	5
Banana Nut (Healthy Choice)	1 (2.5 oz)	180	6	80	32	—
Banana Nut (Pepperidge Farm)	1	170	6	220	28	—
Banana Nut (Weight Watchers)	1 (2.5 oz)	170	5	—	32	—
Blueberry (Healthy Choice)	1 (2.5 oz)	190	4	110	39	—
Blueberry (Pepperidge Farm)	1	170	7	250	27	1
Blueberry (Sara Lee)	1	200	8	290	34	—
Blueberry (Weight Watchers)	1 (2.5 oz)	170	5	—	32	—
Blueberry Free & Light (Sara Lee)	1	120	0	140	28	—
Cheese Streusel (Sara Lee)	1	220	11	170	27	—
Chocolate Chunk (Sara Lee)	1	220	8	210	33	—
Cholesterol Free Multi Grain Muesli (Pepperidge Farm)	1	200	8	230	30	—
Cholesterol Free Oatbran With Apple (Pepperidge Farm)	1	190	7	200	29	—
Cholesterol Free Raisin Bran (Pepperidge Farm)	1	170	6	280	30	—
Cinnamon Swirl (Pepperidge Farm)	1	190	6	170	30	1

FOOD	PORTION	CAL	FAT	SOD	CARB	FIB
Corn (Pepperidge Farm)	1	180	7	260	27	—
Golden Corn (Sara Lee)	1	240	13	310	31	—
Oat Bran (Sara Lee)	1	210	8	320	35	—
Oat Bran Fancy Fruit Blueberry (Health Valley)	1	140	4	100	32	8
Oat Bran Fancy Fruit Blueberry (Health Valley)	1	180	5	90	5	8
Raisin Bran (Sara Lee)	1	220	7	400	37	—
Raisin Spice Fat Free (Health Valley)	1	140	tr	100	32	5
Rice Bran Fancy Fruit Raisin (Health Valley)	1	210	7	125	7	6
HOME RECIPE						
blueberry, as prep with 2% milk	1 (2 oz)	163	6	251	23	—
blueberry, as prep with whole milk	1 (2 oz)	165	6	251	23	—
corn, as prep w/2% milk	1 (2 oz)	180	7	334	25	—
corn, as prep w/whole milk	1 (2 oz)	183	7	333	25	—
plain, as prep w/2% milk	1 (2 oz)	169	7	266	24	—
plain, as prep w/whole milk	1 (2 oz)	172	7	266	24	—
wheat bran, as prep w/ 2% milk	1 (2 oz)	161	7	335	24	—
wheat bran, as prep w/ whole milk	1 (2 oz)	164	7	335	24	—
MIX						
Apple Cinnamon (Betty Crocker)	1	120	4	140	18	—
Apple Cinnamon No Cholesterol Recipe (Betty Crocker)	1	110	2	140	18	—
Nut (Betty Crocker)	1	120	5	140	17	—
Banana Nut No Cholesterol Recipe (Betty Crocker)	1	110	4	140	17	—

FOOD	PORTION	CAL	FAT	SOD	CARB	FIB
Blueberry Streusel Bake Shop (Betty Crocker)	1	210	8	230	31	—
Blueberry Bakery Style (Duncan Hines)	1	190	6	—	—	—
Bran (Arrowhead)	⅓ cup (1.4 oz)	150	2	160	26	7
Bran & Honey (Duncan Hines)	1	120	4	—	—	—
Bran & Honey Nut Bakery Style (Duncan Hines)	1	200	7	—	—	—
Bran Date (Jiffy)	1	110	—	—	—	—
Cinnamon Streusel (Betty Crocker)	1	200	9	240	17	—
Cinnamon Swirl Bakery Style (Duncan Hines)	1	200	7	—	—	—
Corn (Jiffy)	1	115	—	—	—	—
Corn Muffin (Dromedary)	1	120	4	270	20	—
Corn Muffin (Flako)	1	120	4	360	20	—
Cranberry Orange Nut Bakery Style (Duncan Hines)	1	200	8	—	—	—
Oat Bran (Betty Crocker)	1	190	8	240	25	—
Oat Bran (Estee)	1	100	4	65	15	—
Oat Bran Apple Cinnamon (Hain)	1	140	3	200	28	5
Oat Bran Banana Nut (Hain)	1	140	4	190	26	4
Oat Bran (Raspberry Spice (Hain)	1	140	3	190	27	4
Oat Bran No Cholesterol Recipe (Betty Crocker)	1	180	7	240	25	—
Oat Bran Wheat Free (Arrowhead)	⅓ cup (1.5 oz)	160	4	310	23	7
Pecan Nut Bakery Style (Duncan Hines)	1	220	11	—	—	—
Twice The Blueberries (Betty Crocker)	1	120	4	140	18	—

FOOD	PORTION	CAL	FAT	SOD	CARB	FIB
Twice The Blueberries No Cholesterol Recipe (Betty Crocker)	1	110	3	140	18	—
Wild Blueberry (Betty Crocker)	1	120	4	150	18	—
Wild Blueberry (Duncan Hines)	1	110	3	—	—	—
Wild Blueberry Light (Betty Crocker)	1	70	tr	140	16	—
Wild Blueberry Light No Cholesterol Recipe (Betty Crocker)	1	70	tr	140	16	—
Wild Blueberry No Cholesterol Recipe (Betty Crocker)	1	110	3	150	18	—
blueberry	1 (1.75 oz)	149	4	219	24	—
corn	1 (1.75 oz)	160	5	397	25	—
wheat bran, as prep	1 (1.75 oz)	138	5	233	23	—
READY-TO-EAT						
Apple Oat Bran (Dutch Mill)	1 (2 oz)	180	5	210	31	1
Banana Walnut (Dutch Mill)	1 (2 oz)	220	6	210	33	1
Blueberry (Entenmann's)	1 (2 oz)	200	8	250	29	—
Bran'nola (Arnold)	1 (2.3 oz)	160	1	220	30	2
Carrot (Dutch Mill)	1 (2 oz)	190	7	230	31	1
Corn (Dutch Mill)	1 (2 oz)	190	6	280	31	1
Cranberry Orange (Dutch Mill)	1 (2 oz)	170	6	290	26	1
Extra Crisp (Arnold)	1	130	1	230	26	1
Mini Apple Cinnamon (Hostess)	5 (2 oz)	260	16	180	28	3
Mini Banana Nut (Hostess)	5 (2 oz)	260	16	160	28	tr
Mini Blueberry (Hostess)	5 (2 oz)	240	13	180	30	tr
Mini Chocolate Chip (Hostess)	5 (2 oz)	260	15	170	29	1
Muffin Loaf Blueberry (Hostess)	1 (3.8 oz)	440	19	460	62	2
Oat Bran (Hostess)	1 (1.5 oz)	160	8	150	22	tr

FOOD	PORTION	CAL	FAT	SOD	CARB	FIB
Oat Bran Banana Nut (Hostess)	1 (1.5 oz)	150	6	160	22	1
Raisin (Arnold)	1 (2.3 oz)	160	1	220	33	2
Raisin Bran (Dutch Mill)	1 (2 oz)	230	5	330	37	3
Sourdough (Arnold)	1	130	1	250	25	1
blueberry	1 (2 oz)	158	4	255	27	2
corn	1 (2 oz)	174	5	297	29	—
oat bran, wheat free	1 (2 oz)	154	4	224	28	4
toaster type, blueberry	1	103	3	158	18	—
toaster type, corn	1	114	4	142	19	—
toaster type, wheat bran w/ raisins	1 (36 g)	106	3	178	19	—

MULBERRIES

fresh	1 cup	61	1	14	14	—

MULLET

striped, cooked	3 oz	127	4	61	0	—
striped, raw	3 oz	99	3	55	0	—

MUNG BEANS
DRIED

cooked	1 cup	213	1	4	39	—
SPROUTS						
canned	½ cup	8	tr	—	1	—
cooked	½ cup	13	tr	6	3	—
raw	½ cup	16	tr	3	3	—
stir-fried	½ cup	31	tr	—	7	—

MUNGO BEANS
DRIED

cooked	1 cup	190	1	13	33	—

MUSHROOMS
CANNED

Button (Empress)	2 oz	14	0	260	2	—
Button Sliced (Empress)	2 oz	14	0	260	2	—
Mushrooms (B In B)	¼ cup	12	0	240	2	1
Mushrooms (Libby)	¼ cup	35	0	—	—	—
Mushrooms (Seneca)	¼ cup	35	0	—	—	—
Mushrooms With Garlic (B In B)	¼ cup	12	0	200	2	1

FOOD	PORTION	CAL	FAT	SOD	CARB	FIB
Oriental Straw Mushrooms (Green Giant)	¼ cup	12	0	290	2	1
Pieces & Stems (Empress)	2 oz	14	0	260	2	—
Pieces And Stems (Green Giant)	¼ cup	12	0	220	2	1
Sliced (Green Giant)	¼ cup	12	0	220	2	1
Straw Mushrooms Broken (Empress)	2 oz	10	0	180	2	—
Whole (Green Giant)	¼ cup	12	0	220	2	1
chanterelle	3.5 oz	12	1	165	tr	6
pieces	½ cup	19	tr	—	4	—
whole	1 (0.4 oz)	3	tr	—	1	—
DRIED						
chanterelle	3.5 oz	89	2	32	2	60
Shiitake	4 (0.5 oz)	44	tr	2	11	—
FRESH						
chanterelle	3.5 oz	11	tr	3	tr	6
enoki, raw	1 (4 in)	2	tr	0	tr	—
morel	3.5 oz	9	tr	2	0	7
raw	1 (0.5 oz)	5	tr	1	1	tr
raw, sliced	½ cup	9	tr	1	2	tr
shiitake, cooked	4 (2.5 oz)	40	tr	3	10	—
sliced, cooked	½ cup	21	tr	2	4	1
whole, cooked	1 (0.4 oz)	3	tr	0	1	—
FROZEN						
Breaded Mushrooms Ore-Ida	2.67 oz	120	7	440	12	—

MUSKRAT

FOOD	PORTION	CAL	FAT	SOD	CARB	FIB
roasted	3 oz	199	10	81	0	—

MUSSELS

FOOD	PORTION	CAL	FAT	SOD	CARB	FIB
FRESH						
blue, cooked	3 oz	147	4	313	6	—
blue, raw	1 cup	129	3	429	6	—
blue, raw	3 oz	73	2	243	3	—

MUSTARD

FOOD	PORTION	CAL	FAT	SOD	CARB	FIB
Grey Poupon Country Dijon	1 tsp	6	0	120	0	0
Grey Poupon Dijon	1 tsp	6	0	120	0	0
Grey Poupon Parisian	1 tsp	6	0	55	0	0
Gulden's Diablo	1 tsp	8	0	—	—	—

FOOD	PORTION	CAL	FAT	SOD	CARB	FIB
Gulden's Mild	1 tsp	6	0	—	—	—
Gulden's Spicy Brown	1 tsp	8	0	—	—	—
Hain Stone Ground	1 tbsp	14	1	185	1	—
Hain Stone Ground No Salt Added	1 tbsp	14	1	10	1	—
Heinz Mild Yellow	1 tbsp	8	tr	175	1	—
Heinz Spicy Brown	1 tbsp	14	1	115	1	—
Kosciuszko	1 tbsp	11	1	—	—	—
Kraft Horseradish Mustard	1 tbsp	14	1	135	1	—
Kraft Pure Prepared	1 tbsp	4	1	160	1	—
McIlhenny Coarse Ground	1 tsp (0.2 oz)	4	tr	39	tr	tr
McIlhenny Spicy	1 tsp (0.2 oz)	6	tr	28	tr	1
Plochman's Yellow Mustard	1 tbsp	11	1	—	—	—
Plochman's Dijon Mustard	1 tbsp	11	1	—	—	—
Plochman's Spicy Brown Mustard	1 tbsp	11	1	—	—	—
Plochman's Stone Ground Mustard	1 tbsp	11	1	—	—	—
dry mustard seed, yellow	1 tsp	15	1	tr	1	—
yellow, ready-to-use	1 tsp	5	tr	63	tr	—

MUSTARD GREENS
FRESH

FOOD	PORTION	CAL	FAT	SOD	CARB	FIB
chopped, cooked	½ cup	11	tr	11	1	—
raw, chopped	½ cup	7	tr	7	1	—
FROZEN						
chopped, cooked	½ cup	14	tr	19	2	—

NATTO

FOOD	PORTION	CAL	FAT	SOD	CARB	FIB
natto	½ cup	187	10	6	13	—

NAVY BEANS
CANNED

FOOD	PORTION	CAL	FAT	SOD	CARB	FIB
Hanover	½ cup	100	0	—	—	—
Luck's Seasoned w/ Pork	7.5 oz	230	7	—	—	—
Trappey's	½ cup	90	1	410	16	—
Trappey's Jalapeno	½ cup	90	1	480	15	—
navy	1 cup	296	1	1173	54	—

FOOD	PORTION	CAL	FAT	SOD	CARB	FIB
DRIED						
Hurst Brand	1 cup	277	1	—	—	—
cooked	1 cup	259	1	2	48	—
SPROUTS						
cooked	3.5 oz	78	1	—	—	—
raw	½ cup	35	tr	—	—	—

NECTARINE

Dole	1	70	1	0	16	3
fresh	1	67	1	0	16	2

NEUFCHATEL CHEESE
see CREAM CHEESE

NON-DAIRY CREAMERS
see COFFEE WHITENERS

NON-DAIRY WHIPPED TOPPINGS
see WHIPPED TOPPINGS

NOODLES
see also PASTA DINNERS

FOOD	PORTION	CAL	FAT	SOD	CARB	FIB
CANNED						
Van Camp's Noodle Weenee	1 cup	245	9	1245	33	—
DRY						
Chinese (Azumaya)	4 oz	293	1	530	60	—
Chow Mein Narrow (La Choy)	½ cup	150	8	320	16	tr
Chow Mein Wide (La Choy)	½ cup	150	8	300	16	tr
Egg (Creamette)	2 oz	221	3	—	—	—
Egg (Golden Grain)	2 oz	210	2	10	39	2
Egg (Mueller's)	2 oz (57 g)	220	3	8	40	—
Egg (Skinner)	2 oz	220	3	—	—	—
Egg, not prep (Creamette)	2 oz	220	3	20	40	—
Fine Medium Wide & Extra Wide (P&R)	2 oz	220	3	—	—	—
Japanese (Azumaya)	4 oz	289	1	542	59	—
No Yolks (Shofar)	2 oz	210	0	30	41	3
Noodle Trio (Mueller's)	2 oz (57 g)	220	2	18	40	—
Rice (La Choy)	½ cup	130	5	420	21	tr
Spinach Egg Light 'N Fluffy (Skinner)	2 oz	220	3	—	—	—

FOOD	PORTION	CAL	FAT	SOD	CARB	FIB
Veggie Egg, uncooked (Hodgson Mill)	2 oz	200	2	25	37	2
Whole Wheat Spinach Egg, uncooked (Hodgson Mill)	2 oz	190	2	45	32	5
Whole Wheat Egg, uncooked (Hodgson Mill)	2 oz	190	2	20	34	4
cellophane	1 cup	492	tr	14	121	—
chow mein	1 cup	237	14	197	26	—
egg	1 cup (38 g)	145	2	8	27	—
egg, cooked	1 cup	212	2	11	40	—
japanese soba	2 oz	192	tr	451	43	—
japanese soba, cooked	½ cup	56	tr	34	12	—
japanese somen	2 oz	203	tr	1049	42	—
japanese somen, cooked	½ cup	115	tr	142	24	—
spinach/egg	1 cup	145	2	27	27	—
spinach/egg, cooked	1 cup	211	3	20	39	—
DRY MIX						
Kraft Egg Noodle With Chicken Dinner	¾ cup	240	9	1050	32	—
La Choy Ramen Noodles Beef, as prep	1 cup	200	8	865	33	4
La Choy Ramen Noodles Chicken, as prep	1 cup	200	7	740	29	4
Lipton Noodles & Sauce						
Alfredo	½ cup	131	3	530	20	tr
Beef	½ cup	120	2	513	22	0
Butter	½ cup	142	4	461	22	0
Butter And Herb	½ cup	136	3	458	22	0
Carbonara Alfredo	½ cup	126	3	465	20	0
Cheese	½ cup	136	2	470	24	0
Chicken	½ cup	125	2	391	22	tr
Chicken Broccoli	½ cup	124	2	425	22	—
Creamy Chicken	½ cup	125	2	390	22	—
Parmesan	½ cup	138	4	409	20	0
Romanoff	½ cup	136	3	504	23	—
Sour Cream And Chive	½ cup	142	3	442	23	0
Stroganoff	½ cup	110	2	406	19	0
Tomato Alfredo	½ cup	126	3	562	20	—

FOOD	PORTION	CAL	FAT	SOD	CARB	FIB
Maruchan Instant Lunch Oriental Noodles Chicken	1 pkg (14 oz)	290	13	1220	36	2
Minute Microwave Chicken Flavored	½ cup	157	5	471	23	—
Minute Microwave Parmesan	½ cup	178	6	491	24	—
Noodle Roni						
Chicken & Mushroom	½ cup	160	4	550	25	—
Fettuccini	½ cup	300	18	560	29	—
Herb & Butter	½ cup	160	7	290	19	—
Parmesano	½ cup	240	13	140	23	—
Romanoff	½ cup	240	11	730	28	—
Stroganoff	½ cup	350	17	1190	37	—
Ultra Slim-Fast						
Noodles & Alfredo Sauce	2.3 oz	240	4	1110	47	4
Noodles & Beef	2.3 oz	230	3	1070	45	4
Noodles & Cheese	2.3 oz	230	4	770	44	4
Noodles & Chicken Sauce	2.3 oz	220	3	980	45	4
Noodles & Tomato Herb Sauce	2.3 oz	220	3	1090	46	5
TAKE-OUT						
noodle pudding	½ cup	132	7	222	11	—

NUTMEG

FOOD	PORTION	CAL	FAT	SOD	CARB	FIB
ground	1 tsp	12	1	tr	1	—

NUTRITIONAL SUPPLEMENTS
see also BREAKFAST BAR, BREAKFAST DRINKS

FOOD	PORTION	CAL	FAT	SOD	CARB	FIB
DIET						
Dynatrim Dutch Chocolate as prep w/ 1% milk	8 oz	220	4	300	33	6
Dynatrim Strawberry Royale, as prep w/ 1% milk	8 oz	220	4	300	33	6
Dynatrim Vanilla, as prep w/ 1% milk	8 oz	220	4	300	33	6
Figurines						
Chocolate	1 bar	100	5	45	11	—

FOOD	PORTION	CAL	FAT	SOD	CARB	FIB
Chocolate Caramel	1 bar	100	6	55	10	—
Chocolate Peanut Butter	1 bar	100	6	45	10	—
S'Mores	1 bar	100	5	54	11	—
Vanilla	1 bar	100	5	45	11	—
Nestle Sweet Success						
Bar Chewy Chocolate Brownie	1 (1.6 oz)	120	4	35	28	3
Bar Chewy Chocolate Chip	1 (1.6 oz)	120	4	35	23	3
Bar Chewy Chocolate Peanut Butter	1 (1.6 oz)	120	4	35	23	3
Bar Chewy Chocolate Raspberry	1 (1.6 oz)	120	4	35	23	3
Bar Chewy Oatmeal Raisin	1 (1.6 oz)	120	4	30	23	3
Chocolate Mocha Supreme	1 can (10 fl oz)	200	3	220	38	6
Chocolate Mocha Supreme, as prep w/ skim milk	9 fl oz	180	tr	356	30	6
Chocolate Raspberry Truffle	1 can (10 fl oz)	200	3	220	38	6
Chocolate Raspberry, as prep w/ skim milk	9 fl oz	180	1	360	30	6
Classic Chocolate Chip, as prep w/ skim milk	9 fl oz	180	1	288	30	6
Creamy Milk Chocolate	1 can (10 fl oz)	200	3	240	38	6
Creamy Milk Chocolate	1 carton (12 fl oz)	220	2	300	45	6
Creamy Milk Chocolate, as prep w/ skim milk	9 fl oz	180	1	336	30	6
Creamy Vanilla Delight, as prep w/ skim milk	9 fl oz	180	tr	312	33	6
Dark Chocolate Fudge	1 can (10 fl oz)	200	3	220	38	6
Dark Chocolate Fudge	1 carton (12 fl oz)	220	2	310	45	6

FOOD	PORTION	CAL	FAT	SOD	CARB	FIB
Nestle Sweet Success *(cont.)*						
Dark Chocolate Fudge, as prep w/ skim milk	9 fl oz	180	1	356	30	6
Rich Chocolate Almond	1 can (10 fl oz)	200	3	240	38	6
Rich Chocolate Almond	1 carton (12 fl oz)	220	2	300	45	6
Rich Chocolate Almond, as prep w/ skim milk	9 fl oz	180	tr	356	30	6
Smooth Vanilla Creme	1 can (10 fl oz)	200	3	220	38	6
Sego						
Chocolate Malt	10 fl oz	225	1	450	43	—
Vanilla	10 fl oz	225	5	360	34	—
Very Chocolate Chocolate	10 fl oz	225	1	450	43	—
Sego Lite						
Chocolate	10 fl oz	150	3	480	20	—
Dutch Chocolate	10 fl oz	150	3	480	20	—
French Vanilla	10 fl oz	150	4	390	17	—
Strawberry	10 fl oz	150	4	390	17	—
Vanilla	10 fl oz	150	4	390	17	—
Slim-Fast Nutrition Bar						
Dutch Chocolate	1	130	4	90	17	6
Peanut Butter	1	140	6	100	15	7
Slim-Fast Powder						
Chocolate Malt, as prep w/ skim milk	8 oz	190	tr	230	32	2
Chocolate, as prep w/ skim milk	8 oz	190	1	210	32	2
Strawberry, as prep w/ skim milk	8 oz	190	1	220	32	2
Vanilla, as prep w/ skim milk	8 oz	190	1	220	32	2
Ultra Slim-Fast						
Cafe Mocha, as prep w/ skim milk	8 oz	200	tr	280	38	6
Chocolate Royale, as prep w/ skim milk	8 oz	200	1	230	36	5
Crunch Bar Cocoa Almond	1	110	3	30	19	3
Crunch Bar Cocoa Raspberry	1	100	3	30	21	3

FOOD	PORTION	CAL	FAT	SOD	CARB	FIB
Crunch Bar Vanilla Almond	1	110	4	30	18	3
Dutch Chocolate, as prep w/ water	8 oz	220	tr	260	40	5
French Vanilla, as prep w/ skim milk	8 oz	190	tr	250	36	4
French Vanilla, as prep w/ water	8 oz	220	tr	260	40	4
Fruit Juice Mix, as prep w/ fruit juice	8 oz	200	tr	80	43	6
Pina Colada, as prep w/ skim milk	8 oz	180	tr	250	36	6
Ready-to-Drink Chocolate Royale	11 oz	230	3	220	42	5
Ready-to-Drink Chocolate Royale	12 oz	250	1	240	45	5
Ready-to-Drink French Vanilla	11 oz	230	5	190	38	5
Ready-to-Drink French Vanilla	12 oz	220	tr	240	38	5
Ready-to-Drink Strawberry Supreme	12 oz	220	1	240	38	5
Strawberry, as prep w/ skim milk	8 oz	190	1	250	36	4
Strawberry Supreme, as prep w/ water	8 oz	220	tr	260	40	4
REGULAR						
EggPro	4 oz	200	4	105	33	—
Fi-Bar						
Apple	1 (1 oz)	90	3	12	15	5
Cocoa Almond	1	130	4	20	21	4
Cocoa Peanut	1	130	4	20	20	4
Cranberry & Wild Berries	1 (1 oz)	100	3	20	13	4
Lemon	1 (1 oz)	90	3	12	15	5
Mandarin Orange	1 (1 oz)	99	4	12	15	5
Raspberry	1 (1 oz)	100	3	20	13	4
Strawberry	1 (1 oz)	100	3	20	13	4
Treat Yourself Right Almond	1	152	6	38	22	5
Treat Yourself Right Peanutty Butter	1	152	5	56	18	5
Vanilla Almond	1	130	4	20	21	4
Vanilla Peanut	1	130	4	20	20	4

FOOD	PORTION	CAL	FAT	SOD	CARB	FIB
Fi-Bar Nuggets						
Almond Cappuccino Crunch	1 pkg	136	6	—	18	—
Almond Butter Crunch	1 pkg	163	11	—	12	—
Coconut Almond Crunch	1 pkg	136	6	—	18	—
Peanut Butter Crunch	1 pkg	160	10	—	12	—
Gookinaid Lemonade	1 cup (8 fl oz)	45	0	70	12	—
Malsovit Mealwafers	2	152	8	—	—	—
Meal On The Go Apple	1 bar (3 oz)	294	5	114	50	5
Meal On The Go Banana w/ Pecans	1 bar (3 oz)	289	10	109	50	8
Meal On The Go Original	1 bar (3 oz)	286	9	119	52	7
Nutra/Balance						
Frozen Pudding Butterscotch	4 oz	225	8	220	31	—
Frozen Pudding Chocolate	4 oz	225	8	220	31	—
Frozen Pudding Tapioca	4 oz	225	8	220	31	—
Frozen Pudding Vanilla	4 oz	225	8	220	31	—
NutraShake						
Chocolate	4 oz	200	6	55	31	—
Strawberry	4 oz	200	6	55	31	—
Vanilla	4 oz	200	6	55	31	—
With Fibre Vanilla	6 oz	300	2	110	60	—
Nutri-Care Strawberry	1 pkg (1.13 oz)	120	1	—	—	—
Nutri-Care Strawberry, as prep w/ 1 cup whole milk	1 pkg (1.13 oz)	280	9	—	—	—
Nutri-Care Strawberry, as prep w/ 1 cup 2% milk	1 pkg (1.13 oz)	260	5	—	—	—
Vita-J						
Apple Juice	11.5 fl oz	8	0	25	2	—
Fruit Punch	11.5 fl oz	8	0	25	2	—
Grapefruit Cocktail w/ Raspberry	11.5 fl oz	8	0	25	2	—
Orange Juice	11.5 fl oz	8	0	25	2	—

FOOD	PORTION	CAL	FAT	SOD	CARB	FIB
NUTS MIXED						
see also individual names						
Cashews & Peanuts Honey Roasted (Eagle)	1 oz	170	8	130	8	—
Cashews & Peanuts Honey Roasted (Planters)	1 oz	170	12	170	9	—
Mixed (Eagle)	1 oz	180	16	130	6	—
Mixed Deluxe (Eagle)	1 oz	180	17	130	6	—
Mixed Lightly Salted (Planters)	1 oz	170	15	80	6	—
Mixed With Peanuts (Guy's)	1 oz	180	16	140	3	—
Peanuts & Cashews Honey Roasted (Planters)	1 oz	170	12	140	10	—
Tasty Mix (Guy's)	1 oz	130	7	510	14	—
dry roasted, w/ peanuts	1 oz	169	15	3	7	—
dry roasted, w/ peanuts, salted	1 oz	169	15	223	7	—
oil roasted, w/ peanuts	1 oz	175	16	3	6	—
oil roasted, w/ peanuts, salted	1 oz	175	16	217	6	—
oil roasted, w/o peanuts	1 oz	175	16	3	6	—
oil roasted, w/o peanuts, salted	1 oz	175	16	233	6	—
OCTOBER BEANS						
CANNED						
Seasoned w/ Pork Luck's	7.25 oz	230	6	—	—	—
OCTOPUS						
fresh, steamed	3 oz	140	2	—	4	—
OHELOBERRIES						
fresh	1 cup	39	tr	2	10	—
OIL						
see also FAT						
All Blend (Hain)	1 tbsp	120	14	0	0	—
Almond (Hain)	1 tbsp	120	14	0	0	—

FOOD	PORTION	CAL	FAT	SOD	CARB	FIB
Apricot Kernel (Hain)	1 tbsp	120	14	0	0	—
Avocado (Hain)	1 tbsp	120	14	0	0	—
Bertolli (Classico)	1 tbsp	120	14	—	—	—
Bertolli (Extra Light)	1 tbsp	120	14	—	—	—
Bertolli (Extra Virgin)	1 tbsp	120	14	—	—	—
Canola (Hain)	1 tbsp	120	14	0	0	—
Canola (Hollywood)	1 tbsp	120	14	0	0	—
Canola Organic (Hain)	1 tbsp	120	14	0	0	—
Coconut (Hain)	1 tbsp	120	14	0	0	—
Crisco	1 tbsp	120	14	—	—	—
Crisco Corn Oil	1 tbsp	120	14	—	—	—
Flax Seed (Arrowhead)	1 tbsp (0.5 fl oz)	120	14	0	0	0
Garlic & Oil (Hain)	1 tbsp	120	14	0	0	—
Hazelnut (Arrowhead)	1 tbsp (0.5 fl oz)	120	14	0	0	0
Italica	1 tbsp	120	9	—	0	—
Mazola	1 cup (221 g)	1955	221	0	0	—
Mazola	1 tbsp (14 g)	120	14	0	0	—
Mazola No Stick	2.5-second spray (0.2 g)	2	tr	0	0	—
Olive (Hain)	1 tbsp	120	14	0	0	—
Olive (Progresso)	1 tbsp	119	14	0	0	0
Olive Extra Light (Progresso)	1 tbsp	119	14	0	0	0
Olive Extra Virgin (Progresso)	1 tbsp	119	14	0	0	0
Orville Redenbacher's	1 tbsp	120	14	0	0	0
Pam	1-sec spray (0.266 g)	2	tr	0	0	—
Pam Butter	1-sec spray (0.266 g)	2	tr	0	0	—
Pam Olive Oil	1-sec spray (0.266 g)	2	tr	0	0	—
Pam Pump	1-spray (0.43 g)	4	tr	0	0	—
Peanut (Hain)	1 tbsp	120	14	0	0	—
Peanut (Hollywood)	1 tbsp	120	14	0	0	—
Planters Peanut	1 tbsp	120	14	0	0	—
Planters Popcorn	1 tbsp	120	13	0	0	—
Pompeian	1 tbsp	130	14	—	—	—
Puritan	1 tbsp	120	14	—	—	—
Rice Bran (Hain)	1 tbsp	120	14	0	0	—
Safflower (Hain)	1 tbsp	120	14	0	0	—
Safflower (Hollywood)	1 tbsp	120	14	0	0	—
Safflower Hi-Oleic (Hain)	1 tbsp	120	14	0	0	—

FOOD	PORTION	CAL	FAT	SOD	CARB	FIB
Safflower Organic (Hain)	1 tbsp	120	14	0	0	—
Sesame (Hain)	1 tbsp	120	14	0	0	—
Smart Beat	1 tbsp	120	14	0	0	—
Smart Beat Canola	1 tbsp (14 g)	120	14	0	0	—
Soy (Hain)	1 tbsp	120	14	0	0	—
Sunflower Hain	1 tbsp	120	14	0	0	—
Sunflower (Hollywood)	1 tbsp	120	14	0	0	—
Sunflower Organic (Hain)	1 tbsp	120	14	0	0	—
Walnut (Hain)	1 tbsp	120	14	0	0	—
Weight Watchers Butter Spray	1-sec spray	2	tr	0	0	—
Weight Watchers Cooking Spray	1-sec spray	2	tr	0	0	—
Wesson						
Canola	1 tbsp	120	14	0	0	0
Corn	1 tbsp	120	14	0	0	0
Lite Cooking Spray	.5-sec spray	0	0	0	0	0
Olive	1 tbsp	120	14	0	0	0
Sunflower	1 tbsp	120	14	0	0	0
Vegetable	1 tbsp	120	14	0	0	0
almond	1 cup	1927	218	—	0	—
almond	1 tbsp	120	14	—	0	—
apricot kernel	1 cup	1927	218	—	0	—
apricot kernel	1 tbsp	120	14	—	0	—
avocado	1 cup	1927	218	—	0	—
avocado	1 tbsp	124	14	—	0	—
babassu palm	1 tbsp	120	14	—	0	—
canola	1 cup	1927	218	—	0	—
canola	1 tbsp	124	14	—	0	—
coconut	1 tbsp	117	14	—	0	—
corn	1 cup	1927	218	—	0	—
corn	1 tbsp	120	14	—	0	—
cottonseed	1 cup	1927	218	—	0	—
cottonseed	1 tbsp	120	14	—	0	—
cupu assu	1 tbsp	120	14	—	0	—
grapeseed	1 tbsp	120	14	—	0	—
hazelnut	1 cup	1927	218	—	0	—
hazelnut	1 tbsp	120	14	—	0	—
mustard	1 cup	1927	218	—	0	—
mustard	1 tbsp	124	14	—	0	—
oat	1 tbsp	120	14	—	0	—
olive	1 cup	1909	216	tr	0	—
olive	1 tbsp	119	14	0	0	—

FOOD	PORTION	CAL	FAT	SOD	CARB	FIB
palm	1 cup	1927	218	—	0	—
palm	1 tbsp	120	14	—	0	—
palm kernel	1 cup	1879	218	—	0	—
palm kernel	1 tbsp	117	14	—	0	—
peanut	1 cup	1909	216	tr	0	—
peanut	1 tbsp	119	14	tr	0	—
poppyseed	1 tbsp	120	14	—	0	—
pumpkin seed	3.5 oz	925	100	—	0	—
rice bran	1 tbsp	120	14	—	0	—
safflower	1 cup	1927	218	—	0	—
safflower	1 tbsp	120	14	—	0	—
sesame	1 tbsp	120	14	—	0	—
sheanut	1 tbsp	120	14	—	0	—
soybean	1 cup	1927	218	tr	0	—
soybean	1 tbsp	120	14	0	0	—
sunflower	1 cup	1927	218	—	0	—
sunflower	1 tbsp	120	14	—	0	—
teaseed	1 tbsp	120	14	—	0	—
tomatoseed	1 tbsp	120	14	—	0	—
vegetable soybean & cottonseed	1 cup	1927	218	—	0	—
vegetable soybean & cottonseed	1 tbsp	120	14	—	0	—
walnut	1 cup	1927	218	—	0	1
walnut	1 tbsp	120	14	—	0	—
wheat germ	1 tbsp	120	14	—	0	—
FISH OIL						
Cod Liver (Hain)	1 tbsp	120	14	0	0	—
Cod Liver Cherry (Hain)	1 tbsp	120	14	0	0	—
Cod Liver Mint (Hain)	1 tbsp	120	14	0	0	—
cod liver	1 tbsp	123	14	—	0	—
herring	1 tbsp	123	14	—	0	—
menhaden	1 tbsp	123	14	—	0	—
salmon	1 tbsp	123	14	—	0	—
sardine	1 tbsp	123	14	—	0	—
shark	3½ oz	945	100	—	0	—
whale	3½ oz	945	100	—	0	—

OKRA

CANNED

FOOD	PORTION	CAL	FAT	SOD	CARB	FIB
Cocktail Hot (Trappey's)	1 piece (1 oz)	8	tr	139	2	1
Cocktail Mild (Trappey's)	1 piece (1 oz)	9	tr	207	1	1

FOOD	PORTION	CAL	FAT	SOD	CARB	FIB
Creole Gumbo (Trappey's)	½ cup	25	0	—	—	—
Cut (Trappey's)	½ cup	25	0	—	—	—
Pickled McIlhenny	2 pieces (1 oz)	7	tr	18	1	1
FRESH						
raw	8 pods	36	tr	8	7	—
raw, sliced	½ cup	19	tr	4	4	—
sliced, cooked	½ cup	25	tr	4	6	—
sliced, cooked	8 pods	27	tr	5	6	—
FROZEN						
Breaded Okra Ore-Ida	3 oz	170	10	600	17	—
Cut (Hanover)	½ cup	25	0	—	—	—
Whole (Hanover)	½ cup	35	0	—	—	—
sliced, cooked	1 pkg (10 oz)	94	1	8	21	—
sliced, cooked	½ cup	34	tr	3	8	—

OLIVES

FOOD	PORTION	CAL	FAT	SOD	CARB	FIB
California Ripe	2 jumbo	188	9	—	—	—
California Ripe	3 sm	4	tr	29	tr	3
Olive Appetizer (Progresso)	½ cup	180	21	1600	6	—
Olive Condite (Progresso)	½ cup	130	14	870	5	—
Ripe Extra Large (S&W)	3.5 oz	163	18	760	1	—
Ripe Pitted Large (S&W)	3.5 oz	163	18	760	1	—
Salad Olives (Progresso)	½ cup	120	15	2400	1	—
Spanish Green (Tee Pee)	2 oz	98	10	—	1	—
green	3 extra lg	15	2	312	tr	tr
green	4 med	15	2	312	tr	tr
ripe	1 colossal	12	1	136	1	—
ripe	1 jumbo	7	1	75	tr	—
ripe	1 lg	5	tr	38	tr	tr
ripe	1 sm	4	tr	28	tr	tr

ONION
CANNED

FOOD	PORTION	CAL	FAT	SOD	CARB	FIB
Lightly Spiced Cocktail Onions (Vlasic)	1 oz	4	0	365	1	—
Whole Small (S&W)	½ cup	35	0	345	9	—
chopped	½ cup	21	tr	416	5	—
whole	1 (2.2 oz)	12	tr	234	3	—

FOOD	PORTION	CAL	FAT	SOD	CARB	FIB
DRIED						
flakes	1 tbsp	16	tr	1	4	—
powder	1 tsp	7	tr	1	2	—
FRESH						
Antioch Farms Vidalla	1 med	60	0	10	14	3
Dole	1 med	60	0	10	14	3
Dole Green Onions chopped	1 tbsp	2	tr	0	tr	tr
chopped, cooked	½ cup	47	tr	3	11	—
raw, chopped	1 tbsp	4	tr	0	1	tr
raw, chopped	½ cup	30	tr	2	7	—
scallions, raw, chopped	1 tbsp	2	tr	1	tr	tr
scallions, raw, sliced	½ cup	16	tr	8	4	1
welsh, raw	3.5 oz	34	tr	—	7	—
FROZEN						
Chopped (Ore-Ida)	2 oz	20	tr	5	4	—
Chopped (Southland)	2 oz	15	0	—	—	—
Crispy Onion Rings (Mrs. Paul's)	2.5 oz	190	12	230	19	—
Onion Ringers (Ore-Ida)	2 oz	150	9	90	17	—
Polybag Whole Small (Birds Eye)	½ cup	30	0	10	8	2
Small With Cream Sauce (Birds Eye)	½ cup	100	3	340	12	1
chopped, cooked	1 tbsp	4	tr	2	1	—
chopped, cooked	½ cup	30	tr	12	7	—
rings	7 (2.5 oz)	285	19	263	27	—
rings, cooked	2 (0.7 oz)	81	5	75	8	—
whole, cooked	3.5 oz	28	tr	8	7	—
TAKE-OUT						
rings, breaded & fried	8 to 9	275	16	430	31	—
OPOSSUM						
roasted	3 oz	188	9	—	0	—
ORANGE						
CANNED						
Mandarin (Empress)	5.5 oz	100	0	10	25	—
Mandarin From Japan (Empress)	5.5 oz	35	0	—	8	—
Mandarin Natural Style (S&W)	½ cup	60	0	10	15	—

FOOD	PORTION	CAL	FAT	SOD	CARB	FIB
Mandarin Segments (Dole)	½ cup	70	tr	10	19	—
Mandarin Selected Sections in Heavy Syrup (S&W)	½ cup	76	0	10	20	—
Mandarin Unsweetened (S&W)	½ cup	28	0	10	7	—
Pineapple Mandarin Segments (Dole)	½ cup	60	tr	5	15	—
FRESH						
Dole	1	50	0	0	13	6
california valencia	1	59	tr	0	14	3
california navel	1	65	tr	1	16	3
florida	1	69	tr	1	17	4
peel	1 tbsp	6	tr	0	2	—
sections	1 cup	85	tr	0	21	4
JUICE						
BAMA	8.45 fl oz	120	0	60	29	—
Bright & Early Chilled	8 fl oz	120	0	30	30	—
Bright & Early Frozen	8 fl oz	120	0	10	30	—
Hawaiian Punch	6 oz	100	0	—	—	—
Hi-C	1 can (11.5 fl oz)	180	0	40	45	—
Hi-C	8 fl oz	130	0	25	32	—
Hi-C Box	8.45 fl oz	130	0	30	33	—
Juice Works	6 oz	90	0	—	—	—
Kool-Aid Koolers	1 (8.45 oz)	115	0	2	30	—
Kool-Aid Orange	8 oz	98	0	—	25	—
Kool-Aid Sugar Sweetened Orange	8 oz	79	0	—	20	—
Libby's	6 oz	80	0	0	20	—
Minute Maid						
Box	8.45 fl oz	120	0	25	28	—
Calcium Rich Chilled	8 fl oz	120	0	25	27	—
Calcium Rich Frozen	8 fl oz	120	0	0	27	—
Chilled	8 fl oz	110	0	25	27	—
Country Style Chilled	8 fl oz	110	0	25	27	—
Country Style Frozen	8 fl oz	110	0	0	27	—
Juices To Go	1 bottle (10 fl oz)	110	0	25	27	—
Juices To Go	1 bottle (16 fl oz)	160	0	35	39	—

FOOD	PORTION	CAL	FAT	SOD	CARB	FIB
Minute Maid *(cont.)*						
Juices To Go	1 can (11.5 fl oz)	140	0	30	34	—
Orange Punch Box	8.45 fl oz	130	0	25	33	—
Premium Choice Chilled	8 fl oz	110	0	0	27	—
Pulp Free Chilled	8 fl oz	110	0	25	27	—
Pulp Free Frozen	8 fl oz	110	0	0	27	—
Reduced Acid Frozen	8 fl oz	110	0	0	27	—
Mott's Orange Fruit Juice Blend	10 oz	144	0	—	—	—
Mott's Orange Fruit Juice Blend	9.5 oz	139	0	—	—	—
Ocean Spray	8 fl oz	120	0	35	31	0
S&W 100% Unsweetened	½ cup	83	0	2	18	—
S&W 100% Unsweetened	6 oz	83	0	2	18	—
Sippin' Pak 100% Pure	8.45 fl oz	110	0	25	26	—
Sipps Orange	8.45 oz	130	0	—	—	—
Tang Breakfast Crystals Sugar Free, as prep	6 oz	5	0	2	0	—
Tang Breakfast Crystals, as prep	6 oz	86	0	1	22	—
Tang Fruit Box	8.45 oz	127	0	1	31	—
Tree Top	6 oz	90	0	5	22	—
Veryfine 100%	8 oz	121	0	<10	24	—
Veryfine Orange Drink	8 oz	140	0	<70	33	—
canned	1 cup	104	tr	6	25	—
chilled	1 cup	110	1	2	25	—
fresh	1 cup	111	tr	2	26	—
frzn, as prep	1 cup	112	tr	2	27	1
frzn, not prep	6 oz	339	tr	7	81	2
mandarin orange	3.5 oz	47	tr	—	10	—
orange drink	6 oz	94	0	31	24	—

ORANGE EXTRACT

Virginia Dare	1 tsp	22	0	—	—	—

OREGANO

ground	1 tsp	5	tr	tr	1	—

ORGAN MEATS
see BRAINS, GIBLETS, GIZZARDS, HEART, KIDNEY, LIVER, SWEETBREADS

FOOD	PORTION	CAL	FAT	SOD	CARB	FIB

ORIENTAL FOOD
see also DINNER, NOODLES, RICE

CANNED

Chun King Divider Pak

FOOD	PORTION	CAL	FAT	SOD	CARB	FIB
Beef Chow Mein	7 oz	100	2	—	—	—
Beef Chow Mein	8 oz	110	2	—	—	—
Beef Pepper Oriental	7 oz	110	4	—	—	—
Chicken Chow Mein	7 oz	110	4	—	—	—
Chicken Chow Mein	8 oz	120	4	—	—	—
Pork Chow Mein Mein	7 oz	120	4	—	—	—
Shrimp Chow Mein	7 oz	100	2	—	—	—

Chun King Stir Fry Entree

FOOD	PORTION	CAL	FAT	SOD	CARB	FIB
Chow Mein w/ Beef	6 oz	290	19	—	—	—
Chow Mein w/ Chicken	6 oz	220	11	—	—	—
Egg Foo Young	5 oz	140	8	—	—	—
Pepper Steak	6 oz	250	17	—	—	—
Sukiyaki	6 oz	290	19	—	—	—

La Choy Bi-Pack

FOOD	PORTION	CAL	FAT	SOD	CARB	FIB
Beef Pepper	¾ cup	80	2	950	10	2
Chow Mein Chicken	¾ cup	80	3	970	8	1
Chow Mein Pork	¾ cup	80	4	950	7	2
Chow Mein Shrimp	¾ cup	70	1	860	6	1
Sweet & Sour Chicken	¾ cup	120	2	440	18	2
Teriyaki Chicken	¾ cup	85	2	850	8	1
La Choy Dinner Chow Mein Chicken	¾ pkg	300	17	1800	29	2

La Choy Entree

FOOD	PORTION	CAL	FAT	SOD	CARB	FIB
Beef Pepper Oriental	¾ cup	100	4	1340	12	2
Chow Mein Beef	¾ cup	40	2	960	5	2
Chow Mein Chicken	¾ cup	70	4	850	2	4
Chow Mein Meatless	¾ cup	25	tr	860	5	2
Chow Mein Shrimp	¾ cup	35	1	940	4	2
Sweet And Sour Chicken	¾ cup	240	2	1420	47	1
Sweet And Sour Pork	¾ cup	250	4	1540	48	1
chow mein chicken	1 cup	95	tr	725	18	—

FRESH

FOOD	PORTION	CAL	FAT	SOD	CARB	FIB
Won Ton Wraps (Azumaya)	1 (8 g)	23	tr	50	5	—

FOOD	PORTION	CAL	FAT	SOD	CARB	FIB
egg roll wrapper	1	83	tr	162	16	—
wonton wrappers	1	23	tr	46	5	—
FROZEN						
Benihana Oriental Lites Chicken in Spicy Garlic Sauce	9 oz	270	4	—	—	—
Birds Eye						
Chicken Teriyaki Easy Recipe, not prep	½ pkg	160	4	600	28	4
Chinese Stir Fry Internationals, not prep	3.3 oz	35	0	125	6	2
Japanese Stir Fry Internationals, not prep	3.3 oz	30	0	310	6	2
Oriental Beef Easy Recipe, not prep	½ pkg	100	7	620	11	8
Chun King						
Beef Pepper Oriental	13 oz	319	3	1300	53	—
Chicken Chow Mein	13 oz	370	6	1560	53	—
Cruncky Walnut Chicken	13 oz	310	5	1700	49	—
Egg Rolls Chicken	1 (3.6 oz)	220	8	600	32	—
Egg Rolls Meat & Shrimp	1 (3.6 oz)	220	8	680	31	—
Egg Rolls Shrimp	1 (3.6 oz)	200	6	480	31	—
Fried Rice w/ Chicken	8 oz	260	4	1460	41	—
Fried Rice w/ Pork	8 oz	270	6	1210	44	—
Imperial Chicken	13 oz	300	1	1540	54	—
Restaurant Style Egg Rolls Pork	1 (3 oz)	180	6	450	23	—
Sweet & Sour Pork	13 oz	400	5	1460	78	—
Dining Light Chicken Chow Mein	9 oz	180	2	650	31	—
Healthy Choice Chicken Chow Mein	8.5 oz	220	3	440	31	—
La Choy Restaurant Style						
Egg Roll Pork	1 (3 oz)	150	5	480	20	—
Egg Roll Shrimp	1 (3 oz)	130	4	260	19	—
Egg Roll Almond Chicken	1 (3 oz)	120	3	290	19	—

FOOD	PORTION	CAL	FAT	SOD	CARB	FIB
Egg Roll Sweet & Sour Chicken	1 (3 oz)	150	4	280	24	—
La Choy Snack Egg Roll						
Chicken	1 (1.45 oz)	90	3	140	12	—
Lobster	1 (1.45 oz)	75	2	150	12	—
Meat & Shrimp	1 (1.45 oz)	80	3	115	11	—
Shrimp	1 (1.45 oz)	75	2	120	12	—
Lean Cuisine Chicken Chow Mein With Rice	1 pkg (9 oz)	210	5	510	28	2
Stir Fry Kit With Yoshida Oriental Sauce Tyson	10.6 oz	330	10	1740	37	—
Stouffer's Chicken Chow Mein With Rice	1 pkg (10.6 oz)	260	4	940	43	3
Stouffer's Chicken Oriental	1 pkg (9.75 oz)	320	9	930	45	2
Stouffer's Teriyaki Stir-Fry	1 pkg (9 oz)	260	5	550	39	4
Tyson Sweet & Sour Kit With Sweet & Sour Sauce	14.85 oz	440	9	1300	71	—
Worthington Vegetarian Egg Rolls (Worthington)	1 (85 g)	160	6	530	20	—
HOME RECIPE						
chop suey w/ beef & pork	1 cup	300	17	1053	13	—
chow mein chicken	1 cup	255	10	718	10	—
MIX						
Kikkoman Chow Mein Seasoning	1½ oz pkg	98	tr	—	—	—
Kikkoman Teriyaki Baste & Glaze	1 tbsp	24	tr	310	5	—
La Choy Dinner Classics Egg Foo Young	2 patties + 3 oz sauce	170	7	1390	20	1
La Choy Dinner Classics Pepper Steak	¾ cup	180	9	760	9	1
La Choy Dinner Classics Sweet & Sour	¾ cup	310	6	860	30	tr

FOOD	PORTION	CAL	FAT	SOD	CARB	FIB
TAKE-OUT						
chicken teriyaki	¾ cup	399	27	2190	7	—
chop suey w/ pork	1 cup	375	29	1378	29	2
chow mein pork	1 cup	425	24	1673	21	3
chow mein shrimp	1 cup	221	10	1658	21	3
fried rice	6.6 oz	249	6	—	48	2
fried rice w/ egg	6.7 oz	395	20	—	49	2
wonton soup	1 cup	205	3	322	26	1
wonton, fried	½ cup (1 oz)	111	8	147	8	1

OYSTERS
CANNED

FOOD	PORTION	CAL	FAT	SOD	CARB	FIB
Bumble Bee Whole	½ cup (3.5 oz)	100	4	490	6	0
Empress Whole	4 oz	100	4	390	8	—
S&W Fancy Whole	2 oz	95	3	—	4	—
eastern	1 cup	170	6	277	10	—
eastern	3 oz	58	2	95	3	—
FRESH						
eastern, cooked	3 oz	117	4	190	7	—
eastern, cooked	6 med	58	2	94	3	—
eastern, raw	1 cup	170	6	277	10	—
eastern, raw	6 med	58	2	94	3	—
pacific, raw	1 med	41	1	53	2	—
pacific, raw	3 oz	69	2	90	4	—
steamed	1 med	41	1	53	2	—
steamed	3 oz	138	4	180	8	—
FROZEN						
Carnation Jumbo or Extra Select Breaded Oysters (King & Prince)	3.5 oz	130	2	—	—	—
TAKE-OUT						
battered & fried	6 (4.9 oz)	368	18	677	40	—
breaded & fried	6 (4.9 oz)	368	18	677	40	—
eastern, breaded & fried	3 oz	167	11	355	10	—
eastern, breaded & fried	6 med (88 g)	173	11	367	10	—
oysters rockefeller	3 oysters	66	2	80	5	—
stew	1 cup	278	18	928	15	tr

PANCAKE/WAFFLE SYRUP
see also SYRUP

FOOD	PORTION	CAL	FAT	SOD	CARB	FIB
Alaga Breakfast	2 tbsp	108	0	—	—	—
Alaga Butter Lite	2 tbsp	54	0	—	—	—

FOOD	PORTION	CAL	FAT	SOD	CARB	FIB
Alaga Honey Flavor	2 tbsp	124	0	—	—	—
Alaga Lite	2 tbsp	54	0	—	—	—
Aunt Jemima	2 tbsp	110	0	30	27	—
Aunt Jemima Butter Lite	2 tbsp	50	0	90	13	—
Aunt Jemima Lite	2 tbsp	50	0	90	13	—
Brer Rabbit Dark	2 tbsp	120	0	0	31	—
Brer Rabbit Light	2 tbsp	120	0	0	31	—
Estee	1 tbsp	8	0	35	1	—
Golden Griddle	1 cup (321 g)	885	0	225	229	—
Golden Griddle	1 tbsp (20 g)	50	0	55	14	—
Karo	1 tbsp (21 g)	60	0	35	15	—
Log Cabin Country Kitchen	1 oz	103	0	22	27	—
Log Cabin Lite	1 oz	49	0	92	13	—
Tastee	2 tbsp	121	0	—	—	—
Tastee Maple	2 tbsp	113	0	—	—	—
Weight Watchers	1 tbsp	25	0	40	7	—
Whitfield White Label	2 tbsp	121	0	—	—	—
Whitfield Yellow Label	2 tbsp	125	0	—	—	—
Whitfield Yellow Label Butter Flavor	2 tbsp	117	0	—	—	—
Whitfield Yellow Label Maple Flavor	2 tbsp	117	0	—	—	—
low calorie	1 tbsp	12	0	—	3	0
maple	2 tbsp	122	0	19	32	—

PANCAKES
FROZEN

FOOD	PORTION	CAL	FAT	SOD	CARB	FIB
Blueberry (Aunt Jemima)	3.48 oz	220	4	826	42	2
Blueberry (Downyflake)	3	290	9	920	48	—
Blueberry (Kid Cuisine)	3.47 oz	210	9	410	25	—
Blueberry Microwave (Pillsbury)	3	250	4	540	49	—
Buttermilk						
(Aunt Jemima)	3.48 oz	210	3	860	41	—
(Downyflake)	3	280	9	920	45	—
(Kid Cuisine)	4.17 oz	180	4	410	31	—
(Weight Watchers)	2 (2.5 oz)	140	3	270	22	—
Batter, as prep (Aunt Jemima)	3.6 oz	180	2	778	36	2
Microwave (Pillsbury)	3	260	4	590	51	—

FOOD	PORTION	CAL	FAT	SOD	CARB	FIB
Harvest Wheat Microwave (Pillsbury)	3	240	4	420	48	—
Lite Buttermilk (Aunt Jemima)	3.48 oz	140	3	660	28	—
Lite Pancakes & Lite Links (Quaker)	1 pkg (6 oz)	310	10	970	43	—
Lite Pancakes & Lite Syrup (Quaker)	1 pkg (6 oz)	260	3	860	53	—
Original (Aunt Jemima)	3.48 oz	211	4	801	40	2
Original Microwave (Pillsbury)	3	240	4	550	47	—
Original Batter, as prep (Aunt Jemima)	3.6 oz	183	2	763	37	2
Pancakes & Sausages (Quaker)	1 pkg (6 oz)	420	16	1140	57	—
Pancakes And Sausages (Downyflake)	1 pkg (5.5 oz)	430	23	1170	47	—
Pancakes And Sausages (Great Starts)	6 oz	460	22	920	52	—
Pancakes With Bacon (Great Starts)	4½ oz	400	20	1000	43	—
Pancakes w/ LeanLinks (Healthy Starts)	6 oz	360	8	490	48	—
Pancakes/Links (Morningstar Farms)	1 pkg (4 oz)	240	8	700	31	—
Pancakes With Links (Weight Watchers)	4 oz	220	10	—	21	—
Regular (Downyflake)	3	280	9	920	45	—
Rolled Pancakes w/ Apples (Kid Cuisine)	3.85 oz	210	7	310	30	—
Silver Dollar Pancakes And Sausage (Great Starts)	3¾ oz	310	14	680	37	—
Whole Wheat Pancakes With Lite Links (Great Starts)	5.5 oz	350	16	600	39	—
buttermilk	1 4-in diam (1.3 oz)	83	1	183	16	—
plain	1 4-in diam (1.3 oz)	83	1	183	16	—
HOME RECIPE						
blueberry	1 (4-in diam)	84	4	157	11	—

FOOD	PORTION	CAL	FAT	SOD	CARB	FIB
plain	1 (4-in diam)	86	4	157	11	—
MIX						
Apple Cinnamon Shake 'N Pour Bisquick	3 (4-in diam)	240	3	880	47	—
Bluberry (Hungry Jack)	3 (4-in diam)	320	15	820	41	—
Blueberry Shake 'N Pour (Bisquick)	3 (4-in diam)	270	3	840	54	—
Buckwheat (Hodgson Mill)	⅓ cup (1.8 oz)	160	1	550	35	1
Buckwheat Pancake & Waffle Mix (Aunt Jemima)	3 (4-in diam)	230	8	820	35	5
Buttermilk						
(Betty Crocker)	3 (4-in diam)	280	10	810	39	—
(Hungry Jack)	3 (4-in diam)	240	11	820	29	—
Complete (Hungry Jack)	3 (4-in diam)	180	1	710	39	—
Complete Packets (Hungry Jack)	3 (4-in diam)	180	3	680	35	—
Complete Pancake & Waffle Mix (Aunt Jemima)	3 (4-in diam)	230	3	950	46	2
Pancake & Waffle Mix (Aunt Jemima)	3 (4-in diam)	220	8	760	30	1
Shake 'N Pour (Bisquick)	3 (4-in diam)	250	3	880	49	—
Complete Pancake & Waffle Mix (Aunt Jemima)	3 (4-in diam)	250	4	1020	50	2
Extra Lights (Hungry Jack)	3 (4-in diam)	210	7	490	30	—
Extra Lights Complete (Hungry Jack)	3 (4-in diam)	190	2	700	37	—
Fast Shake Blueberry (Little Crow)	1 serving (2.5 oz)	251	3	685	50	—
Fast Shake Buttermilk (Little Crow)	1 serving (2.5 oz)	258	3	770	50	—
Fast Shake Original (Little Crow)	1 serving (2.5 oz)	266	4	738	50	—
Multigrain Pancake & Waffle Mix (Arrowhead)	¼ cup (1.2 oz)	120	1	260	24	3
Original Pancake & Waffle Mix (Aunt Jemima)	3 (4-in diam)	200	7	660	28	1

FOOD	PORTION	CAL	FAT	SOD	CARB	FIB
Original Shake 'N Pour (Bisquick)	3 (4-in diam)	250	3	880	49	—
Pancake Mix (Estee)	3 (3-in) pancakes	100	0	135	21	—
Pancake Mix, not prep (Health Valley)	1 oz	100	1	170	20	3
Panshakes (Hungry Jack)	3 (4-in diam)	250	6	880	43	—
Whole Wheat Pancake & Waffle Mix (Aunt Jemima)	3 (4-in diam)	270	9	950	38	4
buckwheat	1 (4-in diam)	62	2	160	9	—
buttermilk	1 4-in diam (1.3 oz)	74	1	239	14	tr
plain	1 4-in diam (1.3 oz)	74	1	239	14	tr
sugar free, low sodium	1 (3-in diam)	44	tr	58	9	—
whole wheat	1 (4-in diam)	92	3	252	13	—
TAKE-OUT						
buckwheat	1 (4-in diam)	55	2	125	6	—
potato	1 (4-in diam)	78	6	238	4	tr
w/ butter & syrup	3	519	14	1103	91	—

PANCREAS
see SWEETBREADS

PAPAYA
FRESH

Papaya Produce Marketing Assoc	½	80	0	—	—	—
cubed	1 cup	54	tr	4	14	—
papaya	1	117	tr	8	30	—
JUICE						
Goya Nectar	6 oz	110	0	10	27	—
Kern's Nectar	6 oz	110	0	10	28	—
Libby's Nectar	6 oz	110	0	10	28	—
nectar	1 cup	142	tr	14	36	—

PAPRIKA

paprika	1 tsp	6	tr	1	1	—

PARSLEY

Dole, chopped	1 tbsp	10	tr	4	1	tr
dry	1 tbsp	1	tr	2	tr	—
dry	1 tsp	1	tr	1	tr	—
fresh, chopped	½ cup	11	tr	17	2	—

FOOD	PORTION	CAL	FAT	SOD	CARB	FIB
PARSNIPS						
FRESH						
cooked	1 (5.6 oz)	130	tr	17	31	—
cooked, sliced	½ cup	63	tr	8	15	—
raw, sliced	½ cup	50	tr	7	12	—
PASSION FRUIT						
purple	1	18	tr	5	4	—
JUICE						
purple	1 cup	126	tr	—	34	—
yellow	1 cup	149	tr	15	36	—
PASTA						
see also NOODLES, PASTA DINNERS, PASTA SALAD						
DRY						
Acini de Pepe (San Giorgio)	2 oz	210	1	—	—	—
Alphabets (P&R)	2 oz	210	1	—	—	—
Alphabets (San Giorgio)	2 oz	210	1	—	—	—
Alphabets (Skinner)	2 oz	210	1	—	—	—
Baby Pastina (San Giorgio)	2 oz	210	1	—	—	—
Bows Medium & Small (P&R)	2 oz	220	3	—	—	—
Capellini (Delmonico)	2 oz	210	1	—	—	—
Capellini (P&R)	2 oz	210	1	—	—	—
Capellini (Pomi)	2 oz	210	1	<5	41	—
Capellini (San Giorgio)	2 oz	210	1	—	—	—
Dinosaurs (Mueller's)	2 oz (57 g)	210	1	3	42	—
Ditalini (San Giorgio)	2 oz	210	1	—	—	—
Egg (Prince)	2 oz	221	3	3	40	1
Elbow Macaroni (Delmonico)	2 oz	210	1	—	—	—
Elbow Macaroni (San Giorgio)	2 oz	210	1	—	—	—
Elbow Macaroni (Skinner)	2 oz	210	1	—	—	—
Elbow Macaroni Regular & Large (P&R)	2 oz	210	1	—	—	—
Elbow Macaroni, not prep (Creamette)	2 oz	210	1	5	42	—
Elbow Spaghetti (Delmonico)	2 oz	210	1	—	—	—

FOOD	PORTION	CAL	FAT	SOD	CARB	FIB
Elbow Style (Weight Watchers)	2 oz	160	1	35	30	—
Elbows (Ronzoni)	¾ cup (2 oz)	210	1	0	40	—
Fettuccini (P&R)	2 oz	210	1	—	—	—
Fettucini (Ronzoni)	¾ cup (2 oz)	210	1	0	40	—
Fettucini (Skinner)	2 oz	210	1	—	—	—
Fetuccini Egg (P&R)	2 oz	220	3	—	—	—
Fideo Enrollacio (Skinner)	2 oz	210	1	—	—	—
Flakes (San Giorgio)	2 oz	210	1	—	—	—
Fusilli (Ronzoni)	¾ cup (2 oz)	210	1	0	40	—
Fusilli Cut (San Giorgio)	2 oz	210	1	—	—	—
Fusilli Cut (P&R)	2 oz	210	1	—	—	—
Jungle Animals (Mueller's)	2 oz (57 g)	210	1	3	42	—
Kluski (San Giorgio)	2 oz	220	3	—	—	—
Lasagna						
(Delmonico)	2 oz	210	1	—	—	—
(Skinner)	2 oz	210	1	—	—	—
Jumbo (P&R)	2 oz	210	1	—	—	—
No Boil (DeFino)	1 oz	102	tr	2	20	—
Spinach Whole Wheat (Health Valley)	2 oz	170	1	15	40	7
Whole Wheat (Health Valley)	2 oz	170	1	10	40	7
Lasagne (Mueller's)	2 oz (57 g)	210	1	4	42	—
Lasagne (Ronzoni)	¾ cup (2 oz)	210	1	0	40	—
Linguini (P&R)	2 oz	210	1	—	—	—
Linguini (San Giorgio)	2 oz	210	1	—	—	—
Linguini (Skinner)	2 oz	210	1	—	—	—
Linguini Egg (Creamette)	2 oz	221	3	—	—	—
Manicotti (P&R)	2 oz	210	1	—	—	—
Manicotti (Ronzoni)	¾ cup (2 oz)	210	1	0	40	—
Manicotti (San Giorgio)	2 oz	210	1	—	—	—
Manicotti (Skinner)	2 oz	210	1	—	—	—
Monsters (Mueller's)	2 oz (57 g)	210	1	3	42	—
Mostaccioli (Delmonico)	2 oz	210	1	—	—	—
Mostaccioli (Ronzoni)	¾ cup (2 oz)	210	1	0	40	—
Mostaccioli (Skinner)	2 oz	210	1	—	—	—
Mostaccioli Rigati (San Giorgio)	2 oz	210	1	—	—	—

FOOD	PORTION	CAL	FAT	SOD	CARB	FIB
Orzo (San Giorgio)	2 oz	210	1	—	—	—
Outer Space (Mueller's)	2 oz	210	1	3	42	—
Pasta						
(Anthony)	2 oz	210	1	0	42	tr
(Gioia)	2 oz	210	1	0	42	tr
(Golden Grain)	2 oz	203	1	26	41	0
(Luxury)	2 oz	210	1	0	42	tr
(Merlino's)	2 oz	210	1	0	42	tr
(Penn Dutch)	2 oz	210	1	0	42	tr
(Prince)	2 oz	210	1	0	42	tr
(Red Cross)	2 oz	210	1	0	42	tr
(Ronco)	2 oz	210	1	0	42	tr
(Vimco)	2 oz	210	1	0	42	tr
Perciatelli (P&R)	2 oz	210	1	—	—	—
Perciatelli (San Giorgio)	2 oz	210	1	—	—	—
Pot Pie Bows (San Giorgio)	2 oz	220	3	—	—	—
Pot Pie Squares (San Giorgio)	2 oz	220	3	—	—	—
Racing Wheels (San Giorgio)	2 oz	210	1	—	—	—
Rainbow (Prince)	2 oz	210	1	5	42	1
Ribbon Pasta Whole Wheat (Pritikin)	2 oz	220	2	—	—	—
Ribbons No Boil (DeFino)	2 oz	204	2	3	40	—
Rigatoni (Delmonico)	2 oz	210	1	—	—	—
Rigatoni (Ronzoni)	¾ cup (2 oz)	210	1	0	40	—
Rigatoni (San Giorgio)	2 oz	210	1	—	—	—
Rigatoni (Skinner)	2 oz	210	1	—	—	—
Rings (P&R)	2 oz	210	1	—	—	—
Rippled Lasagna (San Giorgio)	2 oz	210	1	—	—	—
Ripplets (Skinner)	2 oz	210	1	—	—	—
Rotelle (Creamette)	2 oz	210	1	—	—	—
Rotelle, uncooked (Ronzoni)	¾ cup (2 oz)	210	1	0	40	—
Rotini (Delmonico)	2 oz	210	1	—	—	—
Rotini (San Giorgio)	2 oz	210	1	—	—	—
Rotini, uncooked (Ronzoni)	¾ cup (2 oz)	210	1	0	40	—
Rotini Rainbow (Creamette)	2 oz	210	1	—	—	—

FOOD	PORTION	CAL	FAT	SOD	CARB	FIB
Shell Macaroni (Skinner)	2 oz	210	1	—	—	—
Shells, uncooked (Ronzoni)	¾ cup (2 oz)	210	1	0	40	—
Shells Jumbo (P&R)	2 oz	210	1	—	—	—
Shells Jumbo (Ronzoni)	¾ cup (2 oz)	210	1	0	40	—
Shells Large Medium & Small (P&R)	2 oz	210	1	—	—	—
Shells Large Medium Small & Jumbo (San Giorgio)	2 oz	210	1	—	—	—
Shells Regular & Jumbo (Delmonico)	2 oz	210	1	—	—	—
Spaghetti						
Amaranth (Health Valley)	2 oz	170	1	10	40	9
(Delmonico)	2 oz	210	1	—	—	—
(Mueller's)	2 oz (57 g)	210	1	3	42	—
(San Giorgio)	2 oz	210	1	—	—	—
(Skinner)	2 oz	210	1	—	—	—
Regular & Thin (P&R)	2 oz	210	1	—	—	—
Spinach Whole Wheat (Health Valley)	2 oz	170	1	15	40	7
Whole Wheat Spinach, uncooked (Hodgson Mill)	2 oz	190	2	25	35	5
uncooked (Ronzoni)	¾ cup (2 oz)	210	1	0	40	—
Spaghetti Egg (Creamette)	2 oz	221	3	—	—	—
Spaghetti Oat Bran (Health Valley)	2 oz	120	1	2	23	4
Spaghetti Thin (Creamette)	2 oz	210	1	—	—	—
Spaghetti Wheels (Hanover)	½ cup	90	0	—	—	—
Spaghetti Whole Wheat (Health Valley)	2 oz	170	1	10	40	7
Spaghetti Whole Wheat (Pritikin)	2 oz	220	2	—	—	—
Spaghetti, not prep (Creamette)	2 oz	210	1	5	42	—

FOOD	PORTION	CAL	FAT	SOD	CARB	FIB
Spaghettini (Delmonico)	2 oz	210	1	—	—	—
Spaghettini (San Giorgio)	2 oz	210	1	—	—	—
Spaghettini (Weight Watchers)	2 oz	160	1	35	30	—
Spinach Egg (Prince)	2 oz	220	3	65	40	1
Spinach Ribbons, not prep (Creamette)	2 oz	210	1	70	42	—
Teddy Bears (Mueller's)	2 oz (57 g)	210	1	3	42	—
Tubettini (Ronzoni)	¾ cup (2 oz)	210	1	0	40	—
Tubettini (San Giorgio)	2 oz	210	1	—	—	—
Twirls (Skinner)	2 oz	210	1	—	—	—
Twists Tri Color (Mueller's)	2 oz (57 g)	210	1	10	41	—
Veggie Bows, uncooked (Hodgson Mill)	2 oz	200	1	15	41	1
Veggie Rotini, uncooked (Hodgson Mill)	2 oz	200	1	15	41	1
Veggie Wagon Wheels, uncooked (Hodgson Mill)	2 oz	200	1	15	41	1
Vermicelli (Delmonico)	2 oz	210	1	—	—	—
Veremicelli (P&R)	2 oz	210	1	—	—	—
Vermicelli (San Giorgio)	2 oz	210	1	—	—	—
Vermicelli (Skinner)	2 oz	210	1	—	—	—
Whole Wheat Spirals, uncooked (Hodgson Mill)	2 oz	190	1	10	34	6
Ziti (Creamette)	2 oz	210	1	—	—	—
Ziti Cut (Delmonico)	2 oz	210	1	—	—	—
Ziti Cut (San Giorgio)	2 oz	210	1	—	—	—
corn, cooked	1 cup	176	1	1	39	—
elbows	1 cup	389	2	8	78	—
elbows, cooked	1 cup	197	tr	1	40	—
protein-fortified, cooked	1 cup	188	tr	6	36	—
shells	1 cup	389	2	4	78	—
shells, cooked	1 cup	197	tr	1	40	—
spaghetti	2 oz	211	tr	4	43	—

FOOD	PORTION	CAL	FAT	SOD	CARB	FIB
spaghetti, cooked	1 cup	197	tr	1	40	—
spaghetti, protein-fortified, cooked	1 cup	229	tr	7	44	—
spinach spaghetti	2 oz	212	tr	20	43	—
spinach spaghetti, cooked	1 cup	183	tr	20	37	—
spirals	1 cup	389	2	8	78	—
spirals, cooked	1 cup	197	tr	1	40	—
vegetable	1 cup	308	tr	36	63	—
vegetable, cooked	1 cup	171	tr	9	36	—
whole wheat	1 cup	365	1	8	79	—
whole wheat spaghetti	2 oz	198	tr	5	43	—
whole wheat spaghetti, cooked	1 cup	174	tr	4	37	—
whole wheat, cooked	1 cup (4.9 oz)	174	tr	4	37	—
FRESH						
Angel's Hair (Contadina)	1¼ cup (2.8 oz)	240	3	30	43	2
Fettuccine (Contadina)	1¼ cup (2.9 oz)	250	4	30	45	2
Fettuccine Cholesterol Free (Contadina)	1 cup (2.9 oz)	240	3	16	46	2
Linguine (Contadina)	1¼ cup (3 oz)	260	4	30	47	2
Linguine Cholesterol Free (Contadina)	1¼ cup (3.1 oz)	250	3	20	49	2
Ravioli Beef And Garlic (Contadina)	1¼ cup (4 oz)	350	14	350	39	3
Ravioli Cheese (Contadina)	1 cup (3.1 oz)	280	12	350	31	2
Ravioli Chicken And Rosemary (Contadina)	1¼ cup (4 oz)	330	12	420	43	3
Ravioli Light Cheese (Contadina)	1 cup (3.1 oz)	240	5	340	35	2
Ravioli Light Garden Vegetable (Contadina)	1¼ cup (3.8 oz)	290	6	370	43	3
Tagliatelli Spinach (Contadina)	1¼ cup (3.1 oz)	270	4	110	46	4
Tortelli Spinach Three Cheese (Contadina)	¾ cup (3.1 oz)	280	5	380	38	3
Tortellini (Contadina)						
Cheese	¾ cup (3 oz)	260	6	330	39	3
Cheese And Basil	1 cup (4 oz)	360	11	380	49	3
Chicken And Prosciutte	1 cup (3.8 oz)	360	13	440	46	3

FOOD	PORTION	CAL	FAT	SOD	CARB	FIB
Chicken And Vegetable	¾ cup (2.9 oz)	260	7	220	39	2
Light Garlic And Cheese	1 cup (3.6 oz)	280	5	390	50	3
Spicy Italian Sausage And Bell Pepper	1 cup (3.6 oz)	330	10	280	47	3
plain made w/ egg, cooked	2 oz	75	tr	3	14	—
spinach made w/ egg, cooked	2 oz	74	tr	3	14	—
HOME RECIPE						
made w/ egg, cooked	2 oz	74	tr	47	13	—
made w/o egg, cooked	2 oz	71	tr	42	14	—

PASTA DINNERS
see also DINNER, PASTA SALAD

CANNED
Chef Boyardee

FOOD	PORTION	CAL	FAT	SOD	CARB	FIB
ABC's & 1,2,3's In Cheese Flavor Sauce	7.5 oz	180	1	940	37	—
ABC's & 1,2,3's w/ Mini Meatballs	7.5 oz	260	11	1005	32	2
Beef Ravioli	7.5 oz	190	4	1160	31	2
Beefaroni	7.5 oz	220	7	1145	31	2
Cheese Ravioli In Meat Sauce	7.5 oz	200	3	1010	37	—
Dinosaurs In Cheese Flavor Sauce	7.5 oz	180	1	880	36	—
Dinosaurs w/ Meatballs	7.5 oz	240	9	900	32	4
Elbows in Beef Sauce	7.5 oz	210	7	1000	29	—
Lasagna	7.5 oz	230	9	1080	31	—
Lasagna In Garden Vegetable Sauce	7.5 oz	170	1	940	34	—
Macaroni & Cheese	7.5 oz	180	5	970	27	1
Microwave Main Meal Beans & Pasta	10.5 oz	200	1	1030	44	10
Micowave Main Meal Beef Ravioli Suprema	10.5 oz	290	4	1390	52	5
Microwave Main Meal Cheese Ravioli Suprema	10.5 oz	290	4	1360	52	5

FOOD	PORTION	CAL	FAT	SOD	CARB	FIB
Chef Boyardee *(cont.)*						
Microwave Main Meal Fettuccine	10.5 oz	290	9	1010	46	6
Microwave Main Meal Lasagna	10.5 oz	290	8	1000	41	5
Microwave Main Meal Meat Tortellini	10.5 oz	220	4	980	53	6
Microwave Main Meal Noodles w/ Chicken	10.5 oz	170	1	1120	27	3
Microwave Main Meal Peas & Pasta	10.5 oz	190	2	1020	39	6
Microwave Main Meal Spaghetti Suprema	10.5 oz	200	7	1000	37	7
Microwave Main Meal Zesty Macaroni	10.5 oz	290	8	1300	40	5
Microwave Main Meal Ziti In Sauce	10.5 oz	210	tr	1030	52	7
Pasta Rings & Meatballs	7.5 oz	220	8	990	33	4
Rigatoni	7.5 oz	210	6	1080	31	—
Rings & Franks	7.5 oz	190	5	980	31	3
Shells In Meat Sauce	7.5 oz	210	6	1090	32	—
Shells In Mushroom Sauce	7.5 oz	170	1	1080	35	—
Spaghetti & Meat Balls	7.5 oz	230	7	1060	29	—
Tic Tac Toes In Cheese Flavor Sauce	7.5 oz	170	1	930	36	3
Tic Tac Toes w/ Mini Meatballs	7.5 oz	250	10	1035	32	3
Turtles In Sauce	7.5 oz	160	1	870	33	2
Turtles w/ Meatballs	7.5 oz	210	8	990	30	2
Franco-American						
Beef RavioliO's In Meat Sauce	½ can (7.5 oz)	250	8	920	35	—
CircusO's Pasta In Tomato And Cheese Sauce	½ can (7.4 oz)	170	2	860	33	—
CircusO's Pasta With Meatballs In Tomato Sauce	½ can (7.4 oz)	210	8	950	25	—
Macaroni & Cheese	½ can (7.4 oz)	170	6	870	24	—

FOOD	PORTION	CAL	FAT	SOD	CARB	FIB
Spaghetti In Tomato Sauce w/ Cheese	½ can (7.4 oz)	180	2	840	36	—
Spaghetti w/ Meatballs In Tomato Sauce	½ can (7.4 oz)	220	8	870	28	—
SpaghettiO's With Meatballs	½ can (7.4 oz)	220	9	950	25	—
SpaghettiO's In Tomato & Cheese Sauce	½ can (7.4 oz)	170	2	860	33	—
SpaghettiO's w/ Sliced Franks	½ can (7.4 oz)	220	9	1000	26	—
SportyO's In Tomato & Cheese Sauce	½ can (7.5 oz)	170	2	860	33	—
SportyO's Pasta With Meatballs In Tomato Sauce	½ can (7.4 oz)	210	8	950	25	—
TeddyO's In Tomato & Cheese Sauce	½ can (7.5 oz)	170	2	900	33	—
TeddyO's Pasta With Meatballs	½ can (7.4 oz)	210	8	950	25	—
Healthy Choice Lasagna w/ Meat Sauce	½ can (7.5 oz)	220	5	530	29	—
Healthy Choice Spaghetti Rings	½ can (7.5 oz)	140	0	460	30	—
Healthy Choice Spaghetti w/ Meat Sauce	½ can (7.5 oz)	150	3	390	21	—
Van Camp's Spaghetti Weenee	1 cup	243	7	1128	35	—
DRY MIX						
Golden Grain Macaroni & Cheese	½ cup	310	15	620	36	—
Hain Pasta & Sauce						
Creamy Parmesan	¼ pkg	150	3	400	22	—
Creamy Swiss	¼ pkg	170	4	360	26	—
Fettuccine Alfredo	¼ pkg	180	4	420	27	—
Italian Herb	¼ pkg	110	2	160	17	—
Primavera	¼ pkg	140	4	430	20	—
Tangy Cheddar	¼ pkg	180	6	350	24	—
Kraft						
Dinomac Macaroni And Cheese Dinner	¾ cup	310	14	560	36	—

FOOD	PORTION	CAL	FAT	SOD	CARB	FIB
Kraft *(cont.)*						
Egg Noodle & Cheese Dinner	¾ cup	340	17	670	37	—
Macaroni & Cheese Deluxe Dinner	¾ cup	260	8	590	36	—
Macaroni & Cheese Dinner	¾ cup	290	13	530	34	—
Macaroni & Cheese Dinner Family Size	¾ cup	290	13	490	34	—
Mild American Style Spaghetti Dinner	1 cup	300	7	630	50	—
Pasta & Cheese Fettuccini Alfredo	½ cup	180	9	590	19	—
Pasta & Cheese 3-Cheese With Vegetables	½ cup	180	8	630	19	—
Pasta & Cheese Cheddar Broccoli	½ cup	180	8	620	19	—
Pasta & Cheese Chicken With Herbs	½ cup	170	7	550	21	—
Pasta & Cheese Parmesan	½ cup	180	8	630	19	—
Pasta & Cheese Sour Cream With Chives	½ cup	180	8	360	22	—
Spaghetti With Meat Sauce Dinner	1 cup	360	14	880	47	—
Spirals Macaroni & Cheese Dinner	¾ cup	340	18	600	36	—
Tangy Italian Style Spaghetti Dinner	1 cup	310	8	670	49	—
Teddy Bears Macaroni And Cheese Dinner	¾ cup	310	14	560	36	—
Wild Wheels Macaroni And Cheese Dinner	¾ cup	310	14	560	36	—
Lipton Pasta & Sauce						
Cheddar Broccoli	½ cup	132	2	458	24	—
Creamy Garlic	½ cup	146	2	447	26	—
Creamy Mushroom	½ cup	143	3	424	25	0
Herb Tomato	½ cup	130	1	356	26	—

FOOD	PORTION	CÁL	FAT	SOD	CARB	FIB
Minute Microwave Cheddar Cheese Broccoli and Pasta, as prep	½ cup	160	5	538	23	—
Terrazza Pasta E. Fagioli, as prep	½ cup	150	3	135	33	—
Ultra Slim-Fast Macaroni & Cheese	2.3 oz	230	3	770	46	4
Uncle Ben Country Inn						
Pasta And Sauce Angel Hair Parmesan	1 serv (2.2 oz)	245	5	926	39	3
Pasta And Sauce Broccoli & White Cheddar	1 serv (2.2 oz)	240	5	799	40	2
Pasta And Sauce Butter & Herb	1 serv (2 oz)	230	6	885	36	1
Pasta And Sauce Creamy Garlic	1 serv (2.4 oz)	261	5	599	45	2
Pasta And Sauce Fettuccine Alfredo	1 serv (2.2 oz)	310	6	656	41	2
Pasta And Sauce Herb Linguine	1 serv (2.2 oz)	240	3	654	43	2
Pasta And Sauce Mushroom Fettuccine	1 serv (2.2 oz)	250	6	638	41	2
Pasta And Sauce Vegetable Alfredo	1 serv (2.2 oz)	240	5	548	42	2
Velveeta Bits Of Bacon Shells And Cheese Dinner	½ cup	240	10	690	27	—
Velveeta Shells And Cheese Dinner	½ cup	210	8	170	25	—
Velveeta Touch of Mexico Shells And Cheese Dinner	½ cup	210	8	630	27	—
FROZEN						
Banquet						
Family Entree Chicken & Vegetable Primavera	7 oz	140	3	—	18	—
Lasagne w/ Meat Sauce	7 oz	270	10	—	30	—
Macaroni & Cheese	7 oz	240	8	1270	40	—

FOOD	PORTION	CAL	FAT	SOD	CARB	FIB
Banquet *(cont.)*						
Macaroni & Cheese	9 oz	260	11	—	28	—
Mostaccioli w/ Meat Sauce	7 oz	170	3	—	28	—
Spaghetti & Meat Sauce	8.75 oz	160	4	650	26	—
Banquet Cookin' Bag Chicken & Vegetables Primavera	4 oz	100	2	—	14	—
Banquet Entree Spaghetti w/ Meat Sauce	8.5 oz	220	8	1180	35	—
Birds Eye Easy Recipe Chicken Primavera, not prep	½ pkg	80	3	540	14	7
Birds Eye Easy Recipe Chicken Alfredo, not prep	½ pkg	160	7	430	22	3
Budget Gourmet						
Cheese Manicotti	1 pkg (10 oz)	440	24	740	36	—
Cheese Tortellini	1 pkg (5.5 oz)	200	8	530	25	—
Cheese Ravioli	1 pkg (9.5 oz)	290	13	750	34	—
Italian Sausage Lasagna	1 pkg (10 oz)	430	23	830	34	—
Lasagne With Meat Sauce	1 pkg (9.4 oz)	290	11	720	30	—
Linguini With Shrimp And Clams	1 pkg (10 oz)	270	9	1160	35	—
Linguini With Shrimp And Clams	1 pkg (9.5 oz)	280	10	710	34	—
Macaroni And Cheese	1 pkg (5.75 oz)	230	12	570	22	—
Macaroni And Cheese With Cheddar And Parmesan	1 pkg (10.5 oz)	330	8	760	49	—
Pasta Alfredo With Broccoli	1 pkg (5.5 oz)	210	10	630	22	—
Penne Pasta With Chunky Tomato Sauce And Italian Sausage	1 pkg (10 oz)	320	9	590	34	—
Rigatoni In Cream Sauce With Broccoli And Chicken	1 pkg (10.8 oz)	290	7	710	44	—

FOOD	PORTION	CAL	FAT	SOD	CARB	FIB
Spaghetti With Chunky Tomato And Meat Sauce	1 pkg (10 oz)	300	8	470	44	—
Three Cheese Lasagna	1 pkg (10 oz)	390	17	640	26	—
Vegetable Lasagna	1 pkg (10.5 oz)	390	10	770	36	—
Ziti In Marinara Sauce	1 pkg (6.25 oz)	200	9	600	23	—
Dining Light						
Cheese Cannelloni	9 oz	310	9	650	38	—
Cheese Lasagna	9 oz	260	6	800	36	—
Fettucini	9 oz	290	12	1020	33	—
Lasagna	9 oz	240	5	800	36	—
Spaghetti	9 oz	220	8	440	25	—
Green Giant						
Garden Gourmet Creamy Mushroom	1 pkg	220	11	860	29	3
Garden Gourmet Pasta Dijon	1 pkg	260	17	630	21	4
Garden Gourmet Pasta Florentine	1 pkg	230	9	840	27	4
Garden Gourmet Rotini Cheddar	1 pkg	230	10	570	32	5
One Serve Cheese Tortellini	1 pkg	260	9	660	37	—
One Serve Macaroni And Cheese	1 pkg	230	9	590	28	—
One Serve Pasta Marinara	1 pkg	180	5	440	29	—
One Serve Pasta Parmesan With Green Peas	1 pkg	170	5	510	23	—
Pasta Accents Creamy Cheddar	½ cup	100	5	310	12	—
Pasta Accents Garden Herb	½ cup	80	3	220	11	—
Pasta Accents Garlic Seasoning	½ cup	110	5	280	13	—
Pasta Accents Pasta Primavera	½ cup	110	5	180	13	—
Healthy Choice						
Baked Cheese Ravioli	9 oz	240	2	460	40	—
Cheese Manicotti	9.25 oz	230	4	450	34	—
Chicken Fettucini	8.5 oz	240	4	370	29	—

FOOD	PORTION	CAL	FAT	SOD	CARB	FIB
Healthy Choice (cónt.)						
Fettucini Alfredo	8 oz	240	7	370	36	—
Fettucini w/ Turkey and Vegetables	12.5 oz	350	6	480	45	—
Lasagna w/ Meat Sauce	10 oz	260	5	420	37	—
Linguini w/ Shrimp	9.5 oz	230	2	420	40	—
Macaroni & Cheese	9 oz	280	6	520	45	—
Pasta Primavera	11 oz	280	3	360	51	—
Pasta w/ Shrimp	12.5 oz	270	4	490	44	—
Rigatoni In Meat Sauce	9.5 oz	240	4	470	36	—
Rigatoni w/ Chicken	12.5 oz	360	4	430	50	—
Spaghetti w/ Meat Sauce	10 oz	280	6	480	42	—
Stuffed Pasta Shells in Tomato Sauce	12 oz	330	3	470	53	—
Teriyaki Pasta w/ Chicken	12.6 oz	350	3	370	58	—
Zesty Tomato Sauce over Ziti Pasta	12 oz	350	5	530	59	—
Zucchini Lasagna	11.5 oz	240	3	390	37	—
Kid Cuisine						
Macaroni & Cheese w/ Mini Franks	9 oz	360	15	920	48	—
Mega Meal Macaroni & Cheese	12.45 oz	470	13	1270	75	—
Mini-Cheese Ravioli	8.75 oz	290	8	780	51	—
Spaghetti w/ Meat Sauce	9.25 oz	310	8	760	50	—
Le Menu						
LightStyle 3-Cheese Stuffed Shells	10 oz	280	8	690	34	—
LightStyle Cheese Tortellini	10 oz	230	6	460	35	—
Manicotti With Three Cheeses	11.75 oz	390	15	870	44	—
Le Menu Entree						
LightStyle Garden Vegetables Lasagna	10.5 oz	260	8	500	35	—
LightStyle Lasagna With Meat Sauce	10 oz	290	8	510	36	—
LightStyle Meat Sauce & Cheese Tortellini	8 oz	250	8	480	34	—

FOOD	PORTION	CAL	FAT	SOD	CARB	FIB
LightStyle Spaghetti With Beef Sauce And Mushrooms	9 oz	280	6	450	45	—
Lean Cuisine						
Angel Hair Pasta	1 pkg (10 oz)	210	4	420	35	4
Cheddar Bake With Pasta	1 pkg (9 oz)	220	6	560	29	3
Cheese Cannelloni	1 pkg (9.1 oz)	270	8	500	28	3
Cheese Ravioli	1 pkg (8.5 oz)	250	8	500	32	4
Chicken Fettucini	1 pkg (9 oz)	270	6	580	33	2
Classic Cheese Lasagna	1 pkg (11.5 oz)	290	6	560	38	5
Fettucini Alfredo	1 pkg (9 oz)	270	7	590	38	2
Fettucini Primavera	1 pkg (10 oz)	260	8	580	33	4
Lasagne With Meat Sauce	1 pkg (10.25 oz)	270	6	560	34	5
Macaroni And Beef	1 pkg (10 oz)	280	8	550	40	3
Macaroni And Cheese	1 pkg (9 oz)	270	7	550	39	2
Marinara Twist	1 pkg (10 oz)	240	3	440	42	4
Rigatoni	1 pkg (9 oz)	180	4	560	25	4
Spaghetti And Meatballs	1 pkg (9.5 oz)	290	7	520	40	4
Spaghetti With Meat Sauce	1 pkg (11.5 oz)	290	6	550	45	4
Tuna Lasagna	1 pkg (9.75 oz)	230	6	540	29	3
Zucchini Lasagna	1 pkg (11 oz)	240	4	470	33	4
Morton Macaroni & Cheese	6.5 oz	290	14	760	30	—
Morton Spaghetti & Meat Sauce	8.5 oz	170	2	930	33	—
Mrs. Paul's Light Seafood Entree Seafood Rotini	9 oz	240	6	570	34	—
Mrs. Paul's Light Seafood Entree Seafood Lasagna	9.5 oz	290	8	750	39	—
Mrs. Paul's Seafood Rotini	9 oz	240	6	570	34	—
Stouffer's						
Beef Ravioli	1 pkg (9.5 oz)	370	14	680	43	5
Cheese Tortellini With Alfredo Sauce	1 pkg (8.9 oz)	550	33	720	38	5
Cheese Tortellini With Tomato Sauce	1 pkg (9.25 oz)	290	6	740	40	4

FOOD	PORTION	CAL	FAT	SOD	CARB	FIB
Stouffer's *(cont.)*						
Cheese Manicotti	1 pkg (9 oz)	340	16	810	32	7
Cheese Ravioli With Tomato Sauce	1 pkg (9.5 oz)	360	16	720	42	4
Cheese Shells With Tomato Sauce	1 pkg (9.25 oz)	340	16	920	29	5
Fettucini Alfredo	1 pkg (10 oz)	480	29	850	40	3
Four Cheese Lasagna	1 pkg (10.75 oz)	410	19	840	37	3
Homestyle Chicken Fettucini	1 pkg (10.5 oz)	380	15	1250	32	3
Lasagne With Meat Sauce	1 cup (7 oz)	260	10	560	24	4
Lasagna With Meat Sauce	1 pkg (10.5 oz)	360	13	780	34	5
Lunch Express Cheese Lasagna Casserole	1 pkg (9.5 oz)	270	7	590	38	5
Lunch Express Cheese Ravioli	1 pkg (8.5 oz)	310	12	620	38	2
Lunch Express Chicken Alfredo	1 pkg (9.6 oz)	360	17	620	34	3
Lunch Express Chicken Fettucini	1 pkg (10.25 oz)	250	6	540	32	4
Lunch Express Fettucini Primavera	1 pkg (10.25 oz)	420	25	690	33	4
Lunch Express Lasagna With Meat Sauce	1 pkg (10 oz)	350	12	940	42	4
Lunch Express Macaroni & Cheese With Broccoli	1 pkg (10.4 oz)	360	19	900	32	3
Lunch Express Macaroni And Cheese And Broccoli	1 pkg (9.5 oz)	240	7	450	30	5
Lunch Express Pasta and Chicken Marinara	1 pkg (9.1 oz)	270	6	540	38	4
Lunch Express Pasta and Tuna Casserole	1 pkg (9.6 oz)	280	6	590	39	4
Lunch Express Pasta And Turkey Dijon	1 pkg (9.9 oz)	270	6	570	37	6

FOOD	PORTION	CAL	FAT	SOD	CARB	FIB
Lunch Express Rigatoni With Meat Sauce	1 pkg (10.75 oz)	340	12	710	44	3
Lunch Express Spaghetti With Meat Sauce	1 pkg (9.6 oz)	320	10	580	43	5
Lunch Express Swedish Meatballs With Pasta	1 pkg (10.25 oz)	530	32	1010	41	3
Macaroni And Beef	1 pkg (11.5 oz)	340	12	1530	40	4
Macaroni And Cheese	1 cup (6 oz)	330	17	940	31	2
Noodles Romanoff	1 pkg (12 oz)	460	23	1400	48	4
Spaghetti With Meat Sauce	1 pkg (12.9 oz)	430	13	760	57	6
Spaghetti With Meatballs	1 pkg (12.6 oz)	420	15	680	51	5
Tuna Noodle Casserole	1 pkg (10 oz)	330	14	1130	31	3
Turkey Tettrazini	1 pkg (10 oz)	360	19	1140	28	2
Vegetable Lasagna	1 cup (8 oz)	280	12	280	29	2
Vegetable Lasagna	1 pkg (10.5 oz)	370	19	820	31	3
Swanson						
Homestyle Lasagna With Meat Sauce	10.5 oz	400	15	1070	39	—
Homestyle Macaroni & Cheese	10 oz	390	19	1150	37	—
Homestyle Spaghetti With Italian Style Meatballs	13 oz	490	18	940	60	—
Macaroni & Cheese	12.25 oz	370	15	1070	48	—
Macaroni & Cheese	7 oz	200	8	740	24	—
Spaghetti & Meatballs	12.5 oz	390	17	1100	46	—
Tyson Parmigiana	1 kg (11.25 oz)	380	17	1100	37	—
Ultra Slim-Fast Pasta Primavera	12 oz	340	9	730	52	5
Ultra Slim-Fast Spaghetti With Beef & Mushroom Sauce	12 oz	370	10	990	49	0
Weight Watchers						
Angel Hair Pasta	10 oz	200	4	330	28	—
Baked Cheese Ravioli	9 oz	240	6	370	27	—

FOOD	PORTION	CAL	FAT	SOD	CARB	FIB
Weight Watchers (cont.)						
Cheese Manicotti	9.25 oz	260	8	510	31	—
Cheese Tortellini	9 oz	310	6	570	50	—
Chicken Fettucini	8.25 oz	280	9	590	25	—
Fettucini Alfredo	8 oz	230	7	550	28	—
Garden Lasagna	11 oz	260	7	430	30	—
Italian Cheese Lasagna	11 oz	290	6	510	29	—
Lasagna	10.25 oz	240	6	510	29	—
Spaghetti With Meat Sauce	10 oz	240	7	490	28	—
HOME RECIPE						
macaroni & cheese	1 cup	430	22	1086	40	—
spaghetti w/ meatballs & tomato sauce	1 cup	330	12	1009	39	—
SHELF STABLE						
Healthy Choice Lasagna w/ Meat Sauce	7.5 oz cup	220	5	530	29	—
Healthy Choice Spaghetti Rings	7.5 oz cup	140	0	460	30	—
Healthy Choice Spaghetti w/ Meat Sauce	7.5 oz cup	150	3	390	21	—
TAKE-OUT						
lasagna	1 piece (2.5 in × 2.5 in)	374	21	668	25	2
macaroni & cheese	1 cup	230	10	730	26	—
manicotti	¾ cup (6.4 oz)	273	12	414	28	2
rigatoni w/ sausage sauce	¾ cup	260	12	106	28	3
spaghetti w/ meatballs & cheese	1 cup	407	19	696	38	—

PASTA SALAD
FROZEN

FOOD	PORTION	CAL	FAT	SOD	CARB	FIB
Hanover Primavera	½ cup	50	0	—	—	—
Hanover Italian	½ cup	60	0	—	—	—
Hanover Milano	½ cup	60	0	—	—	—
Hanover Oriental	½ cup	80	0	—	—	—
MIX						
Kraft Pasta Salad And Dressing Broccoli And Vegetables	½ cup	210	16	290	15	—

FOOD	PORTION	CAL	FAT	SOD	CARB	FIB
Kraft Pasta Salad And Dressing Garden Primavera	½ cup	170	7	450	21	—
Kraft Pasta Salad And Dressing Homestyle	½ cup	240	16	300	21	—
Kraft Pasta Salad And Dressing Light Italian	½ cup	130	3	420	20	—
Kraft Pasta Salad And Dressing Light Rancher's Choice	½ cup	170	7	350	23	—
Lipton Robust Italian Suddenly Salad	½ cup	126	1	118	25	tr
Classic Pasta, as prep	½ cup	160	6	530	23	—
Creamy Macaroni, as prep	½ cup	200	10	280	21	—
Creamy Macaroni, as prep low fat recipe	½ cup	140	4	310	21	—
Italian Pasta, as prep	½ cup	160	6	480	22	—
Pasta Primavera, as prep	½ cup	190	10	340	20	—
Pasta Primavera, as prep low fat recipe	½ cup	150	5	370	21	—
Tortellini Italiano, as prep	½ cup	160	7	450	21	—
TAKE-OUT						
elbow macaroni salad	3.5 oz	160	5	590	26	—
italian style pasta salad	3.5 oz	140	7	480	15	—
mustard macaroni salad	3.5 oz	190	10	560	23	—
pasta salad w/ vegetables	3.5 oz	140	4	210	21	—

PASTRY

see BROWNIE, CAKE, DANISH PASTRY

PÂTÉ

CANNED						
Liver Sells	2.08 oz	190	16	470	4	—
chicken liver	1 oz	238	4	—	2	—
chicken liver	1 tbsp (13 g)	109	2	—	1	—
goose liver, smoked	1 oz	131	12	—	1	—

FOOD	PORTION	CAL	FAT	SOD	CARB	FIB
goose liver, smoked	1 tbsp (13 g)	60	6	—	1	—
liver	1 oz	90	8	198	tr	—
liver	1 tbsp (13 g)	41	4	91	tr	—

PEACH

FOOD	PORTION	CAL	FAT	SOD	CARB	FIB
Clingstone Halves (S&W)	½ cup	100	0	10	25	—
Clingstone Halves Diet (S&W)	½ cup	30	0	5	8	—
Clingstone Halves Unsweetened (S&W)	½ cup	30	0	5	8	—
Clingstone Sliced Diet (S&W)	½ cup	30	0	5	8	—
Clingstone Slices Unsweetened (S&W)	½ cup	30	0	5	8	—
Freestone Halves Diet (S&W)	½ cup	30	0	10	7	—
Freestone Halves in Heavy Syrup (S&W)	½ cup	100	0	10	26	—
Freestone Slices in Heavy Syrup (S&W)	½ cup	100	0	10	26	—
Freestone Slices Diet (S&W)	½ cup	30	0	10	7	—
Halves (Hunt's)	4 oz	90	tr	7	23	tr
Sliced Yellow Cling Natural Style (S&W)	½ cup	90	0	10	20	—
Slices (Hunt's)	4 oz	90	tr	7	23	tr
Yellow Cling Natural Lite (S&W)	½ cup	50	0	10	13	—
Yellow Cling Sliced Premium in Heavy Syrup (S&W)	½ cup	100	0	10	25	—
Yellow Cling Whole Spiced in Heavy Syrup (S&W)	½ cup	90	0	10	23	—
halves in heavy syrup	1 half	60	tr	5	16	—
halves in light syrup	1 half	44	tr	4	12	—
halves, juice pack	1 half	34	tr	3	9	—
halves, water pack	1 half	18	tr	3	5	—
spiced in heavy syrup	1 cup	180	tr	9	49	—
spiced in heavy syrup	1 fruit	66	tr	3	18	—
DRIED						
Mariani	¼ cup	140	0	—	—	—
halves	1 cup	383	1	12	98	13
halves	10	311	1	9	80	11

FOOD	PORTION	CAL	FAT	SOD	CARB	FIB
halves, cooked w/ sugar	½ cup	139	tr	3	36	—
halves, cooked w/o sugar	½ cup	99	tr	3	25	—
FRESH						
Dole	2	70	0	0	19	1
peach	1	37	tr	0	10	1
sliced	1 cup	73	tr	1	19	—
FROZEN						
Big Valley	3.5 oz	45	tr	0	10	—
slices, sweetened	1 cup	235	tr	16	60	—
JUICE						
Dole Pure & Light	6 oz	100	tr	20	20	—
Goya Nectar	6 oz	110	0	30	27	—
Kern's Nectar	6 oz	110	0	5	28	—
Libby's Nectar	6 oz	100	0	5	24	—
Libby's Ripe Nectar	8 oz	130	0	5	32	—
Smucker's	8 oz	120	0	10	30	—
nectar	1 cup	134	tr	17	35	—
PEANUT BUTTER						
Arrowhead Creamy	2 tbsp (1.1 oz)	200	15	0	6	1
Arrowhead Crunchy	2 tbsp (1.1 oz)	200	15	0	6	1
BAMA Creamy	2 tbsp	200	17	140	6	—
BAMA Crunchy	2 tbsp	200	17	115	6	—
BAMA Jelly & Peanut Butter	2 tbsp	150	7	75	20	—
Erewhon Chunky	2 tbsp (32 g)	190	14	75	7	—
Erewhon Chunky Unsalted	2 tbsp (32 g)	190	14	10	7	—
Erewhon Creamy	2 tbsp (32 g)	190	14	75	7	—
Erewhon Creamy Unsalted	2 tbsp (32 g)	190	14	10	7	—
Estee Chunky	1 tbsp	100	8	3	3	—
Estee Creamy	1 tbsp	100	8	3	3	—
Health Valley Chunky No Salt	2 tbsp	170	14	2	6	2
Health Valley Creamy No Salt	2 tbsp	170	14	2	6	3
Hollywood Creamy	1 tbsp	35	3	25	1	1
Hollywood Crunchy	1 tbsp	35	3	25	1	1
Hollywood Unsalted	1 tbsp	35	3	0	1	1
Home Brand	2 tbsp	210	17	—	—	—
Home Brand Natural Lightly Salted	2 tbsp	210	17	—	—	—

FOOD	PORTION	CAL	FAT	SOD	CARB	FIB
Home Brand Natural Unsalted	2 tbsp	210	17	—	—	—
Home Brand No-Sugar Added	2 tbsp	180	16	—	—	—
Jif Creamy	2 tbsp	180	16	155	6	2
Jif Extra Crunchy	2 tbsp	180	16	130	6	2
Jif Simply Creamy	2 tbsp	180	16	65	5	2
Jif Simply Extra Crunchy	2 tbsp	180	16	50	5	2
Peter Pan Creamy	2 tbsp	190	16	150	6	2
Peter Pan Creamy Salt Free	2 tbsp	190	17	0	5	2
Peter Pan Crunchy	2 tbsp	190	16	150	6	2
Peter Pan Crunchy Salt Free	2 tbsp	190	17	0	5	2
Reese's Peanut Butter Flavored Chips	¼ cup (1.5 oz)	230	13	90	19	—
Skippy Creamy	1 cup (263 g)	1540	135	1240	38	—
Skippy Creamy, w/ 2 slices white bread	1 sandwich	340	19	430	33	—
Skippy Reduced Fat Creamy	2 tbsp	190	12	200	13	1
Skippy Super Chunk	1 cup (260 g)	1540	138	1120	36	—
Skippy Super Chunk	2 tbsp (32 g)	190	17	130	4	—
Skippy Super Chunk, w/ 2 slices white bread	1 sandwich	340	19	410	32	—
Smucker's Goober Grape	2 tbsp	180	10	120	18	—
Smucker's Honey Sweetened	2 tbsp	200	16	155	7	—
Smucker's Natural	2 tbsp	200	16	125	6	—
Smucker's Natural No-Salt Added	2 tbsp	200	16	<10	6	—
Teddie Natural Peanut Butter w/ No Salt Added	2 tbsp	200	17	—	—	—
chunky	1 cup	1520	129	1255	56	17
chunky	2 tbsp	188	16	156	7	2
chunky, w/o salt	1 cup	1520	129	44	56	17
chunky, w/o salt	2 tbsp	188	16	5	7	2
smooth	1 cup	1517	128	1234	53	15
smooth	2 tbsp	188	16	153	7	2
smooth, w/o salt	1 cup	1517	129	44	53	15
smooth, w/o salt	2 tbsp	188	16	5	7	2

FOOD	PORTION	CAL	FAT	SOD	CARB	FIB
PEANUTS						
Cocktail Lightly Salted (Planters)	1 oz	170	14	80	5	2
Cocktail Unsalted (Planters)	1 oz	170	14	0	5	—
Dry Roasted (Frito-Lay)	1.2 oz	190	16	300	7	—
Dry Roasted (Guy's)	1 oz	170	14	310	3	—
Dry Roasted Lightly Salted (Planters)	1 oz	160	15	110	5	3
Dry Roasted Unsalted (Planters)	1 oz	170	15	250	5	—
Fresh Roast Lightly Salted (Planters)	1 oz	160	14	120	5	2
Fresh Roast Salted (Planters)	1 oz	170	14	110	5	2
Honey Roasted						
(Eagle)	1 oz	170	13	130	7	—
(Planters)	1 oz	170	13	—	—	—
(Weight Watchers)	0.7 oz	100	6	100	7	—
Cinnamon (Eagle)	1 oz	170	13	90	7	—
Dry Roasted (Planters)	1 oz	160	13	90	7	—
Maple (Eagle)	1 oz	170	13	90	7	—
Honey Toasted (Lance)	1 pkg (39 g)	230	17	240	11	—
Low Salt (Eagle)	1 oz	170	15	90	5	—
Party Peanuts (Fisher)	1 oz	160	14	—	—	—
Peanuts (Beer Nuts)	1 pkg (1 oz)	180	14	60	7	—
Peanuts (Planters)	1 bag (0.5 oz)	80	7	55	3	—
Roasted w/ Shell (Lance)	1 pkg (50 g)	190	15	0	8	—
Salted (Frito-Lay)	1 oz	170	15	170	6	—
Salted (Lance)	1 pkg (32 g)	190	15	105	7	—
Salted (Little Debbie)	1 pkg (1.2 oz)	230	21	45	3	2
Salted Tube (Lance)	1 pkg (42 g)	240	20	120	9	—
Spanish (Planters)	1 oz	170	15	100	3	—
Spanish Raw (Planters)	1 oz	160	14	5	5	—
Spanish Salted (Guy's)	1 oz	170	14	170	3	—
Virginia Fancy (Eagle)	1 oz	90	8	65	3	—
cooked	½ cup	102	7	240	7	—
dry roasted	1 cup	855	73	1187	31	12
dry roasted	1 oz	164	14	228	6	2
oil roasted	1 cup	837	71	624	27	13
oil roasted	1 oz	163	14	121	5	2
oil roasted, w/o salt	1 cup	837	71	9	27	13

FOOD	PORTION	CAL	FAT	SOD	CARB	FIB
oil roasted, w/o salt	1 oz	163	14	2	5	2
spanish oil, roasted	1 oz	162	14	121	5	2
spanish oil, roasted w/o salt	1 oz	162	14	2	5	2
unroasted	1 oz	159	14	5	5	—
valencia oil, roasted	1 cup	848	74	1111	23	9
valencia oil, roasted	1 oz	165	14	216	5	2
valencia oil, roasted w/o salt	1 cup	848	74	9	23	9
valencia oil, roasted w/o salt	1 oz	165	14	2	5	2
virginia oil, roasted	1 cup	826	70	619	28	—
virginia oil, roasted	1 oz	161	14	121	5	—

PEAR
CANNED

FOOD	PORTION	CAL	FAT	SOD	CARB	FIB
Bartlett Halves in Heavy Syrup (S&W)	½ cup	100	0	—	25	—
Bartlett Halves Peeled Unsweetened (S&W)	½ cup	35	0	10	10	—
Halves (Hunt's)	4 oz	90	tr	6	22	tr
Halves Peeled Diet (S&W)	½ cup	35	0	10	10	—
Quartered Peeled Diet (S&W)	½ cup	35	0	10	10	—
Sliced Natural Light Bartlett (S&W)	½ cup	60	0	10	15	—
Sliced Natural Style (S&W)	½ cup	80	0	10	20	—
halves, in heavy syrup	1 cup	188	tr	13	49	—
halves, in heavy syrup	1 half	68	tr	4	15	—
halves, in light syrup	1 half	45	tr	4	12	—
halves, juice pack	1 cup	123	tr	10	32	—
halves, water pack	1 half	22	tr	41	6	—

DRIED

FOOD	PORTION	CAL	FAT	SOD	CARB	FIB
Mariani	¼ cup	150	0	—	—	—
halves	1 cup	472	1	10	125	—
halves	10	459	1	10	122	—
halves, cooked w/ sugar	½ cup	196	tr	4	52	—
halves, cooked w/o sugar	1/2 cup	163	tr	4	43	—

FRESH

FOOD	PORTION	CAL	FAT	SOD	CARB	FIB
Dole	1	100	1	1	25	4
asian	1 (4.3 oz)	51	tr	0	13	—

FOOD	PORTION	CAL	FAT	SOD	CARB	FIB
pear	1	98	1	1	25	4
sliced w/ skin	1 cup	97	1	1	25	4
JUICE						
Goya Nectar	6 oz	120	0	15	29	—
Kern's Nectar	6 oz	110	0	5	26	—
Libby's Nectar	6 oz	110	0	0	28	—
nectar	1 cup	149	tr	9	39	—

PEAS
CANNED

FOOD	PORTION	CAL	FAT	SOD	CARB	FIB
Baked Pea Beans (Van De Kamp's)	8 oz	270	6	750	50	11
Crowder Peas Seasoned w/Pork (Luck's)	7.5 oz	200	7	—	—	—
Early June or Sweet (Owatonna)	½ cup	70	0	—	—	—
Field Peas (Trappey's)	½ cup	90	1	410	16	—
Field Peas With Snaps (Trappey's)	½ cup	90	1	410	15	—
Libby	½ cup	60	0	—	—	—
Natural Pack (Libby)	½ cup	60	1	—	—	—
Natural Pack (Seneca)	½ cup	60	0	—	—	—
Petit Pois (S&W)	½ cup	70	0	330	12	—
Seneca	½ cup	60	0	—	—	—
Small Pea Beans (Friends)	8 oz	360	4	1040	62	—
Sweet (Green Giant)	½ cup	50	0	320	11	4
Sweet (S&W)	½ cup	70	0	330	12	—
Sweet Water Pack (S&W)	½ cup	40	0	5	8	—
Veri-Green Sweet (S&W)	½ cup	70	0	320	14	—
green	½ cup	59	tr	186	11	—
green, low sodium	½ cup	59	tr	2	11	—
DRIED						
Hurst Brand Split	1 cup	277	tr	—	—	—
Hurst Brand Whole	1 cup	272	1	—	—	—
split, cooked	1 cup	231	1	4	41	—
FRESH						
Dole Sugar Peas	½ cup	30	tr	3	5	2
edible-pod, cooked	½ cup	34	tr	3	6	2
edible-pod, raw	½ cup	30	tr	3	5	2
green, cooked	½ cup	67	tr	2	13	—
green, raw	½ cup	58	tr	3	11	—

FOOD	PORTION	CAL	FAT	SOD	CARB	FIB
FROZEN						
Big Valley	3.3 oz	80	0	90	13	—
Chinese Pea Pods (Chun King)	1.5 oz	20	0	<10	3	—
Green (Birds Eye)	½ cup	80	0	130	13	4
Harvest Fresh Early June (Green Giant)	½ cup	60	1	140	12	3
Harvest Fresh Sugar Snap (Green Giant)	½ cup	30	0	100	8	2
Harvest Fresh Sweet (Green Giant)	½ cup	50	0	95	12	3
In Butter Sauce (Birds Eye)	½ cup	80	2	170	12	3
In Butter Sauce (Green Giant)	½ cup	80	2	410	14	4
Le Sueur Early Select (Green Giant)	½ cup	60	0	115	13	4
Le Sueur Early In Butter Sauce (Green Giant)	½ cup	80	2	440	14	3
One Serve In Butter Sauce (Green Giant)	1 pkg	90	2	500	16	5
Petite (Hanover)	½ cup	70	0	—	—	—
Polybag Deluxe Tender Tiny (Birds Eye)	½ cup	60	0	120	11	4
Polybag Green (Birds Eye)	½ cup	70	0	125	12	2
Snow Pea Pods (La Choy)	½ pkg (3 oz)	35	tr	10	6	—
Snow Peas (Hanover)	½ cup	35	0	—	—	—
Sugar Snap Deluxe (Birds Eye)	½ cup	45	0	5	9	4
Sugar Snap Sweet Select (Green Giant)	½ cup	30	0	0	8	2
Sweet (Green Giant)	½ cup	50	0	95	11	4
Sweet (Hanover)	½ cup	70	0	—	—	—
Tender Tiny Deluxe (Birds Eye)	½ cup	60	0	120	11	4
edible-pod, cooked	1 pkg (10 oz)	132	1	12	23	—
edible-pod, cooked	½ cup	42	tr	4	7	—
green, cooked	½ cup	63	tr	70	11	—
SHELF STABLE						
Mini Sweet (Green Giant)	½ cup	60	tr	240	12	4

FOOD	PORTION	CAL	FAT	SOD	CARB	FIB
SPROUTS						
raw	½ cup	77	tr	12	17	—
TAKE-OUT						
pea & potato curry	1 serving (7 oz)	284	22	—	19	6
pea curry	1 serving (4.4 oz)	438	42	—	11	4
PECANS						
Halves (Planters)	1 oz	190	20	0	5	—
Honey Roasted (Eagle)	1 oz	200	19	130	5	—
Pieces (Planters)	1 oz	190	20	0	5	—
dried	1 oz	190	19	0	5	2
dry roasted	1 oz	187	18	0	6	—
dry roasted, salted	1 oz	187	18	260	6	—
halves, dried	1 cup	721	73	1	20	7
oil roasted	1 oz	195	20	0	5	—
oil roasted, salted	1 oz	195	20	252	5	—
PECTIN						
Certo	1 tbsp	2	0	—	—	—
Slim Set	1 pkg	208	0	42	44	14
Slim Set	1 tbsp	3	0	1	1	tr
Sure-Jell	¼ pkg	38	0	—	—	—
Sure-Jell Light	¼ pkg	33	0	—	—	—
PEPPER						
Lemon (Ac'cent)	½ tsp	0	0	0	0	0
Lemon Pepper (Lawry's)	1 tsp	6	tr	340	1	tr
Seasoned (Ac'cent)	½ tsp	0	0	0	0	0
Spice Lemon Pepper (Nile Spice)	⅛ tsp	0	0	5	0	—
black	1 tsp	5	tr	1	1	—
cayenne	1 tsp	6	tr	1	1	—
red	1 tsp	6	tr	1	1	—
white	1 tsp	7	tr	tr	2	—
PEPPERS						
CANNED						
Banana Mild (Trappey's)	3 peppers (1 oz)	6	tr	100	1	1
Banana Sliced Hot (Trappey's)	25 slices (1 oz)	6	tr	529	1	1
Cherry Hot (Trappey's)	2 peppers (1 oz)	7	tr	373	1	1
Cherry Hot (Trappey's)	2 peppers (1 oz)	10	tr	225	2	1

FOOD	PORTION	CAL	FAT	SOD	CARB	FIB
Dulcito Italian Peperoncini Mild (Trappey's)	3 peppers (1 oz)	8	tr	178	2	1
Filet (Hebrew National)	¼ pepper (1 oz)	9	0	310	2	—
Filet Peppers (Schorr's)	1 oz	9	0	310	2	—
Green Chilies Chopped (Old El Paso)	2 tbsp	8	tr	70	2	—
Green Chilies Whole (Old El Paso)	1	8	tr	105	1	—
Hot Banana Pepper Rings (Vlasic)	1 oz	4	0	465	1	—
Hot Cherry (Hebrew National)	⅓ pepper (1 oz)	11	0	270	2	—
Hot Cherry (Progresso)	½ cup	190	20	130	3	—
Hot Cherry (Vlasic)	1 oz	10	0	425	2	—
Hot Cherry Pickled (Progresso)	½ cup	130	12	110	3	—
In Vinegar Hot (Trappey's)	15 peppers (1 oz)	9	tr	573	2	tr
Jalapeno Hot (Trappey's)	1 pepper (1 oz)	11	tr	658	2	1
Jalapeno Hot Sliced (Trappey's)	21 slices (1 oz)	4	tr	296	1	1
Jalapeno Mexican Hot (Vlasic)	1 oz	8	0	380	2	—
Jalapeno Nacho Slices (McIlhenny)	12 slices (1.1 oz)	7	tr	70	1	1
Mexican Tiny Hot (Vlasic)	1 oz	6	0	430	2	—
Mild Cherry (Vlasic)	1 oz	8	0	410	2	—
Mild Greek Peperoncini Salad Peppers (Vlasic)	1 oz	4	0	450	1	—
Piccalilli (Progresso)	½ cup	190	20	220	4	—
Red Filet (Hebrew National)	¼ pepper (1 oz)	9	0	310	2	—
Roasted (Progresso)	½ cup	20	tr	2	5	2
Serano Hot (Trappey's)	3 peppers (1 oz)	7	tr	37	1	tr
Sweet (Rosoff's)	¼ pepper (1 oz)	9	0	310	2	—
Sweet Fried (Progresso)	½ jar	37	tr	17	4	1
Tempero Greek Peperoncini Mild (Trappey's)	1 pepper (1 oz)	7	tr	470	1	1

FOOD	PORTION	CAL	FAT	SOD	CARB	FIB
Torrido Santa Fe Grande Hot (Trappey's)	1 pepper (1 oz)	10	tr	492	2	tr
Tuscan (Progresso)	½ cup	20	0	5	7	—
chili green hot	1 (2.6 oz)	18	tr	—	4	—
chili green hot, chopped	½ cup	17	tr	—	4	—
chili red hot	1 (2.6 oz)	18	tr	—	4	—
chili red hot, chopped	½ cup	17	tr	—	4	—
green halves	½ cup	13	tr	958	3	—
jalapeno, chopped	½ cup	17	tr	995	3	—
red halves	½ cup	13	tr	958	3	—
DRIED						
green	1 tbsp	1	tr	1	tr	—
red	1 tbsp	1	tr	1	tr	—
FRESH						
Dole Bell	1 med	25	1	0	5	2
chili green hot, raw	1	18	tr	3	4	—
chili green hot, raw, chopped	½ cup	30	tr	5	7	—
chili red hot, raw	1 (1.6 oz)	18	tr	3	4	—
chili red, raw, chopped	½ cup	30	tr	5	7	—
green, chopped, cooked	½ cup	19	tr	1	5	—
green, cooked	1 (2.6 oz)	20	tr	1	5	—
green, raw	1 (2.6 oz)	20	tr	1	5	1
green, raw, chopped	½ cup	13	tr	1	3	1
red, chopped, cooked	½ cup	19	tr	1	5	—
red, cooked	1 (2.6 oz)	20	tr	1	5	—
red, raw	1 (2.6 oz)	20	tr	1	5	1
red, raw, chopped	½ cup	13	tr	1	3	1
yellow, raw	1 (6.5 oz)	50	tr	3	12	—
yellow, raw	10 strips	14	tr	1	3	—
FROZEN						
Green Diced (Southland)	2 oz	10	0	—	—	—
Sweet Red & Green Cut (Southland)	2 oz	15	0	—	—	—
green, chopped, not prep	1 oz	6	tr	1	1	—
red, chopped	1 oz	6	tr	1	1	—

FOOD	PORTION	CAL	FAT	SOD	CARB	FIB

PERCH
FRESH
cooked	1 fillet (1.6 oz)	54	1	36	0	—
cooked	3 oz	99	1	67	0	—
ocean perch atlantic, cooked	1 fillet (1.8 oz)	60	1	48	0	—
ocean perch atlantic, cooked	3 oz	103	2	82	0	—
ocean perch atlantic, raw	3 oz	80	1	64	0	—
raw	3 oz	77	1	52	0	—
red, raw	3.5 oz	114	4	80	0	—

FROZEN
Battered (Van De Kamp's)	2 pieces	310	21	500	18	—
Fishmarket Fresh Ocean Perch (Gorton's)	5 oz	140	3	100	2	—
Ocean Perch Light Fillet (Van De Kamp's)	1 piece	280	14	450	21	—
Ocean Perch Natural Fillets (Van De Kamp's)	4 oz	130	5	65	0	—

PERSIMMONS
dried, japanese	1	93	tr	1	25	—
fresh	1	32	tr	0	8	—
fresh, japanese	1	118	tr	3	31	—

PHEASANT
FRESH
breast w/o skin, raw	½ breast (6.4 oz)	243	6	60	0	—
leg w/o skin, raw	1 (3.6 oz)	143	5	48	0	—
w/ skin, raw	½ pheasant (14 oz)	723	37	161	0	—
w/o skin, raw	½ pheasant (12.4 oz)	470	13	131	0	—

PHYLLO DOUGH
Ekizian	½ lb	865	17	573	151	—
phyllo dough	1 oz	85	2	137	15	—
sheet	1	57	1	92	10	—

FOOD	PORTION	CAL	FAT	SOD	CARB	FIB
PICKLES						
Barrel Cured Kosher Dill (Hebrew National)	1 pkg	23	0	1570	4	—
Barrel Cured Kosher Hot Dill (Hebrew National)	1 pkg	23	0	1570	4	—
Bread & Butter Chips (Vlasic)	1 oz	30	0	160	7	—
Bread & Butter Chunks (Vlasic)	1 oz	25	0	120	6	—
Bread & Butter Stixs (Vlasic)	1 oz	18	0	110	5	—
Bread 'N Butter Slices (Claussen)	1 slice	7	tr	—	—	—
Deli Bread & Butter (Vlasic)	1 oz	25	0	120	6	—
Deli Dill Halves (Vlasic)	1 oz	4	0	290	1	—
Dill Spears (Claussen)	1 spear	4	tr	—	—	—
Garlic (Schorr's)	⅓ pickle (1 oz)	3	0	250	1	—
Half Sour (Hebrew National)	½ pickle (1 oz)	4	0	210	1	—
Half Sour (Rosoff's)	⅓ pickle (1 oz)	4	0	210	1	—
Half Sour (Schorr's)	½ spear (1 oz)	4	0	200	1	—
Half Sour (Schorr's)	⅓ pickle (1 oz)	4	0	210	1	—
Half Sour Spears (Rosoff's)	½ spear (1 oz)	4	0	200	1	—
Half-The-Salt Hamburger Dill Chips (Vlasic)	1 oz	2	0	175	1	—
Half-The-Salt Kosher Crunch Dills (Vlasic)	1 oz	4	0	125	1	—
Half-The-Salt Kosher Dill Spears (Vlasic)	1 oz	4	0	120	1	—
Half-The-Salt Sweet Butter Chips (Vlasic)	1 oz	30	0	80	7	—
Hot & Spicy Garden Mix (Vlasic)	1 oz	4	0	380	1	—
Hot N' Sweet (McIhenny)	4 (1 oz)	42	tr	28	10	tr
Kosher (Hebrew National)	⅓ pickle (1 oz)	4	0	260	1	—
(Rosoff's)	⅓ pickle (1 oz)	4	0	260	1	—

FOOD	PORTION	CAL	FAT	SOD	CARB	FIB
Kosher						
Baby Dills (Vlasic)	1 oz	4	0	210	1	—
Chips (Hebrew National)	3 slices (1 oz)	4	0	300	1	—
Crunchy Dills (Vlasic)	1 oz	4	0	210	1	—
Deli (Schorr's)	½ pickle (1 oz)	4	0	160	1	—
Dill Gherkins (Vlasic)	1 oz	4	0	210	1	—
Dill Spears (Vlasic)	1 oz	4	0	175	1	—
Halves (Claussen)	1 half	9	tr	—	—	—
Halves (Hebrew National)	⅓ pickle (1 oz)	4	0	290	1	—
Halves (Rosoff's)	⅓ pickle (1 oz)	4	0	290	1	—
Halves (Schorr's)	⅓ pickle (1 oz)	4	0	290	1	—
Large (Hebrew National)	⅙ pickle (1 oz)	4	0	300	1	—
Slices (Claussen)	1 slice	1	tr	—	—	—
Snack Chunks (Vlasic)	1 oz	4	0	220	1	—
Spears (Hebrew National)	½ spear (1 oz)	4	0	260	1	—
Spears (Schorr's)	½ spear (1 oz)	4	0	260	1	—
Whole (Claussen)	1	9	tr	—	—	—
Whole (Schorr's)	⅓ pickle (1 oz)	4	0	260	1	—
No Garlic Dill Spears (Vlasic)	1 oz	4	0	210	1	—
No Garlic Dills (Claussen)	1	17	tr	—	—	—
Original Dills (Vlasic)	1 oz	2	0	375	1	—
Polish Snack Chunk Dills (Vlasic)	1 oz	4	0	300	1	—
Relish (Claussen)	1 tbsp	14	tr	—	—	—
Sour Garlic (Hebrew National)	⅓ pickle (1 oz)	3	0	250	1	—
Zesty Crunchy Dills (Vlasic)	1 oz	4	0	250	1	—
Zesty Dill Snack Chunks (Vlasic)	1 oz	4	0	290	1	—
Zesty Dill Spears (Vlasic)	1 oz	4	0	230	1	—
dill	1 (2.3 oz)	12	tr	833	3	—
dill low sodium	1 (2.3 oz)	12	tr	12	3	1
dill low sodium, sliced	1 slice	1	tr	1	tr	tr
dill sliced	1 slice	1	tr	77	tr	tr

FOOD	PORTION	CAL	FAT	SOD	CARB	FIB
gherkins	3.5 oz	21	tr	960	4	—
kosher dill	1 (2.3 oz)	12	tr	833	3	1
piccalilli	1.4 oz	13	tr	—	2	1
polish dill	1 (2.3 oz)	12	tr	833	3	1
quick sour	1 (1.2 oz)	4	tr	423	1	—
quick sour, low sodium	1 (1.2 oz)	4	tr	6	1	—
quick sour, sliced	1 slice	1	tr	85	tr	—
sweet	1 (1.2 oz)	41	tr	328	11	tr
sweet gherkin	1 sm (½ oz)	20	tr	107	5	—
sweet, low sodium	1 (1.2 oz)	41	tr	6	11	tr
sweet, sliced	1 slice	7	tr	56	2	tr
PIE						
see also PIE CRUST						
CANNED FILLING						
Mincemeat Condensed (None Such)	¼ pkg	220	2	310	50	—
Mincemeat Old Fashioned (S&W)	½ cup	206	2	206	49	—
Mincemeat Ready-to-Use (None Such)	⅓ cup	200	1	360	48	—
Mincemeat Ready-to-Use With Brandy & Rum (None Such)	⅓ cup	220	2	260	48	—
Pumpkin Pie Mix (Libby)	½ cup	100	0	150	25	2
pumpkin pie mix	1 cup	282	tr	561	71	—
FROZEN						
Apple						
(Banquet)	1 slice (3.3 oz)	250	11	290	37	—
(McMillin's)	4 oz	430	23	340	51	—
(Mrs. Smith's)	⅒ of 10-in pie (4.6 oz)	280	12	310	43	1
(Mrs. Smith's)	⅙ of 8-in pie (4.3 oz)	270	11	300	41	1
(Mrs. Smith's)	⅛ of 9-in pie (4.6 oz)	370	18	430	50	2
(Pet-Ritz)	⅙ pie (4.33 oz)	330	12	385	53	—
(Weight Watchers)	1 slice (3.5 oz)	165	4	90	30	—
Apple Cranberry (Mrs. Smith's)	⅙ of 8-in pie (4.3 oz)	280	11	290	43	1
Apple Homestyle (Sara Lee)	1 slice (4 oz)	280	12	220	42	—
Apple Homestyle High (Sara Lee)	1 slice (4.9 oz)	400	23	450	46	—

FOOD	PORTION	CAL	FAT	SOD	CARB	FIB
Apple Lattice Ready to Serve (Mrs. Smith's)	⅕ of 8-in pie (4.6 oz)	310	13	350	45	2
Apple SmartStyle (Mrs. Smith's)	⅕ of 8-in pie (4 oz)	220	5	180	44	2
Apple Streusel Free & Light (Sara Lee)	1 slice (2.9 oz)	170	2	140	36	—
Banana (Banquet)	1 slice (2.3 oz)	180	10	150	21	—
Banana Cream (Mrs. Smith's)	¼ of 8-in pie (3.4 oz)	250	9	170	40	1
Banana Cream (Pet-Ritz)	⅙ pie (2.33 oz)	170	9	155	22	—
Berry (McMillin's)	4 oz	430	23	410	52	—
Berry (Mrs. Smith's)	⅙ of 8-in pie (4.3 oz)	280	11	340	44	0
Blackberry (Banquet)	1 slice (3.3 oz)	270	11	350	40	—
Blackberry (Mrs. Smith's)	⅙ of 8-in pie (4.3 oz)	280	11	320	43	1
Blueberry (Banquet)	1 slice (3.3 oz)	270	11	350	40	—
Blueberry (Mrs. Smith's)	⅙ of 8-in pie	260	11	320	39	1
Blueberry (Pet-Ritz)	⅙ pie (4.33 oz)	370	12	330	50	—
Blueberry Cheese Yogurt SmartStyle (Mrs. Smith's)	¼ of 7-in pie (4.2 oz)	270	8	260	48	1
Blueberry Homestyle (Sara Lee)	1 slice (4 oz)	300	12	210	45	—
Boston Cream (Mrs. Smith's)	⅙ of 8-in pie (2.4 oz)	170	5	140	29	0
Cherry						
(Banquet)	1 slice (3.3 oz)	250	11	260	36	—
(McMillin's)	4 oz	430	24	350	51	—
(Mrs. Smith's)	⅒ of 10-in pie (4.6 oz)	410	18	—	—	—
(Mrs. Smith's)	⅙ of 8-in pie	270	11	320	41	1
(Mrs. Smith's)	⅛ of 9-in pie (4.6 oz)	320	13	350	48	1
(Pet-Ritz)	⅙ pie (4.33 oz)	300	12	330	48	—
Cherry Homestyle (Sara Lee)	1 slice (4 oz)	270	13	270	37	—
Cherry Lattice Ready to Serve	⅕ of 8-in pie (4.6 oz)	320	13	340	47	1
Cherry SmartStyle (Mrs. Smith's)	⅕ of 8 in pie (4 oz)	230	4	180	47	1
Cherry Streusel Free & Light (Sara Lee)	1 slice (3.6 oz)	160	2	140	34	—

FOOD	PORTION	CAL	FAT	SOD	CARB	FIB
Chocolate (Banquet)	1 slice (2.3 oz)	190	10	110	24	—
Chocolate Cream (Mrs. Smith's)	¼ of 8-in pie (3.4 oz)	290	14	180	37	1
Chocolate Cream (Pet-Ritz)	⅙ pie (2.33 oz)	190	8	145	27	—
Chocolate Mocha (Weight Watchers)	1 (2.75 oz)	180	4	150	30	—
Chocolate Pudding (McMillin's)	4 oz	420	21	350	54	—
Coconut (Banquet)	1 slice (2.3 oz)	190	11	120	22	—
Coconut Cream (Mrs. Smith's)	¼ of 8-in pie (3.4 oz)	280	14	160	36	0
Coconut Cream (Pet-Ritz)	⅙ pie (2.33 oz)	190	8	145	27	—
Coconut Custard (Mrs. Smith's)	⅕ of 8-in pie (5 oz)	280	12	350	35	0
Coconut Pudding (McMillin's)	4 oz	450	26	420	50	—
Dutch Apple (Mrs. Smith's)	1/10 of 10-in pie (4.6 oz)	320	12	270	50	1
Dutch Apple (Mrs. Smith's)	⅙ of 8-in pie	310	13	270	48	1
Dutch Apple (Mrs Smith's)	⅛ of 9-in pie (4.5 oz)	300	12	240	48	2
Dutch Apple Homestyle (Sara Lee)	1 slice (4 oz)	300	12	310	45	—
Egg Custard (Pet-Ritz)	⅙ pie (4.0 oz)	200	8	—	28	—
French Silk Cream (Mrs. Smith's)	⅙ of 8-in pie (4.8 oz)	410	21	250	55	1
Hearty Pumpkin (Mrs. Smith's)	⅙ of 8-in pie (5.2 oz)	280	10	350	46	2
Hyannis Boston Cream Pie (Pepperidge Farm)	1	230	10	125	34	2
Lemon (Banquet)	1 slice (2.3 oz)	170	9	120	23	—
Lemon Cream (Mrs. Smith's)	¼ of 8-in pie (3.4 oz)	270	13	150	36	0
Lemon Cream (Pet-Ritz)	⅙ pie (2.33 oz)	190	9	150	26	—
Lemon Meringue (Mrs. Smith's)	⅙ of 8-in pie (4.8 oz)	300	8	220	54	0
Mince (Mrs. Smith's)	⅙ of 8 in pie (4.3 oz)	300	11	400	48	2
Mince (Pet-Ritz)	⅙ pie (4.33 oz)	280	9	—	48	—

FOOD	PORTION	CAL	FAT	SOD	CARB	FIB
Mince Homestyle (Sara Lee)	1 slice (4 oz)	300	13	340	43	—
Mincemeat (Banquet)	1 slice (3.3 oz)	260	11	370	38	—
Mississippi Mud (Pepperidge Farm)	1	310	23	45	23	—
Neapolitan Cream (Pet-Ritz)	⅙ pie (2.33 oz)	180	10	185	17	—
Peach (Banquet)	1 slice (3.3 oz)	245	11	280	35	—
Peach (McMillin's)	4 oz	430	24	370	52	—
Peach (Mrs. Smith's)	⅙ of 8-in pie	260	11	310	38	1
Peach (Mrs. Smith's)	⅛ of 9-in pie (4.6 oz)	310	13	350	46	1
Peach (Pet-Ritz)	⅙ pie (4.33 oz)	320	12	320	51	—
Peach Cheese Yogurt SmartStyle (Mrs. Smith's)	¼ of 7 in pie (4.2 oz)	270	8	240	46	1
Peach Homestyle (Sara Lee)	1 slice (3.4 oz)	280	12	170	41	—
Pecan (Mrs. Smith's)	⅛ of 10-in pie (4.5 oz)	500	23	460	68	1
Pecan Homestyle (Sara Lee)	1 slice (3.4 oz)	400	18	290	56	—
Pumpkin (Banquet)	1 slice (3.3 oz)	200	8	350	29	—
Pumpkin (Mrs. Smith's)	⅕ of 8-in pie (5.2 oz)	270	8	350	44	1
Pumpkin (Mrs. Smith's)	⅛ of 10-in pie (5.1 oz)	250	8	330	42	1
Pumpkin Custard (Pet-Ritz)	⅙ pie (4.33 oz)	250	9	—	39	—
Pumpkin Homestyle (Sara Lee)	1 slice (4 oz)	240	10	250	34	—
Raspberry Homestyle (Sara Lee)	1 slice (4 oz)	280	13	150	39	—
Red Raspberry (Mrs. Smith's)	⅙ of 8-in pie (4.3 oz)	280	11	310	43	0
Strawberry (Banquet)	1 slice (2.3 oz)	170	9	120	22	—
Strawberry (McMillin's)	4 oz	400	20	370	50	—
Strawberry Banana Yogurt SmartStyle (Mrs. Smith's)	¼ of 7-in pie (4.2 oz)	240	5	190	48	1
Strawberry Rhubarb (Mrs. Smith's)	⅕ of 8-in pie (4.8 oz)	520	23	450	73	1
Strawberry Rhubarb (Mrs. Smith's)	⅙ of 8-in pie (4.3 oz)	280	11	380	44	0

FOOD	PORTION	CAL	FAT	SOD	CARB	FIB
Strawberry SmartStyle (Mrs. Smith's)	⅕ of 8-in pie (4 oz)	210	4	150	43	2
Strawberry Cream (Pet-Ritz)	⅙ pie (2.33 oz)	170	9	145	20	—
Sweet Potato (Pet-Ritz)	⅙ pie (3.33 oz)	150	7	110	21	—
apple	⅛ of 9-in pie (4.4 oz)	297	14	333	43	2
blueberry	⅛ of 9-in pie (4.4 oz)	289	13	406	44	—
cherry	⅛ of 9-in pie (4.4 oz)	325	14	308	50	1
chocolate creme	⅙ of 8-in pie (4 oz)	344	22	153	38	—
coconut creme	⅙ of 7-in pie (2.2 oz)	191	11	163	24	1
lemon meringue	⅙ of 8-In pie (4.5 oz)	303	10	165	53	1
peach	⅙ of 8-in pie (4.1 oz)	261	12	316	39	—
HOME RECIPE						
apple	⅛ of 9-in pie (5.4 oz)	411	19	327	58	3
banana cream	⅛ of 9-in pie (5.2 oz)	398	20	355	49	—
blueberry	⅛ of 9-in pie (5.2 oz)	360	18	272	49	—
butterscotch	⅛ of 9-in pie (4.5 oz)	355	18	335	42	—
cherry	⅛ of 9-in pie (6.3 oz)	486	22	343	69	—
coconut creme	⅛ of 9-in pie (4.7 oz)	396	21	356	46	—
custard	⅛ of 9-in pie (4.5 oz)	262	11	256	34	2
lemon meringue	⅛ of 9-in pie (4.5 oz)	362	16	307	50	2
mince	⅛ of 9-in pie (5.8 oz)	477	18	419	79	—
pecan	⅛ of 9-in pie (4.3 oz)	502	27	320	64	4
pumpkin	⅛ of 9-in pie (5.4 oz)	316	14	349	41	4
vanilla cream	⅛ of 9-in pie (4.4 oz)	350	18	327	41	—

FOOD	PORTION	CAL	FAT	SOD	CARB	FIB
MIX						
Banana Cream as prep w/ whole milk (Jello-O)	⅙ of 8-in pie	103	3	161	18	—
Boston Cream Classic Dessert (Betty Crocker)	⅛ pie	270	6	390	50	—
Chocolate Cream Pie No Bake Dessert (Jell-O)	⅛ pie	260	17	—	—	—
Chocolate Mousse (Jello-O)	⅛ pie	259	17	426	25	—
Coconut Cream (Jell-O)	⅛ pie	258	16	304	27	—
Coconut Cream, as prep w/ whole milk (Jell-O)	⅙ of 8-in pie	111	4	140	16	—
Key Lime Pie Filling (Royal)	mix for 1 serving	50	0	120	13	—
Lemon (Jell-O)	⅙ of 8-in pie	175	2	95	38	—
Lemon Meringue No-Bake (Royal)	⅛ pie	210	5	170	38	—
Lemon Pie Filling (Royal)	mix for 1 serving	50	0	120	13	0
Pumpkin (Jell-O)	⅛ pie	253	13	448	31	—
banana cream no-bake	⅛ of 9-in pie (3.2 oz)	231	12	267	29	—
chocolate mousse no-bake	⅛ of 9-in pie (3.3 oz)	247	15	437	28	—
coconut creme no-bake	⅛ of 9-in pie (3.3 oz)	259	17	309	27	—
READY-TO-EAT						
Apple Homestyle (Entenmann's)	1 serving (2.1 oz)	140	7	150	21	—
Coconut Custard (Entenmann's)	1 serving (1.8 oz)	140	8	160	16	—
coconut custard	⅙ of 8-in pie (3.6 oz)	271	14	348	32	—
custard	⅙ of 9-in pie	330	17	436	36	—
pecan	⅙ of 8-in pie (4 oz)	452	21	480	65	4
pumpkin	⅙ of 8-in pie (3.8 oz)	229	10	308	30	3
SNACK						
Apple (Drake's)	1 (2 oz)	210	10	135	29	—
Apple (Tastykake)	1 pkg (113 g)	300	12	340	46	2

FOOD	PORTION	CAL	FAT	SOD	CARB	FIB
Banana Creme (Tastykake)	1 pkg (120 g)	380	16	430	54	2
Blueberry (Drake's)	1 (2 oz)	210	10	135	30	—
Blueberry (Tastykake)	1 pkg (113 g)	310	9	410	55	2
Cherry (Drake's)	1 (2 oz)	220	10	135	30	—
Cherry (Tastykake)	1 pkg (113 g)	300	10	310	49	2
Coconut Creme (Tastykake)	1 pkg (113 g)	380	20	420	46	2
French Apple (Tastykake)	1 pkg (120 g)	350	11	220	63	2
Lemon (Drake's)	1 (2 oz)	210	11	115	27	—
Lemon (Tastykake)	1 pkg (113 g)	320	13	380	48	2
Lemon Lime (Tastykake)	1 pkg (113 g)	320	13	310	49	1
Marshmallow Banana (Little Debbie)	1 pkg (1.4 oz)	160	5	95	27	0
Marshmallow Banana (Little Debbie)	1 pkg (2 oz)	240	8	140	40	0
Marshmallow Banana (Little Debbie)	1 pkg (2.7 oz)	320	11	190	54	0
Marshmallow Chocolate (Little Debbie)	1 pkg (1.4 oz)	160	5	95	27	1
Marshmallow Chocolate (Little Debbie)	1 pkg (2 oz)	240	9	135	40	1
Marshmallow Chocolate (Little Debbie)	1 pkg (2.7 oz)	320	11	190	53	1
Oatmeal Creme (Little Debbie)	1 pkg (1.3 oz)	170	8	200	25	1
Oatmeal Creme (Little Debbie)	1 pkg (2.5 oz)	300	11	330	48	1
Oatmeal Creme (Little Debbie)	1 pkg (3 oz)	360	14	400	58	2
Peach (Tastykake)	1 pkg (113 g)	300	12	360	47	—
Pecan (Lance)	1 (38 g)	350	15	70	51	—
Pineapple Cheese (Tastykake)	1 pkg (120 g)	340	13	410	54	2
Pumpkin (Tastykake)	1 pkg (4 oz)	320	14	520	46	2
Raisin Creme (Little Debbie)	1 pkg (1.2 oz)	140	5	120	23	1
Raisin Creme (Little Debbie)	1 pkg (2.5 oz)	290	12	240	47	0
Strawberry (Tastykake)	1 pkg (113 g)	340	11	300	57	1

FOOD	PORTION	CAL	FAT	SOD	CARB	FIB
Tasty Klair (Tastykake)	1 pkg (113 g)	400	20	320	51	2
apple	1 (3 oz)	266	14	325	33	—
cherry	1 (3 oz)	266	14	325	33	—
fried, apple	1 (6.4 oz)	404	21	479	55	3
fried, blueberry	1 (6.4 oz)	404	21	479	55	3
fried, cherry	1 (6.4 oz)	404	21	479	55	3
fried, lemon	1 (6.4 oz)	404	21	479	55	3
fried, peach	1 (6.4 oz)	404	21	479	55	3
fried, strawberry	1 (6.4 oz)	404	21	479	55	3
lemon	1 (3 oz)	266	14	325	33	—

PIE CRUST
see also PIE

FROZEN

FOOD	PORTION	CAL	FAT	SOD	CARB	FIB
Oronoque	⅙ pie (1.23 oz)	170	12	170	14	—
Oronoque Deep Dish	⅙ pie (1.41 oz)	200	13	200	16	—
Pepperidge Farm Patty Shells	1	210	15	180	16	—
Pepperidge Farm Puff Pastry Sheets	¼ sheet	260	17	290	22	—
Pet-Ritz Deep Dish	⅙ pie (1 oz)	130	8	120	12	—
Pet-Ritz Graham Cracker	⅙ pie (0.83 oz)	110	6	80	8	—
Pet-Ritz Regular	⅙ pie (0.83 oz)	110	7	110	11	—
Pet-Ritz Tart Shells	1	150	10	150	12	—
baked	⅛ of 9-in pie (0.6 oz)	82	5	104	8	—
baked	9-in shell (4.4 oz)	647	41	815	63	—
puff pastry, baked	1 shell (1.4 oz)	223	15	101	18	—

HOME RECIPE

FOOD	PORTION	CAL	FAT	SOD	CARB	FIB
9-inch crust	1	900	60	1100	79	—
baked	⅛ of 9-in crust (0.8 oz)	119	8	122	11	—
baked	9-in shell (6.3 oz)	949	62	975	86	—

MIX

FOOD	PORTION	CAL	FAT	SOD	CARB	FIB
Betty Crocker	⅟₁₆ pkg	120	8	140	10	—
Betty Crocker Sticks	⅟₁₆ pkg	120	8	140	10	—
Flako	⅙ of 9-in crust	250	15	390	24	—
Pillsbury Stick	⅙ of a 2-crust pie	270	17	420	25	—
Pillsbury Mix	⅙ of 2-crust pie	270	17	420	25	—
as prep	⅛ of 9-in pie (0.7 oz)	100	6	146	10	—

FOOD	PORTION	CAL	FAT	SOD	CARB	FIB
as prep	9-in crust (5.6 oz)	801	49	1167	81	—
READY-TO-EAT						
Generic Label Graham Cracker	⅛ pie (0.7 oz)	110	5	110	14	1
Honeymaid Graham (Nabisco)	1 slice (0.75 oz)	110	6	100	15	—
Nilla (Nabisco)	1 slice (0.75 oz)	110	6	50	14	—
Oreo (Nabisco)	1 slice (0.75 oz)	110	6	140	14	—
Ready Crust Chocolate	1 (3 in diam)	110	5	135	15	—
Ready Crust Chocolate	⅛ of 9-in crust	100	5	120	14	—
Ready Crust Graham	1 (3 in diam)	110	5	145	15	—
Ready Crust Graham	⅛ of 9-in crust	100	5	130	13	—
chocolate cookie crumb, baked	⅛ of 9-in pie (1 oz)	139	9	185	15	—
chocolate cookie crumb, baked	9-in crust (7.7 oz)	1130	69	1502	122	—
chocolate cookie crumb, chilled	⅛ of 9-in pie (1 oz)	142	9	188	15	—
chocolate cookie crumb, chilled	9-in crust (7.8 oz)	1127	69	1499	121	—
graham cracker, baked	⅛ of 9-in pie (1 oz)	148	8	171	20	—
graham cracker, baked	9-in crust (8.4 oz)	1181	60	1365	156	—
graham cracker, chilled	⅛ of 9-in pie (1 oz)	150	8	173	20	—
graham cracker, chilled	9-in crust (8.6 oz)	1182	60	1365	155	—
vanilla wafer cracker crumbs, baked	⅛ of 9-in pie (0.8 oz)	119	8	116	11	—
vanilla wafer cracker crumbs, baked	9-in crust (6.1 oz)	937	64	909	89	—
vanilla wafer cracker crumbs, chilled	⅛ of 9-in pie (0.8 oz)	117	8	113	11	—
vanilla wafer cracker crumbs, chilled	9-in crust (6.2 oz)	934	64	906	88	—
REFRIGERATED						
Pillsbury All Ready	⅛ of 2-crust pie	240	15	200	24	—

PIEROGI
FROZEN

FOOD	PORTION	CAL	FAT	SOD	CARB	FIB
Potato And Cheddar Cheese (Mrs. T's)	1 (1.3 oz)	60	tr	170	11	—

FOOD	PORTION	CAL	FAT	SOD	CARB	FIB
Potato And Onion (Mrs. T's)	1 (1.3 oz)	50	tr	140	10	—
Potato Cheese (Golden)	3 (4 oz)	250	8	260	38	—
Potato Onion (Golden)	3 (4 oz)	210	6	220	36	—
Sauerkraut (Mrs. T's)	1	60	0	—	—	—
TAKE-OUT						
pierogi	¾ cup (4.4 oz)	307	19	369	24	—

PIG'S EARS AND FEET

ears, frzn, simmered	1 ear (3.7 oz)	183	12	183	0	—
feet, pickled	1 lb	923	73	—	tr	—
feet, pickled	1 oz	58	5	—	tr	—
feet, simmered	2.5 oz	138	9	—	0	—

PIGEON PEAS
DRIED

cooked	1 cup	204	1	9	39	—
cooked	½ cup	102	tr	5	20	—

PIGNOLIA
see PINE NUTS

PIKE
FRESH

northern, cooked	½ fillet (5.4 oz)	176	1	76	0	—
northern, cooked	3 oz	96	1	42	0	—
northern, raw	3 oz	75	1	33	0	—
roe, raw	3.5 oz	130	2	—	2	—
walleye, baked	3 oz	101	1	56	0	—
walleye fillet, baked	4.4 oz	147	2	81	0	—

PILLNUTS

canarytree, dried	1 oz	204	23	1	1	—

PIMIENTOS

Dromedary	1 oz	10	0	5	2	—
canned	1 slice	0	0	0	tr	—
canned	1 tbsp	3	tr	2	1	—

PINE NUTS

pignolia, dried	1 oz	146	14	1	4	—
pignolia, dried	1 tbsp	51	5	0	1	—
pinyon, dried	1 oz	161	17	20	5	—

FOOD	PORTION	CAL	FAT	SOD	CARB	FIB
PINEAPPLE						
CANNED						
All Cuts Juice Pack (Dole)	½ cup	70	tr	10	18	—
All Cuts Syrup Pack (Dole)	½ cup	90	tr	10	23	—
Chunk (Empress)	4 oz	70	0	—	18	—
Crushed (Empress)	4 oz	70	0	—	18	—
Hawaiian Slice In Heavy Syrup (S&W)	½ cup	90	0	0	23	—
Hawaiian Slice Juice Pack (S&W)	½ cup	70	0	10	17	—
Sliced (Empress)	4 oz	70	0	—	18	—
Sliced Unsweetened (S&W)	½ cup	60	0	10	15	—
chunks, in heavy syrup	1 cup	199	tr	3	52	—
chunks, juice pack	1 cup	150	tr	4	39	—
crushed, in heavy syrup	1 cup	199	tr	3	52	—
slices, in heavy syrup	1 slice	45	tr	1	12	—
slices, in light syrup	1 slice	30	tr	1	8	—
slices, juice pack	1 slice	35	tr	1	9	—
slices, water pack	1 slice	19	tr	1	5	—
tidbits, in heavy syrup	1 cup	199	tr	3	52	—
tidbits, in juice	1 cup	150	tr	4	19	—
tidbits, in water	1 cup	79	tr	3	20	—
FRESH						
Chiquita	1 cup	90	1	—	—	—
Dole	2 slices	90	1	10	21	2
diced	1 cup	77	tr	1	19	2
slice	1 slice	42	tr	1	10	1
FROZEN						
chunks, sweetened	½ cup	104	tr	2	27	—
JUICE						
Bright & Early Frozen	8 fl oz	120	0	10	30	—
Dole	6 oz	100	tr	280	25	—
Dole New Breakfast Juice	6 oz	100	tr	5	25	—
Libby's Nectar	6 oz	110	0	30	27	—
Minute Maid Box	8.45 fl oz	130	0	25	33	—
Minute Maid Frozen	8 fl oz	130	0	0	31	—
Mott's	9.5 oz	169	0	—	—	—
S&W Unsweetened	6 oz	100	0	0	25	—
Tree Top	6 oz	100	0	0	24	—

FOOD	PORTION	CAL	FAT	SOD	CARB	FIB
Veryfine 100%	8 oz	125	0	10	31	—
canned	1 cup	139	tr	2	34	—
frzn, as prep	1 cup	129	tr	3	32	—
frzn, not prep	6 oz	387	tr	6	96	—

PINK BEANS
CANNED
Goya Spanish Style	7.5 oz	140	tr	800	32	10

DRIED
cooked	1 cup	252	1	3	47	—

PINTO BEANS
CANNED
Gebhardt	4 oz	100	tr	600	19	5
Goya Spanish Style	7.5 oz	140	1	860	31	10
Green Giant	½ cup	90	1	280	20	5
Green Giant Picante	½ cup	100	1	580	21	6
Luck's Seasoned w/ Pork w/ Onions	7.5 oz	220	6	—	—	—
Old El Paso	½ cup	100	0	320	19	15
Progresso	½ cup	110	tr	410	21	7
Trappey's	½ cup	90	1	410	17	—
Trappey's Hearty Texas	½ cup	110	2	440	18	—
Trappey's Jalapinto	½ cup	90	1	480	15	—
pinto	1 cup	186	1	998	35	—

DRIED
Arrowhead	¼ cup (1.5 oz)	150	1	0	27	8
Bean Cuisine	½ cup	115	1	5	—	5
Hurst Brand	1 cup	265	tr	—	—	—
cooked	1 cup	235	1	3	44	—

FROZEN
cooked	3 oz	152	tr	—	29	—

SPROUTS
cooked	3.5 oz	22	tr	—	4	—
raw	3.5 oz	62	1	—	12	—

PINYON
see PINE NUTS

PISTACHIOS
California Natural Dole	1 oz	90	7	250	3	—
Dry Roasted Planters	1 oz	170	15	—	—	—
Lance	1 pkg (32 g)	100	8	100	4	—
Red Salted Planters	1 oz	170	14	250	6	—
Shelled & Roasted Dole	1 oz	163	14	—	7	—

FOOD	PORTION	CAL	FAT	SOD	CARB	FIB
dried	1 cup	739	62	7	32	14
dried	1 oz	164	14	2	7	3
dry roasted	1 oz	172	15	2	8	—
dry roasted, salted	1 cup	776	68	1040	35	—
dry roasted, salted	1 oz	172	15	260	8	—

PITANGA
fresh	1	2	tr	0	1	—
fresh	1 cup	57	1	5	13	—

PIZZA
FROZEN
Celeste

Canadian Style Bacon	1 (9.25 oz)	550	26	—	—	—
Cheese	1 (6.5 oz)	500	24	—	—	—
Deluxe	1 (8.25 oz)	600	32	—	—	—
Pepperoni	1 (6.25 oz)	540	29	—	—	—
Sausage	1 (7.5 oz)	580	32	—	—	—
Sausage & Mushroom	1 (9.25 oz)	600	32	—	—	—
Supreme	1 (9 oz)	690	39	—	—	—
Fox Deluxe						
Golden Topping	½ pizza	240	11	600	25	—
Hamburger	½ pizza	260	12	700	26	—
Pepperoni	½ pizza	250	13	640	26	—
Sausage	½ pizza	260	13	630	26	—
Sausage & Pepperoni	½ pizza	260	13	640	26	—
Healthy Choice						
French Bread Cheese	1 (5.3 oz)	270	2	420	45	—
French Bread Deluxe	1 (6.25 oz)	330	8	490	41	—
French Bread Italian Turkey Sausage	1 (6.45 oz)	320	7	440	42	—
French Bread Pepperoni	1 (6.25 oz)	320	8	490	41	—
Jeno's						
4-Pack Cheese	1 pizza	160	8	460	17	—
4-Pack Combination	1 pizza	180	9	470	17	—
4-Pack Hamburger	1 pizza	180	9	500	17	—
4-Pack Pepperoni	1 pizza	170	9	460	17	—
4-Pack Sausage	1 pizza	180	9	460	17	—
Crisp 'n Tasty Canadian Bacon	½ pizza	250	11	880	27	—

FOOD	PORTION	CAL	FAT	SOD	CARB	FIB
Jeno's *(cont.)*						
Crisp 'n Tasty Cheese	½ pizza	270	14	770	28	—
Crisp 'n Tasty Hamburger	½ pizza	290	15	810	28	—
Crisp 'n Tasty Pepperoni	½ pizza	280	15	760	27	—
Crisp 'n Tasty Sausage	½ pizza	300	16	850	28	—
Crisp 'n Tasty Sausage & Pepperoni	½ pizza	300	16	840	27	—
Microwave Pizza Rolls Pepperoni & Cheese	6	240	13	440	23	—
Microwave Pizza Rolls Sausage & Cheese	6	250	13	440	24	—
Pizza Rolls Cheese	6	240	12	350	23	—
Pizza Rolls Hamburger	6	240	13	280	21	—
Pizza Rolls Pepperoni & Cheese	6	230	13	390	22	—
Pizza Rolls Sausage & Pepperoni	6	230	13	380	22	—
Kid Cuisine						
Cheese	1 (6.85 oz)	380	12	390	57	—
Hamburger	1 (6.85 oz)	330	10	700	50	—
Mega Meal Cheese	1 (9.7 oz)	430	7	700	75	—
Lean Cuisine						
French Bread Cheese	1 pkg (6 oz)	350	8	400	48	4
French Bread Deluxe	1 pkg (6.1 oz)	350	6	560	45	5
French Bread Pepperoni	1 pkg (5.25 oz)	330	7	590	46	4
MicroMagic						
Deep Dish Combination	1 (6.5 oz)	605	34	1280	60	—
Deep Dish Pepperoni	1 (6.5 oz)	615	32	1300	65	—
Deep Dish Sausage	1 (6.5 oz)	590	31	1250	62	—
Mr. P's						
Combination	½ pizza	260	13	640	26	—
Golden Topping	½ pizza	240	11	600	25	—
Hamburger	½ pizza	260	12	700	26	—

FOOD	PORTION	CAL	FAT	SOD	CARB	FIB
Pepperoni	½ pizza	250	13	640	26	—
Sausage	½ pizza	260	13	630	26	—
Pappalo's						
French Bread Cheese	1 pizza	360	15	830	40	—
French Bread Combination	1 pizza	430	21	1120	41	—
French Bread Pepperoni	1 pizza	410	20	1130	41	—
French Bread Sausage	1 pizza	410	18	1000	41	—
Thin Crust Combination	⅙ pizza	260	10	590	29	—
Thin Crust Hamburger	⅙ pizza	240	8	470	28	—
Thin Crust Pepperoni	⅙ pizza	270	11	600	28	—
Thin Crust Sausage	⅙ pizza	250	9	490	28	—
Combination	⅙ pizza	340	15	700	34	—
Hamburger	⅙ pizza	310	12	580	34	—
Pepperoni	⅙ pizza	330	14	710	34	—
Sausage	⅙ pizza	360	18	550	34	—
Pepperidge Farm						
Croissant Pastry Cheese	1	430	23	640	41	—
Croissant Pastry Deluxe	1	440	23	790	43	—
Croissant Pastry Pepperoni	1	420	22	690	43	—
Pillsbury						
Microwave Cheese	½ pizza	240	10	540	28	—
Microwave Combination	½ pizza	310	15	780	29	—
Microwave French Bread	1 pizza	370	15	680	41	—
Microwave French Bread Pepperoni	1 pizza	430	19	940	46	—
Microwave French Bread Sausage	1 pizza	410	16	860	48	—
Microwave French Bread Sausage & Pepperoni	1 pizza	450	21	950	47	—
Microwave Pepperoni	½ pizza	300	15	790	29	—
Microwave Sausage	½ pizza	280	13	680	29	—

FOOD	PORTION	CAL	FAT	SOD	CARB	FIB
Stouffer's						
French Bread Bacon Cheddar	1 piece (5.8 oz)	440	22	940	44	4
French Bread Cheese	1 piece (5.2 oz)	350	14	660	42	3
French Bread Cheeseburger	1 piece (6 oz)	440	26	1110	31	5
French Bread Deluxe	1 piece (6.2 oz)	440	22	980	42	5
French Bread Double Cheese	1 piece (5.9 oz)	420	19	790	44	5
French Bread Garden Vegetable	1 piece (5.8 oz)	340	12	540	45	4
French Bread Pepperoni	1 piece (5.6 oz)	420	20	930	42	3
French Bread Pepperoni & Mushroom	1 piece (6.1 oz)	430	21	1000	43	3
French Bread Sausage	1 piece (6 oz)	420	20	900	41	4
French Bread Sausage & Pepperoni	1 piece (6.25 oz)	460	25	1130	45	4
French Bread Vegetable Deluxe	1 piece (6.4 oz)	380	17	830	43	5
French Bread White Pizza	1 piece (5.1 oz)	460	28	760	43	5
Lunch Express Deluxe	1 pkg (6.6 oz)	460	25	1000	40	4
Lunch Express Double Cheese	1 pkg (5.9 oz)	420	19	710	41	3
Lunch Express Pepperoni	1 pkg (5.75 oz)	440	23	960	39	4
Lunch Express Sausage	1 pkg (6.5 oz)	460	25	1090	40	3
Lunch Express Sausage and Pepperoni	1 pkg (6.4 oz)	500	27	1140	41	4
Tombstone						
Double Top Double Cheese	⅙ pie (4.6 oz)	350	19	740	25	2
Double Top Pepperoni With Double Cheese	⅙ pie (4.6 oz)	370	21	820	25	2

FOOD	PORTION	CAL	FAT	SOD	CARB	FIB
Double Top Sausage & Pepperoni With Double Cheese	⅙ pie (4.6 oz)	360	20	800	25	2
For One ½ Less Fat Cheese	1 pie (6.5 oz)	360	10	920	45	3
For One ½ Less Fat Pepperoni	1 pie (6.7 oz)	400	20	1040	45	4
For One ½ Less Fat Supreme	1 pie (7.7 oz)	400	13	1090	45	4
For One ½ Less Fat Vegetable	1 pie (7.2 oz)	360	10	730	46	5
For One Extra Cheese	1 pie (6.9 oz)	540	30	910	41	3
For One Italian Sausage	1 pie (7 oz)	560	33	1130	40	2
For One Pepperoni	1 pie (6.9 oz)	580	35	1170	41	3
For One Sausage & Pepperoni	1 pie (7 oz)	590	37	1200	40	3
For One Supreme	1 pie (7.6 oz)	570	34	1130	41	3
Tombstone 12 in						
Canadian Bacon	⅕ pie (5.4 oz)	370	16	840	36	2
Deluxe	⅙ pie (4.6 oz)	320	16	640	29	2
Extra Cheese	⅕ pie (5.1 oz)	370	17	680	36	2
Hamburger	⅕ pie (5.3 oz)	320	16	660	29	2
Light Supreme	⅕ pie (4.8 oz)	270	9	710	30	3
Light Vegetable	⅕ pie (4.6 oz)	240	7	500	31	3
Pepperoni	⅕ pie (5.3 oz)	340	18	750	29	2
Sausage	⅕ pie (5.3 oz)	320	16	650	29	2
Sausage & Mushroom	⅕ pie (4.5 oz)	320	16	630	29	2
Sausage & Pepperoni	⅕ pie (5.3 oz)	340	16	740	29	2
Special Order Four Cheese	⅙ pie (5.1 oz)	380	18	830	38	3
Special Order Four Meat	⅙ pie (4.6 oz)	340	17	880	31	3
Special Order Pepperoni	⅙ pie (5.3 oz)	420	21	1010	38	3
Special Order Super Supreme	⅙ pie (4.7 oz)	340	17	860	32	3
Special Order Three Sausage	⅙ pie (4.5 oz)	330	16	790	32	3
Supreme	⅕ pie (4.6 oz)	330	17	720	29	2
ThinCrust Four Meat	¼ pie (5.1 oz)	410	25	940	25	2

FOOD	PORTION	CAL	FAT	SOD	CARB	FIB
Tombstone 12 in *(cont.)*						
ThinCrust Italian Sausage	¼ pie (5.1 oz)	400	24	880	25	2
ThinCrust Pepperoni	¼ pie (5 oz)	420	27	950	25	2
ThinCrust Supreme	¼ pie (5.3 oz)	400	24	880	26	2
ThinCrust Taco	¼ pie (5.1 oz)	380	23	850	26	2
ThinCrust Three Cheese	¼ pie (4.8 oz)	380	22	730	25	2
Tombstone 9 in						
Deluxe	⅓ pie (4.5 oz)	320	16	620	20	2
Extra Cheese	⅓ pie (5.6 oz)	420	19	730	42	3
Hamburger	⅓ pie (4.1 oz)	310	16	620	28	2
Pepperoni	⅓ pie (4.1 oz)	340	19	740	28	2
Pepperoni & Sausage	⅓ pie (5.3 oz)	360	21	820	28	2
Sausage	⅓ pie (4.1 oz)	310	16	610	28	2
Special Order Four Meat	⅙ pie (5.2 oz)	390	19	1000	36	3
Special Order Pepperoni	⅙ pie (4.9 oz)	390	20	950	36	3
Special Order Super Supreme	⅙ pie (5.4 oz)	390	20	980	36	3
Special Order Three Sausage	⅙ pie (5 oz)	370	18	890	36	3
Totino's						
Microwave Cheese	1 pizza	250	8	760	34	—
Microwave Pepperoni	1 pizza	280	12	880	34	—
Microwave Sausage	1 pizza	320	16	870	33	—
Microwave Sausage Pepperoni Combination	1 pizza	310	15	970	31	—
My Classic Deluxe Cheese	⅙ pizza	210	9	420	23	—
My Classic Deluxe Combination	⅙ pizza	270	14	630	23	—
My Classic Deluxe Pepperoni	⅙ pizza	260	13	630	23	—
Pan Pepperoni	⅙ pizza	330	14	730	34	—
Pan Sausage	⅙ pizza	320	13	630	34	—
Pan Sausage & Pepperoni Combination	⅙ pizza	340	15	720	34	—
Pan Three Cheese	⅙ pizza	290	10	510	33	—
Party Bacon	½ pizza	370	20	1030	35	—

FOOD	PORTION	CAL	FAT	SOD	CARB	FIB
Party Canadian Bacon	½ pizza	310	14	1150	35	—
Party Cheese	½ pizza	340	17	1000	34	—
Party Combination	½ pizza	380	21	1230	35	—
Party Hamburger	½ pizza	370	19	1060	35	—
Party Mexican Style	½ pizza	380	21	970	35	—
Party Pepperoni	½ pizza	370	20	1310	35	—
Party Sausage	½ pizza	390	21	1180	35	—
Party Vegetable	½ pizza	300	13	910	36	—
Slices Cheese	1	170	7	350	20	—
Slices Combination	1	200	10	630	20	—
Slices Pepperoni	1	190	9	530	20	—
Slices Sausage	1	200	10	540	20	—
Weight Watchers						
Cheese	1 (6.03 oz)	300	7	310	36	—
Deluxe Combination	1 (7.32 oz)	320	9	370	36	—
Deluxe French Bread	1 (5.94 oz)	260	7	480	29	—
Pepperoni	1 (6.08 oz)	320	8	550	36	—
Sausage	1 (6.43 oz)	340	10	380	37	—
SAUCE						
Contadina Pizza Sauce	¼ cup	35	2	350	6	1
Contadina Pizza Sauce Flavored With Pepperoni	¼ cup	40	2	420	6	1
Contadina Pizza Sauce With Italian Cheeses	¼ cup	40	2	420	6	1
Contadina Pizza Squeeze	¼ cup	35	2	350	6	1
Ragu Pizza Quick Traditional	3 tbsp (1.7 oz)	35	2	330	3	—
TAKE-OUT						
cheese	⅛ of 12-in pie	140	3	336	21	—
cheese	12-in pie	1121	26	2680	164	—
cheese, meat & vegetables	⅛ of 12-in pie	184	5	382	21	—
cheese, meat & vegetables	12-in pie	1472	43	3054	170	—
pepperoni	⅛ of 12-in pie	181	7	267	20	—
pepperoni	12-in pie	1445	56	2133	157	—

PLANTAINS

FOOD	PORTION	CAL	FAT	SOD	CARB	FIB
All Natural Plantain Chips (Top Banana)	1 oz	150	8	85	17	—
FRESH						
sliced, cooked	½ cup	89	tr	4	24	—

FOOD	PORTION	CAL	FAT	SOD	CARB	FIB
uncooked	1 (6.3 oz)	218	1	7	57	—
TAKE-OUT						
ripe, fried	2.8 oz	214	7	—	38	4

PLUMS
CANNED

FOOD	PORTION	CAL	FAT	SOD	CARB	FIB
Halves Purple Fancy Unpeeled In Extra Heavy Syrup (S&W)	½ cup	135	0	25	35	—
Halves Unpeeled Diet (S&W)	½ cup	52	0	0	13	—
Whole Purple Fancy Unpeeled In Extra Heavy Syrup (S&W)	½ cup	135	0	25	35	—
Whole Unpeeled Diet (S&W)	½ cup	52	0	0	13	—
purple in heavy syrup	1 cup	320	tr	50	60	—
purple in heavy syrup	3	119	tr	26	31	—
purple in light syrup	1 cup	158	tr	50	41	—
purple in light syrup	3	83	tr	26	22	—
purple, juice pack	1 cup	146	tr	3	38	—
purple, juice pack	3	55	tr	1	14	—
purple, water pack	1 cup	102	tr	2	27	—
purple, water pack	3	39	tr	1	10	—
FRESH						
Dole	2	70	1	0	17	1
plum	1	36	tr	0	9	—
sliced	1 cup	91	1	1	21	—
JUICE						
Kern's Nectar	6 oz	110	0	10	26	—

POI

FOOD	PORTION	CAL	FAT	SOD	CARB	FIB
poi	½ cup	134	tr	14	33	—

POKEBERRY SHOOTS
FRESH

FOOD	PORTION	CAL	FAT	SOD	CARB	FIB
cooked	½ cup	16	tr	—	3	—
raw	½ cup	18	tr	—	3	—

POLLACK

FOOD	PORTION	CAL	FAT	SOD	CARB	FIB
atlantic fillet, baked	5.3 oz	178	2	166	0	—
atlantic, baked	3 oz	100	1	94	0	—
FROZEN						
Mrs. Paul's Light Fillets	1 fillet (4.5 oz)	240	11	530	18	—

FOOD	PORTION	CAL	FAT	SOD	CARB	FIB
POMEGRANATES						
FRESH						
pomegranate	1	104	tr	5	26	—
POMPANO						
florida, cooked	3 oz	179	10	65	0	—
florida, raw	3 oz	140	8	55	0	—
POPCORN						
see also CHIPS, PRETZELS, SNACKS						
Cape Cod	½ oz	80	5	150	6	—
Cape Cod Light	½ oz	60	3	95	8	—
Cheetos Cheddar Cheese	0.5 oz	80	6	160	6	—
Chesters	0.5 oz	70	3	200	9	—
Chesters Cheddar Cheese	0.5 oz	80	5	200	7	—
Chesters Microwave	3 cups	110	7	170	13	—
Chesters Microwave Butter Flavored	3 cups	120	7	180	13	—
Chesters Microwave Cheese Flavored	3 cups	110	8	230	11	—
Cracker Jack	1 oz	120	3	85	22	—
Eagle	½ oz	80	6	150	6	—
Jiffy Pop						
Bag Butter	3 cups	90	5	140	11	2
Bag Lite	3 cups	70	3	110	11	2
Bag Regular	3 cups	100	6	140	11	2
Glazed Popcorn Clusters	1 oz	120	2	120	25	1
Microwave Butter	4 cups	140	7	270	17	3
Microwave Regular	4 cups	140	7	270	17	3
Pan Butter	4 cups	130	6	270	16	2
Pan Regular	4 cups	130	6	270	16	2
Lance Cheese	1 pkg (25 g)	130	8	280	13	—
Lance Plain	1 pkg (25 g)	140	9	210	13	—
Lance White Cheddar Cheese	1 pkg (25 g)	140	9	170	12	—
Newman's Own						
Oldstyle Picture Show	3½ cups	80	1	0	16	—
Oldstyle Picture Show Microwave Natural Butter	3 cups	150	8	200	18	4

FOOD	PORTION	CAL	FAT	SOD	CARB	FIB
Newman's Own *(cont.)*						
Oldstyle Picture Show Microwave Light Butter	3 cups	90	3	100	18	4
Oldstyle Picture Show Microwave Light Natural	3 cups	90	3	100	18	4
Oldstyle Picture Show Microwave No Salt	3 cups	150	8	0	18	4
Orville Redenbacher's						
Gourmet Hot Air	3 cups	40	tr	0	10	3
Gourmet Original	3 cups	80	4	0	10	3
Gourmet White	3 cups	80	4	0	10	3
Microwave Gourmet	3 cups	100	6	200	11	3
Microwave Gourmet Butter	3 cups	100	6	240	11	3
Microwave Gourmet Butter Toffee	2.5 cups	210	12	85	26	2
Microwave Gourmet Caramel	2.5 cups	240	14	90	29	2
Microwave Gourmet Cheddar Cheese	3 cups	130	8	280	14	3
Microwave Gourmet Frozen	3 cups	100	6	200	11	3
Microwave Gourmet Frozen Butter	3 cups	100	6	240	11	3
Microwave Gourmet Light	3 cups	70	3	115	8	3
Microwave Gourmet Light Butter	3 cups	70	3	110	8	3
Microwave Gourmet Salt Free	3 cups	100	6	0	11	3
Microwave Gourmet Salt Free Butter	3 cups	100	6	0	11	3
Microwave Gourmet Sour Cream 'n Onion	3 cups	160	12	270	12	3
Pillsbury Microwave Butter	3 cups	210	13	410	20	—
Pillsbury Microwave Original	3 cups	210	13	410	20	—
Pillsbury Microwave Salt Free	3 cups	170	7	0	23	—

FOOD	PORTION	CAL	FAT	SOD	CARB	FIB
Pop Secret						
Butter Flavor	3 cups	100	6	170	11	2
Butter Flavor Singles	6 cups	250	16	310	23	4
Natural Flavor	3 cups	100	6	170	11	2
Natural Flavor Salt Free	3 cups	100	6	5	11	2
Pop Qwiz Butter Flavor	3 cups	100	6	170	11	2
Pop Qwiz Natural Flavor	3 cups	100	6	170	11	2
Butter Flavor	3 cups	70	3	115	12	2
Butter Flavor Singles	6 cups	140	6	190	23	4
Natural Flavor	3 cups	70	3	160	12	2
Natural Flavor Singles	6 cups	150	6	320	23	4
Smartfood Cheddar Cheese	0.5 oz	80	5	130	7	—
Snyder's Butter	1 oz	140	9	140	13	3
Ultra Slim-Fast Lite N' Tasty	½ oz	60	2	150	10	2
Weight Watchers Microwave	1 oz	100	1	5	22	—
Weight Watchers Ready-to-Eat Butter	0.7 oz	90	3	100	13	—
Weight Watchers Ready-to-Eat White Cheddar Cheese	0.7 oz	90	4	120	11	—
Wise Tender Eating	0.5 oz	70	6	120	4	—
Wise With Real Premium White Cheddar Cheese	0.5 oz	70	5	170	4	—
air-popped	1 cup	30	tr	tr	6	—
popped w/ vegetable oil	1 cup	55	3	86	6	—
sugar syrup coated	1 cup	135	1	tr	30	—

POPOVER

FOOD	PORTION	CAL	FAT	SOD	CARB	FIB
home recipe, as prep w/ 2% milk	1 (1.4 oz)	87	3	82	11	—
home recipe, as prep w/ whole milk	1 (1.4 oz)	90	3	82	11	—
mix, as prep	1 (1.2 oz)	67	2	143	10	—

POPPY SEEDS

FOOD	PORTION	CAL	FAT	SOD	CARB	FIB
poppy seeds	1 tsp	15	1	1	1	—

FOOD	PORTION	CAL	FAT	SOD	CARB	FIB

PORK
see also BACON, BACON SUBSTITUTES, CANADIAN BACON, HAM, LUNCHEON MEAT/COLD CUTS, SAUSAGE

The values for cooked pork may differ slightly from values for raw pork. When meat is cooked some moisture and fat is lost, changing the nutritive value slightly. As a rule of thumb, it can be assumed that a 4 oz raw portion will equal a 3 oz cooked portion of meat.

FRESH

FOOD	PORTION	CAL	FAT	SOD	CARB	FIB
blade chop, roasted	1 (3.1 oz)	321	27	54	0	—
center loin chop, broiled	1 (3.1 oz)	275	24	61	0	—
center loin chop lean & fat, braised	1 chop (2.6 oz)	266	19	—	—	—
center loin chop lean & fat, broiled	1 chop (3.1 oz)	275	19	—	—	—
center loin chop lean & fat, panfried	1 chop (3.1 oz)	333	27	—	—	—
center loin chop lean & fat, roasted	1 chop (3.1 oz)	268	19	—	—	—
center loin chop lean only, braised	1 chop (2.1 oz)	166	8	—	—	—
center loin chop lean only, broiled	1 chop (2.5 oz)	166	8	—	—	—
center loin chop lean only, panfried	1 chop (2.4 oz)	178	11	—	—	—
center loin chop lean only, roasted	1 chop (2.4 oz)	180	10	—	—	—
center loin lean & fat, braised	3 oz	301	22	—	—	—
center loin lean & fat, panfried	3 oz	318	26	—	—	—
center loin lean only, broiled	3 oz	196	9	—	—	—
center loin lean only, panfried	3 oz	226	14	—	—	—
center loin lean only, roasted	3 oz	204	11	—	—	—
center loin, roasted	3 oz	259	18	54	0	—
ham fresh rump half lean & fat, roasted	3 oz	233	23	—	—	—

FOOD	PORTION	CAL	FAT	SOD	CARB	FIB
ham fresh rump half lean only, roasted	3 oz	187	9	—	—	—
ham fresh shank half lean & fat, roasted	3 oz	258	19	—	—	—
ham fresh shank half lean only, roasted	3 oz	183	9	—	—	—
ham fresh whole lean & fat, roasted	3 oz	250	18	—	—	—
ham fresh whole lean only, roasted	3 oz	187	9	—	—	—
leg loin & shoulder lean only, roasted	3 oz	198	11	—	—	—
loin blade chop lean & fat, braised	1 chop (2.4 oz)	275	23	—	—	—
loin blade chop lean & fat, braised	1 chop (3.1 oz)	321	27	—	—	—
loin blade chop lean & fat, panfried	1 chop (3.1 oz)	368	33	—	—	—
loin blade chop lean only, braised	1 chop (1.8 oz)	156	10	—	—	—
loin blade chop lean only, broiled	1 chop (2.1 oz)	177	13	—	—	—
loin blade chop lean only, panfried	1 chop (2.2 oz)	175	12	—	—	—
loin blade chop lean only, roasted	1 chop (2.5 oz)	198	14	—	—	—
loin blade lean & fat, braised	3 oz	348	29	—	—	—
loin blade lean & fat, broiled	3 oz	334	29	—	—	—
loin blade lean & fat, panfried	3 oz	352	31	—	—	—
loin blade lean & fat, roasted	3 oz	310	26	—	—	—
loin blade lean only, broiled	3 oz	255	18	—	—	—
loin blade lean only, panfried	3 oz	240	17	—	—	—
loin blade lean only, roasted	3 oz	238	16	—	—	—
loin chop lean & fat, braised	1 chop (2.3 oz)	267	20	—	—	—
loin chop lean & fat, broiled	1 chop (2.7 oz)	295	23	—	—	—

FOOD	PORTION	CAL	FAT	SOD	CARB	FIB
loin chop lean & fat, panfried	1 chop (2.9 oz)	337	29	—	—	—
loin chop lean & fat, roasted	1 chop (2.8 oz)	274	21	—	—	—
loin chop lean only, braised	1 chop (1.8 oz)	147	8	—	—	—
loin chop lean only, broiled	1 chop (2.1 oz)	165	10	—	—	—
loin chop lean only, panfried	1 chop (2 oz)	157	9	—	—	—
loin chop lean only, roasted	1 chop (2.3 oz)	167	9	—	—	—
loin chop lean & fat, braised	1 chop (2.5 oz)	261	20	—	—	—
loin chop lean & fat, roasted	1 chop (2.9 oz)	262	20	—	—	—
loin lean & fat, braised	3 oz	312	24	—	—	—
loin lean & fat, broiled	3 oz	294	23	—	—	—
loin lean only, braised	3 oz	232	12	—	—	—
loin lean only, broiled	3 oz	218	13	—	—	—
loin lean only, roasted	3 oz	204	12	—	—	—
loin w/ fat, roasted	3 oz	271	21	53	0	—
lungs, braised	3 oz	84	3	—	—	—
pancreas, braised	3 oz	186	9	—	—	—
rib chop lean only, braised	1 chop (1.8 oz)	147	8	—	—	—
rib chop lean only, broiled	1 chop (2.1 oz)	162	9	—	—	—
rib chop lean only, panfried	1 chop (2 oz)	160	9	—	—	—
rib chop lean only, roasted	1 chop (2.2 oz)	162	9	—	—	—
rib chop lean & fat, braised	1 chop (2.2 oz)	246	18	—	—	—
rib chop lean & fat, broiled	1 chop (2.6 oz)	264	20	—	—	—
rib chop lean & fat panfried	1 chop (2.9 oz)	343	29	—	—	—
rib chop lean & fat, roasted	1 chop (2.6 oz)	252	19	—	—	—
shoulder arm picnic cured lean & fat, roasted	3 oz	238	18	—	—	—

FOOD	PORTION	CAL	FAT	SOD	CARB	FIB
shoulder arm picnic cured lean only, roasted	3 oz	145	6	1046	0	—
shoulder arm picnic lean only, braised	3 oz	211	10	—	—	—
shoulder arm picnic lean only, roasted	3 oz	194	11	—	—	—
shoulder arm picnic lean & fat, braised	3 oz	293	22	—	—	—
shoulder arm & picnic lean & fat, roasted	3 oz	281	22	—	—	—
shoulder blade boston steak lean & fat, braised	1 steak (5.6 oz)	594	46	—	—	—
shoulder blade boston steak lean & fat, broiled	1 steak (6.5 oz)	647	53	—	—	—
shoulder blade boston steak lean & fat, roasted	1 steak (6.5 oz)	594	47	—	—	—
shoulder blade boston steak lean only, braised	1 steak (4.6 oz)	382	23	—	—	—
shoulder blade boston steak lean only, broiled	1 steak (5.3 oz)	413	28	—	—	—
shoulder blade boston steak lean only, roasted	1 steak (5.5 oz)	404	27	—	—	—
shoulder blade roll cured lean & fat	3 oz	304	25	1412	0	—
shoulder boston blade lean & fat, braised	3 oz	316	24	—	—	—
shoulder boston blade lean & fat, broiled	3 oz	297	24	—	—	—
shoulder boston blade lean & fat, roasted	3 oz	273	21	—	—	—
shoulder boston blade lean only, braised	3 oz	250	15	—	—	—
shoulder boston blade lean only, broiled	3 oz	233	16	—	—	—
shoulder boston blade lean only, roasted	3 oz	218	14	—	—	—
shoulder whole lean only, roasted	3 oz	207	13	—	—	—

FOOD	PORTION	CAL	FAT	SOD	CARB	FIB
shoulder whole, roasted	3 oz	277	22	58	0	—
sirloin chop lean & fat, braised	1 chop (2.4 oz)	250	18	—	—	—
sirloin chop lean & fat, broiled	1 chop (2.8 oz)	278	21	—	—	—
sirloin chop lean & fat, roasted	1 chop (2.8 oz)	244	17	—	—	—
sirloin chop lean only, braised	1 chop (1.9 oz)	149	7	—	—	—
sirloin chop lean only, broiled	1 chop (2.3 oz)	165	9	—	—	—
sirloin chop lean only, roasted	1 chop (2.5 oz)	175	10	—	—	—
spareribs, braised	3 oz	338	26	79	0	—
spleen, braised	3 oz	127	3	—	0	—
tail, simmered	3 oz	336	30	—	—	—
tenderloin lean only, roasted	3 oz	141	4	57	0	—

POSOLE
see HOMINY

POT PIE
FROZEN

FOOD	PORTION	CAL	FAT	SOD	CARB	FIB
Beef (Morton)	7 oz	430	31	—	—	—
Beef (Swanson)	7 oz	370	19	730	36	—
Beef Hungry Man (Swanson)	16 oz	610	31	1360	58	—
Beef Pie (Stouffer's)	1 pkg (10 oz)	450	26	1140	36	3
Chicken (Swanson)	7 oz	380	22	760	35	—
Chicken Homestyle (Swanson)	8 oz	410	21	1030	41	—
Chicken Hungry Man (Swanson)	16 oz	630	35	1600	57	—
Chicken Pie (Stouffer's)	1 pkg (10 oz)	520	33	1000	37	3
Chicken Pie (Stouffer's)	½ pkg (8 oz)	460	30	850	35	3
Turkey (Stouffer's)	1 cup (8 oz)	500	31	910	36	3
Turkey (Stouffer's)	1 pkg (10 oz)	530	33	1040	36	3
Turkey (Swanson)	7 oz	380	21	720	36	—
Turkey Hungry Man (Swanson)	16 oz	650	36	1470	57	—

FOOD	PORTION	CAL	FAT	SOD	CARB	FIB
Vegetable Pie w/ Beef (Banquet)	7 oz	510	33	870	39	—
Vegetable Pie w/ Beef (Morton)	7 oz	430	31	740	27	—
Vegetable Pie w/ Chicken (Banquet)	7 oz	550	36	860	39	—
Vegetable Pie w/ Chicken (Morton)	7 oz	420	28	740	27	—
Vegetable Pie w/ Turkey (Banquet)	7 oz	510	31	860	39	—
Vegetable Pie w/ Turkey (Morton)	7 oz	420	28	740	27	—
HOME RECIPE						
beef, baked	⅛ of 9-in pie (7.4 oz)	515	30	596	39	—
chicken	⅛ of 9-in pie (8.1 oz)	545	31	594	42	—

POTATO
see also CHIPS

FOOD	PORTION	CAL	FAT	SOD	CARB	FIB
CANNED						
Hunt's Whole New	4 oz	70	tr	230	15	tr
Libby	½ cup	45	0	—	—	—
S&W New Potatoes Extra Small	½ cup	45	0	310	9	—
Seneca	½ cup	45	0	—	—	—
potatoes	½ cup	54	tr	—	12	—
FRESH						
Yukon Gold	1 (5.3 oz)	110	0	—	—	—
baked, skin only	1 skin (2 oz)	115	tr	12	27	2
baked, w/ skin	1 (6.5 oz)	220	tr	16	51	—
baked, w/o skin	1 (5 oz)	145	tr	8	34	2
baked, w/o skin	½ cup	57	tr	3	13	1
boiled	½ cup	68	tr	3	16	1
microwaved	1 (7 oz)	212	tr	16	49	—
microwaved w/o skin	½ cup	78	tr	5	18	—
raw, w/o skin	1 (3.9 oz)	88	tr	7	20	—
FROZEN						
Au Gratin (Stouffer's)	½ cup (2.25 oz)	130	6	590	15	1
Baked Potato Broccoli & Ham (Weight Watchers)	11.5 oz	280	17	520	39	—
Baked Potato Broccoli and Cheese (Weight Watchers)	10.5 oz	270	6	570	43	—

FOOD	PORTION	CAL	FAT	SOD	CARB	FIB
Baked Potato Chicken Divan (Weight Watchers)	11.25 oz	280	7	480	38	—
Baked Potato Homestyle Turkey (Weight Watchers)	11.75 oz	250	7	510	26	—
Baked Potato w/ Broccoli & Cheese Sauce (Healthy Choice)	10 oz	240	5	510	41	—
Baked With Broccoli and Cheese (Budget Gourmet)	1 pkg (10.5 oz)	300	10	740	40	—
Broccoli & Cheese Over Baked Potato (Stouffer's)	1 pkg (10.1 oz)	320	15	770	30	4
Broccoli & Cheese Over Baked Potato Lunch Express (Stouffer's)	1 pkg (10.25 oz)	250	9	490	28	6
Cheddar Browns (Ore-Ida)	3 oz	90	2	330	14	—
Cheddar Cheese & Bacon Over Baked Potato (Stouffer's)	1 pkg (9.4 oz)	380	22	900	31	5
Cheddared Potatoes (Budget Gourmet)	1 pkg (5.5 oz)	260	16	600	22	—
Cheddared Potatoes With Broccoli (Budget Gourmet)	1 pkg (5 oz)	150	7	410	14	—
Cottage Fries (Ore-Ida)	3 oz	130	4	15	21	—
Crispers! (Ore-Ida)	3 oz	220	13	490	24	—
Crispy Crowns! (Ore-Ida)	3 oz	190	11	390	21	—
Crispy Crunchers (Ore-Ida)	3 oz	180	9	410	23	—
Deep Fries Crinkle Cuts (Ore-Ida)	3 oz	160	7	10	23	—
Deep Fries French Fries (Ore-Ida)	3 oz	170	7	10	23	—
Deluxe Cheddar (Lean Cuisine)	1 pkg (10.4 oz)	270	10	550	30	3
Dinner Fries Country Style (Ore-Ida)	3 oz	110	2	10	20	—

FOOD	PORTION	CAL	FAT	SOD	CARB	FIB
French Fries (MicroMagic)	1 pkg (3 oz)	290	13	30	40	—
Golden Crinkles (Ore-Ida)	3 oz	120	3	10	21	—
Golden Fries (Ore-Ida)	3 oz	120	3	10	20	—
Golden Patties (Ore-Ida)	1 (2.5 oz)	130	7	210	16	—
Golden Twirls (Ore-Ida)	3 oz	160	7	15	22	—
Hash Browns Shredded (Ore-Ida)	3 oz	70	tr	15	15	—
Hash Browns Southern Style (Ore-Ida)	3 oz	70	tr	15	16	—
Lites Crinkle Cuts (Ore-Ida)	3 oz	90	2	10	17	—
Microwave Crinkle Cuts (Ore-Ida)	3.5 oz	190	8	10	27	—
Microwave Hash Browns (Ore-Ida)	2 oz	110	6	210	13	—
Microwave Tater Tots (Ore-Ida)	4 oz	210	9	370	28	—
O'Brien Potatoes (Ore-Ida)	3 oz	60	tr	10	13	—
One Serve Potatoes and Broccoli In Cheese Sauce (Green Giant)	1 pkg	130	5	720	19	—
One Serve Potatoes Au Gratin (Green Giant)	1 pkg	200	10	560	20	—
Pixie Crinkles (Ore-Ida)	3 oz	140	5	15	21	—
Potato Pancakes (Golden)	1 (1.33 oz)	71	3	187	10	—
Scalloped (Stouffer's)	½ cup (2.25 oz)	130	6	450	17	2
Shoestrings (Ore-Ida)	3 oz	150	6	15	23	—
Skinny Fries (MicroMagic)	1 pkg (3 oz)	350	15	40	49	—
Stuffed Potatoes w/ Cheddar Cheese (Oh Boy!)	1 (6 oz)	150	4	490	23	—
Stuffed Potatoes w/ Real Bacon (Oh Boy!)	1 (6 oz)	120	3	360	21	—
Stuffed Potatoes w/ Sour Cream & Chives (Oh Boy!)	1 (6 oz)	110	2	360	21	—
Tater Tots (Ore-Ida)	3 oz	160	8	280	21	—

FOOD	PORTION	CAL	FAT	SOD	CARB	FIB
Tater Tots With Bacon (Ore-Ida)	3 oz	150	7	390	21	—
Tater Tots With Onion (Ore-Ida)	3 oz	150	7	370	21	—
Three Cheese Potatoes (Budget Gourmet)	1 pkg (5.75 oz)	220	11	470	23	—
Toaster Hash Browns (Ore-Ida)	1 (1.75 oz)	100	5	230	12	—
Topped Broccoli & Cheese (Ore-Ida)	1 (5.63 oz)	160	4	400	25	—
Topped Vegetable Primavera (Ore-Ida)	1 (6.13 oz)	160	5	390	23	—
Twice Baked Butter Flavor (Ore-Ida)	1 (5 oz)	200	8	460	28	—
Twice Baked Cheddar Cheese (Ore-Ida)	1 (5 oz)	210	9	570	28	—
Twice Baked Sour Cream & Chives (Ore-Ida)	1 (5 oz)	190	8	430	27	—
Wedges Home Style (Ore-Ida)	3 oz	110	2	10	19	—
Zesties! (Ore-Ida)	3 oz	160	8	300	21	—
french fries	10 strips	111	4	15	17	2
french fries thick cut	10 strips	109	4	23	17	—
hashed brown	½ cup	170	9	27	22	—
potato puffs	½ cup	138	7	462	19	—
potato puffs, as prep	1	16	1	52	2	—
HOME RECIPE						
au gratin	½ cup	160	9	528	14	—
hash brown	½ cup	163	11	19	17	2
mashed	½ cup	111	4	309	18	—
o'brien	1 cup	157	3	421	30	—
potato dumpling	3.5 oz	334	1	1	74	3
potato pancakes	1 (1.3 oz)	101	7	188	11	—
scalloped	½ cup	105	5	409	13	—
MIX						
Au Gratin, as prep (Betty Crocker)	½ cup	140	5	580	21	—
Cheddar 'N Bacon, as prep (Betty Crocker)	½ cup	140	5	520	21	—
Cheddar And Bacon Casserole (French's)	½ cup	130	5	390	18	—
Cheesy Scalloped, as prep (Betty Crocker)	½ cup	140	5	560	20	—

FOOD	PORTION	CAL	FAT	SOD	CARB	FIB
Creamy Stroganoff (French's)	½ cup	130	4	520	20	—
Creamy Italian Scalloped (French's)	½ cup	120	3	430	19	—
Crispy Top Scalloped w/ Savory Onion (French's)	½ cup	140	5	390	20	—
Hash Browns, as prep (Betty Crocker)	½ cup	160	6	460	24	—
Hash Browns, as prep w/o salt (Betty Crocker)	½ cup	160	6	100	24	—
Homestyle American Cheese, as prep (Betty Crocker)	½ cup	140	5	610	20	—
Homestyle Broccoli Au Gratin, as prep (Betty Crocker)	½ cup	130	5	540	19	—
Homestyle Cheddar Cheese, as prep (Betty Crocker)	½ cup	140	5	530	20	—
Homestyle Cheesy Scalloped, as prep (Betty Crocker)	½ cup	140	5	590	20	—
Julienne, as prep (Betty Crocker)	½ cup	130	5	580	18	—
Mashed Potato Flakes (Hungry Jack)	½ cup	40	7	380	17	—
Mashed, not prep (Country Store)	⅓ cup	70	0	10	15	—
Potato Buds, as prep (Betty Crocker)	½ cup	130	6	360	17	—
Potato Buds, as prep w/o salt (Betty Crocker)	½ cup	130	6	90	17	—
Potatoes & Cheese 2-Cheese (Kraft)	½ cup	130	4	540	19	—
Potatoes & Cheese Au Gratin (Kraft)	½ cup	130	5	570	19	—
Potatoes & Cheese Broccoli Au Gratin (Kraft)	½ cup	120	5	530	20	—
Potatoes & Cheese Scalloped (Kraft)	½ cup	140	5	500	20	—

FOOD	PORTION	CAL	FAT	SOD	CARB	FIB
Potatoes & Cheese Scalloped With Ham (Kraft)	½ cup	150	5	510	20	—
Potatoes & Cheese Sour Cream With Chives (Kraft)	½ cup	150	5	610	20	—
Real Cheese Scalloped (French's)	½ cup	140	5	380	19	—
Real Sour Cream and Chives (French's)	½ cup	150	7	550	19	—
Scalloped & Ham, as prep (Betty Crocker)	½ cup	160	6	620	22	—
Scalloped, as prep (Betty Crocker)	½ cup	140	5	570	20	—
Smokey Cheddar, as prep (Betty Crocker)	½ cup	140	5	680	21	—
Sour Cream 'N Chive, as prep (Betty Crocker)	½ cup	140	5	520	21	—
Spuds Mashed (French's)	½ cup	140	7	380	17	—
Tangy Au Gratin (French's)	½ cup	130	5	460	20	—
Twice Baked Bacon And Cheddar, as prep (Betty Crocker)	½ cup	210	11	600	21	—
Twice Baked Herbed Butter, as prep (Betty Crocker)	½ cup	220	13	540	20	—
Twice Baked Mild Cheddar With Onion, as prep (Betty Crocker)	½ cup	190	10	640	20	—
Twice Baked Sour Cream & Chive, as prep (Betty Crocker)	½ cup	200	11	570	19	—
au gratin, as prep	4.5 oz	127	6	601	18	—
instant mashed flakes, as prep w/ whole milk & butter	½ cup	118	6	349	16	—
instant mashed flakes, not prep	½ cup	78	tr	24	18	—
instant mashed granules, not prep	½ cup	372	1	67	86	—

FOOD	PORTION	CAL	FAT	SOD	CARB	FIB
instant mashed granules, as prep w/ whole milk & butter	½ cup	114	5	270	15	—
scalloped, as prep	4.5 oz	127	6	467	18	—
REFRIGERATED						
Simply Potatoes Au Gratin	¼ pkg (3 oz)	130	8	370	13	—
Simply Potatoes Hash Browns	⅕ pkg (4 oz)	100	tr	410	23	—
Simply Potatoes Hash Browns Onion	⅕ pkg (4 oz)	120	tr	380	26	—
Simply Potatoes Hash Browns Southwest Style	⅕ pkg (4 oz)	100	tr	410	23	—
Simply Potatoes Mashed	⅕ pkg (4 oz)	90	2	150	15	—
Simply Potatoes Scalloped	¼ pkg (3 oz)	100	5	390	11	—
SHELF STABLE						
Augratin Potatoes Pantry Express	½ cup	120	5	430	17	2
TAKE-OUT						
au gratin w/ cheese	½ cup	178	10	548	17	—
baked, topped w/ cheese sauce	1	475	29	381	47	—
baked, topped w/ cheese sauce & bacon	1	451	26	973	44	—
baked, topped w/ cheese sauce & broccoli	1	402	14	484	47	—
baked, topped w/ cheese sauce & chili	1	481	22	701	56	—
baked, topped w/ sour cream & chives	1	394	22	182	50	—
curry	1 serv (6 oz)	292	16	—	36	4
french fried in beef tallow	1 lg	358	19	187	44	—
french fried in beef tallow	1 reg	237	12	124	29	—
french fried in vegetable oil	1 lg	355	19	187	44	—
french fried in vegetable oil	1 reg	235	12	124	29	—

FOOD	PORTION	CAL	FAT	SOD	CARB	FIB
hash brown	½ cup	151	9	290	16	—
mashed w/ whole milk & margarine	⅓ cup	66	tr	182	13	—
mustard potato salad	3.5 oz	120	6	393	16	—
potato salad	½ cup	179	10	661	14	—
potato salad	⅓ cup	108	6	312	13	—
potato salad w/ vegetables	3.5 oz	120	3	390	20	—
scalloped	½ cup	127	5	435	18	—

POTATO STARCH
Manischewitz	1 cup	570	0	1	137	—
potato starch	3.5 oz	335	tr	8	83	—

POUT
FRESH
ocean, baked	3 oz	86	1	66	0	—
ocean fillet, baked	4.8 oz	139	2	107	0	—

PRESERVE
see JAM/JELLY/PRESERVES

PRETZELS
see also CHIPS, POPCORN, SNACKS
A & Eagle	1 oz	110	2	570	22	—
A & Eagle Beer	1 oz	110	2	610	22	—
Estee Unsalted	7	50	tr	0	11	—
J&J Soft	1 (2.25 oz)	170	0	140	37	—
J&J Soft Bites	5 bites	110	0	95	23	—
Lance Twist	1 pkg (42 g)	150	1	700	30	—
Mister Salty						
Dutch	1 oz	110	1	440	22	—
Fat Free Sticks	1 oz	100	0	380	23	—
Fat Free Twists	1 oz	100	0	380	23	—
Mini	1 oz	110	1	450	21	—
Twists	1 oz	110	2	580	21	—
Very Thin Sticks	1 oz	110	1	600	22	—
Mr. Phipps Chips	8 (0.5 oz)	60	1	310	10	—
Fat Free	8 (0.5 oz)	50	0	315	11	—
Lightly Salted	8 (0.5 oz)	60	1	200	11	—
Sesame	8	60	2	250	10	—
Quinlan						
Beers	1 oz	110	1	—	—	—
Butter Tiny Thins	1 oz	108	1	—	—	—
Cheese Tiny Thins	1 oz	109	2	—	—	—
Logs	1 oz	103	tr	—	—	—

FOOD	PORTION	CAL	FAT	SOD	CARB	FIB
Party Thins	1 oz	109	tr	—	—	—
Philly Style	1 oz	107	tr	—	—	—
Rods	1 oz	100	tr	—	—	—
Sour Cheese Tiny Thins	1 oz	100	0	—	—	—
Sour Thins Dough Hard	1 oz	100	0	—	—	—
Sticks	1 oz	105	tr	—	—	—
Thins	1 oz	104	tr	—	—	—
Tiny Thins	1 oz	109	2	—	—	—
Tiny Thins No-Salt	1 oz	115	2	—	—	—
Ultra Thins	1 oz	106	tr	—	—	—
Rold Gold						
Bavarian	3 pieces (1 oz)	120	2	430	22	—
Pretzels Chips	1 oz	110	1	310	22	—
Pretzels Chips Cheese	1 oz	120	3	240	22	—
Rods	3 pieces (1 oz)	110	2	410	23	—
Snack Mix	½ cup (1 oz)	140	6	330	18	—
Sour Dough	1½ pieces (1 oz)	110	2	230	22	—
Thin Twist	10 pieces (1 oz)	110	1	510	23	—
Tiny Twist	15 pieces (1 oz)	110	1	420	23	—
Seyfert's Butter						
Rods	1 oz	110	1	530	21	—
Snyder's						
Logs	1 oz	310	0	360	22	—
Minis	1 oz	310	0	460	22	—
Minis Unsalted	1 oz	310	0	70	22	—
Nibblers	1 oz	310	0	460	22	—
Oat Bran	1 oz	120	1	300	14	—
Old Fashioned Hard	1 oz	111	0	655	23	—
Old Fashioned Hard Unsalted	1 oz	100	0	89	23	—
Old Tyme	1 oz	310	0	310	22	—
Old Tyme Unsalted	1 oz	110	0	70	22	—
Rods	1 oz	310	0	320	22	—
Sourdough Hard Buttermilk Ranch	1 oz	130	5	250	19	0
Sourdough Hard Cheddar Cheese	1 oz	160	7	320	13	0
Sourdough Hard Honey Mustard & Onion	1 oz	130	5	250	19	0
Stix	1 oz	310	0	900	22	—
Very Thins	1 oz	310	0	720	22	—

FOOD	PORTION	CAL	FAT	SOD	CARB	FIB
Ultra Slim-Fast Lite N'Tasty	1 oz	100	tr	460	21	4
Wege Sourdough	1 oz	102	tr	548	23	—
Wege Unsalted	1 oz	102	tr	60	23	—
Wege Whole Wheat	1 oz	109	1	25	21	—
sticks	10	10	tr	48	2	—
twist	1 (.5 oz)	65	1	258	13	—
twists, thin	10 (2 oz)	240	2	966	48	—

PRICKLY PEAR
fresh	1	42	1	6	10	—

PRUNES
CANNED
in heavy syrup	1 cup	245	tr	6	65	—
in heavy syrup	5	90	tr	2	24	—

DRIED
Mariani Pitted	¼ cup	140	1	—	—	—
Mariani Whole	¼ cup	140	1	—	—	—
Sunsweet Orange Essence Pitted Prunes	6 (1.4 oz)	100	0	5	26	3
cooked, w/ sugar	½ cup	147	tr	2	39	7
cooked, w/o sugar	½ cup	113	tr	2	30	6
dried	1 cup	385	1	6	101	12
dried	10	201	tr	3	53	6

JUICE
Mott's	6 oz	130	0	—	—	—
Mott's Country Style	6 oz	130	0	—	—	—
S&W Unsweetened	6 oz	120	0	20	31	—
canned	1 cup	181	tr	11	45	3

PUDDING
see also CUSTARD, PUDDING POPS
HOME RECIPE
bread w/ raisins	½ cup	180	5	185	31	—
corn	½ cup	97	1	—	—	—
corn	⅔ cup	181	9	92	21	—
yorkshire, as prep w/ skim milk	3.5 oz	93	4	—	12	1
yorkshire, as prep w/ whole milk	3.5 oz	104	5	—	12	1

MIX
Banana Cream (Royal)	mix for 1 serv	80	0	110	20	0

FOOD	PORTION	CAL	FAT	SOD	CARB	FIB
Banana Cream Instant (Royal)	mix for 1 serv	90	0	390	22	—
Butterscotch (My*T*Fine)	mix for 1 serv	90	0	190	22	—
Butterscotch (Royal)	mix for 1 serv	90	0	180	25	0
Butterscotch Instant (Royal)	mix for 1 serv	90	0	400	22	—
Cherry Vanilla Instant (Royal)	mix for 1 serv	90	0	300	23	0
Chocolate (Estee)	½ cup	70	tr	75	13	—
Chocolate (My*T*Fine)	mix for 1 serv	100	0	135	23	0
Chocolate (Royal)	mix for 1 serv	90	0	90	22	0
Chocolate Instant (Royal)	mix for 1 serv	110	0	450	23	0
Chocolate Instant, as prep w/ skim milk (Weight Watchers)	½ cup	100	0	430	18	—
Chocolate Almond (My*T*Fine)	mix for 1 serv	100	1	135	23	—
Chocolate Almond Instant (Royal)	mix for 1 serv	120	1	440	26	—
Chocolate Chocolate Chip, Instant (Royal)	mix for 1 serv	110	1	590	26	0
Chocolate Fudge (My*T*Fine)	mix for 1 serv	100	0	140	24	1
Chocolate Peanut Butter Instant (Royal)	mix for 1 serv	110	1	480	26	0
Chocolate Sugar Free Instant (Royal)	mix for 1 serv	50	0	420	11	—
Creme Caramel Flan And Sauce, as prep (Knorr)	½ cup + 1 tbsp sauce	190	4	70	34	—
Dark 'n Sweet Chocolate (Royal)	mix for 1 serv	90	0	95	22	1
Dark 'n Sweet Instant (Royal)	mix for 1 serv	110	0	460	25	0
Lemon (My*T*Fine)	mix for 1 serv	90	0	170	22	—
Lemon Instant (Royal)	mix for 1 serv	90	0	320	23	—
Pistachio Instant (Royal)	mix for 1 serv	90	1	360	22	0
Strawberry Instant (Royal)	mix for 1 serv	100	0	330	24	—
Toasted Coconut Instant (Royal)	mix for 1 serv	100	2	450	22	—

FOOD	PORTION	CAL	FAT	SOD	CARB	FIB
Vanilla (Estee)	½ cup	70	tr	75	13	—
Vanilla (My*T*Fine)	mix for 1 serv	90	0	120	22	0
Vanilla (Royal)	mix for 1 serv	80	0	160	20	0
Vanilla Chocolate Chip Instant (Royal)	mix for 1 serv	90	1	350	22	0
Vanilla Instant (Royal)	mix for 1 serv	90	0	325	23	—
Vanilla Instant, as prep w/ skim milk (Weight Watchers)	½ cup	90	0	510	19	—
Vanilla Tapioca (My*T*Fine)	mix for 1 serv	80	0	160	19	—
MIX WITH 2% MILK						
Banana Instant Sugar Free (Jell-O)	½ cup	84	2	392	11	—
Chocolate Instant Sugar Free (Jell-O)	½ cup	92	3	381	13	—
Chocolate Sugar Free (Jell-O)	½ cup	91	3	164	13	—
Pistachio Instant Sugar Free (Jell-O)	½ cup	94	3	393	12	—
Vanilla Instant Sugar Free (Jell-O)	½ cup	82	2	199	11	—
MIX WITH SKIM MILK						
Butterscotch (D-Zerta)	½ cup	68	0	65	12	—
Chocolate (D-Zerta)	½ cup	65	0	68	11	—
Dietetic (Emes)	½ cup (4 fl oz)	71	1	110	13	—
Vanilla (D-Zerta)	½ cup	69	0	65	12	—
MIX WITH WHOLE MILK						
Banana Cream Instant (Jell-O)	½ cup	165	4	409	28	—
Butter Pecan Instant (Jell-O)	½ cup	170	5	409	28	—
Butterscotch (Jell-O)	½ cup	169	4	191	30	—
Butterscotch Instant (Jell-O)	½ cup	164	4	447	28	—
Chocolate Instant (Jell-O)	½ cup	176	5	476	31	—
Chocolate Tapioca Americana (Jell-O)	½ cup	169	5	168	28	—
Chocolate Fudge Instant (Jell-O)	½ cup	175	5	439	31	—
Coconut Cream Instant (Jell-O)	½ cup	178	6	322	27	—
French Vanilla (Jell-O)	½ cup	169	4	185	30	—

FOOD	PORTION	CAL	FAT	SOD	CARB	FIB
French Vanilla Instant (Jell-O)	½ cup	165	4.	405	28	—
Golden Egg Custard Americana (Jell-O)	½ cup	167	6	—	—	—
Lemon Instant (Jell-O)	½ cup	168	4	362	29	—
Milk Chocolate Instant (Jell-O)	½ cup	179	5	468	31	—
Pineapple Cream Instant (Jell-O)	½ cup	165	4	361	29	—
Pistachio Instant (Jell-O)	½ cup	170	5	408	28	—
Rice Americana (Jell-O)	½ cup	175	4	157	30	—
Vanilla (Jell-O)	½ cup	156	4	198	26	—
Vanilla Instant (Jell-O)	½ cup	168	4	407	29	—
Vanilla Tapioca Americana (Jell-O)	½ cup	160	4	170	27	—
chocolate	½ cup	150	4	167	25	—
chocolate instant	½ cup	155	4	440	27	—
rice	½ cup	155	4	140	27	—
tapioca	½ cup	145	4	152	25	—
vanilla	½ cup	145	4	178	25	—
vanilla instant	½ cup	150	4	375	27	—
READY-TO-USE						
Banana (Snack Pack)	4.25 oz	145	6	180	22	0
Butterscotch (Snack Pack)	4.25 oz	170	6	210	27	0
Butterscotch (Swiss Miss)	4 oz	180	6	135	29	0
Butterscotch (Ultra Slim-Fast)	4 oz	100	tr	230	21	2
Butterscotch Sugar Free (Diamond Crystal)	½ cup	80	tr	—	—	—
Chocolate (Jell-O)	1 (4 oz)	171	6	121	28	—
Chocolate (Snack Pack)	4.25 oz	170	6	120	26	0
Chocolate (Swiss Miss)	4 oz	180	6	160	29	0
Chocolate (Ultra Slim-Fast)	4 oz	100	tr	240	21	2
Chocolate Caramel Swirl (Jell-O)	1 (4 oz)	175	6	122	28	—
Chocolate Fudge (Jell-O)	1 (4 oz)	171	6	121	28	—

FOOD	PORTION	CAL	FAT	SOD	CARB	FIB
Chocolate Fudge (Snack Pack)	4.25 oz	165	6	125	27	0
Chocolate Fudge (Swiss Miss)	4 oz	220	6	180	38	0
Chocolate Fudge Light (Jell-O)	1 (4 oz)	101	1	113	22	—
Chocolate Fudge Light (Swiss Miss)	4 oz	100	1	120	20	0
Chocolate Fudge Milk Chocolate Swirl (Jell-O)	1 (4 oz)	171	6	123	29	—
Chocolate Light (Jell-O)	1 (4 oz)	104	2	113	21	—
Chocolate Light (Snack Pack)	4.25 oz	100	2	120	20	0
Chocolate Light (Swiss Miss)	4 oz	100	1	120	20	0
Chocolate Marshmallow (Snack Pack)	4.25 oz	165	6	125	26	0
Chocolate Sugar Free (Diamond Crystal)	½ cup	70	tr	—	—	—
Chocolate Sundae (Swiss Miss)	4 oz	220	7	140	36	0
Chocolate Vanilla Light (Jell-O)	1 (4 oz)	104	2	116	21	—
Chocolate Vanilla Swirl (Jell-O)	1 (4 oz)	175	6	125	28	—
Chocolate Vanilla Swirl (Jell-O)	1 (5.5 oz)	240	8	173	39	—
Lemon (Snack Pack)	4.25 oz	150	4	75	30	tr
Lemon Dream (Imagine Foods)	1 (4 oz)	120	0	5	30	—
Milk Chocolate (Jell-O)	1 (4 oz)	173	6	126	29	—
Tapioca (Jell-O)	1 (5.5 oz)	229	6	186	40	—
Tapioca (Swiss Miss)	4 oz	160	5	170	27	0
Tapioca (Jell-O)	1 (4 oz)	167	4	135	29	—
Tapioca (Snack Pack)	4.25 oz	150	5	125	23	0
Tapioca Light (Snack Pack)	4.25 oz	100	2	105	18	0
Vanilla (Jell-O)	1 (4 oz)	182	7	133	28	—
Vanilla (Jell-O)	1 (5.5 oz)	250	9	183	38	—
Vanilla (Snack Pack)	4.25 oz	170	6	150	27	0
Vanilla (Swiss Miss)	4 oz	190	7	140	30	0

FOOD	PORTION	CAL	FAT	SOD	CARB	FIB
Vanilla (Ultra Slim-Fast)	4 oz	100	tr	230	21	2
Vanilla Chocolate Parfait Light (Swiss Miss)	4 oz	100	1	110	20	0
Vanilla Chocolate Swirl (Jell-O)	1 (4 oz)	178	6	129	28	—
Vanilla Light (Jell-O)	1 (4 oz)	104	2	118	20	—
Vanilla Light (Swiss Miss)	4 oz	100	1	105	20	0
Vanilla Parfait (Swiss Miss)	4 oz	180	6	150	29	0
Vanilla Sugar Free (Diamond Crystal)	½ cup	80	tr	—	—	—
Vanilla Sundae (Swiss Miss)	4 oz	200	7	180	36	0
TAKE-OUT						
blancmange	1 serv (4.7 oz)	154	5	—	25	tr
bread pudding	1 serv (6.7 oz)	564	18	—	94	6
queen of puddings	1 serv (4.4 oz)	266	10	—	41	tr
rice pudding	1 serv (3 oz)	110	4	—	17	tr
rice w/ raisins	½ cup	246	6	270	42	4
tapioca	½ cup	169	6	154	21	—

PUDDING POPS

see also ICE CREAM AND FROZEN DESSERTS, PUDDING

FOOD	PORTION	CAL	FAT	SOD	CARB	FIB
Jell-O						
Chocolate	1 pop	79	2	82	13	—
Chocolate Caramel Swirl	1 pop	74	2	63	12	—
Chocolate Fudge	1 pop	79	2	82	13	—
Chocolate Peanut Butter Swirl	1 bar	78	3	70	12	—
Chocolate Swirl	1 pop	80	2	83	13	—
Chocolate Vanilla Swirl	1 pop	78	2	66	13	—
Milk Chocolate	1 pop	80	2	83	13	—
Vanilla	1 pop	77	2	50	13	—
Jell-O Deluxe						
Chocolate Covered	1 pop	201	10	212	27	—
Peanuts and Chocolate	1 bar	185	9	83	24	—

FOOD	PORTION	CAL	FAT	SOD	CARB	FIB
PUMMELO						
fresh	1	228	tr	7	59	—
sections	1 cup	71	tr	2	18	—
PUMPKIN						
CANNED						
Libby's Solid Pack	½ cup	60	1	5	15	4
Owatonna	½ cup	40	1	—	—	—
pumpkin	½ cup	41	tr	6	10	—
FRESH						
cooked, mashed	½ cup	24	tr	2	6	—
flowers, cooked	½ cup	10	tr	4	2	—
flowers, raw	1	0	0	0	tr	—
leaves, cooked	½ cup	7	tr	3	1	—
leaves, raw	½ cup	4	tr	2	tr	—
raw, cubed	½ cup	15	tr	1	4	—
SEEDS						
dried	1 oz	154	13	5	5	—
roasted	1 cup	1184	96	40	31	—
roasted	1 oz	148	12	5	4	—
salted & roasted	1 cup	1184	96	1294	31	—
salted & roasted	1 oz	148	12	144	4	—
whole roasted	1 cup	285	12	12	34	—
whole roasted	1 oz	127	6	5	15	—
whole salted, roasted	1 cup	285	12	268	34	—
whole salted, roasted	1 oz	127	6	191	15	—
PURSLANE						
cooked	1 cup	21	tr	51	4	—
raw	1 cup	7	tr	20	1	—
QUAHOGS						
see CLAMS						
QUAIL						
FRESH						
breast w/o skin, raw	1 (2 oz)	69	2	31	0	—
w/ skin, raw	1 quail (3.8 oz)	210	13	58	0	—
w/o skin, raw	1 quail (3.2 oz)	123	4	47	0	—
QUICHE						
HOME RECIPE						
lorraine	⅛ of 8-in pie	600	48	653	29	—
TAKE-OUT						
cheese	1 slice (3 oz)	283	20	—	16	1

FOOD	PORTION	CAL	FAT	SOD	CARB	FIB
lorraine	1 slice (3 oz)	352	25	—	18	1
mushroom	1 slice (3 oz)	256	18	—	17	1
QUINCE						
fresh	1	53	tr	4	14	—
QUINOA						
Arrowhead	¼ cup (1.4 oz)	140	2	0	25	4
quinoa	½ cup	318	5	—	59	—
RABBIT						
domestic w/o bone, roasted	3 oz	167	7	40	0	—
wild w/o bone, stewed	3 oz	147	3	38	0	—
RACCOON						
roasted	3 oz	217	12	—	0	—
RADICCHIO						
raw, shredded	½ cup	5	tr	4	1	—
RADISHES						
DRIED						
chinese	½ cup	157	tr	161	37	—
daikon	½ cup	157	tr	161	37	—
FRESH						
Dole	7	20	0	35	3	0
chinese, raw	1 (12 oz)	62	tr	71	14	—
chinese, raw, sliced	½ cup	8	tr	9	2	—
chinese, sliced, cooked	½ cup	13	tr	10	3	—
daikon, raw	1 (12 oz)	62	tr	71	14	—
daikon, raw, sliced	½ cup	8	tr	9	2	—
daikon, sliced, cooked	½ cup	13	tr	10	3	—
red, raw	10	7	tr	11	2	—
red, sliced	½ cup	10	tr	14	2	—
white icicle, raw	1 (.5 oz)	2	tr	3	tr	—
white icicle, raw, sliced	½ cup	7	tr	8	1	—
SPROUTS						
raw	½ cup	8	tr	1	1	—
RAISINS						
Cinderella Seedless	½ cup	250	0	—	—	—
Dole Golden	½ cup	260	0	25	63	—
Dole Seedless	½ cup	260	0	25	63	—
golden seedless	1 cup	437	1	17	115	8
seedless	1 cup	434	1	17	115	8
seedless	1 tbsp	27	tr	—	7	—

FOOD	PORTION	CAL	FAT	SOD	CARB	FIB
sultanas	1 oz	88	0	—	23	2

RASPBERRIES
CANNED
in heavy syrup	½ cup	117	tr	4	30	—

FRESH
Dole	1 cup	45	0	0	10	9
raspberries	1 cup	61	1	0	14	—
raspberries	1 pint	154	2	0	36	—

FROZEN
Red (Big Valley)	3.5 oz	55	1	0	14	—
Whole In Lite Syrup (Birds Eye)	½ cup	100	1	0	25	4
sweetened	1 cup	256	tr	1	65	—
sweetened	1 pkg (10 oz)	291	tr	1	74	—

JUICE
Crystal Geyser Juice Squeeze Mountain Raspberry	1 bottle (12 fl oz)	135	0	20	32	—
Dole Pure & Light	6 oz	90	tr	15	24	—
Kool-Aid Sugar Free	8 oz	2	0	24	0	—
Smucker's	8 oz	120	0	10	30	—
Smucker's Juice Sparkler	10 oz	130	tr	5	32	—

RED BEANS
CANNED
B&M Small Baked	8 oz	223	5	725	36	11
Green Giant	½ cup	90	1	340	19	5
Hunt's Small	4 oz	90	tr	560	18	6
Van Camp's	1 cup	194	1	928	38	—

DRIED
Bean Cuisine	½ cup	115	1	5	—	5

MIX
Mahatma Red Beans & Rice	1 cup	190	1	790	40	7
Pasta & Beans Barcelona Red Beans With Radiatore (Bean Cuisine)	½ cup	170	4	379	170	—

RELISH
Dill (Vlasic)	1 oz	2	0	415	1	—
Hamburger (Vlasic)	1 oz	40	0	255	9	—

FOOD	PORTION	CAL	FAT	SOD	CARB	FIB
Hot Dog (Vlasic)	1 oz	40	1	255	8	—
Hot Piccalilli (Vlasic)	1 oz	35	0	165	8	—
India (Vlasic)	1 oz	30	0	205	8	—
Jalapeno (Old El Paso)	2 tbsp	16	0	100	4	1
Sandwich Spred (Hellman's)	1 tbsp (15 g)	55	5	170	2	—
Sweet (Vlasic)	1 oz	30	0	220	8	—
cranberry orange	½ cup	246	tr	44	64	—
hamburger	1 tbsp	19	tr	164	5	—
hamburger	½ cup	158	1	1338	42	—
hot dog	1 tbsp	14	tr	164	4	—
hot dog	½ cup	111	1	1332	28	—
piccalilli	1.4 oz	13	tr	—	2	1
sweet	1 tbsp	19	tr	122	5	—
sweet	½ cup	159	1	990	43	—

RHUBARB

FOOD	PORTION	CAL	FAT	SOD	CARB	FIB
Big Valley, frzn Big Valley	3.5 oz	16	1	0	4	—
fresh	½ cup	13	tr	2	3	—
frzn	½ cup	60	tr	1	3	—
frzn, as prep w/ sugar	½ cup	139	tr	2	37	—

RICE

see also BRAN, CEREAL, FLOUR, RICE CAKES, WILD RICE

BROWN

FOOD	PORTION	CAL	FAT	SOD	CARB	FIB
Arrowhead Basmati	½ cup (1.5 oz)	150	1	0	33	2
Arrowhead Quick Regular	⅓ cup (1.5 oz)	150	1	0	32	2
Arrowhead Quick Spanish Style	¼ pkg (1.4 oz)	150	1	250	30	2
Arrowhead Quick Vegetable Herb	¼ pkg (1.4 oz)	150	1	160	30	3
Arrowhead Quick Wild Rice & Herb	¼ pkg (1.3 oz)	140	1	220	28	3
Minute Precooked, as prep	½ cup	121	1	7	26	1
Pritikin Pilaf	½ cup	90	tr	—	—	—
Pritikin Spanish	½ cup	100	tr	—	—	—
S&W Quick Natural Long Grain	3.5 oz	110	0	0	25	—
S&W Quick Natural Long Grain, cooked	3.5 oz	119	0	0	26	—
Uncle Ben	1 serv (1.6 oz)	158	1	1	34	1
long-grain, cooked	½ cup	109	tr	5	23	2

FOOD	PORTION	CAL	FAT	SOD	CARB	FIB
medium-grain, cooked	½ cup	109	tr	1	23	—
CANNED						
Old El Paso Spanish	½ cup	70	1	400	15	1
Van Camp's Spanish	1 cup	160	4	1270	27	—
DRY MIX						
Chun King Entree Stir Fry	.25 oz	20	0	—	—	—
Goodman's Rice & Vermicelli For Beef	¾ cup	160	1	860	33	0
Goodman's Rice & Vermicelli For Chicken	¾ cup	160	1	920	33	1
Hain Rice Almondine	½ cup	130	5	260	17	—
Hain Rice Oriental 3-Grain Goodness	½ cup	120	5	300	15	—
Kikkoman Fried Rice Seasoning Mix	1 oz pkg	91	tr	—	—	—
Knorr Risotto Milanese With Saffron	½ cup	130	3	420	24	—
Knorr Risotto Tomato	½ cup	110	tr	460	23	—
Knorr Risotto With Mushrooms	½ cup	110	tr	430	24	—
Knorr Risotto With Onion	½ cup	110	tr	390	24	—
Knorr Risotto With Peas And Corn	½ cup	110	1	470	23	—
La Choy Chinese Fried Rice	¾ cup	190	1	820	41	tr
Lipton						
Golden Saute Fried Rice Beef	½ cup	124	2	516	24	—
Golden Saute Fried Rice Chicken	½ cup	129	2	509	24	—
Golden Saute Fried Rice Oriental	½ cup	127	2	675	24	—
Rice And Sauce Beef	½ cup	119	1	602	26	0
Rice And Sauce Cajun	½ cup	123	tr	596	26	tr
Rice And Sauce Cheddar Broccoli	½ cup	125	1	487	25	—
Rice And Sauce Chicken	½ cup	124	1	469	25	0
Rice And Sauce Chicken Broccoli	½ cup	129	2	495	25	—

FOOD	PORTION	CAL	FAT	SOD	CARB	FIB
Rice And Sauce Creamy Chicken	½ cup	142	2	417	27	—
Rice And Sauce Herbs & Butter	½ cup	123	2	446	24	0
Rice And Sauce Long Grain And Wild Rice Original	½ cup	121	tr	530	26	0
Rice And Sauce Mushroom	½ cup	123	1	497	26	0
Rice And Sauce Pilaf	½ cup	122	1	410	26	0
Rice And Sauce Skillet Style Spanish	½ cup	104	1	426	21	—
Rice And Sauce Spanish	½ cup	118	1	536	25	0
Rice Asparagus With Hollandaise	½ cup	123	1	462	25	tr
Mahatma						
Broccoli & Cheese	1 cup	200	2	620	41	2
Jambalaya	1 cup (2 oz)	190	1	700	43	tr
Long Grain & Wild	1 cup (2 oz)	190	1	1240	41	2
Pilaf	1 cup (2 oz)	190	0	820	43	tr
Spanish	1 cup (2 oz)	180	1	760	42	2
Yellow Rice Mix	1 cup	190	0	970	43	tr
Minute						
Fried Rice With Vermicelli, as prep	½ cup	158	5	549	25	—
Rib Roast With Vermicelli, as prep	½ cup	151	4	722	25	—
Rice Drumstick With Vermicelli, as prep	½ cup	153	4	686	25	—
Minute Microwave						
Broccoli Almondine	½ cup	143	4	394	24	—
Cheddar Cheese Broccoli	½ cup	164	5	534	26	—
French Pilaf	½ cup	133	3	423	24	—
Long Grain Brown and Wild	½ cup	140	3	312	25	—
Rice With Savory Cheese Sauce, as prep	½ cup	162	5	435	26	—
Near East Lentil Pilaf, as prep w/ butter	¾ cup (4.9 oz)	180	1	480	30	4

FOOD	PORTION	CAL	FAT	SOD	CARB	FIB
Near East Pilaf Chicken Flavor, as prep w/ butter	½ cup	160	4	460	25	—
Nile Spice Rozdali Vegetable Curry	½ cup	154	4	130	25	—
Old El Paso Mexican	½ cup	140	2	370	28	—
Rice-A-Roni						
Beef	½ cup	140	4	610	24	—
Beef & Mushroom	½ cup	150	3	740	26	—
Chicken	½ cup	150	3	560	26	—
Chicken & Broccoli	½ cup	150	3	710	25	—
Chicken & Mushroom	½ cup	180	7	840	26	—
Chicken & Vegetables	½ cup	140	3	790	25	—
Fried Rice	½ cup	110	5	700	21	—
Herb & Butter	½ cup	130	4	790	22	—
Long Grain & Wild Chicken w/ Almonds	½ cup	140	4	690	24	—
Long Grain & Wild Original	½ cup	130	3	660	23	—
Long Grain & Wild Pilaf	½ cup	130	3	550	23	—
Pilaf	½ cup	150	4	620	25	—
Risotto	½ cup	200	6	1130	32	—
Spanish	½ cup	150	4	1090	25	—
Stroganoff	½ cup	200	8	810	27	—
Yellow Rice	½ cup	140	4	780	25	—
Success						
Beef Oriental	½ cup	190	1	920	43	2
Broccoli & Cheese	½ cup	200	2	690	41	2
Brown & Wild	½ cup	190	1	830	40	3
Classic Chicken	½ cup	150	1	720	32	1
Long Grain & Wild	½ cup	190	0	890	42	1
Pilaf	½ cup	200	0	630	44	2
Spanish	½ cup	190	1	780	43	1
Ultra Slim-Fast Oriental Style	2.3 oz	240	1	900	58	4
Ultra Slim-Fast Rice & Chicken Sauce	2.3 oz	240	1	1080	56	4
Uncle Ben						
Brown & Wild Fast Cooking	1 serv (1.3 oz)	120	1	383	26	1
Country Inn Broccoli Almondine	1 serv (1.2 oz)	124	2	367	25	1

FOOD	PORTION	CAL	FAT	SOD	CARB	FIB
Country Inn Broccoli And White Cheddar	1 serv (1.2 oz)	131	3	288	24	1
Country Inn Broccoli Au Gratin	1 serv (1.1 oz)	116	2	342	22	1
Country Inn Chicken Stock	1 serv (1.2 oz)	123	1	269	24	1
Country Inn Chicken With Wild Rice	1 serv (1.1 oz)	108	1	359	23	1
Country Inn Creamy Chicken & Mushroom	1 serv (1.3 oz)	138	3	380	24	1
Country Inn Creamy Chicken & Wild Rice	1 serv (1.3 oz)	135	1	340	27	1
Country Inn Green Bean Almondine	1 serv (1.2 oz)	128	2	280	25	1
Country Inn Herbed Au Gratin	1 serv (1.2 oz)	119	2	361	24	1
Country Inn Homestyle Chicken And Vegetables	1 serv (1.3 oz)	139	3	298	24	1
Country Inn Rice Florentine	1 serv (1.2 oz)	212	2	354	24	1
Country Inn Vegetable Pilaf	1 serv (1.2 oz)	115	1	357	25	1
Long Grain & Wild Chicken Stock Sauce	1 serv (1.3 oz)	133	2	601	25	1
Long Grain & Wild Fast Cooking	1 serv (1 oz)	101	tr	450	22	1
Long Grain & Wild Garden Vegetable Blend	1 serv (1.3 oz)	128	1	601	26	1
Long Grain & Wild Original	1 serv (1 oz)	96	tr	363	21	1
FROZEN						
Birds Eye French Style	½ cup	170	3	450	33	1
Birds Eye Rice And Broccoli Au Gratin	½ pkg	150	4	490	24	1
Budget Gourmet Oriental Rice With Vegetables	1 pkg (5.75 oz)	230	12	420	28	—
Budget Gourmet Rice Pilaf With Green Beans	1 pkg (5.5 oz)	230	11	510	30	—

FOOD	PORTION	CAL	FAT	SOD	CARB	FIB
Green Giant						
Garden Gourmet Asparagus Pilaf	1 pkg	190	4	610	37	3
Garden Gourmet Sherry Wild Rice	1 pkg	210	4	580	40	3
One Serve Rice 'N Broccoli In Cheese Sauce	1 pkg	180	6	550	25	—
One Serve Rice, Peas And Mushrooms With Sauce	1 pkg	130	2	410	27	—
Rice Originals Italian Rice & Spinach In Cheese Sauce	½ cup	140	4	400	22	—
Rice Originals Pilaf	½ cup	110	1	530	21	—
Rice Originals Rice 'N Broccoli In Cheese Sauce	½ cup	120	4	510	18	—
Rice Originals Rice Medley	½ cup	100	1	310	19	—
Rice Originals White And Wild	½ cup	130	2	540	24	—
TAKE-OUT						
pilaf	½ cup	84	3	362	11	3
risotto	6.6 oz	426	18	—	65	3
spanish	¾ cup	363	27	1339	19	—
WHITE						
Arrowhead Basmati	¼ cup (1.5 oz)	150	0	0	34	tr
Minute Boil In Bag Long Grain, as prep	½ cup	94	0	4	21	—
Minute Long Grain And Wild, as prep	½ cup	149	4	574	25	—
Minute Long Grain, as prep	⅔ cup	150	3	31	27	1
Minute, as prep	⅔ cup	141	2	21	27	1
S&W Long Grain, cooked	3.5 oz	106	0	0	23	—
Superfino Arborio Rice	½ cup	100	0	5	22	—
Uncle Ben Boil-In-Bag	1 serv (0.9 oz)	94	tr	9	22	tr
Uncle Ben Converted	1 serv (1.2 oz)	123	tr	1	27	tr
Uncle Ben In An Instant	1 serv (1.1 oz)	111	tr	10	25	tr
glutinous, cooked	½ cup	116	tr	6	25	—

FOOD	PORTION	CAL	FAT	SOD	CARB	FIB
long-grain instant, cooked	½ cup	80	tr	2	17	tr
long-grain parboiled, cooked	½ cup	100	tr	3	22	tr
long-grain, cooked	½ cup	131	tr	2	28	tr
medium-grain, cooked	½ cup	132	tr	0	29	—
short-grain, cooked	½ cup	133	tr	0	29	—
starch	3.5 oz	343	0	61	85	—

RICE CAKES

FOOD	PORTION	CAL	FAT	SOD	CARB	FIB
7 Grain (Pritikin)	1	35	0	—	—	—
Hain						
5-Grain	1	40	tr	10	8	—
Plain	1	40	tr	10	8	—
Plain No Salt Added	1	40	tr	5	8	—
Sesame	1	40	tr	10	8	—
Sesame No Salt	1	40	tr	5	8	—
Hain Mini						
Apple Cinnamon	½ oz	60	tr	10	12	0
Barbeque	½ oz	70	3	50	10	0
Cheese	½ oz	60	2	100	10	0
Honey Nut	½ oz	60	tr	30	11	0
Nacho Cheese	½ oz	70	2	90	10	0
Plain	½ oz	60	tr	20	12	0
Plain No Salt Added	½ oz	60	tr	5	12	0
Ranch	½ oz	70	3	90	9	—
Teriyaki	½ oz	50	tr	75	12	0
Plain (Pritikin)	1	35	0	—	—	—
Sesami (Pritikin)	1	35	0	—	—	—

ROCKFISH

FRESH

FOOD	PORTION	CAL	FAT	SOD	CARB	FIB
pacific, cooked	1 fillet (5.2 oz)	180	3	114	0	—
pacific, cooked	3 oz	103	2	65	0	—
pacific, raw	3 oz	80	1	51	0	—

ROE

see INDIVIDUAL FISH NAMES

FOOD	PORTION	CAL	FAT	SOD	CARB	FIB
baked	1 oz	58	2	—	1	—
baked	3 oz	173	7	—	2	—

FOOD	PORTION	CAL	FAT	SOD	CARB	FIB

ROLL
see also BISCUIT, CROISSANT, ENGLISH MUFFIN, MUFFIN, POPOVER, SCONE

FROZEN

FOOD	PORTION	CAL	FAT	SOD	CARB	FIB
All Butter Cinnamon Roll w/o Icing (Sara Lee)	1	230	11	220	31	—
All Butter Cinnamon Roll w/ Icing (Sara Lee)	1	280	11	220	43	—
Cinnamon Roll (Pepperidge Farm)	1 (2.25 oz)	220	14	190	34	—
Cinnamon Rolls (Weight Watchers)	1 (2.1 oz)	180	5	170	31	—
HOME RECIPE						
dinner, as prep w/ 2% milk	1 (2½ in)	111	3	145	19	—
dinner, as prep w/ whole milk	1 (2½ in)	112	3	145	19	—
raisin & nut	1 (2 oz)	196	7	185	30	—
MIX						
Hot Roll Mix (Dromedary)	2	239	5	410	41	—
Hot Roll Mix (Pillsbury)	2	240	4	430	42	—
READY-TO-EAT						
8-inch Francisco Arnold	1 (2.5 oz)	210	3	260	39	—
Augusto Pan Cubano (Arnold)	1	230	3	500	43	2
Bakery Light (Arnold)	1 (1.5 oz)	80	2	190	21	4
Big Marty Poppy (Martin's)	1	170	2	320	31	3
Big Marty Sesame (Martin's)	1	170	2	320	31	3
Bran'nola Buns (Arnold)	1 (1.5 oz)	100	1	160	20	3
Brown & Serve (Roman Meal)	2 (2 oz)	140	3	275	24	2
Brown 'N Serve Club (Pepperidge Farm)	1	100	1	190	19	1
Brown 'N Serve French (Pepperidge Farm)	½ roll	180	2	380	36	1
Brown 'N Serve Hearth (Pepperidge Farm)	1	50	1	100	10	tr

FOOD	PORTION	CAL	FAT	SOD	CARB	FIB
Buns (Wonder)	1	70	1	160	13	1
Dark Bread (Hollywood)	1	40	tr	—	—	—
Deli Kaiser (Arnold)	1	170	2	—	34	—
Deli Onion (Arnold)	1	170	2	—	34	—
Dinner (August Bros.)	1	90	1	170	18	—
Dinner (Pepperidge Farm)	1	60	2	95	8	tr
Dinner (Roman Meal)	2 (2 oz)	136	2	282	24	2
Dinner Country Style Classic (Pepperidge Farm)	1	50	1	90	9	0
Dinner Light Pan Special Formula (Hollywood)	1	60	tr	—	—	—
Dinner Plain (Arnold)	1 (0.7 oz)	50	1	80	9	1
Dinner Sesame (Arnold)	1 (0.7 oz)	50	1	80	9	1
Dutch Egg (Arnold)	1	130	3	180	21	2
Finger Poppy Seed (Pepperidge Farm)	1	50	2	80	8	tr
Finger Sesame Seed (Pepperidge Farm)	1	60	2	85	9	tr
Frankfurt (Country Kitchen)	1	120	2	—	—	—
Frankfurter w/ Poppy Seeds (Pepperidge Farm)	1	130	2	280	23	1
Frankfurter Dijon (Pepperidge Farm)	1	160	5	230	23	2
Frankfurter Side Sliced (Pepperidge Farm)	1	140	3	270	24	1
Frankfurter Top Sliced (Pepperidge Farm)	1	140	3	270	24	1
French Francisco (Arnold)	1 (2.5 oz)	210	3	260	39	—
French Mini Francisco (Arnold)	1	130	2	140	24	—
French Style (Pepperidge Farm)	1	100	1	230	20	1
Hamburger						
(Arnold)	1	120	2	190	20	2
(Pepperidge Farm)	1	130	2	240	22	1

FOOD	PORTION	CAL	FAT	SOD	CARB	FIB
Hamburger *(cont.)*						
(Roman Meal)	1 (1.6 oz)	111	2	229	19	2
(Shop 'n Save)	1	120	2	—	—	—
Hamburger Light (Wonder)	1	80	1	210	14	5
Heat & Serve Butter Crescent (Pepperidge Farm)	1	110	6	150	13	tr
Heat & Serve Golden Twist (Pepperidge Farm)	1	110	5	150	14	tr
Hoagie (Martin's)	1	240	3	430	41	3
Hoagie Sesame (Martin's)	1	240	3	430	41	4
Hoagie Soft (Pepperidge Farm)	1	210	5	320	34	1
Hot Dog (Arnold)	1 (1.5 oz)	110	2	160	21	1
Hot Dog Bran'nola (Arnold)	1 (1.5 oz)	110	2	170	18	1
Hot Dog New England Style (Arnold)	1	110	2	160	20	1
Hotdog (Roman Meal)	1 (1.5 oz)	103	2	214	18	2
Hotdog Light (Wonder)	1	80	1	210	14	5
Italian 8-inch Savoni (Arnold)	1	210	3	—	38	3
Kaiser (August Bros.)	1	170	1	310	35	2
Kaiser Francisco (Arnold)	1 (2 oz)	180	—	230	34	—
Old Fashioned (Pepperidge Farm)	1	50	2	85	7	tr
Onion (August Bros.)	1	160	1	310	33	2
Onion Premium (Arnold)	1 (2.6 oz)	180	1	340	38	2
Onion Soft (Arnold)	1	140	—	200	28	2
Parker House (Pepperidge Farm)	1	60	1	80	9	tr
Party (Pepperidge Farm)	1	30	1	50	5	tr
Party Petite (Arnold)	2	70	2	70	10	1
Potato (Arnold)	1	140	2	210	25	2
Potato Dinner (Martin's)	1	100	1	135	18	1
Potato Long (Martin's)	1	140	1	200	27	2
Potato Party (Martin's)	1	50	1	70	10	1

FOOD	PORTION	CAL	FAT	SOD	CARB	FIB
Potato Sandwich (Martin's)	1	140	1	200	26	2
Potato Sandwich (Pepperidge Farm)	1	160	4	260	28	1
Salad Roll (Matthew's)	1	110	2	190	19	2
Sandwich (Matthew's)	1	110	2	180	19	2
Sandwich (Roman Meal)	1 (2.7 oz)	181	3	392	31	3
Sandwich (Roman Meal)	1 (2.7 oz)	181	3	392	31	3
Sandwich Onion w/ Poppy Seeds (Pepperidge Farm)	1	150	3	260	26	1
Sandwich Salad (Pepperidge Farm)	1	110	4	150	16	—
Sandwich Soft Sesame (Arnold)	1	130	3	220	23	2
Sandwich Whole Wheat 100% Stoneground (Martin's)	1	160	2	290	28	5
Sandwich w/ Sesame Seeds (Pepperidge Farm)	1	140	3	230	23	1
Sesame Cubano (Augusto Bros.)	1	170	1	310	35	2
Sliced Light Special Formula (Hollywood)	1	80	tr	—	—	—
Soft Family (Pepperidge Farm)	1	100	2	190	18	1
Sourdough Brown N' Serve (Arnold)	1 (1 oz)	100	1	120	19	—
Sourdough Francisco (Arnold)	1 (1 oz)	100	1	120	19	—
Sourdough French (Pepperidge Farm)	1	100	1	240	19	1
Sub Old Country (Levy)	1	180	2	230	34	—
Wheat Old Fashioned (Arnold)	2	80	3	98	11	—
brown & serve	1 (1 oz)	85	2	148	14	—
cheese	1 (2.3 oz)	238	12	236	29	—
cinnamon raisin	1 (2¾ in)	223	10	229	31	1
dinner	1 (1 oz)	85	2	148	14	—

FOOD	PORTION	CAL	FAT	SOD	CARB	FIB
egg	1 (2½ in)	107	2	191	18	1
french	1 (1.3 oz)	105	2	232	19	—
hamburger	1 (1.5 oz)	123	2	241	22	—
hamburger, multi-grain	1 (1.5 oz)	113	2	197	19	2
hamburger, reduced calorie	1 (1.5 oz)	84	1	190	18	3
hard	1 (3½ in)	167	2	310	30	—
hot cross bun	1	202	4	—	38	1
hotdog	1 (1.5 oz)	123	2	241	22	—
hotdog, multi-grain	1 (1.5 oz)	113	2	197	19	2
hotdog, reduced calorie	1 (1.5 oz)	84	1	190	18	3
kaiser	1 (3½ in)	167	2	310	30	—
oat bran	1 (1.2 oz)	78	2	136	13	1
rye	1 (1 oz)	81	1	253	15	—
submarine	1 (4.7 oz)	155	2	313	30	—
wheat	1 (1 oz)	77	2	96	13	—
whole wheat	1 (1 oz)	75	1	135	15	—
REFRIGERATED						
Pillsbury Best Quick Cinnamon Rolls w/ Icing	1	110	5	260	17	—
Pillsbury Butterflake	1	140	5	530	20	—
Pillsbury Crescent	1	100	6	230	11	—
cinnamon w/ frosting	1	109	4	250	17	—
crescent	1 (1 oz)	98	4	341	14	—

ROMAN BEANS
CANNED

Progresso	½ cup	110	tr	420	18	12

ROSE APPLE

fresh	3.5 oz	32	tr	—	7	—

ROSE HIP

fresh	3.5 oz	91	0	146	19	—

ROSELLE

fresh	1 cup	28	tr	3	6	—

ROSEMARY

dried	1 tsp	4	tr	1	1	—

ROUGHY

orange baked	3 oz	75	1	69	0	—

FOOD	PORTION	CAL	FAT	SOD	CARB	FIB
RUTABAGA						
FRESH						
cooked, mashed	½ cup	41	tr	22	9	—
raw, cubed	½ cup	25	tr	14	6	—
SABLEFISH						
baked	3 oz	213	17	61	0	—
fillet, baked	5.3 oz	378	30	108	0	—
SMOKED						
sablefish	1 oz	72	6	206	0	—
sablefish	3 oz	218	17	626	0	—
SAFFLOWER						
seeds, dried	1 oz	147	11	—	10	—
SAFFRON						
saffron	1 tsp	2	tr	1	tr	—
SAGE						
ground	1 tsp	2	tr	tr	tr	—
SALAD						
see also PASTA SALAD						
MIX						
Suddenly Salad Caesar, as prep	½ cup	170	8	450	20	—
Suddenly Salad Ranch And Bacon, as prep	½ cup	210	11	320	22	—
Suddenly Salad Ranch And Bacon, as prep low fat recipe	½ cup	160	5	350	23	—
TAKE-OUT						
chef, w/o dressing	1½ cups	386	28	279	9	—
tossed, w/o dressing	1½ cups	32	tr	53	7	—
tossed, w/o dressing	¾ cup	16	0	27	3	—
tossed, w/o dressing w/ cheese & egg	1½ cups	102	6	119	5	—
tossed, w/o dressing w/ chicken	1½ cups	105	2	209	4	—
tossed, w/o dressing w/ pasta & seafood	1½ cups (14.6 oz)	380	21	1572	32	—
tossed, w/o dressing w/ shrimp	1½ cups	107	2	487	7	—
waldorf	½ cup	79	6	49	6	1

FOOD	PORTION	CAL	FAT	SOD	CARB	FIB

SALAD DRESSING
HOME RECIPE

FOOD	PORTION	CAL	FAT	SOD	CARB	FIB
french	1 tbsp	88	10	92	1	—
vinegar & oil	1 tbsp	72	8	tr	tr	—

MIX
Good Seasons

FOOD	PORTION	CAL	FAT	SOD	CARB	FIB
Bleu Cheese And Herbs, as prep	1 tbsp	72	8	148	1	—
Buttermilk Farm, as prep	1 tbsp	58	6	137	1	—
Cheese Garlic, as prep	1 tbsp	72	8	167	1	—
Cheese Italian, as prep	1 tbsp	72	8	127	1	—
Classic Dill	1 pkg	28	tr	2273	5	—
Garlic And Herbs, as prep	1 tbsp	71	8	187	1	—
Italian, as prep	1 tbsp	71	8	172	1	—
Italian Lite, as prep	1 tbsp	27	3	177	1	—
Italian No Oil, as prep	1 tbsp	7	0	32	2	—
Lemon And Herbs, as prep	1 tbsp	71	8	143	1	—
Lite Cheese Italian, as prep	1 tbsp	27	3	137	1	—
Lite Ranch, as prep	1 tbsp	29	2	115	2	—
Lite Zesty Italian, as prep	1 tbsp	26	3	133	1	—
Mild Italian, as prep	1 tbsp	73	8	192	1	—
Ranch, as prep	1 tbsp	57	6	112	1	—
Zesty Italian, as prep	1 tbsp	71	8	121	1	—

Hain No Oil

FOOD	PORTION	CAL	FAT	SOD	CARB	FIB
1000 Island	1 tbsp	12	0	150	3	—
Bleu Cheese	1 tbsp	14	1	190	1	—
Buttermilk	1 tbsp	11	tr	150	1	—
Caesar	1 tbsp	6	tr	200	1	—
French	1 tbsp	12	0	340	3	—
Garlic & Cheese	1 tbsp	6	tr	180	1	—
Herb	1 tbsp	2	0	140	1	—
Italian	1 tbsp	2	0	170	1	—

READY-TO-USE

FOOD	PORTION	CAL	FAT	SOD	CARB	FIB
Catalina	1 tbsp	15	1	120	3	—
Catalina French	1 tbsp	60	5	180	4	—

FOOD	PORTION	CAL	FAT	SOD	CARB	FIB
Diamond Crystal Blue Cheese	1 tbsp	20	1	—	—	—
Diamond Crystal Home Style	1 tbsp	20	1	—	—	—
Diamond Crystal Thousand Island	1 tbsp	20	1	—	—	—
Estee						
Blue Cheese	1 tbsp	8	tr	50	1	—
Dijon Creamy	1 tbsp	8	tr	100	tr	—
French	1 tbsp	4	0	10	1	—
Garlic Creamy	1 tbsp	2	0	10	0	—
Italian Creamy	1 tbsp	4	0	12	1	—
Red Wine Vinegar	1 tbsp	2	0	10	0	—
Thousand Island	1 tbsp	8	0	30	2	—
Hain						
1000 Island	1 tbsp	50	5	85	0	—
Creamy Caesar	1 tbsp	60	6	220	1	—
Creamy Caesar Low Salt	1 tbsp	60	6	15	1	—
Creamy French	1 tbsp	60	6	80	1	—
Creamy Italian	1 tbsp	80	8	100	0	—
Creamy Italian No Salt Added	1 tbsp	80	8	25	1	—
Cucumber Dill	1 tbsp	80	8	210	0	—
Dijon Vinaigrette	1 tbsp	50	5	180	0	—
Garlic & Sour Cream	1 tbsp	70	7	100	0	—
Honey & Sesame	1 tbsp	60	5	210	2	—
Italian Cheese Vinaigrette	1 tbsp	55	6	130	0	—
Old Fashioned Buttermilk	1 tbsp	70	7	100	0	—
Poppyseed Rancher's	1 tbsp	60	7	105	0	—
Savory Herb No Salt Added	1 tbsp	90	10	45	0	—
Swiss Cheese Vinaigrette	1 tbsp	60	7	160	0	—
Traditional Italian	1 tbsp	80	8	330	0	—
Traditional Italian No Salt Added	1 tbsp	60	6	20	1	—
Hain Canola						
Garden Tomato	1 tbsp	60	6	150	1	—
Italian	1 tbsp	50	5	150	1	—

FOOD	PORTION	CAL	FAT	SOD	CARB	FIB
Hain Canola *(cont.)*						
Spicy French Mustard	1 tbsp	50	5	190	1	—
Healthy Sensation						
Blue Cheese	1 tbsp	19	1	144	4	—
French	1 tbsp	21	1	121	4	—
Honey Dijon	1 tbsp	26	1	142	5	—
Italian	1 tbsp	7	tr	141	1	—
Ranch	1 tbsp	15	tr	138	3	—
Thousand Island	1 tbsp	20	tr	134	4	—
Herb Magic						
Cucumber Creamy Reduced Calorie	1 tbsp	8	0	—	—	—
Herb Basket Reduced Calorie	1 tbsp	6	0	—	—	—
Italian Reduced Calorie	1 tbsp	4	0	—	—	—
Sweet & Sour Reduced Calorie	1 tbsp	18	0	—	—	—
Thousand Island Reduced Calorie	1 tbsp	8	0	—	—	—
Vinegarette Reduced Calorie	1 tbsp	6	0	—	—	—
Zesty Tomato Reduced Calorie	1 tbsp	14	0	—	—	—
Hollywood						
Caesar	1 tbsp	70	7	65	2	0
Creamy Italian	1 tbsp	90	9	140	2	0
Dijon Vinaigrette	1 tbsp	60	6	40	2	0
Italian	1 tbsp	90	9	300	1	0
Italian Cheese	1 tbsp	80	8	60	2	0
Poppy Seed Rancher's	1 tbsp	75	8	35	1	0
Thousand Island	1 tbsp	60	6	15	3	0
Kraft						
Bacon Creamy	1 tbsp	30	2	150	2	—
Bacon & Tomato	1 tbsp	70	7	130	1	—
Bacon & Tomato Reduced Calorie	1 tbsp	30	2	150	2	—
Blue Cheese Chunky	1 tbsp	60	6	230	2	—
Buttermilk Creamy	1 tbsp	80	8	120	1	—
Buttermilk Creamy Reduced Calorie	1 tbsp	30	3	125	1	—
Chunky Blue Cheese Reduced Calorie	1 tbsp	30	2	240	2	—

FOOD	PORTION	CAL	FAT	SOD	CARB	FIB
Coleslaw	1 tbsp	70	6	200	4	—
Creamy Garlic	1 tbsp	50	5	170	1	—
Creamy Italian With Real Sour Cream	1 tbsp	50	5	120	1	—
Cucumber Creamy	1 tbsp	70	8	190	1	—
Cucumber Creamy Reduced Calorie	1 tbsp	25	2	220	1	—
Free French Nonfat	1 tbsp	26	0	120	4	—
Free Italian Nonfat	1 tbsp	6	0	210	1	—
Free Ranch Nonfat	1 tbsp	16	0	150	3	—
Free Thousand Island Nonfat	1 tbsp	20	0	135	5	—
French	1 tbsp	60	6	125	2	—
French Reduced Calorie	1 tbsp	20	1	120	3	—
Golden Caesar	1 tbsp	70	7	180	1	—
House Italian	1 tbsp	60	3	115	1	—
House Italian Reduced Calorie	1 tbsp	30	2	115	1	—
Italian Creamy Reduced Calorie	1 tbsp	25	2	120	1	—
Italian Oil-Free	1 tbsp	4	0	220	1	—
Miracle French	1 tbsp	70	6	240	3	—
Oil & Vinegar	1 tbsp	70	7	210	1	—
Onion & Chives Creamy	1 tbsp	70	7	—	—	—
Presto Italian	1 tbsp	70	7	150	1	—
Red Wine Vinegar & Oil	1 tbsp	50	4	—	—	—
Red Wine Vinegar And Oil	1 tbsp	60	4	200	4	—
Russian Creamy	1 tbsp	60	5	150	2	—
Russian Reduced Calorie	1 tbsp	30	1	130	4	—
Russian With Pure Honey	1 tbsp	60	5	130	4	—
Thousand Island	1 tbsp	60	5	150	2	—
Thousand Island & Bacon	1 tbsp	60	6	100	2	—
Thousand Island Reduced Calorie	1 tbsp	20	1	135	3	—
Zesty Italian	1 tbsp	50	5	260	1	—
Zesty Italian Reduced Calorie	1 tbsp	20	2	230	1	—

FOOD	PORTION	CAL	FAT	SOD	CARB	FIB
Magic Mountain						
Bleu Cheese	1 tbsp	5	tr	—	—	—
French	1 tbsp	4	tr	—	—	—
Northern Italian	1 tbsp	2	tr	—	—	—
Herb & Spice No Oil	1 tbsp	2	tr	—	—	—
Newman's Own Italian Light	1 tbsp (0.5 fl oz)	10	tr	170	tr	—
Newman's Own Olive Oil And Vinegar	1 tbsp (0.5 oz)	80	9	80	tr	—
Newman's Own Ranch	1 tbsp (0.5 fl oz)	90	9	80	1	—
Ott's Famous Chef	1 tbsp	40	3	—	—	—
Ott's Italian Chef	1 tbsp	80	9	—	—	—
Pritikin						
Creamy Italian	1 tbsp	12	0	—	—	—
French	1 tbsp	10	0	—	—	—
Italian	1 tbsp	6	0	—	—	—
Ranch	1 tbsp	18	0	—	—	—
Russian	1 tbsp	12	0	—	—	—
Vinaigrette	1 tbsp	10	0	—	—	—
Zesty Tomato	1 tbsp	18	0	—	—	—
Rancher's Choice	1 tbsp	90	6	140	1	—
Rancher's Choice Creamy	1 tbsp	30	3	150	1	—
Roka Blue Cheese	1 tbsp	60	6	170	1	—
Roka Blue Cheese Reduced Calorie	1 tbsp	15	1	280	1	—
S&W						
Blue Cheese Low Calorie	1 tbsp	25	2	200	2	—
Cucumber Creamy Low Calorie	1 tbsp	25	2	190	2	—
French Low Calorie	1 tbsp	18	0	120	3	—
Italian Creamy Low Calorie	1 tbsp	10	1	180	1	—
Italian No-Oil	1 tbsp	2	0	290	0	—
Russian Low Calorie	1 tbsp	25	1	120	4	—
Thousand Island Low Calorie	1 tbsp	25	2	105	2	—
Seven Seas						
Buttermilk	1 tbsp	80	8	130	1	—
Buttermilk Ranch! Light	1 tbsp	50	5	135	1	—
French Creamy	1 tbsp	60	6	240	2	—

FOOD	PORTION	CAL	FAT	SOD	CARB	FIB
French! Light	1 tbsp	35	3	210	2	—
Herb & Spice	1 tbsp	60	6	170	1	—
Italian Creamy	1 tbsp	70	7	240	1	—
Thousand Island! Creamy	1 tbsp	50	5	150	2	—
Thousand Island! Light	1 tbsp	30	2	160	3	—
Seven Seas Free						
Ranch Nonfat	1 tbsp	16	0	120	4	—
Red Wine Vinegar Nonfat	1 tbsp	6	0	190	1	—
Seven Seas Viva						
Free Italian Nonfat	1 tbsp	4	0	220	1	—
Herbs & Spices! Light	1 tbsp	30	3	200	1	—
Italian	1 tbsp	50	5	240	1	—
Italian! Light	1 tbsp	30	3	230	1	—
Ranch	1 tbsp	80	8	135	1	—
Ranch! Light	1 tbsp	50	5	125	2	—
Red Wine Vinegar & Oil	1 tbsp	70	7	290	1	—
Red Wine! Vinegar & Oil Light	1 tbsp	45	4	190	1	—
Ultra Slim-Fast French	1 tbsp	20	tr	150	4	0
Ultra Slim-Fast Italian	1 tbsp	6	tr	170	1	0
W.J. Clark						
Ginger Orange Vinaigrette	1 tbsp	73	7	134	tr	0
Herbs and Romano	1 tbsp	67	6	111	2	0
Lemon Peppercorn	1 tbsp	72	7	135	tr	0
Lime Cilantro Vinaigrette	1 tbsp	73	8	147	tr	0
Poppy Seed	1 tbsp	75	6	106	3	0
Sweet Pepper Basil	1 tbsp	69	7	127	2	0
Tarragon Honey Mustard	1 tbsp	66	6	139	2	0
Walden Farms						
Bleu Cheese	1 tbsp	27	2	270	2	—
Creamy Italian With Parmesan	1 tbsp	35	3	210	3	—
French	1 tbsp	33	2	132	3	—
Italian	1 tbsp	9	tr	300	2	—
Italian No Sugar Added	1 tbsp	6	tr	180	tr	—

FOOD	PORTION	CAL	FAT	SOD	CARB	FIB
Walden Farms *(cont.)*						
Italian Sodium Free	1 tbsp	9	tr	—	2	—
Ranch	1 tbsp	35	2	165	3	—
Thousand Island	1 tbsp	24	2	132	3	—
Weight Watchers						
Caesar	1 pkg (¾ oz)	6	0	280	1	—
Caesar	1 tbsp	4	0	200	1	—
Cucumber Creamy	1 tbsp	18	0	85	4	—
Italian	1 pkg (¾ oz)	8	tr	270	2	—
Italian	1 tbsp	6	tr	200	1	—
Italian Creamy	1 tbsp	12	0	85	3	—
Peppercorn Creamy	1 tbsp	8	0	85	2	—
Ranch Creamy	1 pkg (¾ oz)	35	tr	130	8	—
Ranch Creamy	1 tbsp	25	tr	100	6	—
Russian	1 tbsp	50	5	80	2	—
Thousand Island	1 tbsp	50	5	80	2	—
Wishbone						
Blue Cheese Chunky	1 tbsp	73	8	148	1	—
Blue Cheese Chunky Lite	1 tbsp	40	4	197	2	0
Caesar With Olive Oil Lite	1 tbsp	28	3	172	1	—
Dijon Vinaigrette Classic	1 tbsp	57	6	159	1	0
Dijon Vinaigrette Classic Lite	1 tbsp	30	3	176	1	—
French Deluxe	1 tbsp	57	5	83	2	0
French Fat Free	1 tbsp	6	tr	249	1	—
French Lite	1 tbsp	30	3	67	2	0
French Red	1 tbsp	64	6	170	4	—
French Red Lite	1 tbsp	17	tr	155	3	—
French Sweet 'N Spicy	1 tbsp	613	6	156	3	—
French Sweet 'N Spicy Lite	1 tbsp	17	tr	134	4	—
Italian	1 tbsp	45	5	281	1	—
Italian Creamy	1 tbsp	54	6	149	1	—
Italian Creamy Lite	1 tbsp	26	2	148	2	—
Italian Lite	1 tbsp	6	tr	249	1	—
Italian Robusto	1 tbsp	46	5	288	2	0
Olive Oil Italian Classic	1 tbsp	33	3	190	2	—
Olive Oil Italian Classic Lite	1 tbsp	20	2	155	1	—
Olive Oil Vinaigrette	1 tbsp	30	3	126	2	—

FOOD	PORTION	CAL	FAT	SOD	CARB	FIB
Olive Oil Vinaigrette Lite	1 tbsp	16	1	133	2	—
Ranch	1 tbsp	76	8	103	1	—
Ranch Lite	1 tbsp	42	4	148	3	0
Red Wine Vinaigrette Olive Oil Lite	1 tbsp	20	2	151	1	—
Red Wine Olive Oil Vinaigrette	1 tbsp	34	3	191	2	—
Russian	1 tbsp	54	3	173	7	tr
Russian Lite	1 tbsp	21	tr	142	5	—
Thousand Island	1 tbsp	66	6	168	3	—
Thousand Island Lite	1 tbsp	22	1	135	5	—
blue cheese	1 tbsp	77	8	—	1	—
french	1 tbsp	67	6	214	3	—
french reduced calorie	1 tbsp	22	1	128	4	—
italian	1 tbsp	69	7	116	2	—
italian reduced calorie	1 tbsp	16	2	118	1	—
russian	1 tbsp	76	8	133	2	—
russian reduced calorie	1 tbsp	23	1	141	5	—
sesame seed	1 tbsp	68	7	153	1	—
thousand island	1 tbsp	59	6	109	2	—
thousand island reduced calorie	1 tbsp	24	2	153	3	—

SALMON
CANNED

FOOD	PORTION	CAL	FAT	SOD	CARB	FIB
Bumble Bee Keta	3.5 oz	160	8	490	0	—
Bumble Bee Pink	3.5 oz	160	8	490	0	—
Bumble Bee Pink Skinless & Boneless	3.25 oz	120	5	420	0	—
Bumble Bee Red	3.5 oz	180	10	490	0	—
Bumble Bee Red Skinless & Boneless	3.25 oz	130	6	420	0	—
Deming's Alaska Keta	½ cup	140	5	450	0	—
Deming's Alaska Pink	½ cup	140	6	450	0	—
Deming's Alaska Red Sockeye	½ cup	170	9	450	0	—
Double Q Alaska Pink	½ cup	140	6	450	0	—
Humpty Dumpty Alaska Chum	½ cup	140	2	450	0	—
Libby's Keta	½ cup (3.8 oz)	140	6	—	—	—
Libby's Pink	½ can (3.8 oz)	150	7	—	—	—

FOOD	PORTION	CAL	FAT	SOD	CARB	FIB
S&W Bluepack Fancy Diet	½ cup	188	11	45	0	—
S&W Red Fancy Sockeye Bluepack	½ cup	190	10	590	0	—
chum w/ bone	1 can (13.9 oz)	521	20	1797	0	—
chum w/ bone	3 oz	120	5	414	0	—
pink w/ bone	1 can (15.9 oz)	631	27	2514	0	—
pink w/ bone	3 oz	118	5	471	0	—
sockeye w/ bone	1 can (12.9 oz)	566	27	1987	0	—
sockeye w/ bone	3 oz	130	6	458	0	—
FRESH						
atlantic, baked	3 oz	155	7	48	0	—
chinook, baked	3 oz	196	11	51	0	—
chum, baked	3 oz	131	4	54	0	—
coho, cooked	½ fillet (5.4 oz)	286	12	91	0	—
coho, cooked	3 oz	157	6	50	0	—
coho, raw	3 oz	124	5	39	0	—
pink, baked	3 oz	127	4	73	0	—
roe, raw	3.5 oz	207	10	—	1	—
sockeye, cooked	½ fillet (5.4 oz)	334	17	102	0	—
sockeye, cooked	3 oz	183	9	102	0	—
sockeye, raw	3 oz	143	7	40	0	—
smoked						
chinook	1 oz	33	1	220	0	—
chinook	3 oz	99	4	666	0	—
TAKE-OUT						
salmon cake	1 (3 oz)	241	15	602	6	—

SALSA

FOOD	PORTION	CAL	FAT	SOD	CARB	FIB
Casa Fiesta Chili Salsa	1 oz	9	tr	117	2	—
Chi Chi's Hot	1 oz	8	tr	138	2	—
Chi Chi's Medium	1 oz	8	0	130	2	—
Chi Chi's Mild	1 oz	9	tr	96	2	—
Frito-Lay Hot	1 oz	12	0	180	2	—
Frito-Lay Medium	1 oz	12	0	150	2	—
Frito-Lay Mild	1 oz	12	0	200	2	—
Hain Hot	¼ cup	22	0	480	4	—
Hain Mild	¼ cup	20	0	410	4	—
Heluva Good Cheese Cheese & Salsa	2 tbsp (1.1 oz)	80	6	210	3	0
Heluva Good Cheese Thick & Chunky Hot	2 tbsp (1.2 oz)	10	0	180	2	0
Heluva Good Cheese Thick & Chunky Mild	2 tbsp (1.2 oz)	10	0	180	2	0
Hot Cha Cha Medium	2 tbsp (1 oz)	5	0	0	2	—

FOOD	PORTION	CAL	FAT	SOD	CARB	FIB
Newman's Own Bandito Hot	1 tbsp (0.7 oz)	6	tr	120	tr	—
Newman's Own Bandito Medium	1 tbsp (0.7 oz)	6	tr	45	tr	—
Newman's Own Bandito Mild	1 tbsp (0.7 oz)	6	tr	40	tr	—
Old El Paso						
Picante Hot	2 tbsp	10	tr	160	2	—
Picante Medium	2 tbsp	10	tr	160	2	—
Picante Mild	2 tbsp	10	tr	160	2	—
Thick 'n Chunky Green Chili	2 tbsp	3	0	270	1	0
Thick 'n Chunky Hot	2 tbsp	6	tr	170	1	—
Thick 'n Chunky Medium	2 tbsp	6	tr	170	1	—
Thick 'n Chunky Mild	2 tbsp	6	tr	170	1	—
Thick 'n Chunky Salsa Verde	2 tbsp	10	tr	135	2	1
Ortega Hot Green Chili	1 tbsp	6	0	190	2	—
Ortega Medium Green Chili	1 tbsp	6	0	190	1	—
Ortega Mild Green Chili	1 tbsp	8	0	190	2	—
Pace Thick & Chunky	2 tbsp (1 fl oz)	12	0	321	2	1
Rosarita						
Chunky Hot	3 tbsp (1.5 oz)	25	tr	300	6	tr
Chunky Medium	3 tbsp (1.5 oz)	25	tr	350	6	tr
Chunky Mild	3 tbsp (1.5 oz)	25	tr	340	6	tr
Taco Salsa Chunky Medium	3 tbsp (1.5 oz)	25	tr	310	6	tr
Taco Salsa Chunky Mild	3 tbsp (1.5 oz)	25	tr	300	6	tr

SALSIFY
FRESH
cooked, sliced	½ cup	46	tr	11	10	—
raw, sliced	½ cup	55	tr	13	12	—

SALT SUBSTITUTES
Estee Salt-It	⅛ tsp	0	0	0	0	—
Morton	1 tsp	2	tr	—	—	—
Nu-Salt	1 pkg (1g)	0	0	—	—	—
Papa Dash Lite Lite Lite Salt	¼ tsp (0.5 g)	1	0	87	tr	—
Papa Dash Salt Lover's Blend	¼ tsp (0.7 g)	tr	0	231	tr	—

FOOD	PORTION	CAL	FAT	SOD	CARB	FIB

SALT/SEASONED SALT
see also SALT SUBSTITUTES

FOOD	PORTION	CAL	FAT	SOD	CARB	FIB
Garlic Morton	1 tsp	3	tr	—	—	—
Hain Sea Salt	1 tsp	0	0	2255	0	—
Hain Sea Salt Iodized	1 tsp	0	0	2255	0	—
Iodized (Morton)	1 tsp	tr	0	—	—	—
Kosher (Morton)	1 tsp	0	0	—	—	—
Lite (Morton)	1 tsp	tr	0	—	—	—
Morton Nature's Season Seasoning Blend	1 tsp	3	tr	—	—	—
Non-Iodized (Morton)	1 tsp	0	0	—	—	—
Seasoned (Morton)	1 tsp	4	tr	—	—	—
salt	1 tsp	0	0	2132	0	—

SAPODILLA

FOOD	PORTION	CAL	FAT	SOD	CARB	FIB
fresh	1	140	2	20	34	—
fresh cut up	1 cup	199	3	29	48	—

SAPOTES

FOOD	PORTION	CAL	FAT	SOD	CARB	FIB
fresh	1	301	1	21	76	—

SARDINES
CANNED

FOOD	PORTION	CAL	FAT	SOD	CARB	FIB
Empress Skinless & Boneless Olive Oil	1 can (3.8 oz)	420	38	530	2	—
Empress Skinless & Boneless Soy Oil	1 can (4.4 oz)	500	45	630	2	—
In Mustard Sauce Port Clyde Foods	1 can (3.75 oz)	175	11	—	—	—
In Soybean Oil Port Clyde Foods	1 can (3.75 oz)	225	18	—	—	—
In Tomato Sauce Port Clyde Foods	1 can (3.75 oz)	170	11	—	—	—
S&W Norwegian Brisling	1.5 oz	130	10	220	0	—
Underwood Brisling In Olive Oil	3.75 oz	260	20	450	1	—
Underwood In Mustard Sauce	3.75 oz	220	16	560	2	—
Underwood In Mild Oil, drained	3.75 oz	460	42	120	1	—
Underwood In Soya Oil, drained	3 oz	230	18	400	1	—
Underwood In Tomato Sauce	3.75 oz	220	16	500	2	—

FOOD	PORTION	CAL	FAT	SOD	CARB	FIB
Underwood With Tabasco Brand Pepper Sauce, drained	3 oz	220	16	400	1	—
Viking's Delight Brisling In Olive Oil	1 can (3.75 oz)	460	42	450	1	—
Viking's Delight Brisling In Olive Oil, drained	1 can (3.75 oz)	260	20	450	1	—
atlantic in oil w/ bone	1 can (3.2 oz)	192	11	465	0	—
atlantic in oil w/ bone	2	50	3	121	0	—
pacific in tomato sauce w/ bone	1	68	5	157	0	—
pacific in tomato sauce w/ bone	1 can (13 oz)	658	44	1532	0	—
FRESH						
raw	3.75 oz	135	5	100	0	—

SAUCE

see also GRAVY, PIZZA, SPAGHETTI SAUCE, TOMATO

FOOD	PORTION	CAL	FAT	SOD	CARB	FIB
DRY						
Au Jus, as prep (Knorr)	2 oz	8	tr	160	1	—
Bar-B-Q (Diamond Crystal)	2 oz	35	1	—	—	—
Bearnaise, as prep (Knorr)	2 oz	170	17	340	5	—
Brown (Diamond Crystal)	2 oz	15	tr	—	—	—
Cheese (Diamond Crystal)	2 oz	50	2	—	—	—
Classic Brown Gravy, as prep (Knorr)	2 oz	25	1	300	3	—
Cream (Diamond Crystal)	2 oz	40	1	—	—	—
Demi-Glace, as prep (Knorr)	2 oz	30	1	310	4	—
Etouffee Seasoning Mix (Cajun King)	3.5 oz	383	6	1087	70	—
Hollandaise, as prep (Knorr)	2 oz	170	18	310	5	—
Hunter, as prep (Knorr)	2 oz	25	tr	340	4	—
Italian (Diamond Crystal)	3 oz	50	tr	—	—	—
Jambalaya Seasoning Mix (Cajun King)	3.5 oz	375	9	2855	61	—

FOOD	PORTION	CAL	FAT	SOD	CARB	FIB
Lyonnaise, as prep (Knorr)	2 oz	20	tr	360	3	—
Marinade For Meat (Kikkoman)	1 oz pkg	64	tr	—	—	—
Mushroom, as prep (Knorr)	2 oz	60	3	240	5	—
Napoli, as prep (Knorr)	4 oz	100	3	960	17	—
Pepper, as prep (Knorr)	2 oz	20	1	380	3	—
Sweet & Sour (Kikkoman)	2⅛ oz pkg	228	tr	—	—	—
Sweet 'n Sour Entree Mix (Chun King)	3.8 oz	370	0	—	—	—
Teriyaki (Kikkoman)	1½ oz pkg	125	tr	—	—	—
bearnaise, as prep w/ milk & butter	1 cup	701	68	1265	18	—
cheese, as prep w/ milk	1 cup	307	17	1566	23	—
curry, as prep w/ milk	1 cup	270	15	1276	26	—
mushroom, as prep w/ milk	1 cup	228	10	1533	24	—
sour cream, as prep w/ milk	1 cup	509	30	1007	45	—
stroganoff, as prep	1 cup	271	11	1829	34	—
sweet & sour, as prep	1 cup	294	tr	779	73	—
teriyaki, as prep	1 cup	131	1	4791	28	—
white, as prep w/ milk	1 cup	241	13	796	21	—
JARRED						
7 Spice Chili (McIlhenny)	2 tbsp (1.1 fl oz)	16	tr	191	3	1
Alfredo (Progresso)	½ cup	340	30	1080	6	—
B-B-Q (McIlhenny)	2 tbsp (1.1 oz)	48	2	201	7	tr
BBQ Dijon Honey (Lawry's)	¼ cup	203	1	1768	27	tr
Bandito Diavalo Spicy (Newman's Own)	4 oz	70	2	530	11	—
Bar-B-Que Honey (Hain)	1 tbsp	14	1	120	1	—
Barbecue						
(Estee)	1 tbsp	18	tr	5	3	—
(Kraft)	2 tbsp	45	1	460	10	—
(Maull's)	3.5 oz	123	2	—	—	—
(Ott's)	1 tbsp	14	tr	—	—	—
Homestyle (Hunt's)	1 tbsp	20	tr	170	6	tr
Mesquite Smoke (Kraft)	2 tbsp	45	1	410	10	—
Original (Bull's Eye)	2 tbsp	50	0	—	—	—

FOOD	PORTION	CAL	FAT	SOD	CARB	FIB
Original (Hunt's)	1 tbsp	20	tr	160	5	tr
Southern Style (Hunt's)	1 tbsp	20	tr	170	5	tr
Sweet-N-Mild (Maull's)	3.5 oz	167	2	—	—	—
Sweet-N-Smoky (Maull's)	3.5 oz	160	tr	—	—	—
Barbecue Beer Non-Alcoholic (Maull's)	3.5 oz	128	2	—	—	—
Barbecue Country Style (Hunt's)	1 tbsp	20	tr	140	5	tr
Barbecue Garlic (Kraft)	2 tbsp	40	0	420	9	—
Barbecue Hickory (Hunt's)	1 tbsp	20	tr	160	5	tr
Barbecue Hickory Smoke (Kraft)	2 tbsp	45	1	440	10	—
Barbecue Hickory Smoke Onion Bits (Kraft)	2 tbsp	50	1	340	11	—
Barbecue Hot (Kraft)	2 tbsp	45	1	520	9	—
Barbecue Hot Hickory Smoke (Kraft)	2 tbsp	45	1	360	9	—
Barbecue Italian Seasoning (Kraft)	2 tbsp	50	1	280	10	—
Barbecue Kansas City Style (Hunt's)	1 tbsp	20	tr	85	5	tr
Barbecue Kansas City Style (Kraft)	2 tbsp	50	1	270	11	—
Barbecue New Orleans Style (Hunt's)	1 tbsp	20	tr	150	5	tr
Barbecue Onion Bits (Kraft)	2 tbsp	50	1	340	11	—
Barbecue Select (Heinz)	1 oz	40	0	275	9	—
Barbecue Select Hickory (Heinz)	1 oz	35	0	260	8	—
Barbecue Smokey (Ott's)	1 tbsp	14	tr	—	—	—
Barbecue Smoky (Maull's)	3.5 oz	124	tr	—	—	—
Barbecue Texas Style (Hunt's)	1 tbsp	25	tr	150	6	tr
Barbecue Thick & Rich Cajun Style (Heinz)	1 oz	35	0	360	8	—
Barbecue Thick & Rich Chunky (Heinz)	1 oz	30	0	380	6	—

FOOD	PORTION	CAL	FAT	SOD	CARB	FIB
Barbecue Thick & Rich 1 oz Hawaiian Style (Heinz)	1 oz	40	0	210	10	—
Barbecue Select Hickory (Heinz)	1 oz	35	0	280	8	—
Barbecue Thick & Rich Hickory Smoke (Heinz)	1 oz	35	0	380	8	—
Barbecue Thick & Rich Mesquite Smoke (Heinz)	1 oz	30	0	380	7	—
Barbecue Thick & Rich Mushroom (Heinz)	1 oz	30	0	460	6	—
Barbecue Thick & Rich Old Fashioned (Heinz)	1 oz	35	0	350	8	—
Barbecue Thick & Rich Onion (Heinz)	1 oz	30	0	420	7	—
Barbecue Thick & Rich Original (Heinz)	1 oz	35	0	390	8	—
Barbecue Thick & Rich Texas Hot (Heinz)	1 oz	30	0	390	7	—
Barbecue Thick'n Spicy Chunky (Kraft)	2 tbsp	60	1	420	13	—
Barbecue Thick'n Spicy Hickory Smoke (Kraft)	2 tbsp	50	1	430	12	—
Barbecue Thick'n Spicy Kansas City Style (Kraft)	2 tbsp	60	1	270	13	—
Barbecue Thick'n Spicy Mesquite Smoke (Kraft)	2 tbsp	50	1	430	12	—
Barbecue Thick'n Spicy Original (Kraft)	2 tbsp	50	1	430	12	—
Barbecue Thick'n Spicy With Honey (Kraft)	2 tbsp	60	1	340	13	—
Barbecue Western Style (Hunt's)	1 tbsp	20	tr	170	5	tr
Barbecue w/ Onion Bits (Maull's)	3.5 oz	126	2	—	—	—
Cajun Style (Golden Dipt)	1 oz	90	8	360	5	—
Cocktail (Heluva Good Cheese)	¼ cup (1.6 oz)	40	0	410	10	—
Cocktail (Sauceworks)	1 tbsp	14	0	170	3	—
Creole (Golden Dipt)	1 oz	20	1	190	2	—
Diable (Escoffier)	1 tbsp	20	0	160	4	—
Dijonnaise (Golden Dipt)	1 oz	52	4	130	2	—
Duck Sauce Sweet & Sour (La Choy)	1 tbsp	25	tr	40	7	tr

FOOD	PORTION	CAL	FAT	SOD	CARB	FIB
Enchilada Green (Old El Paso)	2 tbsp	11	0	200	3	0
Enchilada Hot (Old El Paso)	¼ cup	30	1	250	4	—
Enchilada Mild (Old El Paso)	¼ cup	25	1	250	4	—
Enchilada Sauce (Gebhardt)	3 tbsp (1.5 oz)	25	1	170	2	tr
French White (Golden Dipt)	1 oz	55	4	210	3	—
Ginger Teriyaki Marinade (Golden Dipt)	1 oz	120	7	920	12	—
Grilling And Broiling Chardonnay (Knorr)	1.6 oz	50	4	630	4	—
Grilling and Broiling Tequilla Lime (Knorr)	1.6 oz	50	3	690	6	—
Grilling and Broiling Spicy Plum (Knorr)	1.7 oz	60	2	790	11	—
Grilling And Broiling Tuscan Herb (Knorr)	1.6 oz	50	4	600	5	—
Hot Dog (Just Rite)	2 oz	60	3	220	6	tr
Hot Dog (Wolf Brand)	1.25 oz	44	2	199	4	—
Hot Dog Chili Sauce (Gebhardt)	2 tbsp	30	1	180	4	tr
Hot Sauce (Gebhardt)	½ tsp	tr	tr	55	tr	tr
Indi-Pep West Indian Style Pepper Sauce (Trappey's)	1 tsp (0.1 oz)	1	tr	41	tr	tr
Lemon Butter Dill (Golden Dipt)	1 oz	100	9	190	4	—
Lemon Herb Marinade (Golden Dipt)	1 oz	130	14	210	2	—
Manwich Mexican	2.5 oz	35	1	460	9	1
Mexi Pep Louisiana Hot Sauce (Trappey's)	1 tsp (0.1 oz)	tr	tr	59	tr	tr
Microwave Hollandaise (Knorr)	1 oz	50	5	190	1	—
Microwave Mandarin Ginger (Knorr)	1.6 oz	50	4	690	5	—
Microwave Parmesano (Knorr)	1.6 oz	50	4	680	3	—
Microwave Vera Cruz (Knorr)	3.3 oz	70	3	580	9	—

FOOD	PORTION	CAL	FAT	SOD	CARB	FIB
Newburg With Sherry (Snow's)	⅓ cup	120	8	520	10	—
Pepper Sauce (Trappey's)	1 tsp (0.2 oz)	1	tr	85	tr	tr
Picante						
(Pace)	2 tbsp (1 fl oz)	7	0	294	2	tr
(Tabasco)	2 tbsp (1.5 oz)	17	tr	313	3	1
(Wise)	2 tbsp	12	0	130	3	—
Hot (Old El Paso)	2 tbsp	8	tr	310	2	—
Medium (Old El Paso)	2 tbsp	8	tr	310	2	—
Mild (Old El Paso)	2 tbsp	8	tr	310	2	—
Picante Chunky Hot (Old El Paso)	2 tbsp	7	0	270	2	0
Picante Chunky Medium (Old El Paso)	2 tbsp	7	0	270	2	0
Picante Chunky Mild (Old El Paso)	2 tbsp	7	0	270	2	0
Primavera Creamy (Progresso)	½ cup	190	17	410	8	1
Red Devil Buffalo Style Hot Sauce (Trappey's)	1 tsp (0.1 oz)	1	tr	59	tr	tr
Red Devil Cayenne Pepper Sauce (Trappey's)	1 tsp (0.1 oz)	1	tr	44	tr	tr
Rib (Gold's)	1 oz	60	0	250	14	—
Seafood Cocktail (Golden Dipt)	1 tbsp	20	0	210	5	—
Seafood Cocktail Extra Hot (Golden Dipt)	1 tbsp	20	0	210	5	—
Simmer Chef Golden Honey Mustard (Campbell)	½ cup (4 fl oz)	150	2	400	30	1
Simmer Chef Hearty Onion & Mushroom (Campbell)	½ cup (4 fl oz)	50	1	670	9	1
Sloppy Joe (Manwich)	2.5 oz	40	tr	390	10	1
Steak (Estee)	1 tbsp	14	0	35	3	—
Steak (Lea & Perrins)	1 oz	40	tr	220	10	—
Steak (Mrs. Dash)	1 tbsp	17	tr	10	4	—
Stir-Fry (Kikkoman)	1 tbsp	16	tr	369	3	1
Sweet & Sour (Kikkoman)	1 tbsp	19	tr	97	4	tr

FOOD	PORTION	CAL	FAT	SOD	CARB	FIB
Sweet & Sour (La Choy)	1 tbsp	25	tr	40	7	tr
Sweet 'N Sour (Sauceworks)	1 tbsp	25	0	50	5	—
Sweet 'n Sour (Contadina)	2 tbsp	40	1	110	8	—
Tabasco (McIlhenny)	1 tsp	1	tr	30	tr	tr
Taco Hot (Old El Paso)	2 tbsp	10	tr	130	2	—
Taco Medium (Old El Paso)	2 tbsp	10	tr	130	2	—
Taco Mild (Old El Paso)	2 tbsp	10	tr	130	2	—
Tartar						
(Best Foods)	1 tbsp (14 g)	70	8	190	tr	—
(Bright Day)	1 tbsp	50	5	—	—	—
(Golden Dipt)	1 tbsp	70	7	100	2	—
(Hellman's)	1 tbsp (14 g)	70	8	190	tr	—
(Sauceworks)	1 tbsp	50	5	85	2	—
(Weight Watchers)	1 tbsp	35	3	80	3	—
Tartar Lite (Golden Dipt)	1 tbsp	50	4	40	4	—
Tartar Natural Lemon And Herb (Kraft)	1 tbsp	70	8	85	0	—
Teriyaki (Kikkoman)	1 tbsp	15	0	626	3	0
Teriyaki Marinade (Lawry's)	2 tbsp	72	tr	7100	11	tr
Tomatoes & Jalapenos (Old El Paso)	¼ cup	11	tr	150	2	0
Tomatoes & Green Chilies (Old El Paso)	¼ cup	14	tr	480	3	—
Welsh Rarebit Cheese (Snow's)	½ cup	170	11	460	10	—
Worcestershire (Heinz)	1 tbsp	6	0	170	1	—
Worcestershire (Lea & Perrins)	1 tsp	5	tr	55	1	—
Worcestershire Chef Magic (Trappey's)	1 tsp (0.1 oz)	3	tr	39	1	tr
Worcestershire White Wine (Lea & Perrins)	1 tsp	4	tr	40	1	—
barbecue	1 cup	188	5	2038	32	—
teriyaki	1 oz	30	0	1380	6	—
teriyaki	1 tbsp	15	0	690	3	—

SAUERKRAUT
CANNED

FOOD	PORTION	CAL	FAT	SOD	CARB	FIB
Claussen	½ cup	17	tr	—	—	—
Hebrew National Gallon Kraut	½ cup	25	0	800	4	—

FOOD	PORTION	CAL	FAT	SOD	CARB	FIB
Libby	½ cup	20	0	—	—	—
New Kraut (Hebrew National)	½ cup (3.1 oz)	50	1	550	11	—
Rosoff's	½ cup (3.2 oz)	50	1	550	11	—
S&W	½ cup	25	0	850	5	—
Schorr's New Kraut	½ cup (3.2 oz)	50	1	550	11	—
Seneca	½ cup	20	0	—	—	—
SnowFloss Kraut	4 oz	28	0	780	4	1
SnowFloss Kraut Bavarian Style	4 oz	64	0	780	12	1
Vlasic Old Fashioned	1 oz	4	0	280	1	—
canned	½ cup	22	tr	780	5	—
JUICE						
S&W	4 oz	14	0	1120	3	—

SAUSAGE

see also HOT DOG, SAUSAGE SUBSTITUTES

FOOD	PORTION	CAL	FAT	SOD	CARB	FIB
Armour						
Country Sausage Lower Salt	1 oz	110	11	—	—	—
Country Sausage Lower Salt Links	1 oz	110	11	—	—	—
Country Sausage Lower Salt Patties	1.5 oz	160	16	—	—	—
Pork	1 oz	110	11	—	—	—
Pork Links	1 oz	110	11	—	—	—
Pork Patties	1.5 oz	160	16	—	—	—
Bil Mar Foods Breakfast Turkey	1 oz	58	4	—	—	—
Bill Mar Foods Smoked	3 oz	142	10	—	—	—
Brown 'N Serve (Swift Premium)						
Bacon	1	90	8	140	tr	—
Beef	1	90	9	190	tr	—
Light	1	60	5	140	1	—
Regular	1	100	10	150	tr	—
Golden Brown						
Beef	1	80	7	160	tr	—
Light Links	1	60	5	130	1	—
Mild	1	100	10	150	tr	—
Mild Pattie	1	150	14	220	tr	—
Spicy	1	100	9	150	tr	—
Hebrew National Beef Knocks	1 (3 oz)	260	25	670	—	—

FOOD	PORTION	CAL	FAT	SOD	CARB	FIB
Hebrew National Polish Beef	1 link	240	22	680	—	—
Hillshire						
Beer Bratwurst	1 (2 oz)	190	17	500	2	—
Bratwurst Fresh	1 (2 oz)	190	17	410	1	—
Bratwurst Light Fresh	1 (2 oz)	150	11	620	2	—
Bratwurst Spicy	1 (2 oz)	180	17	490	1	—
Flavorseal Kielbasa Polska	2 oz	190	17	540	2	—
Flavorseal Kielbasa Polska Beef	2 oz	190	17	550	2	—
Flavorseal Kielbasa Polska Lite	2 oz	130	11	512	1	—
Flavorseal Kielbasa Polska Mild	2 oz	190	17	530	2	—
Flavorseal Kielbasa Polska Turkey	2 oz	90	5	500	2	—
Flavorseal Smoked	2 oz	190	17	500	2	—
Flavorseal Smoked Beef	2 oz	180	16	490	2	—
Flavorseal Smoked Beef And Cheddar	2 oz	190	15	500	1	—
Flavorseal Smoked Country Recipe	2 oz	180	16	490	2	—
Flavorseal Smoked Hot	2 oz	180	16	510	2	—
Flavorseal Smoked Lite	2 oz	130	11	512	1	—
Flavorseal Smoked Turkey	2 oz	90	5	500	2	—
Flavorseal Smoked w/ Italian Seasoning	2 oz	200	18	500	1	—
Italian Hot	1 (2 oz)	180	17	500	1	—
Italian Hot Light	1 (2 oz)	150	11	620	2	—
Italian Mild	1 (2 oz)	190	17	490	1	—
Italian Mild Light	1 (2 oz)	150	11	620	2	—
Kielbasa Fresh Polska	1 (2 oz)	190	17	410	1	—
Kielbasa Fresh Polska Lower Fat	1 (2 oz)	150	11	620	2	—
Links 80% Fat Free Cheddar Hots	2 oz	150	12	640	1	—
Links 80% Fat Free Kielbasa	2 oz	130	10	630	2	—

FOOD	PORTION	CAL	FAT	SOD	CARB	FIB
Hillshire *(cont.)*						
Links 80% Fat Free Smokies	2 oz	130	10	640	2	—
Links Brats Fully Cooked	2 oz	170	16	380	1	—
Links Bratwurst Smoked	2 oz	190	17	540	1	—
Links Cheddarwurst	2 oz	190	17	480	1	—
Links Cheddarwurst Lite	1 link (2.7 oz)	190	15	680	2	—
Links Hot	2 oz	190	16	530	2	—
Links Hot Beef	2 oz	190	17	560	1	—
Links Hot Lite	1 link (2.7 oz)	190	15	690	2	—
Links Kielbasa Polska	2 oz	190	17	530	2	—
Links Kielbasa Polska Lite	1 link (2.7 oz)	190	15	610	2	—
Links Knockwurst Lite	2 oz	180	16	460	1	—
Links Lit'l Polskas	2 oz	180	16	600	2	—
Links Lit'l Smokies	2 oz	180	16	600	2	—
Links Lit'l Smokies Beef	2 oz	180	16	600	2	—
Links Lit'l Smokies Cheddar	2 oz	180	16	600	2	—
Links Lit'l Smokies Light	2 oz	120	8	600	1	—
Links Polish	2 oz	190	17	520	2	—
Links Smoked	2 oz	190	18	520	1	—
Links Bun Size Cheddarwurst	2 oz	200	18	480	1	—
Links Bun Size Kielbasa	2 oz	180	16	570	2	—
Links Bun Size Smoked	2 oz	180	16	570	2	—
Links Bun Size Smoked Beef	2 oz	180	16	570	2	—
Mexican Style	1 (2 oz)	190	17	410	1	—
Mexican Style Lower Fat	1 (2 oz)	150	11	620	2	—
Jones						
Cello Beef	1 slice (1 oz)	130	13	160	tr	—
Cello Hot Country	1 slice (1 oz)	110	10	170	tr	—
Cello Original	1 slice (1 oz)	100	10	180	tr	—
Dinner Link	1	280	28	310	tr	—

FOOD	PORTION	CAL	FAT	SOD	CARB	FIB
Light Link	1	70	6	210	1	—
Little Link	1	140	14	170	tr	—
Patties	1	150	14	270	tr	—
Scrapple	1 slice	90	6	230	5	—
Scrapple	1 slice (1.5 oz)	90	6	230	5	—
Louis Rich						
Polska Kielbasa	2 oz	80	5	510	1	0
Smoked Sausage With Cheese cooked	1 (1 oz)	47	3	269	1	—
Turkey	2.5 oz	110	6	580	3	0
Turkey & Cheese Smoked	2 oz	90	5	550	2	0
Turkey Links	2 (2 oz)	90	6	470	0	0
Turkey Smoked	2 oz	90	5	510	2	0
Mr. Turkey Polish Kielbasa	3 oz	177	13	—	—	—
Oscar Mayer						
Little Fryers Pork, cooked	1 (3.4 oz)	82	8	219	tr	—
Smokie Links	1 (1.5 oz)	126	11	426	1	—
Smokies Beef	1 (1.5 oz)	124	11	429	1	—
Smokies Cheese	1 (1.5 oz)	126	11	452	1	—
Smokies Little	1 (½ oz)	27	3	92	tr	—
Perdue Breakfast Links Turkey, cooked	1 (1.3 oz)	40	3	106	tr	—
Perdue Breakfast Patties Turkey, cooked	1 (1.3 oz)	61	4	175	tr	—
Perdue Hot Italian Turkey, cooked	1 (2 oz)	94	6	348	0	—
Perdue Sweet Italian Turkey, cooked	1 (2 oz)	94	6	348	0	—
Shofar Knockwurst Beef	1 (3 oz)	260	23	620	tr	0
blutwurst, uncooked	3.5 oz	424	39	680	0	—
bockwurst pork & veal, raw	1 link (2.3 oz)	200	18	—	tr	—
bratwurst pork	1 oz	92	8	315	1	—
bratwurst pork, cooked	1 link (3 oz)	256	22	473	2	—
bratwurst pork & beef	1 link (2.5 oz)	226	19	778	2	—
country-style pork, cooked	1 link (½ oz)	48	4	168	tr	—
country-style pork, cooked	1 patty (1 oz)	100	8	349	tr	—

FOOD	PORTION	CAL	FAT	SOD	CARB	FIB
gelbwurst uncooked	3.5 oz	363	33	640	0	—
italian pork, cooked	1 (2.4 oz)	216	17	618	1	—
italian pork, cooked	1 (3 oz)	268	21	765	1	—
kielbasa pork	1 oz	88	8	305	1	—
knockwurst pork & beef	1 (2.4 oz)	209	19	687	1	—
knockwurst pork & beef	1 oz	87	8	286	1	—
mettwurst, uncooked	3.5 oz	483	45	1090	0	—
plockwurst, uncooked	3.5 oz	312	45	—	0	—
polish pork	1 (8 oz)	739	65	1989	4	—
polish pork	1 oz	92	8	248	tr	—
pork & beef, cooked	1 link (½ oz)	52	5	105	tr	—
pork & beef, cooked	1 patty (1 oz)	107	10	217	1	—
pork, cooked	1 link (½ oz)	48	4	168	tr	—
pork, cooked	1 patty (1 oz)	100	8	349	tr	—
regensburger, uncooked	3½ oz	354	31	—	0	—
smoked beef, cooked	1 sausage (1.4 oz)	134	12	—	—	—
smoked pork	1 link (2.4 oz)	265	22	1020	1	—
smoked pork	1 sm link (½ oz)	62	5	240	tr	—
smoked pork & beef	1 link (2.4 oz)	229	21	151	1	—
smoked pork & beef	1 sm link (½ oz)	54	5	151	tr	—
vienna, canned	1 (½ oz)	45	4	152	tr	—
vienna, canned	7 (4 oz)	315	28	1077	2	—
weisswurst, uncooked	3.5 oz	305	27	620	0	—
TAKE-OUT						
pork	1 link (.5 oz)	48	4	168	tr	—
pork	1 patty (1 oz)	100	8	349	tr	—

SAUSAGE DISHES
FROZEN

FOOD	PORTION	CAL	FAT	SOD	CARB	FIB
Jimmy Dean Microwave Sausage Biscuits	1	210	14	—	—	—
Ovenstuffs French Roll Italian Sausage	1 (4.75 oz)	390	22	910	29	—
Ovenstuffs French Roll Pepperoni	1 (4.75 oz)	370	20	870	30	—
TAKE-OUT						
sausage roll	1 (2.3 oz)	311	24	—	22	1

SAUSAGE SUBSTITUTES

FOOD	PORTION	CAL	FAT	SOD	CARB	FIB
LaLoma Linketts	2 (71 g)	140	8	320	2	—
LaLoma Little Links	2 (46 g)	90	5	180	2	—
Lightlife Lean Links Breakfast	1.25 oz	69	3	250	4	—

FOOD	PORTION	CAL	FAT	SOD	CARB	FIB
Lightlife Lean Links Italian	1.5 oz	83	3	300	5	—
Morningstar Farms						
Breakfast Patties	2 (76 g)	190	12	710	7	—
Breakfast Links	2 (45 g)	90	5	300	3	—
Country Crisp Patties	1 (71 g)	220	15	620	13	—
Grillers	1 (64 g)	180	12	350	5	—
Worthington						
Leanies	1 link (40 g)	100	6	440	2	—
Prosage Links	2 (45 g)	130	9	460	3	—
Saucettes	2 links (67 g)	150	11	430	3	—
Super-Links	1 (48 g)	100	7	440	3	—
Veja-Links	2 (62 g)	140	10	330	4	—

SAVORY
ground	1 tsp	4	tr	tr	1	—

SCALLOP
FRESH
raw	3 oz	75	1	137	2	—

FROZEN
Fried (Mrs. Paul's)	2 oz	160	7	320	18	—
Lightly Breaded (King & Prince)	3.5 oz	120	tr	—	—	—

HOME RECIPE
breaded & fried	2 lg	67	3	144	3	—

TAKE-OUT
breaded & fried	6 (5 oz)	386	19	919	38	—

SCONE
HOME RECIPE
apricot scone	1	232	7	201	39	—

TAKE-OUT
cheese	1 (1.75 oz)	182	9	—	22	1
fruit	1 (1.75 oz)	158	5	—	27	2
plain	1 (1.75 oz)	181	7	—	27	1

SCROD
FROZEN
Microwave Entree Baked (Gorton's)	1 pkg	320	18	420	18	—
Ready-To-Bake (King & Prince)	5 oz	252	16	—	—	—

FOOD	PORTION	CAL	FAT	SOD	CARB	FIB
SCUP						
FRESH						
baked	3 oz	115	3	46	0	—
SEA BASS						
see BASS						
SEA TROUT						
see TROUT						
SEAWEED						
DRIED						
agar	1 oz	87	tr	29	23	—
spirulina	1 oz	83	2	309	7	—
FRESH						
agar	1 oz	tr	tr	3	2	—
irish moss	1 oz	14	tr	19	4	—
kelp	1 oz	12	tr	66	3	—
kombu	1 oz	12	tr	66	3	—
laver	1 oz	10	tr	14	1	—
nori	1 oz	10	tr	14	1	—
spirulina	1 oz	7	tr	28	1	—
tangle	1 oz	12	tr	66	3	—
wakame	1 oz	13	tr	249	3	—
SEMOLINA						
dry	½ cup	303	tr	1	61	3
SESAME						
Sesame Butter (Erewhon)	2 tbsp (32 g)	190	17	20	3	—
Sesame Tahini (Arrowhead)	1 oz	170	17	5	4	—
Sesame Tahini (Erewhon)	2 tbsp (32 g)	200	18	65	3	—
seeds	1 tsp	16	2	1	tr	—
seeds, dried	1 cup	825	72	16	34	—
seeds, dried	1 tbsp	52	5	1	2	—
seeds, roasted & toasted	1 oz	161	14	3	7	—
sesame butter	1 tbsp	95	8	2	4	1
tahini from roasted & toasted kernels	1 tbsp	89	8	17	3	—
tahini from stone ground kernels	1 tbsp	86	7	11	4	—

FOOD	PORTION	CAL	FAT	SOD	CARB	FIB
tahini from unroasted kernels	1 tbsp	85	8	0	3	—

SESBANIA
flower	1	1	0	0	tr	—
flowers	1 cup	5	tr	3	1	—
flowers, cooked	1 cup	23	tr	11	5	—

SHAD
american, baked	3 oz	214	15	56	0	—
roe, raw	3.5 oz	130	2	—	2	—
FRESH						
roe, baked w/ butter & lemon	3.5 oz	126	3	73	2	—

SHALLOTS
dried	1 tbsp	3	0	1	1	—
raw chopped	1 tbsp	7	tr	1	2	—

SHARK
FRESH						
batter-dipped & fried	3 oz	194	12	103	5	—
raw	3 oz	111	4	67	0	—

SHEEPSHEAD FISH
cooked	1 fillet (6.5 oz)	234	3	136	0	—
cooked	3 oz	107	1	62	0	—
raw	3 oz	92	2	61	0	—

SHELLFISH
see INDIVIDUAL NAMES, SHELLFISH SUBSTITUTES

SHELLFISH SUBSTITUTES
Kibun Sea Pasta w/ Shrimp w/ dressing	½ pkg	210	9	—	—	—
Kibun Sea Pasta w/ Shrimp w/o dressing	½ pkg	140	1	—	—	—
Kibun Sea Pasta w/ dressing	½ pkg	220	7	—	—	—
Kibun Sea Pasta w/o dressing	½ pkg	110	1	—	—	—
Kibun Sea Stix Salad Style	4 oz	110	tr	—	—	—
Kibun Sea Stix Whole Leg	4 oz	110	tr	—	—	—
Kibun Sea Tails	4 oz	110	tr	—	—	—

FOOD	PORTION	CAL	FAT	SOD	CARB	FIB
Louis Kemp Crab Delights Chunk Style	2 oz	54	tr	320	5	—
Louis Kemp Lobster Delights	2 oz	60	tr	470	6	—
Louis Kemp Maryland Style Cakes	2.5 oz	154	9	780	10	—
crab imitation	3 oz	87	1	715	1	—
scallop imitation	3 oz	84	tr	676	9	—
shrimp imitation	3 oz	86	1	599	8	—
surimi	1 oz	28	tr	40	2	—
surimi	3 oz	84	1	122	6	—

SHELLIE BEANS
CANNED

FOOD	PORTION	CAL	FAT	SOD	CARB	FIB
shellie beans	½ cup	37	tr	408	8	—

SHERBET
see also ICES AND ICE POPS

FOOD	PORTION	CAL	FAT	SOD	CARB	FIB
All Flavors (Bresler's)	3.5 oz	140	2	—	30	—
Borden (Orange)	½ cup	110	1	40	25	—
Land O'Lakes Fruit	4 oz	130	2	—	—	—
Lime (Sealtest)	½ cup (3 oz)	130	1	30	28	0
Orange (Sealtest)	½ cup (3 oz)	130	1	30	28	0
Rainbow Orange, Red Raspberry, Lime (Sealtest)	½ cup (3 oz)	130	1	25	28	0
Red Raspberry (Sealtest)	½ cup (3 oz)	130	1	25	28	0
orange	1 cup	270	4	88	59	—
orange	½ gal	2158	31	706	469	—
orange, home recipe	½ cup	120	2	30	24	—

SHRIMP
CANNED

FOOD	PORTION	CAL	FAT	SOD	CARB	FIB
Canned Shrimp (Robinson)	2 oz	58	1	—	—	—
Deveined Medium Whole Shrimp (S&W)	2 oz	65	0	—	1	—
canned	1 cup	154	3	216	1	—
canned	3 oz	102	2	143	1	—
FRESH						
cooked	3 oz	84	1	190	0	—
cooked	4 large	22	tr	49	0	—
raw	3 oz	90	1	126	1	—
raw	4 large	30	tr	42	tr	—

FOOD	PORTION	CAL	FAT	SOD	CARB	FIB
FROZEN						
Butterfly Shrimp (Gorton's)	4 oz	160	tr	540	16	—
Cooked in the Shell (King & Prince)	4 oz	70	tr	—	—	—
Gourmet Hand Breaded Shrimp Butterfly (King & Prince)	3.5 oz	150	tr	—	—	—
Gourmet Hand Breaded Shrimp Round (King & Prince)	3.5 oz	150	tr	—	—	—
Light Seafood Entrees Shrimp And Clams With Linguini (Mrs. Paul's)	10 oz	240	5	750	36	—
Microwave Crunchy Shrimp (Gorton's)	5 oz	380	20	870	35	—
Microwave Entree Scampi (Gorton's)	1 pkg	390	30	470	21	—
Shrimp Creole (Cajun Cookin')	12 oz	390	11	1130	55	—
Shrimp Crisps (Gorton's)	4 oz	280	15	740	26	—
Shrimp Del Rey (King & Prince)	3 oz	85	6	—	—	—
Shrimp Etouffee (Cajun Cookin')	17 oz	360	9	1170	52	—
Shrimp Jambalaya (Cajun Cookin')	12 oz	450	20	800	43	—
Shrimp a la Monterey (King & Prince)	3.5 oz	190	7	—	—	—
Supreme Hand Breaded Shrimp Butterfly (King & Prince)	3.5 oz	130	tr	—	—	—
Supreme Hand Breaded Shrimp Round (King & Prince)	3.5 oz	140	tr	—	—	—
Western Style Breaded Shrimp (King & Prince)	3.5 oz	115	tr	—	—	—
READY-TO-USE						
Fried Shrimp (American Original Foods)	4 oz	253	12	—	23	—

FOOD	PORTION	CAL	FAT	SOD	CARB	FIB
TAKE-OUT						
breaded & fried	3 oz	206	10	292	10	—
breaded & fried	4 large	73	4	103	3	—
breaded & fried	6 to 8 (6 oz)	454	25	1447	40	—
jambalaya	¾ cup	188	5	83	26	8
SMELT						
rainbow, cooked	3 oz	106	3	65	0	—
rainbow, raw	3 oz	83	2	51	0	—
SNACKS						
see also CHIPS, FRUIT SNACKS, NUTS MIXED, POPCORN, PRETZELS						
Apple Chips (Weight Watchers)	¾ oz	70	0	110	19	—
Bakem-ets	21 pieces (1 oz)	160	10	850	2	—
Bakem-ets Hot 'N Spicy	21 pieces (1 oz)	150	9	750	1	—
Bugles	1 oz	150	8	290	18	—
Bugles Nacho Cheese	1 oz	160	9	250	17	—
Bugles Ranch	1 oz	150	9	290	16	—
Carrot Lites (Health Valley)	0.5 oz	75	4	5	9	tr
Cheese Balls (Lance)	1 pkg (32 g)	190	13	420	16	—
Cheese Curls (Weight Watchers)	½ oz	70	2	45	10	—
Cheetos (Cheddar Valley)	26 pieces (1 oz)	160	9	240	16	1
Cheetos						
Crunchy	26 pieces (1 oz)	150	9	310	17	1
Curls	15 pieces (1 oz)	150	9	270	17	1
Flamin' Hot	26 pieces (1 oz)	150	9	240	16	1
Light	38 pieces (1 oz)	140	6	280	19	1
Paws	16 pieces (1 oz)	160	10	310	15	1
Puffed Ball	38 pieces (1 oz)	160	10	360	16	1
Puffs	33 pieces (1 oz)	160	9	330	16	1
Cheez Doodles Crunchy	1 oz	160	10	230	16	—
Cheez Doodles Puffed	1 oz	150	9	360	16	—
Cheez Waffies	1 oz	140	8	420	14	—
Chex Snack Mix Barbeque (Ralston)	½ cup (1.1 oz)	130	5	330	20	1
Chex Snack Mix Cool Sour Cream And Onion (Ralston)	½ cup (1 oz)	130	4	310	21	2
Chex Snack Mix Golden Cheddar (Ralston)	½ cup (1 oz)	130	4	310	20	1

FOOD	PORTION	CAL	FAT	SOD	CARB	FIB
Chex Snack Mix Traditional (Ralston)	⅔ cup (1.2 oz)	150	5	410	23	2
Combos						
Cheddar	1 pkg (1.7 oz)	250	13	520	28	1
Cheddar Cheese Cracker	1 oz	140	8	300	16	0
Cheddar Cheese Pretzel	1 oz	130	5	310	18	0
Cheddar Cheese Pretzel	1 pkg (1.8 oz)	240	9	560	33	1
Chili Cheese w/ Corn Shell	1 oz	140	6	420	17	1
Chili Cheese w/ Corn Shell	1 pkg (1.7 oz)	230	11	710	29	2
Mustard Pretzel	1 oz	130	5	300	18	1
Mustard Pretzel	1 pkg (1.8 oz)	230	8	500	35	1
Nacho	1 pkg (1.8 oz)	230	8	580	34	1
Nacho Cheese Pretzel	1 oz	130	5	320	19	1
Nacho Cheese w/ Tortilla Shell	1 oz	140	6	380	17	1
Nacho Cheese w/ Tortilla Shell	1 pkg (1.7 oz)	230	11	640	30	1
Pepperoni And Cheese Pizza	1 oz	140	7	280	17	0
Pepperoni And Cheese Pizza	1 pkg (1.7 oz)	240	11	480	30	1
Pizzeria Pretzel	1 oz	130	5	290	19	1
Pizzeria Pretzel	1 pkg (1.8 oz)	230	8	520	35	1
Tortilla Ranch	1 bag (1.7 oz)	240	12	610	29	1
Tortilla Ranch	1 oz	140	7	350	17	1
Cornnuts						
Barbecue	1 oz	120	4	270	22	2
Nacho Cheese	1 oz	120	4	180	22	2
Original	1 oz	120	4	170	22	2
Picante	1 oz	120	4	260	22	2
Ranch	1 oz	120	4	190	20	2
Crunchy Cheese Twists (Lance)	1 pkg (42 g)	260	16	290	25	—
Doo Dads	1 oz	130	6	360	17	—
Eagle Cheese Crunch	1 oz	160	10	310	16	—
Easy Cheddar Nacho	1 oz	80	6	340	2	—
Easy Cheese American	1 oz	80	6	340	2	—
Easy Cheese Cheddar	1 oz	80	6	360	2	—

FOOD	PORTION	CAL	FAT	SOD	CARB	FIB
Easy Cheese Cheese 'n Bacon	1 oz	80	6	340	2	—
Easy Cheese Sharp Cheddar	1 oz	80	6	360	2	—
Frito-Lay Corn Nuggets Toasted	1.38 oz	170	5	265	29	—
Funyums Onion Rings	11 pieces (1 oz)	140	7	265	18	1
Gold-N-Chees (Lance)	1 pkg (39 g)	180	9	410	23	—
Hain Carrot Chips	1 oz	150	9	160	16	0
Hain Carrot Chips Barbecue	1 oz	140	8	160	16	0
Hain Carrot Chips No Salt Added	1 oz	150	7	30	16	0
Health Valley Cheddar Lites	0.75 oz	40	2	35	4	tr
Health Valley Cheddar Lites With Green Onion	0.75 oz	40	2	35	4	tr
Munchos	16 pieces (1 oz)	160	10	230	15	—
Pork Skins (Lance)	1 pkg (14 g)	80	5	270	0	—
Pork Skins BBQ (Lance)	1 pkg (14 g)	80	5	400	0	—
Ritz Snack Mix Cheese (Nabisco)	1 oz	130	6	350	18	—
Ritz Snack Mix Traditional Nabisco)	1 oz	130	6	300	18	—
Snyder's Cheddar Cheese Twists	1 oz	150	8	200	17	—
Snyder's Kruncheez	1 oz	160	10	170	15	—
Snyder's Onion Toasters	1 oz	150	8	280	17	3
Snyder's Snack Mix	1 oz	170	8	410	11	tr
Snyder's Sopaipillas Apple & Cinnamon	1 oz	150	8	15	18	1
Ultra Slim-Fast Lite N' Tasty Cheese Curls	1 oz	110	3	360	20	3
Wheat Snax (Estee)	1 oz	100	tr	15	22	—

SNAIL
FRESH

cooked	3 oz	233	1	350	13	—
raw	3 oz	117	tr	175	7	—

SNAP BEANS
CANNED

green	½ cup	13	tr	170	3	1
green, low sodium	½ cup	13	tr	1	3	1

FOOD	PORTION	CAL	FAT	SOD	CARB	FIB
italian	½ cup	13	tr	170	3	1
italian, low sodium	½ cup	13	tr	1	3	1
yellow	½ cup	13	tr	170	3	1
yellow, low sodium	½ cup	13	tr	1	3	1
FRESH						
green, cooked	½ cup	22	tr	2	5	—
green, raw	½ cup	17	tr	3	4	1
yellow, raw	½ cup	17	tr	3	4	—
yellow, cooked	½ cup	22	tr	2	5	—
FROZEN						
green, cooked	½ cup	18	tr	9	4	—
italian, cooked	½ cup	18	tr	9	4	—
yellow, cooked	½ cup	18	tr	9	4	—

SNAPPER
FRESH

FOOD	PORTION	CAL	FAT	SOD	CARB	FIB
cooked	1 fillet (6 oz)	217	3	96	0	—
cooked	3 oz	109	1	48	0	—
raw	3 oz	85	1	54	0	—

SODA
see also DRINK MIXERS, MINERAL WATER/BOTTLED WATER

FOOD	PORTION	CAL	FAT	SOD	CARB	FIB
7Up	1 oz	12	0	—	—	—
Cherry	1 oz	13	0	—	—	—
Cherry Diet	1 oz	tr	0	—	—	—
Diet	1 oz	tr	0	—	—	—
Gold	1 oz	13	0	—	—	—
Gold Diet	1 oz	tr	0	—	—	—
Caffeine Free Diet Pepsi	8 fl oz	1	0	tr	tr	—
Caffeine Free Pepsi	8 fl oz	105	0	0	27	—
Coca-Cola Cherry	8 fl oz	104	0	4	28	—
Coca-Cola Classic	8 fl oz	97	0	9	27	—
Coca-Cola Classic Caffeine-Free	8 fl oz	97	0	9	27	—
Coca-Cola Diet Cherry	8 fl oz	1	0	4	tr	—
Coke II Coca-Cola	8 fl oz	105	0	4	29	—
Crush						
Apple	6 oz	90	0	—	—	—
Apple Diet	6 oz	10	0	—	—	—
Cherry	6 oz	100	0	—	—	—
Grape	6 oz	100	0	—	—	—
Orange	6 oz	100	0	—	—	—
Orange Diet	6 oz	12	0	—	—	—
Pineapple	6 oz	100	0	—	—	—
Strawberry	6 oz	90	0	—	—	—

FOOD	PORTION	CAL	FAT	SOD	CARB	FIB
Diet Coke Coca-Cola	8 fl oz	1	0	4	tr	—
Diet Coke Caffeine-Free	6 oz	tr	0	—	—	—
Diet Coke Caffeine-free	8 fl oz	1	0	4	tr	—
Diet Cranberry Apple Salt/Sodium Free (Royal Crown)	8 fl oz	2	0	1	tr	—
Diet Cranberry Salt/ Sodium Free (Royal Crown)	8 fl oz	2	0	1	tr	—
Diet Mountain Dew	8 fl oz	2	0	0	tr	—
Diet Mug Cream	8 fl oz	2	0	29	0	—
Diet Mug Root Beer	8 fl oz	1	0	26	tr	—
Diet Pepsi Pepsi-Cola	8 fl oz	1	0	tr	tr	—
Diet Rite						
Black Cherry Salt/ Sodium Free	8 fl oz	2	0	0	1	—
Cola Caffeine/Sugar Free	8 fl oz	1	0	7	tr	—
Cola Salt/Sodium Free	8 fl oz	1	0	tr	tr	—
Fruit Punch Salt/ Sodium Free	8 fl oz	2	0	0	tr	—
Golden Peach Salt/ Sodium Free	8 fl oz	2	0	0	tr	—
Key Lime Salt/ Sodium Free	8 fl oz	7	0	0	2	—
Pink Grapefruit Salt/ Sodium Free	8 fl oz	2	0	0	1	—
Red Raspberry Salt/ Sodium Free	8 fl oz	3	0	tr	1	—
Tangerine Salt/ Sodium Free	8 fl oz	2	0	0	tr	—
White Grape Salt/ Sodium Free	8 fl oz	1	0	0	tr	—
Diet Royal Crown	8 fl oz	1	0	tr	tr	—
Diet Royal Crown Caffeine Free	8 fl oz	1	0	tr	tr	—
Diet Tropical Chill Soda	8 fl oz	1	0	0	tr	—
Diet Upper 10	8 fl oz	3	0	0	1	—
Diet Upper 10 Salt/ Sodium Free	8 fl oz	3	0	0	1	—
Dr Pepper	1 oz	13	0	—	—	—
Dr Pepper Diet	1 oz	tr	0	—	—	—
Dr. Nehi	8 fl oz	100	0	35	26	—
Fanta Ginger Ale	8 fl oz	86	0	4	23	—

FOOD	PORTION	CAL	FAT	SOD	CARB	FIB
Fanta Grape	8 fl oz	117	0	9	31	—
Fanta Orange	8 fl oz	118	0	9	32	—
Fanta Root Beer	8 fl oz	111	0	4	29	—
Fresca	8 fl oz	3	0	1	tr	—
Health Valley Ginger Ale	12 oz	153	1	30	35	0
Health Valley Rootbeer Old Fashioned	12 oz	120	1	12	26	—
Health Valley Sarsaparilla Rootbeer	12 oz	153	1	27	35	—
Health Valley Wild Berry	12 oz	142	1	27	33	—
Hires Root Beer	6 oz	90	0	—	—	—
Hires Root Beer Sugar-Free	6 oz	2	0	—	—	—
Jolt	12 oz	167	0	—	—	—
Kick Royal Crown	8 fl oz	120	0	35	32	—
Like Cola	1 oz	13	0	—	—	—
Like Cola Sugar Free	1 oz	tr	0	—	—	—
Lucozade	7 oz	136	0	—	36	0
Manischewitz Seltzer No Salt Added No Calories	8 fl oz	0	0	9	0	—
Mellow Yellow	8 fl oz	119	0	9	32	—
Mellow Yellow Diet	8 fl oz	4	0	tr	tr	—
Minute Maid	8 fl oz	110	0	11	29	—
Berry	8 fl oz	111	0	9	30	—
Diet Orange	8 fl oz	2	0	0	0	—
Fruit Punch	8 fl oz	117	0	10	32	—
Grape	8 fl oz	121	0	9	32	—
Grapefruit	8 fl oz	108	0	9	29	—
Orange	8 fl oz	118	0	0	32	—
Pineapple	8 fl oz	109	0	9	30	—
Raspberry	8 fl oz	111	0	9	30	—
Strawberry	8 fl oz	122	0	9	33	—
Mountain Dew	8 fl oz	118	0	21	30	—
Mr. PiBB	6 oz	97	0	7	26	—
Mr. PiBB Diet	8 fl oz	1	0	2	tr	—
Mug Cream	8 fl oz	122	0	21	32	—
Mug Root Beer	8 fl oz	141	0	26	29	—
Nehi						
Cream	8 fl oz	120	0	0	32	—
Fruit Punch	8 fl oz	120	0	35	34	—
Ginger Ale	8 fl oz	90	0	35	24	—
Grape	8 fl oz	120	0	35	32	—
Orange	8 fl oz	130	0	35	35	—
Peach	8 fl oz	130	0	35	34	—

FOOD	PORTION	CAL	FAT	SOD	CARB	FIB
Nehi *(cont.)*						
Pineapple	8 fl oz	130	0	0	36	—
Quinine Water	8 fl oz	90	0	35	23	—
Root Beer	8 fl oz	120	0	35	32	—
Strawberry	8 fl oz	120	0	35	32	—
Wild Red	8 fl oz	120	0	33	32	—
Orangina	6 fl oz	80	0	0	19	—
Pepper Free	1 oz	12	0	—	—	—
Pepper Free Diet	1 oz	tr	0	—	—	—
Pepsi-Cola	8 fl oz	105	0	0	27	—
Raging Razzberry Cola	8 fl oz	117	0	0	31	—
Ramblin' Root Beer	8 fl oz	120	0	4	33	—
Royal Crown Caffeine Free Cola	8 fl oz	110	0	35	29	—
Royal Crown Cherry	8 fl oz	110	0	35	29	—
Royal Crown Cola	8 fl oz	100	0	35	28	—
Royal Mistic 'N Juice						
Black Cherry	12 fl oz	146	0	26	36	—
Peach Vanilla	12 fl oz	146	0	18	36	—
Tangerine Orange	12 fl oz	146	0	30	36	—
Tropical Supreme	12 fl oz	152	0	14	38	—
Wild Berry	12 fl oz	156	0	30	38	—
Royal Mistic						
Caribbean Fruit Punch	16 fl oz	230	0	5	57	—
Grape Strawberry	16 fl oz	230	0	5	57	—
Sparkling Diet With Lime Kiwi	11.1 fl oz	0	0	<90	0	—
Sparkling Diet With Raspberry Boysenberry	11.1 fl oz	0	0	<90	0	—
Sparkling Diet With Royal Peach	11.1 fl oz	0	0	<90	0	—
Sparkling Diet With Wild Cherry	11.1 fl oz	0	0	<90	0	—
Sparkling With Lime Kiwi	11.1 fl oz	112	0	38	28	—
Sparkling With Mandarin Orange Pineapple	11.1 fl oz	120	0	18	30	—
Sparkling With Mango Passion	11.1 fl oz	112	0	34	28	—
Sparkling With Raspberry Boysenberry	11.1 fl oz	112	0	24	28	—

FOOD	PORTION	CAL	FAT	SOD	CARB	FIB
Sparkling With Royal Peach	11.1 fl oz	112	0	30	28	—
Sparkling With Wild Cherry	11.1 fl oz	112	0	28	28	—
Schweppes						
Bitter Lemon	6 oz	78	0	—	—	—
Grapefruit	6 oz	77	0	—	—	—
Seltzer	6 oz	0	0	—	—	—
Seltzer Flavored	6 oz	0	0	—	—	—
Sparkling Orange	6 oz	86	0	—	—	—
Tonic Water	6 oz	64	0	—	—	—
Tonic Water Diet	6 oz	tr	0	—	—	—
Schweppes Club	6 oz	0	0	—	—	—
Schweppes Ginger Ale	6 oz	63	0	—	—	—
Schweppes Ginger Ale Diet	6 oz	tr	0	—	—	—
Schweppes Ginger Beer	6 oz	68	0	—	—	—
Schweppes Grape	6 oz	92	0	—	—	—
Schweppes Lemon Lime	6 oz	71	0	—	—	—
Schweppes Root Beer	6 oz	75	0	—	—	—
Shasta						
Birch Beer Diet	12 oz	4	0	—	—	—
Black Cherry	12 oz	162	0	—	—	—
Cherry Cola	12 oz	140	0	—	—	—
Citrus Mist	12 oz	170	0	—	—	—
Club	12 oz	0	0	—	—	—
Cola	12 oz	147	0	—	—	—
Cola	8 oz	98	0	—	—	—
Cola Diet	8 oz	0	0	—	—	—
Collins	12 oz	118	0	—	—	—
Creme	12 oz	154	0	—	—	—
Dr. Diablo	12 oz	140	0	—	—	—
Free Cola	12 oz	151	0	—	—	—
Fruit Punch	12 oz	173	0	—	—	—
Ginger Ale	12 oz	120	0	—	—	—
Ginger Ale	8 oz	80	0	—	—	—
Ginger Ale Diet	8 oz	0	0	—	—	—
Grape	12 oz	177	0	—	—	—
Lemon Lime	12 oz	146	0	—	—	—
Lemon Lime	8 oz	97	0	—	—	—
Lemon Lime Diet	8 oz	0	0	—	—	—
Orange	12 oz	177	0	—	—	—
Red Berry	12 oz	158	0	—	—	—
Red Pop	12 oz	158	0	—	—	—

FOOD	PORTION	CAL	FAT	SOD	CARB	FIB
Shasta *(cont.)*						
Root Beer	12 oz	154	0	—	—	—
Strawberry	12 oz	147	0	—	—	—
Tonic Water	12 oz	0	0	—	—	—
Slice						
Diet Lemon Lime	8 fl oz	5	0	1	tr	—
Diet Mandarin	8 fl oz	5	0	10	tr	—
Lemon Lime	8 fl oz	100	0	10	26	—
Mandarin Orange	8 fl oz	128	0	10	33	—
Red	8 fl oz	128	0	10	33	—
Sprite	8 fl oz	100	0	31	26	—
Sprite Diet (Sprite)	8 fl oz	3	0	0	0	—
Strawberry Burst Cola (Pepsi-Cola)	8 fl oz	117	0	0	31	—
Sun-Drop	6 oz	90	0	—	—	—
Sun-Drop Diet	6 oz	4	0	—	—	—
TAB	8 fl oz	1	0	4	tr	—
Tropical Chill Cola (Pepsi-Cola)	8 fl oz	117	0	0	31	—
Upper 10 (Royal Crown)	8 fl oz	100	0	35	28	—
Upper 10 Salt Free (Royal Crown)	8 fl oz	100	0	0	29	—
Welch's Sparkling Apple	12 oz	180	0	—	—	—
Welch's Sparkling Grape	12 oz	180	0	—	—	—
Welch's Sparkling Orange	12 oz	180	0	—	—	—
Welch's Sparkling Strawberry	12 oz	180	0	—	—	—
Yoo-Hoo	9 fl oz	150	tr	200	31	tr
club	12 oz	0	0	75	0	—
cola	12 oz	151	tr	14	39	—
cream	12 oz	191	0	43	49	—
diet cola	12 oz	2	0	21	tr	—
diet cola w/ NutraSweet	12 oz	2	0	21	tr	—
diet cola w/ saccharin	12 oz	2	0	57	tr	—
ginger ale	12 oz can	124	0	25	32	—
grape	12 oz	161	0	57	42	—
lemon lime	12 oz	149	0	41	38	—
orange	12 oz	177	0	49	46	—
pepper type	12 oz	151	tr	38	38	—
quinine	12 oz	125	0	15	32	—
root beer	12 oz	152	0	49	39	—
tonic water	12 oz	125	0	15	32	—

FOOD	PORTION	CAL	FAT	SOD	CARB	FIB
SOLDIER BEANS						
DRIED						
Bean Cuisine	½ cup	115	1	5	—	5
SOLE						
FRESH						
lemon, raw	3.5 oz	85	1	80	0	—
raw	3.5 oz	90	1	100	0	—
FROZEN						
A La Monterey (King & Prince)	6 oz	221	13	—	—	—
Fishmarket Fresh (Gorton's)	5 oz	110	1	140	1	—
Light Fillets (Mrs. Paul's)	1 fillet	240	10	450	20	—
Light Fillets (Van De Kamp's)	1 piece	250	12	480	18	—
Microwave Entree In Lemon Butter (Gorton's)	1 pkg	380	24	560	17	—
Microwave Entree In Wine Sauce (Gorton's)	1 pkg	180	8	770	3	—
Natural Fillets (Van De Kamp's)	4 oz	100	2	105	0	—
SORBET						
see ICES AND ICE POPS						
SORGHUM						
sorghum	½ cup	325	3	—	72	—
SOUFFLE						
HOME RECIPE						
cheese	3.5 oz	253	20	—	10	tr
grand marnier	1 cup	109	4	58	14	—
lemon, chilled	1 cup	176	tr	108	34	—
raspberry, chilled	1 cup	173	tr	108	34	—
spinach	1 cup	218	18	763	3	—
SOUP						
CANNED						
Asparagus Cream Of, as prep (Campbell)	8 oz	80	4	820	10	—
Bean And Ham (Healthy Choice)	½ can (7.5 oz)	220	4	480	35	—

FOOD	PORTION	CAL	FAT	SOD	CARB	FIB
Bean And Ham Home Cookin' (Campbell)	10.75 oz	210	4	1000	29	—
Bean Homestyle, as prep (Campbell)	8 oz	130	1	700	25	—
Bean With Bacon, as prep (Campbell)	8 oz	140	4	840	21	—
Bean w/ Bacon Healthy Request, as prep (Campbell)	8 oz	140	4	470	22	—
Beef (Progresso)	1 can (10.5 fl oz)	180	6	840	17	—
Beef, as prep (Campbell)	8 oz	80	2	830	10	—
Beef Barley (Progresso)	1 can (10.5 fl oz)	150	5	870	16	—
Beef Broth (College Inn)	½ can (7 oz)	16	0	960	1	—
Beef Broth (Health Valley)	7.5 oz	10	tr	420	2	0
Beef Broth (Pritikin)	6.9 oz	20	tr	—	—	—
Beef Broth (Swanson)	7.25 oz	18	1	750	1	—
Beef Broth No Salt Added (Health Valley)	7.5 oz	10	tr	5	2	0
Beef Broth, as prep (Campbell)	8 oz	16	0	820	1	—
Beef Chunky Ready-To-Serve (Campbell)	10.75 oz	200	5	1100	24	—
Beef Minestrone (Progresso)	1 can (10.5 fl oz)	180	6	1000	18	—
Beef Noodle (Progresso)	9.5 fl oz	170	4	1030	18	—
Beef Noodle, as prep (Campbell)	8 oz	70	3	830	7	—
Beef Noodle Homestyle, as prep (Campbell)	8 oz	80	4	810	7	—
Beef Stroganoff Chunky Ready-To-Serve (Campbell)	10.75 oz	320	16	1230	28	—
Beef Vegetable (Progresso)	1 can (10.5 fl oz)	170	3	880	18	—
Beef With Vegetables And Pasta Home Cookin' (Campbell)	10.75 oz	140	2	1060	18	—
Beefy Mushroom, as prep (Campbell)	8 oz	60	3	960	5	—
Black Bean (Goya)	7.5 oz	160	4	720	29	9

FOOD	PORTION	CAL	FAT	SOD	CARB	FIB
Black Bean (Health Valley)	7.5 oz	150	2	280	24	16
Black Bean No Salt Added (Health Valley)	7.5 oz	150	2	20	24	16
Borscht (Gold's)	8 oz	100	0	1280	21	—
Borscht Lo-Cal (Gold's)	8 oz	20	tr	1160	5	—
Borscht Low Calorie (Manischewitz)	8 fl oz	20	0	725	4	—
Borscht With Beets (Manischewitz)	8 fl oz	80	0	660	20	—
Broccoli Cream Of, as prep (Campbell)	8 oz	80	5	790	8	—
Broccoli Cream Of, as prep w/ 2% milk (Campbell)	8 oz	140	7	850	14	—
Celery Cream Of, as prep (Campbell)	8 oz	100	7	820	8	—
Cheddar Cheese, as prep (Campbell)	8 oz	110	6	810	10	—
Chickarina (Progresso)	9.5 fl oz	130	5	820	13	—
Chicken Alphabet, as prep (Campbell)	8 oz	80	3	800	10	—
Chicken & Stars, as prep (Campbell)	8 oz	60	2	870	7	—
Chicken 'n Dumplings, as prep (Campbell)	8 oz	80	3	960	9	—
Chicken Barley (Progresso)	9.25 fl oz	100	2	710	12	4
Chicken Barley, as prep (Campbell)	8 oz	70	2	850	10	—
Chicken Broth (College Inn)	½ can (7 oz)	35	3	990	0	0
Chicken Broth (Hain)	8.75 fl oz	70	6	870	0	—
Chicken Broth (Health Valley)	7.5 oz	35	2	410	1	0
Chicken Broth (Pritikin)	6.9 oz	14	0	—	—	—
Chicken Broth (Progresso)	4 fl oz	8	0	360	0	—
Chicken Broth (Swanson)	7.25 oz	30	2	900	2	—
Chicken Broth Healthy Request Ready-To-Serve (Campbell)	8 oz	10	0	400	1	—
Chicken Broth Low Sodium Ready-To-Serve (Campbell)	10.5 oz	30	1	85	2	—

FOOD	PORTION	CAL	FAT	SOD	CARB	FIB
Chicken Broth Lower Salt (College Inn)	½ can (7 oz)	20	2	550	0	0
Chicken Broth No Salt Added (Hain)	8.75 fl oz	60	5	75	0	—
Chicken Broth No Salt Added (Health Valley)	7.5 oz	35	2	0	1	0
Chicken Broth & Noodles, as prep (Campbell)	8 oz	45	1	860	8	—
Chicken Broth, as prep (Campbell)	8 oz	30	2	710	2	—
Chicken Corn Chowder Chunky Ready-To-Serve (Campbell)	10.75 oz	340	21	1200	23	—
Chicken Cream Of, as prep (Campbell)	8 oz	110	7	810	9	—
Chicken Cream Of (Progresso)	9.5 fl oz	190	11	970	12	—
Chicken Gumbo (Pritikin)	7.4 oz	60	1	—	—	—
Chicken Gumbo With Sausage Home Cookin' (Campbell)	10.75 oz	140	4	1090	15	—
Chicken Gumbo, as prep (Campbell)	8 oz	60	2	900	8	—
Chicken Minestrone (Progresso)	1 can (10.5 fl oz)	140	4	1060	14	—
Chicken Minestrone Home Cookin' (Campbell)	10.75 oz	180	6	950	17	—
Chicken Mushroom Creamy, as prep (Campbell)	8 oz	120	8	920	8	—
Chicken Noodle (Hain)	9.5 fl oz	120	4	980	11	—
Chicken Noodle (Progresso)	1 can (10.5 fl oz)	120	4	970	8	—
Chicken Noodle (Weight Watchers)	10.5 oz	80	2	1230	9	—
Chicken Noodle Chunky Ready-To-Serve (Campbell)	10.75 oz	200	7	1140	20	—
Chicken Noodle Healthy Request, as prep (Campbell)	8 oz	60	2	460	8	—

FOOD	PORTION	CAL	FAT	SOD	CARB	FIB
Chicken Noodle Homestyle, as prep (Campbell)	8 oz	70	3	880	8	—
Chicken Noodle No Salt Added (Hain)	9.5 fl oz	120	4	90	12	—
Chicken Noodle, as prep (Campbell)	8 oz	60	2	900	8	—
Chicken Noodle-O's, as prep (Campbell)	8 oz	70	2	820	9	—
Chicken Nuggets w/ Vegetables & Noodles Chunky (Campbell)	10.75 oz	190	6	1060	24	—
Chicken Rice (Progresso)	1 can (10.5 fl oz)	120	4	990	12	—
Chicken Rice Home Cooking' (Campbell)	10.75 oz	150	6	1090	10	—
Chicken Vegetable (Pritikin)	7.25 oz	70	tr	—	—	—
Chicken Vegetable (Progresso)	1 can (10.5 fl oz)	150	4	790	18	—
Chicken Vegetable Beef Low Sodium Ready-To-Serve (Campbell)	10.75 oz	180	5	90	19	—
Chicken Vegetable Chunky Ready-To-Serve (Campbell)	9.5 oz	170	6	1080	19	—
Chicken Vegetable, as prep (Campbell)	8 oz	70	3	850	8	—
Chicken With Noodles Home Cookin' (Campbell)	10.75 oz	140	4	1150	12	—
Chicken With Noodles Low Sodium Ready-To-Serve (Campbell)	10.75 oz	170	5	90	17	—
Chicken w/ Ribbon Pasta (Pritikin)	7.27 oz	60	tr	—	—	—
Chicken w/ Rice (Healthy Choice)	½ can (7.5 oz)	140	4	510	18	—
Chicken With Rice Chunky Ready-To-Serve (Campbell)	9.5 oz	140	4	1060	16	—
Chicken With Rice Healthy Request, as prep (Campbell)	8 oz	60	3	480	7	—

FOOD	PORTION	CAL	FAT	SOD	CARB	FIB
Chicken With Rice, as prep (Campbell)	8 oz	60	3	790	7	—
Chili Beef Chunky Ready-To-Serve (Campbell)	11 oz	290	7	1120	37	—
Chili Beef, as prep (Campbell)	8 oz	140	5	840	20	—
Chunky Beef Vegetable (Healthy Choice)	½ can (7.5 oz)	110	1	490	14	—
Chunky Chicken Noodle And Vegetable (Healthy Choice)	½ can (7.5 oz)	160	4	500	18	—
Chunky Chicken Vegetable (Health Valley)	7.5 oz	125	2	290	20	4
Chunky Five Bean Vegetable (Health Valley)	7.5 oz	110	2	290	21	11
Chunky Five Bean Vegetable No Salt Added (Health Valley)	7.5 oz	110	2	60	21	11
Chunky Vegetable Chicken No Salt Added (Health Valley)	7.5 oz	125	2	60	20	4
Clam Chowder Manhattan Style Chunky Ready-To-Serve (Campbell)	10.75 oz	160	4	1110	24	—
Clam Chowder Manhattan Style, as prep (Campbell)	8 oz	70	2	820	10	—
Clam Chowder New England Chunky Ready-To-Serve (Campbell)	10.75 oz	290	17	1200	26	—
Clam Chowder New England, as prep (Campbell)	8 oz	80	3	870	12	—
Clam Chowder New England, as prep w/ whole milk (Campbell)	8 oz	150	7	930	17	—

FOOD	PORTION	CAL	FAT	SOD	CARB	FIB
Consomme, as prep (Campbell)	8 oz	25	0	750	2	—
Corn Chowder (Progresso)	9.25 fl oz	200	10	840	22	—
Country Vegetable (Healthy Choice)	½ can (7.5 oz)	120	1	540	23	—
Country Vegetable Home Cookin' (Campbell)	10.75 oz	120	2	1070	20	—
Cream of Mushroom Healthy Request, as prep (Campbell)	8 oz	60	2	460	9	—
Cream of Chicken Healthy Request (Campbell)	8 oz	70	2	490	11	—
Creamy Chicken Mushroom Chunky Ready-To-Serve (Campbell)	10.5 oz	270	19	1280	13	—
Creamy Mushroom (Hain)	9.25 fl oz	110	4	740	16	—
Creole Style Chunky Ready-To-Serve (Campbell)	10.75 oz	240	8	910	31	—
Curly Noodle With Chicken, as prep (Campbell)	8 oz	80	3	800	11	—
Escarole In Chicken Broth (Progresso)	9.25 fl oz	30	1	1100	2	—
French Onion, as prep (Campbell)	8 oz	60	2	900	9	—
Green Pea, as prep (Campbell)	8 oz	160	3	820	25	—
Green Split Pea (Health Valley)	7.5 oz	180	tr	290	34	15
Green Split Pea (Progresso)	1 can (10.5 fl oz)	201	3	920	31	—
Green Split Pea No Salt Added (Health Valley)	7.5 oz	180	tr	25	34	15
Ham & Bean (Progresso)	9.5 fl oz	140	2	950	28	8
Ham 'n Butter Bean Chunky Ready-To-Serve (Campbell)	10.75 oz	280	10	1180	34	—

FOOD	PORTION	CAL	FAT	SOD	CARB	FIB
Hearty Beef (Healthy Choice)	½ can (7.5 oz)	120	2	580	17	—
Hearty Beef (Progresso)	9.5 fl oz	160	4	820	15	—
Hearty Chicken (Healthy Choice)	½ can (7.5 oz)	150	5	530	17	—
Hearty Chicken (Progresso)	1 can (10.5 fl oz)	130	4	960	9	—
Hearty Chicken Noodle Healthy Request Ready-To-Serve (Campbell)	8 oz	80	2	470	7	—
Hearty Chicken Rice Healthy Request Ready-To-Serve (Campbell)	8 oz	110	2	400	15	—
Hearty Chicken Vegetable Healthy Request (Campbell)	8 oz	120	2	460	16	—
Hearty Lentil Home Cookin' (Campbell)	10.75 oz	170	2	930	28	—
Hearty Minestrone (Progresso)	9.25 fl oz	110	2	740	16	—
Hearty Minestrone Healthy Request Ready-To-Serve (Campbell)	8 oz	90	3	430	13	—
Hearty Vegetable Beef Healthy Request Ready-To-Serve (Campbell)	8 oz	120	3	490	15	—
Hearty Vegetable Healthy Request Ready-To-Serve (Campbell)	8 oz	110	3	480	17	—
Homestyle Chicken (Progresso)	9.5 fl oz	110	3	740	12	—
Italian Vegetable Pasta (Hain)	9.5 fl oz	160	5	910	25	—
Italian Vegetable Pasta Low Sodium (Hain)	9.5 fl oz	140	6	90	22	—
Lentil (Health Valley)	7.5 oz	220	4	290	33	10
Lentil (Pritikin)	7.4 oz	100	0	—	—	—
Lentil (Progresso)	1 can (10.5 fl oz)	140	4	1000	24	—

FOOD	PORTION	CAL	FAT	SOD	CARB	FIB
Lentil No Salt Added (Health Valley)	7.5 oz	220	4	25	4	10
Lentil With Sausage (Progresso)	9.5 fl oz	170	8	840	21	5
Macaroni & Bean (Progresso)	1 can (10.5 fl oz)	150	4	1020	27	—
Manhattan Clam Chowder (Health Valley)	7.5 oz	110	2	290	15	2
Manhattan Clam Chowder (Pritikin)	7.4 oz	70	tr	—	—	—
Manhattan Clam Chowder (Progresso)	9.5 fl oz	120	2	800	13	—
Manhattan Clam Chowder No Salt Added (Health Valley)	7.5 oz	110	2	60	15	2
Manhattan Clam Chowder, as prep w/ water (Snow's)	7.5 fl oz	70	2	630	9	—
Mediterranean Vegetable Chunky Ready-To-Serve (Campbell)	9.5 oz	170	6	1010	24	—
Minestrone (Hain)	9.5 fl oz	170	2	1060	27	—
Minestrone (Health Valley)	7.5 oz	130	3	290	19	13
Minestrone (Healthy Choice)	½ can (7.5 oz)	160	2	520	30	—
Minestrone (Pritikin)	7.4 oz	110	tr	—	—	—
Minestrone (Progresso)	1 can (10.5 fl oz)	120	3	930	25	—
Minestrone Chunky Ready-To-Serve (Campbell)	9.5 oz	160	4	870	24	—
Minestrone Home Cookin' (Campbell)	10.75 oz	140	3	1220	22	—
Minestrone No Salt Added (Hain)	9.5 fl oz	160	4	35	28	—
Minestrone No Salt Added (Health Valley)	7.5 oz	130	3	90	19	13
Minestrone, as prep (Campbell)	8 oz	80	2	900	13	—
Mushroom (Pritikin)	7.4 oz	60	tr	—	—	—
Mushroom Barley (Hain)	9.5 fl oz	100	2	600	17	—

FOOD	PORTION	CAL	FAT	SOD	CARB	FIB
Mushroom Barley (Health Valley)	7.5 oz	100	2	290	2	9
Mushroom Barley No Salt Added (Health Valley)	7.5 oz	100	2	20	16	9
Mushroom Cream Of (Progresso)	9.25 fl oz	160	10	1120	14	—
Mushroom Cream Of (Weight Watchers)	10.5 oz	90	2	1250	14	—
Mushroom Cream Of Low Sodium Ready-To-Serve (Campbell)	10.5 oz	210	14	55	18	—
Mushroom Cream Of, as prep (Campbell)	8 oz	100	7	820	8	—
Mushroom Golden, as prep (Campbell)	8 oz	70	3	870	9	—
Nacho Cheese, as prep (Campbell)	8 oz	110	8	740	8	—
Nacho Cheese, as prep w/ milk (Campbell)	8 oz	180	12	800	13	—
Natural Goodness Clear Chicken Broth (Swanson)	7.25 oz	20	1	580	1	—
Navy Bean (Pritikin)	7.4 oz	130	tr	—	—	—
New England Chowder (American Original Foods)	4 oz	64	1	—	8	—
New England Chowder, as prep w/ milk (American Original Foods)	4 oz	145	6	—	14	—
New England Clam Chowder (Hain)	9.25 fl oz	180	4	780	26	—
New England Clam Chowder (Pritikin)	7.4 oz	118	tr	—	—	—
New England Clam Chowder, as prep w/ milk (Snow's)	7.5 fl oz	140	6	670	13	—
New England Clam Chowder, as prep w/ whole milk (Gorton's)	¼ can	140	5	740	17	—
New England Corn Chowder, as prep w/ milk (Snow's)	7.5 fl oz	150	6	640	18	—
New England Fish Chowder, as prep w/ milk (Snow's)	7.5 fl oz	130	6	620	11	—

FOOD	PORTION	CAL	FAT	SOD	CARB	FIB
New England Seafood Chowder, as prep w/ milk (Snow's)	7.5 fl oz	130	6	690	11	—
New England Style Clam Chowder (Progresso)	1 can (10.5 fl oz)	220	12	1050	21	—
Noodles & Ground Beef, as prep (Campbell)	8 oz	90	4	820	10	—
Old Fashioned Bean w/ Ham Chunky Ready-To-Serve (Campbell)	11 oz	290	9	1110	38	—
Old Fashioned Chicken Chunky Ready-To-Serve (Campbell)	10.75 oz	180	5	1220	21	—
Old Fashioned Chicken Noodle (Healthy Choice)	½ can (7.5 oz)	90	3	520	9	—
Old Fashioned Vegetable Beef Chunky Ready-To-Serve (Campbell)	10.75 oz	190	6	1100	20	—
Onion Cream Of, as prep (Campbell)	8 oz	100	5	830	12	—
Onion Cream Of, as prep w/ whole milk & water (Campbell)	8 oz	140	7	860	15	—
Oyster Stew, as prep (Campbell)	8 oz	70	5	840	5	—
Oyster Stew, as prep w/ whole milk (Campbell)	8 oz	140	9	890	10	—
Pepper Pot, as prep (Campbell)	8 oz	90	4	970	9	—
Pepper Steak Chunky Ready-To-Serve (Campbell)	10.75 oz	180	3	1050	24	—
Potato Cream Of, as prep (Campbell)	8 oz	80	3	870	12	—
Potato Cream Of, as prep w/ whole milk & water (Campbell)	8 oz	120	4	900	15	—
Potato Leek (Health Valley)	7.5 oz	130	2	290	23	7
Potato Leek No Salt Added (Health Valley)	7.5 oz	130	2	20	23	7
Shav (Gold's)	8 oz	25	0	1380	4	—
Shav (Manischewitz)	1 cup	11	tr	4	—	—

FOOD	PORTION	CAL	FAT	SOD	CARB	FIB
Scotch Broth, as prep (Campbell)	8 oz	80	3	870	9	—
Seafood Soup/ Spicy (Port Clyde Foods)	7.5 oz	68	1	—	—	—
Seasoned Beef Broth (Progresso)	4 fl oz	40	tr	380	tr	—
Shrimp Cream Of, as prep (Campbell)	8 oz	90	6	810	8	—
Shrimp Cream Of, as prep w/ whole milk (Campbell)	8 oz	160	10	860	13	—
Sirloin Burger Chunky Ready-To-Serve (Campbell)	10.75 oz	220	9	1240	23	—
Split Pea (Hain)	9.5 fl oz	170	1	970	28	—
Split Pea (Pritikin)	7.5 oz	130	tr	—	—	—
Split Pea And Ham (Healthy Choice)	½ can (7.5 oz)	170	3	460	25	—
Split Pea Low Sodium Ready-To-Serve (Campbell)	10.75 oz	230	4	30	37	—
Split Pea No Salt Added (Hain)	9.5 fl oz	170	1	40	29	—
Split Pea With Bacon, as prep (Campbell)	8 oz	160	4	780	24	—
Split Pea With Ham (Progresso)	1 can (10.5 fl oz)	160	5	980	24	6
Split Pea w/ Ham Chunky Ready-To-Serve (Campbell)	10.75 oz	230	6	1080	33	—
Split Pea With Ham Home Cookin' (Campbell)	10.75 oz	230	1	1310	38	—
Steak and Potato Chunky Ready-To-Serve (Campbell)	10.75 oz	200	5	1140	24	—
Teddy Bear, as prep (Campbell)	8 oz	70	2	790	11	—
Tomato (Health Valley)	7.5 oz	130	3	290	21	1
Tomato (Progresso)	9.5 fl oz	120	3	1000	20	—
Tomato Beef With Rotini (Progresso)	9.5 fl oz	170	6	930	18	—
Tomato Bisque, as prep (Campbell)	8 oz	120	3	820	22	—

FOOD	PORTION	CAL	FAT	SOD	CARB	FIB
Tomato Garden (Healthy Choice)	½ can (7.5 oz)	130	3	510	22	—
Tomato Garden Home Cookin' (Campbell)	10.75 oz	150	3	930	29	—
Tomato Healthy Request, as prep (Campbell)	8 oz	90	2	430	17	—
Tomato Healthy Request, as prep w/ skim milk (Campbell)	8 oz	130	2	490	22	—
Tomato Homestyle Cream Of, as prep (Campbell)	8 oz	110	3	810	20	—
Tomato Homestyle Cream Of, as prep w/ whole milk (Campbell)	8 oz	180	7	860	25	—
Tomato No Salt Added (Health Valley)	7.5 oz	130	3	40	21	1
Tomato Rice Old Fashioned, as prep (Campbell)	8 oz	110	2	730	22	—
Tomato Tortellini (Progresso)	9.5 fl oz	130	5	1040	16	—
Tomato w/ Tomato Pieces (Pritikin)	7.5 oz	70	0	—	—	—
Tomato With Tomato Pieces Low Sodium Ready-To-Serve (Campbell)	10.5 oz	190	6	45	30	—
Tomato Zesty, as prep (Campbell)	8 oz	100	2	760	20	—
Tomato, as prep (Campbell)	8 oz	90	2	680	17	—
Tomato, as prep w/ 2% milk (Campbell)	8 oz	150	4	740	22	—
Tortellini (Progresso)	9.5 fl oz	90	3	930	11	—
Tortellini Creamy (Progresso)	9.25 fl oz	240	16	910	17	—
Turkey Noodle, as prep (Campbell)	8 oz	70	2	880	9	—
Turkey Rice (Hain)	9.5 fl oz	100	3	970	10	—
Turkey Rice No Salt Added (Hain)	9.5 fl oz	120	4	85	13	—

FOOD	PORTION	CAL	FAT	SOD	CARB	FIB
Turkey Vegetable Chunky Ready-To-Serve (Campbell)	9.4 oz	150	6	1060	16	—
Turkey Vegetable w/ Ribbon Pasta (Pritikin)	7.4 oz	50	tr	—	—	—
Turkey Vegetable, as prep (Campbell)	8 oz	70	3	710	8	—
Vegetable (Health Valley)	7.5 oz	110	1	300	20	8
Vegetable (Pritikin)	7.4 oz	70	0	—	—	—
Vegetable (Progresso)	1 can (10.5 fl oz)	80	2	1190	15	—
Vegetable Beef (Healthy Choice)	½ can (7.5 oz)	130	1	530	21	—
Vegetable Beef Healthy Request, as prep (Campbell)	8 oz	70	2	490	9	—
Vegetable Beef Home Cookin' (Campbell)	10.75 oz	140	3	1160	17	—
Vegetable Beef, as prep (Campbell)	8 oz	70	2	780	10	—
Vegetable Broth (Hain)	9.5 fl oz	45	0	1180	10	—
Vegetable Broth (Swanson)	7.25 fl oz	20	1	920	3	—
Vegetable Broth Low Sodium (Hain)	9.5 fl oz	40	tr	85	8	—
Vegetable Chicken (Hain)	9.5 fl oz	120	4	930	14	—
Vegetable Chicken No Salt Added (Hain)	9.5 fl oz	130	4	100	14	—
Vegetable Chunky Ready-To-Serve (Campbell)	10.75 oz	160	4	1100	28	—
Vegetable Healthy Request, as prep (Campbell)	8 oz	90	2	500	14	—
Vegetable Homestyle, as prep (Campbell)	8 oz	60	2	880	9	—
Vegetable No Salt Added (Health Valley)	7.5 oz	110	1	40	20	8
Vegetable Old Fashioned, as prep (Campbell)	8 oz	60	2	880	9	—
Vegetable Split Pea (Hain)	9.5 fl oz	170	1	970	28	—
Vegetable Split Pea No Salt Added (Hain)	9.5 fl oz	170	1	70	27	—

FOOD	PORTION	CAL	FAT	SOD	CARB	FIB
Vegetable, as prep (Campbell)	8 oz	90	2	830	14	—
Vegetarian Lentil (Hain)	9.5 fl oz	160	3	690	25	—
Vegetarian Lentil No Salt Added (Hain)	9.5 fl oz	160	3	65	24	—
Vegetarian Vegetable (Hain)	9.5 fl oz	140	4	920	22	—
Vegetarian Vegetable No Salt Added (Hain)	9.5 fl oz	150	5	45	23	—
Vegetarian Vegetable, as prep (Campbell)	8 oz	80	2	790	13	—
Won Ton, as prep (Campbell)	8 oz	40	1	850	5	—
Zesty Minestrone (Progresso)	9.5 fl oz	150	8	1130	19	—
asparagus, cream of, as prep w/ milk	1 cup	161	8	1041	16	—
asparagus, cream of, as prep w/ water	1 cup	87	4	981	11	—
beef broth ready-to-serve	1 can (14 oz)	27	1	1294	tr	—
beef broth ready-to-serve	1 cup	16	1	782	tr	—
beef noodle, as prep w/ water	1 cup	84	3	952	9	—
black bean turtle soup	1 cup	218	1	922	40	—
black bean, as prep w/ water	1 cup	116	2	1198	20	—
celery, cream of, as prep w/ water	1 cup	90	6	949	9	—
celery, cream of, as prep w/ milk	1 cup	165	10	1010	15	—
celery, cream of, not prep	1 can (10.75 oz)	219	14	2308	21	—
cheese, as prep w/ milk	1 cup	230	15	1020	16	—
cheese, as prep w/ water	1 cup	155	10	959	11	—
cheese, not prep	1 can (11 oz)	377	25	2331	26	—
chicken broth, as prep w/ water	1 cup	39	1	776	1	—
chicken, cream of, as prep w/ milk	1 cup	191	11	1046	15	—
chicken, cream of, as prep w/ water	1 cup	116	7	986	9	—

FOOD	PORTION	CAL	FAT	SOD	CARB	FIB
chicken gumbo, as prep w/ water	1 cup	56	1	955	8	—
chicken noodle, as prep w/ water	1 cup	75	2	1107	9	—
chicken rice, as prep w/ water	1 cup	251	2	814	7	—
clam chowder Manhattan, as prep w/ water	1 cup	77	2	1029	12	—
clam chowder New England, as prep w/ milk	1 cup	163	7	992	17	—
clam chowder New England, as prep w/ water	1 cup	95	3	914	12	—
consomme w/ gelatin, as prep w/ water	1 cup	29	0	637	2	—
consomme w/ gelatin, not prep	1 can (10.5 oz)	71	0	1550	4	—
escarole ready-to-serve	1 cup	27	2	3865	2	—
french onion, as prep w/ water	1 cup	57	2	1053	8	—
gazpacho ready-to-serve	1 cup	57	2	1183	1	—
minestrone, as prep w/ water	1 cup	83	3	911	11	—
mushroom, cream of, as prep w/ milk	1 cup	203	14	1076	15	—
mushroom, cream of, as prep w/ water	1 cup	129	9	1031	9	—
oyster stew, as prep w/ milk	1 cup	134	8	1040	10	—
oyster stew, as prep w/ water	1 cup	59	4	980	4	—
pepperpot, as prep w/ water	1 cup	103	5	970	9	—
potato, cream of, as prep w/ water	1 cup	73	2	1000	11	—
potato, cream of, as prep w/ milk	1 cup	148	6	1060	17	—
scotch broth, as prep w/ water	1 cup	80	3	1012	9	—
split pea w/ ham, as prep w/ water	1 cup	189	4	1008	28	—

FOOD	PORTION	CAL	FAT	SOD	CARB	FIB
tomato, as prep w/ milk	1 cup	160	6	932	22	—
tomato, as prep w/ water	1 cup	86	2	872	17	—
vegetarian vegetable, as prep w/ water	1 cup	72	2	823	12	—
vichyssoise	1 cup	148	6	1060	17	—
DRY						
13 Bean, uncooked (Hodgson Mill)	1.5 oz	100	1	0	14	12
Asparagus, as prep (Knorr)	8 oz	80	3	770	11	—
Bean Bouillabaisse (Bean Cuisine)	1 cup (7.5 fl oz)	174	tr	5	18	5
Bean & Barley (Arrowhead)	¼ cup (1.9 oz)	170	0	0	35	7
Bean With Bacon 'n Ham Microwave (Campbell)	7.5 oz	230	5	830	38	—
Beef Base (Emes)	1 tsp	18	tr	10	2	—
Beef Bouillon Instant (Wyler's)	1 tsp	6	tr	930	1	—
Beef Bouillon Instant Cube (Wyler's)	1	6	tr	930	1	—
Beef Bouillon Instant Low Sodium (Lite Line)	1 tsp	12	tr	5	2	—
Beef Bouillon, as prep (Knorr)	8 oz	15	1	1220	tr	—
Beef Broth Instant (Weight Watchers)	1 pkg	8	0	910	1	—
Beef Cup Of Soup (Goodman's)	1 pkg (1.5 cups)	180	3	1640	32	2
Beef Flavor Bouillon, as prep (Diamond Crystal)	6 oz	17	tr	—	—	—
Beef Instant Oriental Noodle (Lipton)	8 oz	177	1	912	34	—
Beef Low Fat, as prep (Ramen Noodle)	8 oz	160	1	890	32	—
Beef Mushroom (Lipton)	8 oz	38	1	763	7	—
Beef Noodle (Campbell's Cup)	1 (1.35 oz)	130	2	1270	23	—

FOOD	PORTION	CAL	FAT	SOD	CARB	FIB
Beef Noodle (Ultra Slim-Fast)	6 oz	45	tr	700	7	2
Beef With Vegetables Low Fat, as prep (Cup-A-Ramen)	8 oz	220	2	1600	44	—
Beef With Vegetables, as prep (Cup-A-Ramen)	8 oz	270	10	1530	38	—
Beef, as prep (Diamond Crystal)	6 oz	30	1	—	—	—
Beef, as prep (Ramen Noodle)	8 oz	190	8	1010	26	—
Beefy Onion (Lipton)	8 oz	27	1	635	5	—
Broth & Vegetable Seasoning (George Washington)	1 serv	12	0	—	—	—
Broth & Brown Seasoning (George Washington)	1 serv	6	0	—	—	—
Broth & Golden Seasoning (George Washington)	1 serv	6	0	—	—	—
Broth & Onion Seasoning (George Washington)	1 serv	12	0	—	—	—
Cauliflower, as prep (Knorr)	8 oz	100	3	750	13	—
Cheese & Broccoli (Hain)	¾ cup	310	22	980	19	—
Cheese Savory (Hain)	¾ cup	250	16	890	20	—
Chick 'N Pasta, as prep (Knorr)	8 oz	90	2	850	16	—
Chicken Base (Emes)	1 tsp	18	tr	10	2	—
Chicken Bouillon Instant (Wyler's)	1 tsp	8	tr	900	1	—
Chicken Bouillon Instant Cube (Wyler's)	1	8	tr	900	1	—
Chicken Bouillon Instant Low Sodium (Lite Line)	1 tsp	12	tr	5	2	—
Chicken Bouillon, as prep (Knorr)	8 oz	16	1	1200	tr	—
Chicken Broth (Cup-A-Soup)	6 oz	19	1	605	3	0
Chicken Broth Instant (Weight Watchers)	1 pkg	8	0	900	1	—

FOOD	PORTION	CAL	FAT	SOD	CARB	FIB
Chicken Instant Oriental Noodle (Lipton)	8 oz	180	2	785	33	—
Chicken Leek (Ultra Slim-Fast)	6 oz	50	tr	1070	7	2
Chicken Low Fat, as prep (Ramen Noodle)	8 oz	160	1	940	32	—
Chicken Noodle (Campbell's Cup)	1 (1.35 oz)	140	3	1340	22	—
Chicken Noodle (Lipton)	8 oz	82	2	702	12	—
Chicken Noodle (Ultra Slim-Fast)	6 oz	45	tr	970	6	2
Chicken Noodle (Weight Watchers)	7.5 oz	90	1	450	13	—
Chicken Noodle Cup Of Soup (Goodman's)	1 pkg (1½ cups)	180	3	1360	31	2
Chicken Noodle Hearty (Lipton)	8 oz	81	1	766	14	—
Chicken Noodle Microwave (Campbell)	7.5 oz	100	4	870	11	—
Chicken Noodle w/ White Meat, as prep (Campbell's Cup)	6 oz	90	2	770	12	—
Chicken Noodle, as prep (Campbell)	8 oz	100	2	710	16	—
Chicken Noodle, as prep (Knorr)	8 oz	100	2	710	18	—
Chicken Vegetable (Cup-A-Soup)	6 oz	47	1	566	8	—
Chicken With Rice Microwave (Campbell)	7.5 oz	100	4	820	14	—
Chicken With Vegetables Low Fat, as prep (Cup-A-Ramen)	8 oz	220	2	1500	44	—
Chicken With Vegetables, as prep (Cup-ARamen)	8 oz	270	10	1470	38	—
Chicken, as prep (Ramen Noodle)	8 oz	190	8	970	26	—
Chili Beef Microwave (Campbell)	7.5 oz	190	4	870	32	—
Chunky Beef Stew (Weight Watchers)	7.5 oz	120	2	450	14	—
Country Vegetable (Lipton)	8 oz	80	1	803	16	—
Country Barley, as prep (Knorr)	8 oz	120	2	940	23	—

FOOD	PORTION	CAL	FAT	SOD	CARB	FIB
Cream, as prep (Diamond Crystal)	6 oz	90	3	—	—	—
Creamy Broccoli (Ultra Slim-Fast)	6 oz	75	tr	800	14	2
Creamy Broccoli And Cheese (Cup-A-Soup)	6 oz	70	3	595	10	—
Creamy Chicken w/ White Meat, as prep (Campbell's Cup)	6 oz	90	4	1020	12	—
Creamy Tomato (Ultra Slim-Fast)	6 oz	60	tr	800	10	2
Fine Herb, as prep (Knorr)	8 oz	130	6	990	15	—
Fish Bouillon, as prep (Knorr)	8 oz	10	tr	1130	tr	—
French Onion, as prep (Knorr)	8 oz	50	1	970	9	—
Giggle Noodle (Lipton)	8 oz	72	2	708	12	—
Green Pea (Cup-A-Soup)	6 oz	113	4	553	14	tr
Hearty Chicken And Noodles (Cup-A-Soup)	6 oz	110	2	587	20	—
Hearty Creamy Chicken Lots-A-Noodles (Cup-A-Soup)	7 oz	179	8	639	21	0
Hearty Minestrone, as prep (Knorr)	10 oz	130	2	940	23	—
Hearty Noodle, as prep (Campbell)	8 oz	90	1	840	15	—
Hearty Noodles With Vegetables (Campbell's Cup)	1 (1.7 oz)	180	2	1320	32	—
Hearty Noodles With Vegetables (Lipton)	8 oz	75	2	687	12	—
Hearty Vegetable (Ultra Slim-Fast)	6 oz	50	tr	750	7	2
Island Black Bean (Bean Cuisine)	1 cup (8.6 fl oz)	202	tr	7	24	8
Leek, as prep (Knorr)	8 oz	110	4	800	14	—
Lentil Savory (Hain)	¾ cup	130	2	810	20	—
Lobster Bisque (Golden Dipt)	¼ pkg	30	1	560	5	—
Lots of Lentil (Bean Cuisine)	1 cup (7.7 oz)	166	tr	7	19	6

FOOD	PORTION	CAL	FAT	SOD	CARB	FIB
Manhattan Clam Chowder (Golden Dipt)	¼ pkg	80	2	700	13	—
Matzo Ball & Soup (Goodman's)	1 cup	40	1	1040	9	1
Matzo Ball & Soup 50% Less Salt (Goodman's)	1 serv	50	1	640	10	1
Mesa Maize (Bean Cuisine)	1 cup (9.2 fl oz)	179	tr	9	21	6
Minestrone Savory (Hain)	¾ cup	110	1	870	20	—
Minestrone, as prep (Manischewitz)	6 fl oz	50	tr	160	9	—
Mushroom Cream Of (Cup-A-Soup)	6 oz	71	3	756	9	0
Mushroom Savory (Hain)	¾ cup	210	15	710	11	—
Mushroom Savory No Salt Added (Hain)	¾ cup	250	20	180	15	—
Mushroom, as prep (Knorr)	8 oz	100	4	870	12	—
New England Clam Chowder (Golden Dipt)	¼ pkg	24	2	680	12	—
New England Clam Chowder (Weight Watchers)	7.5 oz	90	0	450	16	—
Noodle (4C)	8 oz	50	2	960	7	—
Noodle With Chicken Broth, as prep (Campbell's Cup)	6 oz	90	2	910	15	—
Noodle, as prep (Campbell)	8 oz	110	2	700	19	—
Noodleman (Goodman's)	1 cup	45	1	990	9	0
Noodleman Low Sodium (Goodman's)	1 cup	50	1	95	9	1
Onion (Cup-A-Soup)	6 oz	27	1	665	5	tr
Onion (Goodman's)	1 cup	30	1	1280	5	1
Onion (Lipton)	8 oz	20	tr	632	4	—
Onion (Ultra Slim-Fast)	6 oz	45	tr	930	7	2
Onion Bouillon Instant (Wylers)	1 tsp	10	tr	910	1	—
Onion Golden (Lipton)	8 oz	62	2	716	11	—
Onion Low Sodium (Goodman's)	1 cup	30	1	115	6	1

FOOD	PORTION	CAL	FAT	SOD	CARB	FIB
Onion Mushroom (Lipton)	8 oz	41	1	684	7	0
Onion Reduced Salt (4C)	8 oz	30	1	760	5	—
Onion Savory (Hain)	¾ cup	50	2	900	6	—
Onion Savory No Salt Added (Hain)	¾ cup	50	1	470	9	—
Onion, as prep (Campbell)	8 oz	30	0	700	7	—
Oriental Hot And Sour, as prep (Knorr)	8 oz	80	3	690	9	—
Oriental Low Fat, as prep (Ramen Noodle)	8 oz	150	1	940	31	—
Oriental With Vegetables Low Fat, as prep (Cup-A-Ramen)	8 oz	220	2	1400	44	—
Oriental With Vegetables, as prep (Cup-A-Ramen)	8 oz	270	10	1210	38	—
Oriental, as prep (Ramen Noodle)	8 oz	190	8	930	26	—
Oxtail Hearty Beef, as prep (Knorr)	8 oz	70	2	1120	10	—
Pork Low Fat, as prep (Ramen Noodle)	8 oz	150	1	1140	31	—
Pork, as prep (Ramen Noodle)	8 oz	200	8	860	26	—
Potato Leek (Ultra Slim-Fast)	6 oz	80	tr	780	15	2
Potato Leek Savory (Hain)	¾ cup	260	18	690	20	—
Potato Leek, as prep (Nile Spice)	10 oz	160	6	450	26	—
Potato Romano, as prep (Nile Spice)	10 oz	150	6	450	23	—
Potato Tomato, as prep (Nile Spice)	10 oz	160	6	440	25	—
Ring-O-Noodle (Lipton)	8 oz	67	2	708	11	—
Rocky Mountain Red Bean (Bean Cuisine)	1 cup (8.6 oz)	202	tr	7	24	8
Sante Fe Corn Chowder (Bean Cuisine)	1 cup (9.2 oz)	179	tr	9	21	6
Seafood Chowder (Golden Dipt)	¼ pkg	70	2	730	12	—

FOOD	PORTION	CAL	FAT	SOD	CARB	FIB
Shrimp Bisque (Golden Dipt)	¼ pkg	30	1	570	5	—
Shrimp With Vegetables Low Fat, as prep (Cup-A-Ramen)	8 oz	230	2	1290	45	—
Shrimp With Vegetables, as prep (Cup-A-Ramen)	8 oz	280	10	1190	40	—
Split Pea Savory (Hain)	¾ cup	310	10	940	16	—
Split Pea as prep (Manischewitz)	6 fl oz	45	tr	320	9	—
Spring Vegetable With Herbs, as prep (Knorr)	8 oz	30	tr	710	6	—
Thick As Fog Split Pea (Bean Cuisine)	1 cup (8.6 fl oz)	189	tr	13	21	1
Tomato (Cup-A-Soup)	6 oz	103	1	524	21	0
Tomato Basil, as prep (Knorr)	8 oz	90	3	940	14	—
Tomato Savory (Hain)	¾ cup	220	14	770	19	—
Tomato, as prep (Diamond Crystal)	6 oz	70	2	—	—	—
Tortellini In Brodo, as prep (Knorr)	8 oz	60	1	820	11	—
Ultima Pasta E Fagioli (Bean Cuisine)	1 cup (8.6 fl oz)	179	tr	8	22	4
Vegetable (Lipton)	8 oz	37	1	640	7	tr
Vegetable Bouillon Instant (Wyler's)	1 tsp	6	tr	910	1	—
Vegetable Cup-Of-Soup (Goodman's)	1 pkg (1½ cups)	180	3	1500	32	2
Vegetable Beef (Weight Watchers)	7.5 oz	90	1	450	13	—
Vegetable Beef Microwave (Campbell)	7½ oz	100	2	830	16	—
Vegetable Savory (Hain)	¾ cup	80	1	730	13	—
Vegetable Savory No Salt Added (Hain)	¾ cup	80	1	330	13	—
Vegetable as prep (Campbell)	8 oz	40	0	710	8	—
Vegetable as prep (Knorr)	8 oz	35	1	840	7	—
Vegetable as prep (Manischewitz)	6 fl oz	50	tr	65	9	—

FOOD	PORTION	CAL	FAT	SOD	CARB	FIB
Vegetarian Vegetable Bouillon, as prep (Knorr)	8 oz	16	2	990	1	—
White Bean Provencal (Bean Cuisine)	1 cup (7.7 fl oz)	166	tr	7	19	6
asparagus, cream of, as prep w/ water	1 cup	59	2	801	9	—
beef broth	1 pkg (0.2 oz)	14	1	1019	1	—
beef broth cube	1 cube (3.6 g)	6	tr	864	1	—
beef broth cube, as prep w/water	1 cup	8	tr	1152	1	—
beef broth, as prep w/ water	1 cup	19	1	1368	2	—
celery cream of as prep w/ water	1 cup	63	2	839	10	—
chicken broth	1 pkg (0.2 oz)	16	1	1116	1	—
chicken broth cube	1 cube (4.8 g)	9	tr	1152	1	—
chicken broth cube, as prep w/ water	1 cup	13	tr	792	2	—
chicken broth, as prep w/water	1 cup	21	1	1484	1	—
chicken, cream of, as prep w/ water	1 cup	107	5	1184	13	—
chicken noodle, as prep w/ water	1 cup	53	1	1284	7	—
french onion, not prep	1 pkg (1.4 oz)	115	2	3493	21	—
leek, as prep w/ water	1 cup	71	2	966	11	—
onion, as prep w/ water	1 cup	28	1	848	5	—
tomato, as prep w/ water	1 cup	102	2	943	19	—
FROZEN						
Asparagus, Cream Of (Kettle Ready)	6 oz	62	5	415	5	—
Barley & Mushroom (Jaclyn's)	7.5 fl oz	90	1	234	16	—
Black Bean With Ham (Kettle Ready)	6 oz	154	6	567	23	—
Boston Clam Chowder (Kettle Ready)	6 oz	131	7	420	13	0
Broccoli, Cream Of (Kettle Ready)	6 oz	94	7	487	6	0
Cauliflower, Cream Of (Kettle Ready)	6 oz	93	7	432	6	—

FOOD	PORTION	CAL	FAT	SOD	CARB	FIB
Cheddar Broccoli Cream Of (Kettle Ready)	6 oz	137	11	595	5	—
Chicken, Cream Of (Kettle Ready)	6 oz	98	6	676	5	—
Chicken Gumbo (Kettle Ready)	6 oz	94	4	380	12	—
Chicken Noodle (Kettle Ready)	6 oz	94	3	599	12	—
Chili (Kettle Ready)	6 oz	161	7	425	14	—
Corn & Broccoli Chowder (Kettle Ready)	6 oz	102	5	451	13	0
Creamy Cheddar (Kettle Ready)	6 oz	158	13	625	7	—
French Onion (Kettle Ready)	6 oz	42	2	508	5	—
Garden Vegetable (Kettle Ready)	6 oz	85	3	460	12	0
Hearty Minestrone (Kettle Ready)	6 oz	104	4	352	15	—
Hearty Beef Vegetable (Kettle Ready)	6 oz	85	3	353	11	—
Manhattan Clam Chowder (Kettle Ready)	6 oz	69	3	564	8	—
Mushroom, Cream Of (Kettle Ready)	6 oz	85	6	422	6	—
New England Clam Chowder (Kettle Ready)	6 oz	116	7	336	11	tr
Potato, Cream Of (Kettle Ready)	6 oz	121	5	404	17	0
Savory Bean With Ham (Kettle Ready)	6 oz	113	4	404	20	—
Split Pea (Jaclyn's)	7.5 fl oz	180	2	183	31	—
Split Pea With Ham (Kettle Ready)	6 oz	155	4	351	25	0
Tomato Florentine (Kettle Ready)	6 oz	106	4	389	15	—
Tortellini In Tomato (Kettle Ready)	6 oz	122	5	548	15	—
Vegetable (Jaclyn's)	7.5 fl oz	90	1	195	18	—
HOME RECIPE						
black bean turtle soup	1 cup	241	1	6	45	—
corn & cheese chowder	¾ cup	215	12	386	21	3
greek	¾ cup	63	2	386	7	2
hot & sour	1 cup	74	2	—	—	—

FOOD	PORTION	CAL	FAT	SOD	CARB	FIB
SHELF STABLE						
Chunky Beef Vegetable (Healthy Choice)	7.5 oz cup	110	1	490	14	—
Chunky Chicken Noodle & Vegetable (Healthy Choice)	7.5 oz cup	160	4	500	18	—
TAKE-OUT						
gazpacho	1 cup	46	tr	63	5	—
oxtail	5 oz	64	3	—	7	—

SOUR CREAM
see also SOUR CREAM SUBSTITUTES

FOOD	PORTION	CAL	FAT	SOD	CARB	FIB
Breakstone	1 tbsp	30	3	5	1	—
Breakstone Light Choice Cultured Half & Half	1 tbsp	25	2	10	1	—
Cabot	1 oz	60	6	15	1	—
Cabot Light	1 oz	33	2	72	2	—
Friendship	2 tbsp (1 oz)	60	5	15	2	0
Friendship Light	2 tbsp (1 oz)	35	3	30	2	0
Heluva Good Cheese	2 tbsp (1.1 oz)	60	5	15	2	0
Heluva Good Cheese Fat-Free	2 tbsp (1.1 oz)	20	0	45	3	0
Heluva Good Cheese Light	2 tbsp (1.1 oz)	40	3	20	3	0
Knudsen Hampshire	1 oz	60	6	10	1	—
Knudsen Light N'Lively Light	1 oz	40	3	20	2	—
Land O'Lakes Light	2 tbsp	40	2	35	4	—
Land O'Lakes Light With Chives	2 tbsp	40	2	150	4	—
Naturally Yours No Fat	2 tbsp (1 fl oz)	15	0	15	1	—
Sealtest	1 tbsp	30	3	5	1	—
Sealtest Light Cultured Half & Half	1 tbsp	25	2	10	1	—
Weight Watchers Light Sour	2 tbsp	35	2	40	2	—
sour cream	1 cup	493	48	123	10	—
sour cream	1 tbsp	26	3	6	1	—

SOUR CREAM SUBSTITUTES

FOOD	PORTION	CAL	FAT	SOD	CARB	FIB
Better Than Sour Cream Sour Supreme (Tofutti)	1 oz	50	5	120	1	—
Formagg	1 oz	40	3	—	—	—
Pet Imitation	1 tbsp	25	2	25	tr	—
nondairy	1 cup	479	45	235	15	—

FOOD	PORTION	CAL	FAT	SOD	CARB	FIB
nondairy	1 oz	59	6	29	2	—

SOURSOP
fresh	1	416	2	87	105	—
fresh, cut up	1 cup	150	1	31	38	—

SOY
see also TOFU, MILK SUBSTITUTES, ICE CREAM AND FROZEN DESSERTS

FOOD	PORTION	CAL	FAT	SOD	CARB	FIB
Soo Moo Beverage (Health Valley)	1 cup	120	6	55	12	0
Soy Sauce (Kikkoman)	1 tbsp	12	0	938	2	0
Soy Sauce (La Choy)	½ tsp	2	tr	230	tr	tr
Soy Sauce Chef Magic (Trappey's)	1 tbsp (0.5 oz)	23	tr	952	4	tr
Soy Sauce Lite (Kikkoman)	1 tbsp	13	0	564	2	—
Soy Sauce Lite (La Choy)	½ tsp	1	tr	110	tr	tr
Soy Sauce Mix (Diamond Crystal)	1 tsp	5	tr	—	—	—
Soyagen All Purpose (LaLoma)	¼ cup	130	6	150	14	—
Soyagen Carob (LaLoma)	¼ cup	140	6	160	16	—
Soyagen No Sucrose (LaLoma)	¼ cup	130	6	210	14	—
Soyamel (Worthington)	1 oz	130	7	150	11	—
Tempeh (Lightlife)	4 oz	182	6	10	9	—
lecithin	1 tbsp	104	14	—	0	—
soy milk	1 cup	79	5	30	4	—
soy sauce	1 tbsp	7	tr	1024	1	—
soy sauce shoyu	1 tbsp	9	tr	1029	2	—
soy sauce tamari	1 tbsp	11	tr	1005	1	—
soya cheese	1.4 oz	128	11	—	tr	0
soybean sprouts, raw	½ cup	43	2	5	3	—
soybean sprouts, steamed	½ cup	38	2	5	3	—
soybean sprouts, stir-fried	1 cup	125	7	14	9	—
soybeans, cooked	1 cup	298	15	1	17	—
soybeans, dry-roasted	½ cup	387	19	2	28	—
soybeans, roasted	½ cup	405	22	140	29	—
soybeans, roasted & toasted	1 cup	490	26	4	33	—
soybeans, roasted & toasted	1 oz	129	7	1	9	—

FOOD	PORTION	CAL	FAT	SOD	CARB	FIB
soybeans, salted, roasted & toasted	1 cup	490	26	176	33	—
soybeans, salted, roasted & toasted	1 oz	129	7	54	9	—

SPAGHETTI
see PASTA, PASTA DINNERS, PASTA SALAD, SPAGHETTI SAUCE

SPAGHETTI SAUCE
see also PIZZA, TOMATO

JARRED

FOOD	PORTION	CAL	FAT	SOD	CARB	FIB
Classico						
Beef & Pork	4 fl oz	80	4	540	7	—
Four Cheese	4 fl oz	70	4	440	7	—
Ripe Olives & Mushrooms	4 fl oz	50	2	470	7	—
Spicy Red Pepper	4 fl oz	50	2	250	6	—
Sweet Peppers & Onions	4 fl oz	50	4	360	7	—
Tomato & Basil	4 fl oz	60	3	340	6	—
Contadina	¼ cup	20	0	280	4	tr
Contadina Italian	¼ cup	15	0	320	4	1
Contadina Thick & Zesty	¼ cup	15	0	330	4	1
Estee	4 oz	60	1	30	9	—
Hunt's						
Chunky	4 oz	50	tr	470	12	2
Homestyle	4 oz	60	2	530	10	2
Homestyle With Meat	4 oz	60	2	570	9	2
Homestyle With Mushrooms	4 oz	50	1	530	10	2
Traditional	4 oz	70	2	530	12	2
With Meat	4 oz	70	2	570	12	2
With Mushrooms	4 oz	70	2	560	12	2
Newman's Own Marinara	4 oz	70	2	560	11	—
Newman's Own Marinara With Mushrooms	4 oz	70	2	560	11	—
Newman's Own Sockarooni	4 oz	70	2	560	11	—
Prego						
Chunky Sausage & Green Peppers	4 oz	160	8	500	19	—

FOOD	PORTION	CAL	FAT	SOD	CARB	FIB
Extra Chunky Garden Combination	4 oz	80	2	420	14	—
Extra Chunky Mushroom And Green Pepper	4 oz	100	4	410	14	—
Extra Chunky Mushroom And Onion	4 oz	100	4	490	13	—
Extra Chunky Mushroom And Tomato	4 oz	110	5	500	14	—
Extra Chunky Mushroom With Extra Spice	4 oz	100	3	450	17	—
Extra Chunky Tomato And Onion	4 oz	110	5	490	14	—
Marinara	4 oz	100	6	620	10	—
Meat Flavored	4 oz	140	6	660	20	—
Mushroom	4 oz	130	5	630	20	—
Onion And Garlic	4 oz	110	4	510	16	—
Regular	4 oz	130	5	630	20	—
Three Cheese	4 oz	100	2	410	17	—
Tomato & Basil	4 oz	100	2	370	18	—
Pritikin	4 oz	60	0	—	—	—
Pritikin w/ Mushrooms	4 oz	60	0	—	—	—
Progresso	½ cup	110	5	660	13	—
Bolognese	½ cup	150	12	520	12	3
Marinara	½ cup	90	5	520	9	—
Meat Flavored	½ cup	110	5	660	13	—
Mushroom	½ cup	110	5	630	13	—
Sicilian	½ cup	30	3	660	2	tr
Ragu						
Fino Italian Garden Medley	½ cup (4.5 oz)	90	3	580	14	2
Fino Italian Garlic & Basil	½ cup (4.5 oz)	90	3	580	15	2
Fino Italian Parmesan	½ cup (4.5 oz)	100	3	580	15	2
Fino Italian Sliced Mushroom	½ cup (4.5 oz)	90	3	580	14	2
Fino Italian Tomato & Herb	½ cup (4.5 oz)	90	3	580	15	2
Fino Italian Zesty Tomato	½ cup (4.5 oz)	90	3	580	14	2
Gardenstyle Chunky Garden Combination	½ cup (4.5 oz)	120	4	540	18	3

FOOD	PORTION	CAL	FAT	SOD	CARB	FIB
Ragu *(cont.)*						
Gardenstyle Chunky Green & Red Pepper	½ cup (4.5 oz)	120	4	570	19	2
Gardenstyle Chunky Mushroom & Onion	½ cup (4.5 oz)	120	4	560	19	3
Gardenstyle Chunky Tomato, Garlic & Onion	½ cup (4.5 oz)	120	4	550	19	3
Gardenstyle Super Mushroom	½ cup (4.5 oz)	120	4	540	19	3
Gardenstyle Chunky Mushroom & Green Pepper	½ cup (4.5 oz)	120	4	570	18	3
Gardenstyle Super Vegetable Primavera	½ cup (4.5 oz)	110	4	480	17	4
Homestyle Mushroom	½ cup (4.5 oz)	120	4	650	18	3
Homestyle Tomato & Herb	½ cup (4.5 oz)	120	4	650	18	3
Homestyle With Meat	½ cup (4.5 oz)	130	4	650	18	3
Light Chunky Mushroom	½ cup (4.5 oz)	50	0	410	10	2
Light Garden Harvest	½ cup (4.4 oz)	50	0	410	11	2
Light No Sugar Added	½ cup (4.4 oz)	60	0	410	9	3
Light Tomato & Herb	½ cup (4.4 oz)	50	0	410	10	2
Old World Style Marinara	½ cup (4.4 oz)	90	5	820	9	3
Old World Style Mushrooms	½ cup (4.4 oz)	80	3	820	10	3
Old World Style Traditional	½ cup (4.4 oz)	80	3	820	10	3
Old World Style With Meat	½ cup (4.4 oz)	90	5	820	9	3
Spaghetti Sauce	4 fl oz	80	4	740	9	—
Thick & Hearty Mushroom	½ cup (4.5 oz)	120	3	580	19	3
Thick & Hearty Spaghetti Sauce	4 oz	100	3	460	15	—
Thick & Hearty Tomato & Herb	½ cup (4.5 oz)	120	3	580	19	3
Thick & Hearty With Meat	½ cup (4.5 oz)	130	5	580	19	3

FOOD	PORTION	CAL	FAT	SOD	CARB	FIB
Weight Watchers With Meat	⅓ cup	45	1	310	7	—
Weight Watchers With Mushrooms	⅓ cup	35	0	300	7	—
marinara sauce	1 cup	171	8	1572	25	—
spaghetti sauce	1 cup	272	12	1236	40	—
REFRIGERATED						
Contadina						
Alfredo	½ cup (4.2 fl oz)	400	38	510	8	0
Four Cheese Sauce With White Wine & Shallots	½ cup (4.2 fl oz)	320	25	480	8	0
Light Alfredo	½ cup (4.2 fl oz)	190	13	560	10	0
Light Chunky Tomato	½ cup (4.4 fl oz)	45	0	470	8	3
Light Garden Vegetable	½ cup (4.4 fl oz)	45	1	540	8	3
Marinara	½ cup (4.4 fl oz)	80	4	470	8	2
Pesto With Basil	¼ cup (2 oz)	310	30	440	5	0
Pesto With Sun Dried Tomatoes	¼ cup (2 oz)	250	24	520	6	3
Plum Tomato With Basil	½ cup (4.4 fl oz)	70	3	450	8	3
Spicy Italian Sausage & Bell Pepper	½ cup (4.4 fl oz)	100	5	540	9	3
TAKE-OUT						
bolognese	5 oz	195	15	—	4	tr

SPANISH FOOD

see also BEANS, CHIPS, DINNER, PEPPERS, SALSA, SNACKS

FOOD	PORTION	CAL	FAT	SOD	CARB	FIB
CANNED						
Enchilada Sauce Hot (El Molino)	2 tbsp	16	1	100	2	—
Enchilada Sauce Mild (Rosarita)	2.5 oz	25	1	230	3	tr
Enchiladas (Gebhardt)	2	310	24	460	20	2
Fajita Marinade (Old El Paso)	⅛ jar	14	0	450	3	0
Green Chili Sauce Mild (El Molino)	2 tbsp	10	0	210	2	—
Menudo (Old El Paso)	½ can	476	52	770	14	2

FOOD	PORTION	CAL	FAT	SOD	CARB	FIB
Mexican Sauce (Pritikin)	4 oz	50	1	—	—	—
Picante Chunky Hot (Rosarita)	3 tbsp (2 fl oz)	18	tr	515	4	tr
Picante Chunky Medium (Rosarita)	3 tbsp (2 fl oz)	16	tr	650	4	tr
Picante Chunky Mild (Rosarita)	3 tbsp (2 oz)	25	tr	630	5	tr
Picante Hot (Chi Chi's)	1 oz	11	tr	263	2	—
Picante Mild (Casa Fiesta)	1 oz	9	tr	117	2	—
Picante Mild (Chi Chi's)	1 oz	11	tr	191	2	—
Picante Mild (Guiltless Gourmet)	1 oz	6	0	133	1	tr
Queso Mild Cheddar (Guiltless Gourmet)	1 oz	22	tr	150	5	tr
Taco Sauce Western Style (Ortega)	1 oz	8	0	—	—	—
Taco Sauce Hot (Chi Chi's)	1 oz	17	tr	247	3	—
Taco Sauce Mild (Casa Fiesta)	1 oz	9	tr	117	2	—
Taco Sauce Mild (Chi Chi's)	1 oz	18	tr	165	4	—
Taco Sauce Red Mild (El Molino)	2 tbsp	10	0	170	2	—
Taco Sauce Thick And Smooth Hot (Ortega)	1 tbsp	8	0	105	2	0
Taco Sauce Thick And Smooth Mild (Ortega)	1 tbsp	8	0	115	2	0
Tamales (Derby)	2	160	7	570	15	1
Tamales (Gebhardt)	2	290	22	730	19	2
Tamales (Old El Paso)	2	190	12	380	16	—
Tamales (Wolf Brand)	7.5 oz	328	25	1181	25	—
Tamales Jumbo (Gebhardt)	2	400	30	1025	26	3
Tamales With Sauce (Van Camp's)	1 cup	293	16	1132	29	—
FROZEN						
Banquet						
Beef & Bean Burrito	9.5 oz	390	12	1460	57	—
Beef Enchilada & Tamale w/ Chili Gravy	10 oz	300	10	1390	44	—
Chimichanga	9.5 oz	480	21	1480	60	—

FOOD	PORTION	CAL	FAT	SOD	CARB	FIB
Enchilada Chicken	11 oz	340	9	1370	54	—
Enchilada Beef	11 oz	370	12	1200	53	—
Enchilada Cheese	11 oz	340	9	1310	—	—
Enchilada Beef w/ Chili Sauce	7 oz	270	13	—	28	—
Tamale Beef	11 oz	420	18	1420	53	—
El Charrito						
Burrito Grande B&B	1 pkg (6 oz)	430	16	—	—	—
Burrito Grande Green Chili B&B	1 pkg (6 oz)	410	14	—	—	—
Burrito Grande Jalapeno	1 pkg (6 oz)	410	15	—	—	—
Burrito Grande Red Chili B&B	1 pkg (6 oz)	410	15	—	—	—
Burrito Green Chili B&B	1 pkg (5 oz)	370	16	—	—	—
Burrito Red Chili B&B	1 pkg (5 oz)	380	18	—	—	—
Burrito Red Hot B&B	1 pkg (5 oz)	540	18	—	—	—
Burrito Red Hot Beef	1 pkg (5 oz)	340	17	—	—	—
Enchilada Beef Dinner	1 pkg (13.75 oz)	620	31	—	—	—
Enchilada Cheese Dinner	1 pkg (13.75 oz)	570	24	—	—	—
Enchilada Chicken Dinner	1 pkg (13.75 oz)	510	17	—	—	—
Enchilada Grande Beef Dinner	1 pkg (21 oz)	950	49	—	—	—
Enchiladas 3 Beef	1 pkg (11 oz)	560	31	—	—	—
Enchiladas 3 Cheese	1 pkg (11 oz)	470	20	—	—	—
Enchiladas 3 Chicken	1 pkg (11 oz)	440	13	—	—	—
Enchiladas 4 Grande Beef	1 pkg (16.5 oz)	890	47	—	—	—
Enchiladas 6 Beef	1 pkg (16.25 oz)	880	49	—	—	—
Enchiladas 6 Beef & Cheese	1 pkg (16.25 oz)	880	42	—	—	—
Enchiladas 6 Cheese	1 pkg (16.25 oz)	780	30	—	—	—
Grande Mexican Dinner	1 pkg (20 oz)	850	47	—	—	—
Mexican Dinner	1 pkg (14.25 oz)	690	35	—	—	—
Queso Dinner	1 pkg (13.25 oz)	490	16	—	—	—

FOOD	PORTION	CAL	FAT	SOD	CARB	FIB
El Charrito *(cont.)*						
Satillo Dinner	1 pkg (13.5 oz)	570	24	—	—	—
Satillo Grande Dinner	1 pkg (20.75 oz)	820	34	—	—	—
Tortillas Corn	2	95	1	—	—	—
Tortillas Flour	2	170	4	—	—	—
Fajita Kit Beef (Tyson)	3.84 oz	160	4	240	21	—
Fajita Kit Chicken (Tyson)	4 oz	80	2	240	2	—
Healthy Choice						
Enchilada Beef	12.75 oz	350	5	430	62	—
Enchilada Chicken	12.75 oz	330	5	440	58	—
Enchiladas Chicken	9.5 oz	280	6	510	46	—
Fajitas Beef	7 oz	210	4	250	26	—
Fajitas Chicken	7 oz	200	3	310	25	—
Le Menu Entree LightStyle Enchilada Chicken	8 oz	280	8	530	32	—
Lean Cuisine Chicken Enchanadas	1 pkg (9.9 oz)	220	6	390	29	4
Lean Cuisine Chicken Enchilada Suiza	1 pkg (9 oz)	290	5	530	48	5
Lightlife Vegetarian Taco	2 oz	51	1	280	4	—
Old El Paso						
Beef and Cheese Chimichanga	11 oz	510	23	1400	53	—
Burrito Beef and Bean Hot	1	310	11	710	41	—
Burrito Beef and Bean Medium	1	330	13	630	41	—
Burrito Beef and Bean Mild	1	320	11	500	42	—
Chimichangas Beef	1 pkg (11 oz)	540	21	1200	65	—
Chimichanges Bean & Cheese	1	380	19	610	40	—
Chimichanges Beef & Pork	1	340	16	700	35	—
Chimichanges Chicken	1	370	21	460	35	—
Enchilada Beef	1 pkg (11 oz)	390	8	1200	56	—
Enchilada Cheese	1 pkg (11 oz)	590	31	1200	51	—
Enchilada Chicken	1 pkg (11 oz)	460	18	770	54	—
Enchiladas w/ Sour Cream Sauce	1	280	19	520	18	—

FOOD	PORTION	CAL	FAT	SOD	CARB	FIB
Patio						
Britos Beef & Bean	1 (3 oz)	210	9	290	28	—
Britos Nacho Beef	1 (3 oz)	220	11	350	25	—
Britos Nacho Cheese	1 (3.63 oz)	250	10	330	32	—
Britos Spicy Chicken & Cheese	1 (3 oz)	210	9	280	28	—
Burritos Hot Beef & Bean Red Chili	1 (5 oz)	340	13	810	44	—
Burritos Medium Beef & Bean	1 (5 oz)	370	16	830	43	—
Burritos Mild Beef & Bean Green Chili	1 (5 oz)	330	12	770	43	—
Enchilada Beef Dinner	13.25 oz	520	24	1810	59	—
Enchilada Cheese Dinner	12 oz	370	10	1970	58	—
Fiesta Dinner	12 oz	460	20	1990	54	—
Mexican Dinner	13.25 oz	540	25	1940	64	—
Tamale Dinner	13 oz	470	21	1850	58	—
Stouffer's Cheese Enchilada	1 pkg (9.75 oz)	370	14	890	48	5
Stouffer's Chicken Enchilada	1 pkg (10 oz)	370	14	970	45	3
Swanson Enchiladas Beef	13.75 oz	480	21	1350	55	—
Swanson Mexican Style Combination	14.25 oz	490	18	1760	62	—
Swanson Mexican Style Hungry Man	20.25 oz	820	41	2080	88	—
Van De Kamp's Mexican Holiday Enchilada Dinner Beef	12 oz	390	15	—	—	—
Van De Kamp's Mexican Holiday Enchilada Dinner Cheese	12 oz	450	20	—	—	—
Weight Watchers						
Enchiladas Ranchero Beef	9.12 oz	190	5	500	18	—
Enchiladas Ranchero Cheese	8.87 oz	260	10	550	25	—
Enchiladas Suiza Chicken	9 oz	230	7	530	25	—
Fajitas Chicken	6.75 oz	210	5	490	24	—

FOOD	PORTION	CAL	FAT	SOD	CARB	FIB
MIX						
Burrito Seasoning Mix (Old El Paso)	⅛ pkg	17	0	275	3	1
Enchilada Seasoning Mix (Old El Paso)	⅛ pkg	6	0	80	1	0
Guacamole Seasoning Mix (Old El Paso)	½ pkg	7	0	240	2	0
Masa Harina De Maiz (Quaker)	2 tortillas	137	2	5	28	3
Masa Trigo (Quaker)	2 tortillas	149	4	794	25	1
Menudo Mix (Gebhardt)	1 tsp	5	tr	310	1	tr
Taco Seasoning Mix (Old El Paso)	½₂ pkg	8	tr	298	2	0
Taco Meat Seasoning Mix Mild (Ortega)	1 filled taco	90	1	999	18	—
Taco Seasoning Mix (Hain)	⅒ pkg	10	0	200	2	—
READY-TO-USE						
Taco Shells						
(Casa Fiesta)	3.5 oz	480	23	10	60	—
(Gebhardt)	1	50	2	tr	7	tr
(Old El Paso)	1	55	3	50	6	1
(Rosarita)	1 shell (11 g)	50	2	tr	7	tr
Super (Old El Paso)	1	100	6	95	11	2
Tastaco Shells (Old El Paso)	1	100	5	10	11	1
Toco Shells Mini (Old El Paso)	3	70	4	60	7	1
Tortilla Wheat Flour (Mariachi)	1	112	3	174	20	—
Tortillas						
Burrito Style Flour (Tyson)	1	170	4	40	29	—
Burrito Style Flour Large Heat Pressed (Tyson)	1	182	4	90	33	—
Burrito Style Flour Small Hand Stretched (Tyson)	1	106	2	50	19	—
Enchilada Style Corn (Tyson)	1	54	tr	4	11	—
Fajita Style Flour (Tyson)	1	89	2	21	15	—
Soft Taco Flour (Tyson)	1	121	3	28	20	—

FOOD	PORTION	CAL	FAT	SOD	CARB	FIB
Whole Wheat (Tyson)	1	120	3	32	20	—
Tortillas Flour (Old El Paso)	1	150	3	360	27	—
Tostada Shells (Old El Paso)	1	65	3	65	6	1
Tostada Shells (Rosarita)	1 shell (14 g)	60	3	tr	8	tr
taco shell, baked	1 med (½ oz)	61	3	48	8	tr
taco shell, baked w/o salt	1 med (½ oz)	61	3	2	8	tr
tortilla corn	1 (6-in diam)	56	1	40	12	1
tortilla corn w/o salt	1 6-in diam (.9 oz)	56	1	3	12	1
tortilla flour w/o salt	1 8-in diam (1.2 oz)	114	3	167	20	1
TAKE-OUT						
burrito w/ apple	1 lg (5.4 oz)	484	20	443	73	—
burrito w/ apple	1 sm (2.6 oz)	231	10	211	35	—
burrito w/ beans	2 (7.6 oz)	448	14	986	71	—
burrito w/ beans & cheese	2 (6.5 oz)	377	12	1166	55	—
burrito w/ beans & chili peppers	2 (7.2 oz)	413	15	1043	58	—
burrito w/ beans & meat	2 (8.1 oz)	508	18	1335	66	—
burrito w/ beans, cheese & beef	2 (7.1 oz)	331	13	990	40	—
burrito w/ beans, cheese & chili peppers	2 (11.8 oz)	663	23	2060	85	—
burrito w/ beef	2 (7.7 oz)	523	21	1492	59	—
burrito w/ beef & chili peppers	2 (7.1 oz)	426	17	1116	49	—
burrito w/ beef, cheese & chili peppers	2 (10.7 oz)	634	25	2091	64	—
burrito w/ cherry	1 lg (5.4 oz)	484	20	443	73	—
burrito w/ cherry	1 sm (2.6 oz)	231	10	211	35	—
chimichanga w/ beef	1 (6.1 oz)	425	20	910	43	—
chimichanga w/ beef & cheese	1 (6.4 oz)	443	23	956	39	—
chimichanga w/ beef & red chili peppers	1 (6.7 oz)	424	19	1169	46	—
chimichanga w/ beef, cheese & red chili peppers	1 (6.3 oz)	364	18	895	38	—
enchilada w/ cheese	1 (5.7 oz)	320	19	784	29	—

FOOD	PORTION	CAL	FAT	SOD	CARB	FIB
enchilada w/ cheese & beef	1 (6.7 oz)	324	18	1320	30	—
enchiladas eggplant	1	142	5	—	—	—
enchirito w/ cheese, beef & beans	1 (6.8 oz)	344	16	1251	34	—
frijoles w/ cheese	1 cup (5.9 oz)	226	8	882	29	—
nachos w/ cheese	6 to 8 (4 oz)	345	19	816	36	—
nachos w/ cheese & jalapeno peppers	6 to 8 (7.2 oz)	607	34	1736	60	—
nachos w/ cheese, beans, ground beef & peppers	6 to 8 (8.9 oz)	568	31	1800	56	—
nachos w/ cinnamon & sugar	6 to 8 (3.8 oz)	592	36	439	63	—
taco	1 sm (6 oz)	370	21	802	27	—
taco salad	1½ cups	279	15	763	24	—
taco salad w/ chili con carne	1½ cups	288	13	886	27	—
tostada w/ beans & cheese	1 (5.1 oz)	223	10	543	27	—
tostada w/ beans, beef & cheese	1 (7.9 oz)	334	17	870	30	—
tostada w/ beef & cheese	(5.7 oz)	315	16	896	23	—
tostada w/ guacamole	2 (9.2 oz)	360	23	789	32	—

SPARE RIBS
see PORK

SPELT
Arrowhead	1 oz	83	1	1	20	4

SPICES
see HERBS/SPICES, INDIVIDUAL NAMES

SPINACH
CANNED
S&W Northwest Premium	½ cup	25	0	395	3	—
Seneca	½ cup	25	0	—	—	—
spinach	½ cup	25	1	29	4	—

FRESH
Dole	3 oz	9	tr	107	tr	8
cooked	½ cup	21	tr	63	3	2
mustard, chopped, cooked	½ cup	14	tr	—	3	—
mustard, raw, chopped	½ cup	17	tr	—	3	—

FOOD	PORTION	CAL	FAT	SOD	CARB	FIB
new zealand, chopped, cooked	½ cup	11	tr	97	2	—
new zealand, raw	½ cup	4	tr	36	1	—
raw, chopped	1 pkg (10 oz)	46	1	160	7	—
raw, chopped	½ cup	6	tr	22	1	1
FROZEN						
Birds Eye Chopped	½ cup	20	0	90	3	3
Birds Eye Creamed	½ cup	90	5	320	9	1
Birds Eye Leaf	½ cup	20	0	90	4	3
Budget Gourmet Au Gratin	1 pkg (5.5 oz)	160	11	600	9	—
Green Giant	½ cup	25	0	100	6	5
Green Giant Creamed	½ cup	70	3	480	10	—
Green Giant Cut Leaf In Butter Sauce	½ cup	40	2	380	6	4
Green Giant Harvest Fresh	½ cup	25	0	170	5	3
Stouffer's Creamed	½ cup (2.25 oz)	150	12	380	8	2
Stouffer's Souffle	½ cup (4 oz)	150	10	480	9	—
cooked	½ cup	27	tr	82	5	—
JUICE						
spinach juice	3½ oz	7	0	73	1	—

SPORTS DRINKS

FOOD	PORTION	CAL	FAT	SOD	CARB	FIB
All Sport Diet Lemon Lime Slice	8 fl oz	1	0	40	0	—
All Sport Lemon Lime Slice	8 fl oz	72	0	55	19	—
All Sport Orange Slice	8 fl oz	74	0	55	19	—
All Sport Punch Slice	8 fl oz	81	0	55	22	—
PowerAde Fruit Punch	8 fl oz	72	0	28	19	—
PowerAde Grape	8 fl oz	73	0	28	19	—
PowerAde Lemon-Lime	8 fl oz	72	0	28	19	—
PowerAde Orange	8 fl oz	72	0	28	19	—

SPOT

FOOD	PORTION	CAL	FAT	SOD	CARB	FIB
FRESH						
baked	3 oz	134	5	32	0	—

SQUAB

FOOD	PORTION	CAL	FAT	SOD	CARB	FIB
breast w/o skin, raw	1 (3.5 oz)	135	5	—	0	—
w/ skin, raw	1 squab (6.9 oz)	584	47	—	0	—
w/o skin, raw	1 squab (5.9 oz)	239	13	—	0	—

FOOD	PORTION	CAL	FAT	SOD	CARB	FIB

SQUASH
see also ZUCCHINI

CANNED

FOOD	PORTION	CAL	FAT	SOD	CARB	FIB
crookneck, sliced	½ cup	14	tr	5	3	—

FRESH

FOOD	PORTION	CAL	FAT	SOD	CARB	FIB
Spaghetti Squash (Nature's Pasta)	1 cup (5.5 oz)	20	0	30	4	2
acorn, cooked, mashed	½ cup	41	tr	3	11	3
acorn, cubed, baked	½ cup	57	tr	4	15	2
butternut, baked	½ cup	41	tr	4	11	2
crookneck, raw, sliced	½ cup	12	tr	1	3	1
crookneck, sliced, cooked	½ cup	18	tr	1	4	1
hubbard, baked	½ cup	51	tr	8	11	3
hubbard, cooked, mashed	½ cup	35	tr	6	8	3
scallop, raw, sliced	½ cup	12	tr	1	3	1
scallop, sliced, cooked	½ cup	14	tr	1	3	1
spaghetti, cooked	½ cup	23	tr	14	5	2

FROZEN

FOOD	PORTION	CAL	FAT	SOD	CARB	FIB
Butternut (Southland)	4 oz	45	0	—	—	—
Prepared Squash (Southland)	3.6 oz	80	2	—	—	—
Winter Cooked (Birds Eye)	½ cup	45	0	0	11	2
butternut, cooked, mashed	½ cup	47	tr	2	12	3
crookneck, sliced, cooked	½ cup	24	tr	6	5	—

SEEDS

FOOD	PORTION	CAL	FAT	SOD	CARB	FIB
dried	1 cup	747	63	24	25	—
dried	1 oz	154	13	5	5	—
roasted	1 cup	1184	96	40	31	—
roasted	1 oz	148	12	5	4	—
salted & roasted	1 cup	1184	96	1294	31	—
salted & roasted	1 oz	148	12	5	4	—
whole, roasted	1 cup	285	12	12	34	—
whole, roasted	1 oz	127	6	5	15	—
whole, salted, roasted	1 cup	285	12	368	34	—
whole, salted, roasted	1 oz	127	6	191	15	—

SQUID

FRESH

FOOD	PORTION	CAL	FAT	SOD	CARB	FIB
fried	3 oz	149	6	260	7	—
raw	3 oz	78	1	37	3	—

FOOD	PORTION	CAL	FAT	SOD	CARB	FIB
SQUIRREL						
roasted	3 oz	147	4	102	0	—
STRAWBERRIES						
CANNED						
in heavy syrup	½ cup	117	tr	5	30	—
FRESH						
Dole	8	50	0	0	13	3
strawberries	1 cup	45	1	2	10	4
strawberries	1 pint	97	1	4	22	—
FROZEN						
Big Valley	3.5 oz	35	tr	0	8	—
Halved In Delicious Syrup (Birds Eye)	½ cup	120	0	0	30	2
Halved In Lite Syrup (Birds Eye)	½ cup	90	0	5	22	2
Whole In Lite Syrup (Birds Eye)	½ cup	80	0	0	20	2
sweetened, sliced	1 cup	245	tr	8	66	—
sweetened, sliced	1 pkg (10 oz)	273	tr	9	74	—
unsweetened	1 cup	52	tr	3	14	—
whole, sweetened	1 cup	200	tr	3	54	—
whole, sweetened	1 pkg (10 oz)	223	tr	3	60	—
JUICE						
Juice Works	6 oz	100	0	—	—	—
Kern's Nectar	6 oz	110	0	0	26	—
Kool-Aid Koolers	1 (8.45 oz)	136	0	3	36	—
Libby's Nectar	6 oz	110	0	0	27	—
Libby's Ripe Nectar	8 oz	150	0	5	36	—
Smucker's	8 oz	130	0	10	31	—
Wyler's Drink Mix Unsweetened Strawberry Split	8 oz	2	0	28	1	—
STUFFING/DRESSING						
HOME RECIPE						
bread, as prep w/ water & fat	½ cup	251	15	627	25	—
bread, as prep w/ water, egg & fat	½ cup	107	7	319	9	—
plain, as prep	½ cup (3.5 oz)	195	8	534	26	3
sausage	½ cup	292	11	258	40	1
MIX						
Arnold All Purpose Seasoned	½ oz	50	0	200	9	1

FOOD	PORTION	CAL	FAT	SOD	CARB	FIB
Arnold Corn	½ oz	50	1	140	9	1
Arnold Herb Seasoned	½ oz	50	tr	150	2	1
Arnold Sage & Onion	½ oz	50	tr	230	9	1
Betty Crocker Chicken	½ cup	180	9	620	21	—
Betty Crocker Traditional Herb	½ cup	180	8	640	22	—
Brownberry Corn	1 oz	103	2	350	19	2
Brownberry Herb	1 oz	100	1	297	19	2
Brownberry Sage & Onion	1 oz	97	1	450	18	2
Golden Grain Bread Stuffing Chicken	½ cup	180	9	730	20	—
Golden Grain Bread Stuffing Corn Bread	½ cup	180	9	870	21	—
Golden Grain Bread Stuffing Herb & Butter	½ cup	180	9	810	20	—
Golden Grain Bread Stuffing With Wild Rice	½ cup	180	9	710	21	—
Pepperidge Farm						
Corn Bread	1 oz	110	1	320	22	—
Country Style	1 oz	100	1	400	21	—
Cube	1 oz	110	1	400	22	—
Distinctive Apple Raisin	1 oz	110	1	410	21	—
Distinctive Classic Chicken	1 oz	110	1	410	20	—
Distinctive Country Garden Herb	1 oz	120	4	300	18	—
Distinctive Vegetable & Almond	1 oz	110	3	250	19	—
Distinctive Wild Rice & Mushroom	1 oz	130	5	310	17	—
Herb Seasoned	1 oz	110	1	380	22	—
Stove Top						
Beef, as prep	½ cup	178	9	586	22	—
Chicken, as prep	½ cup	176	8	561	21	—
Chicken With Rice, as prep	½ cup	182	9	557	22	—
Cornbread, as prep	½ cup	175	8	557	22	—
Flex Serve Chicken, as prep	½ cup	173	9	577	20	—
Flex Serve Cornbread, as prep	½ cup	181	9	591	22	—
Flex Serve Homestyle Herb, as prep	½ cup	173	9	515	20	—

FOOD	PORTION	CAL	FAT	SOD	CARB	FIB
Long Grain & Wild Rice, as prep	½ cup	182	9	553	22	—
Select Wild Rice & Mushroom, as prep	½ cup	172	9	—	—	—
bread dry, as prep	½ cup	178	9	543	22	3
cornbread, as prep	½ cup	179	9	455	22	—

STURGEON
roe, raw	3.5 oz	207	10	—	1	—
FRESH						
cooked	3 oz	115	4	—	0	—
raw	3 oz	90	3	—	0	—
SMOKED						
sturgeon	1 oz	48	1	—	0	—
sturgeon	3 oz	147	4	—	0	—

SUCKER
white, baked	3 oz	101	3	44	0	—

SUGAR
see also FRUCTOSE, SUGAR SUBSTITUTES, SYRUP

C&H White	1 tsp	16	0	—	4	—
Domino White	1 tsp	16	0	0	4	—
Hain Turbinado	1 tbsp	50	0	0	12	—
Hollywood Turbinado	1 tbsp	50	0	0	12	—
brown	1 cup	820	0	97	212	—
powdered, sifted	1 cup	385	0	2	100	0
white	1 cup	770	0	5	199	—
white	1 pkt (6 g)	25	0	tr	6	—
white	1 tbsp	45	0	tr	12	—

SUGAR SUBSTITUTES
see also FRUCTOSE

Equal	1 pkt	4	0	0	tr	—
Estee Swiss Sweet Packet	1 pkt	4	0	0	tr	—
Estee Swiss Sweet Tablet	1	0	0	0	tr	—
S&W Liquid Table Sweetener	⅛ tsp	0	0	0	0	—
Spoon For Spoon	1 tsp	2	0	—	—	—
Sprinkle Sweet	1 tsp	2	0	1	tr	—
SugarTwin	1 pkt (0.8 g)	3	0	5	1	—
SugarTwin	1 tsp (0.4 g)	2	0	3	tr	—
SugarTwin Brown	1 tsp (0.4 g)	2	0	3	tr	—

FOOD	PORTION	CAL	FAT	SOD	CARB	FIB
Sweet'n Low Brown Sugar Substitute	⅒ tsp	2	0	—	—	—
Sweet'n Low Granulated	1 pkt (1g)	4	0	—	—	—
Sweet'n Low Liquid	10 drops	0	0	—	—	—
Sweet One	1 pkt	4	0	0	1	—
Sweet*10	⅛ tsp	0	0	2	0	—
Weight Watchers Sweet'ner	1 pkt	4	0	20	1	—

SUGAR-APPLE

FOOD	PORTION	CAL	FAT	SOD	CARB	FIB
fresh	1	146	tr	15	37	—
fresh, cut up	1 cup	236	1	24	59	—

SUNDAE TOPPINGS
see ICE CREAM TOPPINGS

SUNFISH

FOOD	PORTION	CAL	FAT	SOD	CARB	FIB
pumpkinseed baked,	3 oz	97	1	87	0	—

SUNFLOWER SEEDS

FOOD	PORTION	CAL	FAT	SOD	CARB	FIB
Sunflower Butter (Erewhon)	2 tbsp (32 g)	200	18	20	3	—
Sunflower Nuts Dry Roasted Unsalted (Planters)	1 oz	170	15	0	5	—
Sunflower Seeds (Frito-Lay)	1 oz	160	14	265	6	—
(Planters)	1 oz	160	14	30	5	—
dried	1 cup	821	71	4	27	—
dried	1 oz	162	14	1	5	—
dry roasted	1 cup	745	64	4	31	—
dry roasted	1 oz	165	14	1	7	—
dry roasted, salted	1 cup	745	64	975	31	—
dry roasted, salted	1 oz	165	14	195	7	—
oil roasted	1 cup	830	78	4	20	—
oil roasted, salted	1 cup	830	78	804	20	—
oil roasted, salted	1 oz	175	16	201	4	—
sunflower butter	1 tbsp	93	8	82	4	—
sunflower butter w/o salt	1 tbsp	93	8	1	4	—
toasted	1 cup	826	76	4	28	—
toasted	1 oz	176	16	1	6	—
toasted, salted	1 cup	826	76	817	28	—
toasted, salted	1 oz	176	16	204	6	—

FOOD	PORTION	CAL	FAT	SOD	CARB	FIB
SURF						
CANNED						
Surf (American Original Foods)	4 oz	100	tr	—	7	—
FRESH						
Surf (American Original Foods)	4 oz	90	tr	—	2	—
SUSHI						
TAKE-OUT						
California roll	1 piece (0.8 oz)	28	1	37	4	—
kim chi	⅓ cup (5.8 oz)	18	tr	2143	4	—
sashimi	1 serv (6 oz)	198	7	718	4	—
tuna roll	1 piece (0.7 oz)	23	tr	33	3	—
vegetable roll	1 piece (1.2 oz)	27	1	47	5	—
vinegared ginger	⅓ cup (1.6 oz)	48	tr	6	12	—
wasabi	2 tsp (0.3 oz)	5	tr	124	1	—
yellowtail roll	1 piece (0.6 oz)	25	1	32	3	—
SWAMP CABBAGE						
FRESH						
chopped, cooked	½ cup	10	tr	60	2	—
raw, chopped	1 cup	11	tr	63	2	—
SWEET POTATO						
see also YAM						
CANNED						
in syrup	½ cup	106	tr	38	25	—
pieces	1 cup	183	tr	107	42	—
FRESH						
baked, w/ skin	1 (3.5 oz)	118	tr	12	28	3
leaves, cooked	½ cup	11	tr	4	2	—
mashed	½ cup	172	tr	21	40	3
FROZEN						
Candied Sweet Potatoes (Mrs. Paul's)	4 oz	170	0	40	42	—
Candied Sweets 'N Apples (Mrs. Paul's)	4 oz	160	0	60	38	—
cooked	½ cup	88	tr	7	21	—
HOME RECIPE						
candied	3.5 oz	144	3	73	29	—
SWEETBREADS						
beef, braised	3 oz	230	15	51	0	—

FOOD	PORTION	CAL	FAT	SOD	CARB	FIB
lamb, braised	3 oz	199	13	44	0	—
veal, braised	3 oz	218	12	—	0	—

SWISS CHARD
FRESH

cooked	½ cup	18	tr	158	4	—
raw, chopped	½ cup	3	tr	38	1	—

SWORDFISH

cooked	3 oz	132	4	98	0	—
raw	3 oz	103	3	76	0	—

SYRUP
see also ICE CREAM TOPPINGS, PANCAKE/WAFFLE SYRUP

Blueberry (Estee)	1 tbsp	8	0	25	1	—
Blueberry (Whistling Wings)	1 oz	45	tr	1	10	tr
Blueberry Diet (S&W)	1 tbsp	4	0	25	1	—
Cane (McIlhenny)	2 tbsp (1.4 oz)	130	0	20	32	tr
Corn Syrup Dark (Karo)	1 cup (331 g)	975	0	610	243	—
Corn Syrup Dark (Karo)	1 tbsp (21 g)	60	0	40	15	—
Corn Syrup Light (Karo)	1 cup (331 g)	960	0	480	241	—
Corn Syrup Light (Karo)	1 tbsp (21 g)	60	0	30	15	—
Fruit Syrup All Flavors (Smucker's)	2 tbsp	100	0	<10	26	—
Maple Flavored Diet (S&W)	1 tbsp	4	0	25	1	—
Maple Rich (Home Brands)	1 oz	110	0	—	—	—
Raspberry (Whistling Wings)	1 oz	60	tr	2	14	0
Strawberry Diet (S&W)	1 tbsp	4	0	25	1	—
corn	2 tbsp	122	0	19	32	—
raspberry	3.5 oz	267	0	2	66	—

TAHINI
see SESAME

TAMARIND

fresh	1	5	tr	1	1	—
fresh, cut up	1 cup	287	1	33	75	—

TANGERINE
CANNED

in light syrup	½ cup	76	tr	8	20	—
juice pack	½ cup	46	tr	7	12	—

FOOD	PORTION	CAL	FAT	SOD	CARB	FIB
FRESH						
Dole	2	70	1	2	19	2
sections	1 cup	86	tr	3	22	—
tangerine	1	37	tr	1	9	—
JUICE						
Dole Pure & Light	6 oz	100	tr	20	25	—
Minute Maid Frozen	8 fl oz	120	0	0	29	—
canned, sweetened	1 cup	125	1	2	30	—
fresh	1 cup	106	tr	2	25	—
frzn, sweetened, as prep	1 cup	110	tr	2	27	—
frzn, sweetened, not prep	6 oz	344	1	7	83	—
TAPIOCA						
Minute Tapioca (General Foods)	1 tbsp	32	tr	—	8	—
pearl dry	½ cup	174	0	0	45	1
starch	3.5 oz	344	tr	4	85	—
TARO						
chips	1 oz	141	7	97	19	—
chips	10 (0.8 oz)	115	6	79	16	—
leaves, cooked	½ cup	18	tr	2	3	—
raw, sliced	½ cup	56	tr	6	14	—
shoots, sliced, cooked	½ cup	10	tr	1	2	—
sliced, cooked	½ cup (2.3 oz)	94	tr	10	23	—
tahitian, sliced, cooked	½ cup	30	tr	37	5	—
TARRAGON						
ground	1 tsp	5	tr	1	1	—
TEA/HERBAL TEA						
HERBAL						
Almond Orange (Bigelow)	5 fl oz	tr	tr	tr	tr	—
Almond Sunset (Celestial Seasonings)	8 fl oz	3	tr	2	1	—
Apple Orchard (Bigelow)	5 fl oz	5	tr	tr	1	—
Apple Spice (Bigelow)	5 fl oz	tr	tr	1	tr	—
Bengal Spice (Celestial Seasonings)	8 fl oz	5	tr	3	tr	—
Caffeine Free (Celestial Seasonings)	8 fl oz	2	tr	5	1	—
Chamomile (Bigelow)	5 fl oz	tr	tr	2	—	—

FOOD	PORTION	CAL	FAT	SOD	CARB	FIB
Chamomile (Celestial Seasonings)	8 fl oz	2	tr	1	1	—
Chamomile Mint (Bigelow)	5 fl oz	tr	tr	1	tr	—
Cinnamon Apple Spice (Celestial Seasonings)	8 fl oz	<3	tr	1	tr	—
Cinnamon Orange (Bigelow)	5 fl oz	tr	tr	tr	tr	—
Cinnamon Rose (Celestial Seasonings)	8 fl oz	<4	tr	1	1	—
Country Peach Spice (Celestial Seasonings)	8 fl oz	3	tr	1	1	—
Cranberry Cove (Celestial Seasonings)	8 fl oz	2	tr	1	1	—
Early Riser (Bigelow)	5 fl oz	3	tr	tr	1	—
Emperor's Choice (Celestial Seasonings)	8 fl oz	4	tr	2	1	—
Feeling Free (Bigelow)	5 fl oz	1	tr	1	tr	—
Fruit & Almond (Bigelow)	5 fl oz	1	tr	tr	tr	—
Ginseng Plus (Celestial Seasonings)	8 fl oz	3	tr	4	1	—
Grandma's Tummy Mint (Celestial Seasonings)	8 fl oz	2	tr	7	tr	—
Hibiscus & Rose Hips (Bigelow)	5 fl oz	1	tr	1	tr	—
I Love Lemon (Bigelow)	5 fl oz	1	tr	tr	tr	—
Lemon & C (Bigelow)	5 fl oz	tr	tr	tr	tr	—
Lemon Mist (Celestial Seasonings)	8 fl oz	3	tr	3	tr	—
Lemon Zinger (Celestial Seasonings)	8 fl oz	4	tr	1	1	—
Looking Good (Bigelow)	5 fl oz	1	tr	1	1	—
Mama Bear's Cold Care (Celestial Seasonings)	8 fl oz	6	tr	2	tr	—
Mandarin Orange Spice (Celestial Seasonings)	8 fl oz	5	tr	2	1	—
Mellow Mint (Celestial Seasonings)	8 fl oz	2	tr	5	tr	—
Mint Blend (Bigelow)	5 fl oz	tr	tr	3	tr	—
Mint Magic (Celestial Seasonings)	8 fl oz	1	tr	13	tr	—
Mint Medley (Bigelow)	5 fl oz	1	tr	3	tr	—
Orange & C (Bigelow)	5 fl oz	tr	tr	tr	tr	—

FOOD	PORTION	CAL	FAT	SOD	CARB	FIB
Orange & Spice (Bigelow)	5 fl oz	1	tr	1	tr	—
Orange Zinger (Celestial Seasonings)	8 fl oz	6	tr	1	1	—
Peppermint (Bigelow)	5 fl oz	tr	tr	2	tr	—
Peppermint (Celestial Seasonings)	8 fl oz	2	tr	9	1	—
Peppermint (Celestial Seasonings)	8 fl oz	2	tr	9	1	—
Raspberry Patch (Celestial Seasonings)	8 fl oz	4	tr	1	1	—
Red Zinger (Celestial Seasonings)	8 fl oz	4	tr	2	1	—
Roastaroma (Celestial Seasonings)	8 fl oz	10	tr	3	2	—
Roasted Grains & Carob (Bigelow)	5 fl oz	3	tr	1	1	—
Sleepytime (Celestial Seasonings)	8 fl oz	4	tr	2	1	—
Spearmint (Bigelow)	5 fl oz	tr	tr	tr	tr	—
Spearmint (Celestial Seasonings)	8 fl oz	5	1	6	tr	—
Strawberry Fields (Celestial Seasonings)	8 fl oz	4	tr	1	1	—
Sunburst C (Celestial Seasonings)	8 fl oz	3	tr	6	1	—
Sweet Dreams (Bigelow)	5 fl oz	1	tr	1	tr	—
Take-A-Break (Bigelow)	5 fl oz	3	tr	1	1	—
Tropical Escape (Celestial Seasonings)	8 fl oz	1	tr	7	tr	—
Wild Forest Blackberry (Celestial Seasonings)	8 fl oz	2	tr	1	1	—
ICED						
4C Instant 4C	8 oz	90	0	0	22	—
Arizona Raspberry	8 fl oz	95	0	20	25	—
Bigelow Nice Over Ice	5 fl oz	1	tr	1	tr	—
Celestial Seasonings Iced Delight	8 fl oz	4	tr	14	1	—
Crystal Light Sugar Free	8 oz	3	0	1	0	—
Crystal Light Decaffeinated Sugar Free	8 oz	2	0	—	0	—

FOOD	PORTION	CAL	FAT	SOD	CARB	FIB
Lipton						
Instant	6 oz	0	0	0	0	—
Instant Decaffeinated	6 oz	0	0	0	0	—
Instant Raspberry	8 oz	3	0	1	1	—
Instant Lemon	8 oz	3	0	1	1	—
Lemon	6 oz	55	0	1	14	—
Sugar Free	8 oz	1	0	6	tr	—
Sugar Free Peach	8 oz	5	0	1	1	—
Sugar Free Raspberry	8 oz	5	0	1	1	—
With NutraSweet	8 oz	3	0	1	1	—
With NutraSweet Decaffeinated	8 oz	3	0	1	1	—
Nestea						
Decaffeinated 100% Instant, as prep	8 oz	0	0	0	0	—
Lemon	8 oz	6	0	0	1	—
Mix With Sugar And Lemon, as prep	8 oz	70	0	0	19	—
Ready-To-Drink Sugarfree With Lemon	8 oz	2	0	0	1	—
Ready-To-Drink With Sugar And Lemon	8 oz	70	0	0	17	—
Sugarfree Decaffeinated	2 tsp	6	0	0	1	—
Sugarfree Iced Tea Mix Nestea	8 oz	4	0	0	1	—
100% Instant Tea, as prep Nestea	8 oz	2	0	0	0	—
Nestea Ice Teasers						
Citrus	8 oz	6	0	0	1	—
Lemon	8 oz	6	0	0	1	—
Orange	8 oz	6	0	0	1	—
Tropical	8 oz	6	0	0	1	—
Wild Cherry	8 oz	6	0	0	1	—
Royal Mistic						
Diet	12 fl oz	8	0	34	2	—
Lemon	12 fl oz	144	0	26	36	—
Orange	12 fl oz	144	0	26	36	—
Wild Berry	12 fl oz	144	0	34	36	—
Shasta	12 oz	124	0	—	—	—
Sipps	8.45 oz	100	0	—	—	—
Veryfine With Lemon	8 oz	80	0	<10	16	—

FOOD	PORTION	CAL	FAT	SOD	CARB	FIB
instant artificially sweetened lemon flavored, as prep w/ water	8 oz	5	0	24	1	—
instant sweetened lemon flavor, as prep w/ water	9 oz	87	tr	—	22	—
instant unsweetened lemon flavor, as prep w/ water	8 oz	4	0	14	0	—
REGULAR						
Chinese Fortune (Bigelow)	5 fl oz	1	tr	tr	tr	—
Cinnamon Stick (Bigelow)	5 fl oz	1	tr	tr	tr	—
Cinnamon Vienna (Celestial Seasonings)	8 fl oz	2	tr	1	1	—
Constant Comment (Bigelow)	5 fl oz	1	tr	tr	tr	—
Darjeeling Blend (Bigelow)	5 fl oz	1	tr	tr	tr	—
Earl Grey (Bigelow)	5 fl oz	1	tr	tr	tr	—
Earl Grey Extraordinary (Celestial Seasonings)	8 fl oz	3	tr	tr	1	—
English Breakfast Classic (Celestial Seasonings)	8 fl oz	3	tr	tr	tr	—
English Teatime (Bigelow)	5 fl oz	1	tr	tr	tr	—
Kaffree (Natural Touch)	8 fl oz	0	0	<1	0	—
Lemon (Celestial Seasonings)	8 fl oz	7	tr	1	1	—
Lemon Lift (Bigelow)	5 fl oz	1	tr	tr	tr	—
Mint (Celestial Seasonings)	8 fl oz	4	tr	1	tr	—
Morning Thunder (Celestial Seasonings)	8 fl oz	3	tr	1	tr	—
Naturally Decaffeinated (Celestial Seasonings)	8 fl oz	10	1	1	tr	—
Nestea Tea Bag, as prep	6 oz	0	0	0	0	—
Orange Pekoe (Bigelow)	5 fl oz	1	tr	tr	tr	—
Orange Spice (Celestial Seasonings)	8 fl oz	7	tr	1	1	—

FOOD	PORTION	CAL	FAT	SOD	CARB	FIB
Orange Spice Decaff (Celestial Seasonings)	8 fl oz	7	tr	1	1	—
Organically Grown (Celestial Seasonings)	8 fl oz	12	tr	1	1	—
Peppermint Stick (Bigelow)	5 fl oz	1	tr	1	tr	—
Plantation Mint (Bigelow)	5 fl oz	1	tr	1	tr	—
Raspberry (Celestial Seasonings)	8 fl oz	7	tr	1	1	—
Raspberry Royale (Bigelow)	5 fl oz	1	tr	tr	tr	—
brewed tea	6 oz	2	0	5	tr	—
instant unsweetened, as prep w/ water	8 oz	2	0	8	tr	—

TEFF
Whole Grain (Arrowhead)	¼ cup (1.6 oz)	160	1	5	32	6

TEMPEH
tempeh	½ cup	165	6	5	14	—

THYME
ground	1 tsp	4	tr	1	1	—

TILEFISH
FRESH
cooked	½ fillet (5.3 oz)	220	7	88	0	—
cooked	3 oz	125	4	50	0	—
raw	3 oz	81	2	45	0	—

TOFU
Azumaya Blue Label	3.5 oz	46	1	2	4	—
Azumaya Green Label	3.5 oz	68	2	2	4	—
Azumaya Name Age Fried	3.5 oz	144	4	2	9	—
Azumaya Red Label	3.5 oz	68	1	3	5	—
Jaclyn's Grilled In Black Bean Sauce	10.75 oz	270	8	170	45	—
Jaclyn's Grilled In Peanut Sauce	10.75 oz	260	9	145	44	—
Mori-Nu Silken Extra-Firm	½ box (5.25 oz)	90	3	95	4	—
Mori-Nu Silken Firm	½ box (5.25 oz)	90	4	50	4	—
Mori-Nu Silken Lite	1 in slice (3 oz)	35	1	70	1	—
Mori-Nu Silken Soft	½ box (5.25 oz)	80	4	10	4	—

FOOD	PORTION	CAL	FAT	SOD	CARB	FIB
Nasoya Extra Firm	⅛ block (3 oz)	90	5	10	1	0
Nasoya Firm	⅛ block (3 oz)	80	4	10	2	0
Nasoya Silken	⅛ block (3 oz)	50	2	10	2	0
Nasoya Soft	⅛ block (3 oz)	60	3	5	2	0
Spring Creek						
Baked Barbeque	2 oz	88	4	234	7	—
Baked Cajun	2 oz	87	4	228	5	—
Baked Teriyaki	2 oz	84	4	393	3	—
Great Balls Of Tofu!	2 (3 oz)	107	5	485	5	—
Tofu Salads Missing Egg	2 oz	49	14	167	6	—
Nigari Firm	4 oz	140	8	30	tr	3
Tofu Salads !Onion Dip	2 oz	46	14	155	6	—
Tofu Salads !Taco Dip	2 oz	46	14	175	6	—
firm	½ cup	183	11	17	5	2
firm	¼ block (3 oz)	118	7	11	3	1
fresh, fried	1 piece (½ oz)	35	3	2	1	tr
fuyu, salted & fermented	1 block (⅓ oz)	13	1	316	1	tr
koyadofu, dried, frozen	1 piece (½ oz)	82	5	1	2	tr
okara	½ cup	47	1	6	8	1
regular	½ cup	94	6	9	2	1
regular	¼ block (4 oz)	88	6	8	2	1
YOGURT						
Stir Fruity						
Black Cherry	6 oz	141	2	51	25	—
Blueberry	6 oz	140	1	43	26	—
Lemon Chiffon	6 oz	152	3	43	26	—
Mixed Berry	6 oz	149	2	34	26	—
Orange	6 oz	143	2	51	26	—
Peach	6 oz	160	3	34	27	—
Pina Colada	6 oz	162	3	43	28	—
Raspberry	6 oz	155	2	34	29	—
Spiced Apple	6 oz	167	2	43	31	—
Strawberry	6 oz	140	2	51	25	—
Tropical Fruit	6 oz	170	2	43	32	—

TOFUTTI
see ICE CREAM AND FROZEN DESSERTS

TOMATILLO
fresh	1 (1.2 oz)	11	tr	0	2	—
fresh, chopped	½ cup	21	1	1	4	—

FOOD	PORTION	CAL	FAT	SOD	CARB	FIB

TOMATO
see also PIZZA, SPAGHETTI SAUCE

CANNED

FOOD	PORTION	CAL	FAT	SOD	CARB	FIB
Claussen Kosher	1	9	tr	—	—	—
Contadina						
California Sliced	½ cup	40	tr	—	—	—
Crushed	¼ cup	20	0	150	4	1
Italian Paste	2 tbsp	40	1	320	7	1
Italian Style Pear	½ cup	25	0	220	4	1
Italian Style Stewed	½ cup	40	0	260	8	1
Mexican Style Stewed	½ cup	40	0	220	9	1
Pasta Ready Primavera	½ cup	50	2	600	8	1
Pasta Ready Tomatoes	½ cup	50	2	550	7	1
Pasta Ready With Crushed Red Pepper	½ cup	60	3	690	8	1
Pasta Ready With Mushrooms	½ cup	50	2	640	9	1
Pasta Ready With Olives	½ cup	60	3	640	8	1
Pasta Ready With Three Cheeses	½ cup	70	4	650	8	tr
Paste	2 tbsp	30	0	20	6	1
Peeled Whole	½ cup	25	0	220	4	1
Puree	¼ cup	20	0	15	4	tr
Recipe Ready	½ cup	25	0	200	5	3
Stewed	½ cup	40	0	250	9	1
Health Valley Sauce	1 cup	70	1	460	13	tr
Health Valley Sauce Low Sodium	1 cup	70	1	35	13	1
Hebrew National Pickled	⅓ tomato (1 oz)	4	0	280	1	—
Hunt's						
Crushed Angela Mia	4 oz	35	tr	260	7	tr
Crushed Italian	4 oz	40	tr	460	9	tr
Italian Pear Shaped	4 oz	20	tr	320	5	tr
Paste	2 oz	45	tr	135	11	2
Paste Italian Style	2 oz	50	tr	430	11	2
Paste No Salt Added	2 oz	45	tr	25	11	2
Paste With Garlic	2 oz	50	tr	440	11	2
Peeled Choice-Cut	4 oz	20	tr	460	5	1
Puree	4 oz	45	tr	150	10	2
Sauce	4 oz	30	tr	650	7	2

FOOD	PORTION	CAL	FAT	SOD	CARB	FIB
Sauce Herb	4 oz	70	2	470	12	2
Sauce Italian	4 oz	60	2	460	10	2
Sauce Meatloaf Fixin's	4 oz	20	tr	580	5	tr
Sauce No Salt Added	4 oz	35	tr	20	8	2
Sauce Special	4 oz	35	tr	280	8	2
Sauce With Bits	4 oz	30	tr	620	7	2
Sauce With Garlic	4 oz	70	2	480	10	2
Sauce With Mushrooms	4 oz	25	tr	710	6	2
Stewed	4 oz	35	tr	400	8	tr
Stewed Italian	4 oz	40	tr	370	9	tr
Stewed No Salt Added	4 oz	35	tr	20	8	tr
Whole	4 oz	20	tr	330	5	tr
Whole Italian	4 oz	25	tr	420	6	tr
Whole No Salt Added	4 oz	20	tr	15	5	tr
Rosoff's Pickled	⅓ tomato (1 oz)	5	0	290	1	—
S&W						
Aspic Supreme	½ cup	60	0	860	16	—
Diced In Rich Puree	½ cup	35	0	290	8	—
Italian Stewed Sliced	½ cup	35	0	355	9	—
Italian Style w/ Basil	½ cup	25	0	220	5	—
Mexican Style Stewed	½ cup	40	0	360	8	—
Paste	6 oz	150	0	100	35	—
Peeled Ready Cut	½ cup	25	0	220	6	—
Puree	½ cup	60	0	35	14	—
Sauce	½ cup	40	0	620	9	—
Sauce Chunky	½ cup	45	0	615	10	—
Stewed Sliced	½ cup	35	0	355	9	—
Stewed 50% Salt Reduced	½ cup	35	0	180	9	—
Whole Diet	½ cup	25	0	20	5	—
Whole Peeled	½ cup	25	0	220	6	—
Schorr's Pickled	⅓ tomato (1 oz)	4	0	280	1	—
paste	½ cup	110	1	86	25	6
puree	1 cup	102	tr	532	25	6
puree w/o salt	1 cup	102	tr	49	25	6
red whole	½ cup	24	tr	195	5	—
sauce	½ cup	37	tr	738	9	2
sauce spanish style	½ cup	40	tr	—	9	2
sauce w/ mushrooms	½ cup	42	tr	552	10	—

FOOD	PORTION	CAL	FAT	SOD	CARB	FIB
sauce w/ onion	½ cup	52	tr	672	12	—
stewed	½ cup	34	tr	325	8	—
w/ green chiles	½ cup	18	tr	481	4	—
wedges in tomato juice	½ cup	34	tr	285	8	—
dried						
sun dried	1 cup	140	2	1131	30	—
sun dried	1 piece	5	tr	42	1	—
sun dried in oil	1 cup (4 oz)	235	15	293	26	—
sun dried in oil	1 piece (3 g)	6	tr	8	1	—
FRESH						
cooked	½ cup	32	1	13	7	—
green	1	30	tr	16	6	—
red	1 (4.5 oz)	26	tr	11	6	2
red, chopped	1 cup	35	tr	16	8	2
JUICE						
Campbell	6 oz	40	0	540	8	—
Hunt's	6 oz	30	tr	520	7	2
Hunt's No Salt Added	6 oz	35	tr	25	8	2
Libby's	6 oz	35	0	450	35	—
Mott's Beefamato	6 oz	80	0	—	—	—
Mott's Clamato	6 oz	96	0	—	—	—
S&W California	6 oz	35	0	600	8	—
S&W Diet	½ cup	35	0	20	8	—
beef broth & tomato	5.5 oz	61	tr	220	14	—
clam & tomato	1 can (5.5 oz)	77	tr	664	18	—
tomato juice	½ cup	21	tr	441	5	—
tomato juice	6 oz	32	tr	658	8	—
TAKE-OUT						
stewed	1 cup	80	3	460	13	—

TONGUE

FOOD	PORTION	CAL	FAT	SOD	CARB	FIB
beef, simmered	3 oz	241	18	51	tr	—
lamb, braised	3 oz	234	17	57	0	—
pork, braised	3 oz	230	16	93	0	—

TOPPINGS

see ICE CREAM TOPPINGS

TORTILLA CHIPS

see CHIPS

TREE FERN

FOOD	PORTION	CAL	FAT	SOD	CARB	FIB
chopped, cooked	½ cup	28	tr	3	8	—

TRITICALE

see also FLOUR

FOOD	PORTION	CAL	FAT	SOD	CARB	FIB
dry	½ cup	323	2	5	69	17

FOOD	PORTION	CAL	FAT	SOD	CARB	FIB
TROUT						
FRESH						
Rainbow Clear Springs	3.5 oz	140	7	35	tr	—
baked	3 oz	162	7	57	0	—
rainbow, cooked	3 oz	129	4	29	0	—
seatrout, baked	3 oz	113	4	63	0	—
TRUFFLES						
fresh	3.5 oz	25	1	77	17	—
TUNA						
see also TUNA DISHES						
CANNED						
Bumble Bee						
Chunk Light In Water	2 oz	60	1	250	0	—
Chunk Light In Oil	2 oz	160	12	250	0	—
Chunk White In Oil	2 oz	160	12	250	0	—
Chunk White In Water	2 oz	70	2	250	0	—
Chunk White In Water Bumble Bee	2 oz	60	1	30	0	—
Solid White In Oil	2 oz	130	8	250	0	—
Solid White In Water	2 oz	70	2	250	0	—
Empress Chunk Light	2 oz	60	1	310	0	—
Empress Chunk Light Tongol	2 oz	50	1	55	0	—
Empress Solid White	2 oz	70	2	310	0	—
Progresso	⅓ cup	150	13	400	tr	—
S&W Chunk Light Fancy In Oil	2 oz	140	10	450	0	—
S&W Chunk Light Fancy In Water	2 oz	60	1	500	0	—
S&W Fancy White Albacore in Oil	2 oz	160	12	450	0	—
light in oil	1 can (6 oz)	399	14	606	0	—
light in oil	3 oz	169	7	301	0	—
light in water	1 can (5.8 oz)	192	1	558	0	—
light in water	3 oz	99	1	287	0	—
white in oil	1 can (6.2 oz)	331	14	704	0	—
white in oil	3 oz	158	7	336	0	—
white in water	1 can (6 oz)	234	4	673	0	—
white in water	3 oz	116	2	333	0	—
FRESH						
bluefin, cooked	3 oz	157	5	43	0	—

FOOD	PORTION	CAL	FAT	SOD	CARB	FIB
bluefin, raw	3 oz	122	4	33	0	—
skipjack, baked	3 oz	112	1	40	0	—
yellowfin, baked	3 oz	118	1	40	0	—

TUNA DISHES
FROZEN

FOOD	PORTION	CAL	FAT	SOD	CARB	FIB
Microwave Tuna Sandwich (Mrs. Paul's)	1	200	6	590	23	—
Tuna Melt (Chefwich)	5 oz	360	14	—	—	—
MIX						
Bumble Bee Tuna Mix-ins Classic Italian	⅓ pkg (0.17 oz)	25	0	5	5	—
Bumble Bee Tuna Mix-ins Garden & Herb	⅓ pkg (0.17 oz)	25	0	5	5	—
Bumble Bee Tuna Mix-ins Lemon Herb	⅓ pkg (0.17 oz)	25	0	5	6	—
Bumble Bee Tuna Mix-ins Zesty Tomato	⅓ pkg (0.17 oz)	25	0	5	5	—
Tuna Helper						
Au Gratin, as prep	⅕ pkg (6 oz)	280	11	980	30	—
Buttery Rice, as prep	⅕ pkg (6 oz)	280	11	1040	32	—
Cheesy Noodles, as prep	⅕ pkg (7.75 oz)	240	8	980	27	—
Creamy Mushroom, as prep	⅕ pkg (7 oz)	220	6	740	29	—
Creamy Noodles, as prep	⅕ pkg (8 oz)	300	14	960	29	—
Fettucine Alfredo, as prep	⅕ pkg (7 oz)	300	13	1000	30	—
Romanoff, as prep	⅕ pkg (8 oz)	290	8	820	38	—
Tetrazzini, as prep	⅕ pkg (6 oz)	240	8	780	27	—
Tuna Pot Pie, as prep	⅙ pkg (5.1 oz)	420	27	890	31	—
Tuna Salad, as prep	⅕ pkg (5.5 oz)	420	27	870	29	—
READY-TO-USE						
Salad (Wampler Longacre)	1 oz	61	13	—	—	—
Tuna Salad (The Spreadables)	¼ can	90	6	—	—	—
TAKE-OUT						
tuna salad	1 cup	383	19	824	19	—
tuna salad	3 oz	159	8	342	8	—

FOOD	PORTION	CAL	FAT	SOD	CARB	FIB
tuna salad submarine sandwich w/ lettuce & oil	1	584	28	1294	55	—

TURBOT
FRESH

european, baked	3 oz	104	3	163	0	—

TURKEY
see also DINNER, HOT DOG, TURKEY DISHES, TURKEY SUBSTITUTES

CANNED

Chunky Light (Underwood)	2.08 oz	75	2	330	2	—
White (Swanson)	2.5 oz	80	1	260	1	—
w/ broth	1 can (5 oz)	231	10	663	0	—
w/ broth	½ can (2.5 oz)	116	5	332	0	—

FRESH

Bil Mar Foods Ground	3 oz	163	12	—	—	—
Breast Tenderloins Skinless & Boneless, cooked (Perdue)	1 oz	29	tr	12	0	—
Breast Cutlets Thin-Sliced Skinless & Boneless (Perdue)	1 oz	28	tr	13	0	—
Breast Fillets Skinless & Boneless Fit 'n Easy, cooked (Perdue)	1 oz	28	tr	13	0	—
Breast Hotel Style Prime w/ Skin, cooked (Perdue)	1 oz	43	2	12	0	—
Breast Prime Young (Shady Brook)	3 oz	140	7	—	—	—
Breast Skinless Boneless Fit 'n Easy, cooked (Perdue)	1 oz	28	tr	13	0	—
Breast w/ Skin Fresh Young, cooked (Perdue)	1 oz	44	2	14	0	—
Drumsticks w/ Skin Fresh Young, cooked (Perdue)	1 oz	36	2	19	0	—
Ground (Louis Rich)	3 oz	140	9	105	0	0

FOOD	PORTION	CAL	FAT	SOD	CARB	FIB
Ground All White Meat (Butterball)	3 oz	100	3	55	tr	—
Ground All White (Swift-Eckrich)	3 oz	100	3	55	tr	—
Ground Breast Meat, cooked (Perdue)	1 oz	28	tr	13	0	—
Ground, cooked (Perdue)	1 oz	35	2	17	0	—
Thighs Skinless & Boneless Fit 'n Fresh, cooked (Perdue)	1 oz	36	2	15	0	—
Thighs w/ Skin Fresh Young, cooked (Perdue)	1 oz	48	3	20	0	—
Whole Dark Meat w/ skin, cooked (Perdue)	1 oz	48	3	18	0	—
Whole White Meat Fresh Young w/ skin, cooked (Perdue)	1 oz	44	2	13	0	—
Wings (Shady Brook)	3 oz	130	6	—	—	—
Wings Drummettes w/ Skin Fresh Young, cooked (Perdue)	1 oz	43	2	18	0	—
Wings Portions w/ Skin Fresh Young, cooked (Perdue)	1 oz	51	3	18	0	—
Wings w/ Skin Fresh Young, cooked (Perdue)	1 oz	45	2	20	0	—
back w/ skin, roasted	½ back (9 oz)	637	38	191	0	—
breast w/ skin, roasted	4 oz	212	8	70	0	—
dark meat w/ skin, roasted	3.6 oz	230	12	79	0	—
dark meat w/o skin, roasted	1 cup (5 oz)	262	10	110	0	—
dark meat w/o skin, roasted	3 oz	170	7	72	0	—
ground, cooked	3 oz	188	11	68	0	—
leg w/ skin, roasted	1 (1.2 lbs)	1133	54	420	0	—
leg w/ skin, roasted	2.5 oz	147	7	55	0	—
light meat w/ skin, roasted	4.7 oz	268	11	85	0	—
light meat w/ skin, roasted	from ½ turkey (2.3 lbs)	2069	87	658	0	—
light meat w/o skin, roasted	4 oz	183	4	75	0	—
neck, simmered	1 (5.3 oz)	274	11	84	0	—

FOOD	PORTION	CAL	FAT	SOD	CARB	FIB
skin, roasted	1 oz	141	13	17	0	—
skin, roasted	from ½ turkey (9 oz)	1096	98	132	0	—
w/ skin, neck & giblets, roasted	½ turkey (8.8 lbs)	4123	190	1358	1	—
w/ skin, roasted	½ turkey (4 lbs)	3857	181	1269	0	—
w/ skin, roasted	8.4 oz	498	23	164	0	—
w/o skin, roasted	1 cup (5 oz)	238	7	99	0	—
w/o skin, roasted	7.3 oz	354	10	147	0	—
wing w/ skin, roasted	1 (6.5 oz)	426	23	114	0	—
FROZEN						
Tyson Breast Boneless Skinless	3.5 oz	160	3	65	0	—
roast boneless seasoned light & dark meat, roasted	1 pkg (1.7 lbs)	1213	45	5320	24	—
READY-TO-USE						
Bil Mar Foods						
Breast	1 slice (1 oz)	31	tr	—	—	—
Buffet Style Smoked Ham	1 oz	32	1	—	—	—
Cheese Patties	3 oz	213	13	—	—	—
Ham Smoked	1 oz	32	1	—	—	—
Ham Square Chopped	1 slice (1 oz)	37	2	—	—	—
Luncheon Loaf Square Spiced	1 slice (1 oz)	51	4	—	—	—
Smoked Breast	1 oz	31	tr	—	—	—
Smoked Sliced Breast	1 oz	31	tr	—	—	—
Carl Buddig	1 oz	50	3	340	1	0
Carl Buddig Honey Turkey	1 oz	40	2	360	1	—
Carl Buddig Turkey Ham	1 oz	40	2	430	1	0
Deli Chef Breast & White	1 oz	39	6	—	—	—
Falls BBQ	3 oz	140	8	300	—	—
Falls Gourmet Breast	3 oz	80	1	320	—	—
Falls Premium Breast Cooked	3 oz	100	2	240	—	—
Hansel 'n Gretel						
Doubledecker Turkey-Corned Beef	1 oz	30	1	195	1	—
Doubledecker Turkey-Ham	1 oz	30	1	185	1	—

FOOD	PORTION	CAL	FAT	SOD	CARB	FIB
Hansel 'n Gretel *(cont.)*						
Gourmet Breast	1 oz	28	1	170	1	—
Gourmet Smoked Breast	1 oz	31	1	170	tr	—
Honey Breast	1 oz	28	1	170	1	—
Lessalt Cooked Breast	1 oz	25	1	140	tr	—
Oven Cooked Breast	1 oz	26	tr	180	tr	—
Healthy Choice Breast Skinless Honey Roasted & Smoked	1 oz	30	tr	220	1	—
Healthy Choice Breast Skinless Oven Roasted	1 oz	25	tr	230	tr	—
Healthy Choice Breast Skinless Smoked	1 oz	25	tr	240	tr	—
Hebrew National Deli Thin Hickory Smoked National	1.8 oz	55	1	310	—	—
Hebrew National Deli Thin Lemon Garlic National	1.8 oz	50	1	400	—	—
Hebrew National Deli Thin Oven Roasted National	1.8 oz	80	1	420	—	—
Hillshire						
Breast Honey Cured	1 oz	35	1	340	2	—
Breast Smoked	1 oz	35	1	340	1	—
Deli Select Breast Honey Roasted	1 slice	10	tr	90	tr	—
Deli Select Breast Oven Roasted	1 slice	10	tr	105	tr	—
Deli Select Breast Smoked	1 slice	10	tr	100	tr	—
Deli Select Turkey Ham	1 slice	10	tr	95	tr	—
Flavor Pack 90–99% Fat Free Breast Honey Roasted	1 slice (0.75 oz)	20	tr	200	1	—
Flavor Pack 90–99% Fat Free Breast Oven Roasted	1 slice (0.75 oz)	20	tr	230	1	—
Flavor Pack 90–99% Fat Free Breast Smoked	1 slice (0.75 oz)	20	tr	220	tr	—

FOOD	PORTION	CAL	FAT	SOD	CARB	FIB
Louis Rich						
Bologna	1 slice (28 g)	50	4	250	1	0
Breaded Nuggets	4 (3.2 oz)	260	15	640	15	0
Breaded Patties	1 (3 oz)	220	13	550	13	0
Breaded Sticks	3 (3 oz)	230	15	580	12	0
Breast Honey Roasted	1 slice (1 oz)	30	1	320	1	0
Breast Oven Roasted	1 slice (1 oz)	30	1	310	1	0
Breast Oven Roasted	2 oz	60	2	640	2	0
Breast Smoked	1 slice (1 oz)	25	1	260	0	0
Carving Board Breast Oven Roasted	2 slices (1.6 oz)	40	1	560	0	0
Carving Board Breast Oven Roasted Thin Carved	6 slices (2.1 oz)	60	1	740	0	0
Carving Board Breast Smoked	2 slices (1.6 oz)	40	1	560	0	0
Chopped Ham	1 slice (1 oz)	46	3	290	0	0
Cotto Salami	1 slice (28 g)	40	3	290	0	0
Deli-Thin Breast Oven Roasted	4 slices (1.8 oz)	50	1	580	2	0
Deli-Thin Breast Smoked	4 slices (1.8 oz)	50	1	490	1	0
Dinner Slices Breast Hickory Smoked	1 slice (2.8 oz)	80	1	1060	2	0
Dinner Slices Breast Honey Roasted	1 slice (2.8 oz)	80	1	940	3	0
Dinner Slices Breast Oven Roasted	1 slice (2.8 oz)	70	1	910	1	0
Fat Free Breast Hickory Smoked	1 slice (1 oz)	25	0	300	1	0
Fat Free Breast Oven Roasted	1 slice (28 g)	25	0	310	1	0
Ham	4 slices (1.8 oz)	60	2	580	0	0
Ham Round	1 slice (28 g)	34	1	300	0	0
Ham Square	3 slices (2.2 oz)	70	3	710	1	0
Honey Cured Ham	3 slices (2.2 oz)	70	2	660	2	0
Pastrami	2 slices (1.6 oz)	45	2	520	0	0
Salami	1 slice (28 g)	45	3	290	0	0
Skinless Breast Barbecued	2 oz	60	1	680	2	0
Skinless Breast Hickory Smoked	2 oz	60	1	760	1	0
Skinless Breast Honey Roasted	2 oz	60	1	690	2	0

FOOD	PORTION	CAL	FAT	SOD	CARB	FIB
Louis Rich *(cont.)*						
Skinless Breast Oven Roasted	2 oz	50	1	650	1	0
White Smoked	1 slice (1 oz)	30	1	290	0	0
Mr. Turkey						
BBQ Breast Quarter	1 oz	34	1	—	—	—
Bologna	1 oz	63	5	—	—	—
Bologna Red Rind	1 oz	63	5	—	—	—
Breakfast Smoked Ham	1 oz	33	1	—	—	—
Cotto Salami	1 oz	45	3	—	—	—
Diced White Meat	2 oz	84	2	—	—	—
Nuggets	1 nugget	33	2	—	—	—
Oven Roasted Quarter Breast	1 oz	34	1	—	—	—
Patties	3 oz	195	11	—	—	—
Smoked Breast Quarter	1 oz	35	1	—	—	—
Sticks	1 stick	65	4	—	—	—
Oscar Mayer Breast Roast Thin Sliced	1 slice (.4 oz)	12	tr	151	tr	—
Oscar Mayer Oven Roasted Breast	1 slice (¾ oz)	23	1	290	1	—
Oscar Mayer Smoked Breast	1 slice (¾ oz)	20	tr	300	tr	—
Perdue Done It! Nuggets	1 (.67 oz)	54	3	112	3	—
Tyson Breast	1 slice	20	tr	136	tr	—
Tyson Ham	1 slice	23	tr	182	1	—
Wampler Longacre Baked Ham	1 oz	38	6	—	—	—
Wampler Longacre						
Baked Ham w/ 12% Water	1 oz	33	5	—	—	—
Baked Ham w/ 20% Water	1 oz	39	6	—	—	—
Bologna	1 oz	56	16	—	—	—
Breaded Nuggets	1 oz	87	20	—	—	—
Chunk Ham w/ 12% Water	1 oz	36	6	—	—	—
Chunk Ham w/ 20% Water	1 oz	39	6	—	—	—
Chunk Pastrami	1 oz	35	5	—	—	—
Combination Roll	1 oz	43	10	—	—	—
Dark Smoked Cured	1 oz	45	10	—	—	—

FOOD	PORTION	CAL	FAT	SOD	CARB	FIB
Diced Combination Roll	1 oz	43	10	—	—	—
Diced Ham w/ 20% Water	1 oz	39	6	—	—	—
Diced White Roll	1 oz	43	10	—	—	—
Gourmet Breast	1 oz	31	2	—	—	—
Gourmet Brown & Glazed Breast	1 oz	28	2	—	—	—
Gourmet Brown & Roasted Breast	1 oz	35	3	—	—	—
Gourmet High Yield Skinless Breast	1 oz	28	tr	—	—	—
Gourmet Mini Breast	1 oz	35	4	—	—	—
Gourmet Skinless Brown & Roasted Breast	1 oz	31	1	—	—	—
Gourmet Smoked Breast	1 oz	37	3	—	—	—
Ham w/ 20% Water	1 oz	39	6	—	—	—
Lean-Lite Ham	1 oz	36	5	—	—	—
Lean-Lite Smoked Breast	1 oz	38	4	—	—	—
Mini Gourmet Smoked Breast	1 oz	37	3	—	—	—
Oven Roasted Oven Lite Breast	1 oz	35	3	—	—	—
Pastrami	1 oz	35	5	—	—	—
Premium Breast	1 oz	29	2	—	—	—
Premium Brown & Glazed Breast	1 oz	29	2	—	—	—
Premium Skinless Breast	1 oz	28	tr	—	—	—
Premium Skinless Brown & Roasted Breast	1 oz	26	1	—	—	—
Roasted Thighs	1 oz	38	6	—	—	—
Roll Sliced Breast	1 oz	37	5	—	—	—
Roll White	1 oz	43	10	—	—	—
Salami	1 oz	45	8	—	—	—
Salt Watchers Breast	1 oz	35	tr	—	—	—
Sliced Bologna	1 oz	57	16	—	—	—
Sliced Ham	1 oz	37	5	—	—	—
Sliced Pastrami	1 oz	34	5	—	—	—
Sliced Salami	1 oz	46	9	—	—	—
Smoked Sliced Breast	1 oz	27	tr	—	—	—
Smoked Whole	1 oz	40	4	—	—	—

FOOD	PORTION	CAL	FAT	SOD	CARB	FIB
Wampler Longacre *(cont.)*						
Turkey Deli Chef Breast & White	1 oz	35	5	—	—	—
Turkey No Skin Covering Breast & White	1 oz	39	5	—	—	—
Weight Watchers Deli Thin Smoked Breast	5 slices (⅛ oz)	10	tr	80	tr	—
Weight Watchers Oven Roasted Breast	2 slices (¾ oz)	25	1	200	tr	—
Weight Watchers Oven Roasted Turkey Ham	2 slices (¾ oz)	25	1	210	tr	—
Weight Watchers Roasted And Smoked Breast	2 slices (¾ oz)	25	1	170	tr	—
bologna	1 oz	57	4	249	tr	—
breast	1 slice (¾ oz)	23	tr	301	0	—
diced light & dark, seasoned	1 oz	39	2	241	tr	—
diced light & dark, seasoned	½ lb	313	14	1928	2	—
ham thigh meat	1 pkg (8 oz)	291	12	2260	1	—
ham thigh meat	2 oz	73	3	565	tr	—
pastrami	1 pkg (8 oz)	320	14	2372	4	—
pastrami	2 oz	80	4	698	1	—
patties, battered & fried	1 (2.3 oz)	181	12	512	10	—
patties, battered & fried	1 (3.3 oz)	266	17	752	15	—
patties, breaded & fried	1 (2.3 oz)	181	12	512	10	—
patties, breaded & fried	1 (3.3 oz)	266	17	752	15	—
poultry salad sandwich spread	1 oz	238	4	107	2	—
poultry salad sandwich spread	1 tbsp	109	2	49	1	—
prebasted breast w/ skin, roasted	1 breast (3.8 lbs)	2175	60	6868	0	—
prebasted breast w/ skin, roasted	½ breast (1.9 lbs)	1087	30	3434	0	—
prebasted thigh w/ skin, roasted	1 thigh (11 oz)	494	27	1371	0	—
roll light & dark meat	1 oz	42	2	166	1	—
roll light meat	1 oz	42	2	139	2	—
salami, cooked	1 pkg (8 oz)	446	31	2278	1	—

FOOD	PORTION	CAL	FAT	SOD	CARB	FIB
salami, cooked	2 oz	111	8	569	tr	—
turkey loaf breast meat	1 pkg (6 oz)	187	3	2433	0	—
turkey loaf breast meat	2 slices (1.5 oz)	47	1	608	0	—
turkey sticks, battered & fried	1 stick (2.3 oz)	178	11	536	11	—
turkey sticks, breaded & fried	1 stick (2.3 oz)	178	11	536	11	—

TURKEY DISHES
see also DINNER, TURKEY SUBSTITUTES

FROZEN

Banquet Family Entrees Gravy & Sliced Turkey	6 oz	120	6	—	6	—
Kibun Turkey Pasta Salad w/ dressing	½ pkg	250	12	—	—	—
Kibun Turkey Pasta Salad w/o dressing	½ pkg	140	2	—	—	—
Ovenstuffs Turkey Turnover	1 (4.75 oz)	350	16	700	35	—
gravy & turkey	1 cup (8.4 oz)	160	6	1328	11	—
gravy & turkey	1 pkg (5 oz)	95	4	786	7	—

READY-TO-USE

Salad (Wampler Longacre)	1 oz	71	17	—	—	—
The Spreadables Turkey Salad	¼ can	100	6	—	—	—

TURKEY SUBSTITUTES

Harvest Direct TVP Poultry Chunks	3.5 oz	280	1	15	32	18
Harvest Direct TVP Poultry Ground	3.5 oz	280	1	15	32	18
Worthington Smoked Turkey Slices	4 slices (76 g)	180	12	820	5	—
Worthington Turkee Slices	2 slices (63 g)	130	9	430	3	—

TURMERIC

ground	1 tsp	8	tr	1	1	—

TURNIPS
CANNED

Turnip Greens w/ Diced Turnips Seasoned w/ Pork (Luck's)	7.5 oz	90	6	—	—	—
greens	½ cup	17	tr	325	3	—

FOOD	PORTION	CAL	FAT	SOD	CARB	FIB
FRESH						
cooked, mashed	½ cup (4.2 oz)	47	tr	25	10	—
cubed, cooked	½ cup (3 oz)	33	tr	17	7	—
greens, chopped, cooked	½ cup	15	tr	21	3	2
greens, raw, chopped	½ cup	7	tr	11	2	1
raw, cubed	½ cup (2.4 oz)	25	tr	14	6	—
FROZEN						
Mashed (Southland)	3.6 oz	90	6	—	—	—
Rutabaga-Yellow Turnips (Southland)	4 oz	50	0	—	—	—
greens, cooked	½ cup	24	tr	12	4	2
TURTLE						
raw	3.5 oz	85	1	—	0	—
TUSK FISH						
raw	3.5 oz	79	tr	113	0	—
VANILLA						
Vanilla Milk Chips (Hershey)	¼ cup	240	14	65	25	—
Virginia Dare Vanilla Extract	1 tsp	10	0	—	—	—
VEAL						
see also BEEF, DINNER, VEAL DISHES						
FRESH						
cutlet lean only, braised	3 oz	172	4	57	0	—
cutlet lean only, fried	3 oz	156	4	65	0	—
ground, broiled	3 oz	146	6	70	0	—
loin chop w/ bone lean & fat, braised	1 chop (2.8 oz)	227	14	64	0	—
loin chop w/ bone lean only, braised	1 chop (2.4 oz)	155	6	58	0	—
shoulder w/ bone lean only, braised	3 oz	169	5	83	0	—
sirloin w/ bone lean & fat, roasted	3 oz	171	9	71	0	—
sirloin w/ bone lean only, roasted	3 oz	143	5	72	0	—
VEAL DISHES						
TAKE-OUT						
parmigiana	4.2 oz	279	18	545	6	2

FOOD	PORTION	CAL	FAT	SOD	CARB	FIB

VEGETABLES MIXED
see also individual vegetables

CANNED

FOOD	PORTION	CAL	FAT	SOD	CARB	FIB
Chop Suey Vegetables (La Choy)	½ cup	10	tr	320	2	tr
Cut Tomatoes & Corn (Trappey's)	½ cup	25	0	—	—	—
Garden Medley (Green Giant)	½ cup	40	tr	290	9	1
Garden Salad Marinated (S&W)	½ cup	60	0	670	11	—
Mixed (Hanover)	½ cup	110	0	—	—	—
Mixed Vegetables (Libby)	½ cup	40	0	—	—	—
Mixed Vegetables (Seneca)	½ cup	40	0	—	—	—
Mixed Vegetables Old Fashion Harvest Time (S&W)	½ cup	35	0	380	6	—
Peas & Carrots (Libby)	½ cup	50	0	—	—	—
Peas & Carrots (Seneca)	½ cup	50	0	—	—	—
Peas & Carrots Water Pack (S&W)	½ cup	35	0	5	7	—
Succotash (Libby)	½ cup	80	1	—	—	—
Succotash (Seneca)	½ cup	80	1	—	—	—
Succotash Country Style (S&W)	½ cup	80	1	250	16	—
Sweet Peas & Diced Carrots (S&W)	½ cup	50	0	310	9	—
Sweet Peas w/ Tiny Pearl Onions (S&W)	½ cup	60	1	490	10	—
Vegetable Salad (Hanover)	½ cup	90	0	—	—	—
mixed vegetables	½ cup	39	tr	122	8	—
peas & carrots	½ cup	48	tr	332	11	—
peas & carrots low sodium	½ cup	48	tr	332	11	—
peas & onions	½ cup	30	tr	265	5	—
succotash	½ cup	102	1	325	23	—

FROZEN

American Mixtures (Green Giant)

FOOD	PORTION	CAL	FAT	SOD	CARB	FIB
California	½ cup	25	0	40	6	2

FOOD	PORTION	CAL	FAT	SOD	CARB	FIB
American Mixtures *(cont.)*						
Heartland	½ cup	25	0	35	6	2
New England	½ cup	70	1	75	14	4
San Francisco	½ cup	25	0	35	7	2
Sante Fe	½ cup	70	1	0	16	2
Seattle	½ cup	25	0	35	7	2
Breaded Medley (Ore-Ida)	3 oz	160	9	490	16	—
Broccoli, Cauliflower And Carrots In Butter Sauce (Green Giant)	½ cup	30	1	240	4	—
Broccoli, Cauliflower And Carrots In Cheese Sauce (Green Giant)	½ cup	60	2	490	9	2
Broccoli, Cauliflower And Carrots With Cheese Sauce (Birds Eye)	½ pkg	80	4	390	7	4
Broccoli Cut & Cauliflower Cut (Hanover)	½ cup	20	0	—	—	—
California Florentine Blend (Big Valley)	3.5 oz	25	0	20	6	—
Caribbean Blend (Hanover)	½ cup	20	0	—	—	—
Farm Fresh Broccoli Cauliflower And Carrots (Birds Eye)	¾ cup	35	0	40	7	3
Farm Fresh (Birds Eye)						
Broccoli And Cauliflower	¾ cup	30	0	25	5	3
Broccoli, Carrots And Water Chestnuts	¾ cup	40	0	35	8	3
Broccoli, Cauliflower And Red Peppers	¾ cup	30	0	25	5	3
Broccoli, Corn And Red Peppers	⅔ cup	60	1	15	14	3
Broccoli, Green Beans, Pearl Onions and Red Peppers	¾ cup	35	0	15	7	3
Broccoli, Red Peppers, Onions And Mushrooms	¾ cup	30	0	20	6	3
Brussels Sprouts Cauliflower And Carrots	¾ cup	40	0	30	8	4
Cauliflower, Carrots And Snow Peas	⅔ cup	35	0	30	8	4

FOOD	PORTION	CAL	FAT	SOD	CARB	FIB
Garden Medley (Hanover)	½ cup	20	0	—	—	—
Harvest Fresh Mixed Vegetables (Green Giant)	½ cup	40	0	125	9	2
In Butter Sauce Broccoli, Cauliflower And Carrots (Birds Eye)	½ cup	40	2	180	6	2
In Sauce Peas And Pearl Onions With Seasonings (Birds Eye)	½ cup	70	0	440	13	3
Internationals (Birds Eye)						
Austrian	3.3 oz	70	3	390	6	1
Bavarian	3.3 oz	90	5	260	11	2
California	3.3 oz	90	4	200	10	3
French Country	3.3 oz	70	4	230	6	2
Japanese	3.3 oz	60	3	270	6	2
Italian	3.3 oz	80	5	250	8	2
New England	3.3 oz	100	5	280	12	2
Mandarin Vegetables (Budget Gourmet)	1 pkg (5.25 oz)	160	11	440	13	—
Mixed (Birds Eye)	½ cup	60	0	40	13	2
Mixed (Green Giant)	½ cup	40	0	40	9	2
Mixed (Hanover)	½ cup	50	0	—	—	—
Mixed Fancy (La Choy)	½ cup	12	tr	30	2	1
Mixed in Butter Sauce (Green Giant)	½ cup	60	2	300	11	2
New England Recipe Vegetables (Budget Gourmet)	1 pkg (5.5 oz)	230	13	380	21	—
One Serve Broccoli, Carrots & Rotini In Cheese Sauce (Green Giant)	1 pkg	120	3	520	20	—
One Serve Broccoli, Cauliflower and Carrots (Green Giant)	1 pkg	25	0	45	7	3
Oriental Blend (Hanover)	½ cup	25	0	—	—	—
Peas And Potatoes With Cream Sauce (Birds Eye)	½ cup	100	3	420	16	1
Peppers & Onions (Southland)	2 oz	15	0	—	—	—
Polybag (Birds Eye)	½ cup	60	0	40	12	2

FOOD	PORTION	CAL	FAT	SOD	CARB	FIB
Soup Mix Vegetables (Southland)	3.2 oz	50	0	—	—	—
Spring Vegetables In Cheese Sauce (Budget Gourmet)	1 pkg (5 oz)	130	8	370	9	—
Stew Vegetables (Ore-Ida)	3 oz	50	tr	35	11	—
Stew Vegetables (Southland)	4 oz	60	0	—	—	—
Succotash (Hanover)	½ cup	80	0	—	—	—
Summer Vegetables (Hanover)	½ cup	35	0	—	—	—
Valley Combinations Broccoli & Cauliflower (Green Giant)	½ cup	60	2	340	9	—
Vegetables For Soup (Hanover)	½ cup	60	0	—	—	—
mixed vegetables, cooked	½ cup	54	tr	32	12	2
peas & carrots, cooked	½ cup	38	tr	55	8	—
peas & onions, cooked	½ cup	40	tr	—	8	—
succotash, cooked	½ cup	79	1	38	17	—
HOME RECIPE						
succotash	½ cup	111	1	16	23	—
JUICE						
Smucker's Vegetable Juice Hearty	8 oz	58	tr	714	13	—
Smucker's Vegetable Juice Hot & Spicy	8 oz	58	tr	650	13	—
V8	6 oz	35	0	560	8	—
V8 No Salt Added	6 oz	35	0	45	8	—
V8 Spicy Hot	6 oz	35	0	650	8	—
vegetable juice cocktail	½ cup	22	tr	442	6	—
vegetable juice cocktail	6 oz	34	tr	664	8	—
SHELF STABLE						
Corn, Green Beans, Carrots, Pasta In Tomato Sauce (Pantry Express)	½ cup	80	2	330	17	3
Green Beans, Potatoes And Mushrooms In A Seasoned Sauce (Pantry Express)	½ cup	50	2	430	9	2
Mixed Vegetables (Pantry Express)	½ cup	35	tr	300	8	1

FOOD	PORTION	CAL	FAT	SOD	CARB	FIB
TAKE-OUT						
caponata	¼ cup	28	1	—	—	—
curry	1 serv (7.7 oz)	398	33	—	22	—
pakoras	1 (2 oz)	108	5	—	12	3
ratatouille	8.8 oz	190	16	—	10	5
samosa	2 (4 oz)	519	46	—	25	3
VENISON						
Antelope Chili Meat (Broken Arrow Ranch)	3.5 oz	115	2	76	1	—
Antelope Ground Venison (Broken Arrow Ranch)	3.5 oz	110	2	69	tr	—
Antelope Stew Meat (Broken Arrow Ranch)	3.5 oz	110	2	54	2	—
Nilgai Chili Meat (Broken Arrow Ranch)	3.5 oz	115	2	76	1	—
Nilgai Leg (Broken Arrow Ranch)	3.5 oz	100	1	55	1	—
Nilgai Stew Meat (Broken Arrow Ranch)	3.5 oz	110	2	54	2	—
Venison & Beef Smoked Sausage (Broken Arrow Ranch)	6 oz	432	30	—	4	—
Venison Meat Chunks (Broken Arrow Ranch)	6 oz	175	2	—	0	—
Venison Salami (Broken Arrow Ranch)	6 oz	252	8	—	0	—
roasted	3 oz	134	3	46	0	—
VINEGAR						
Apple Cider (White House)	2 tbsp	2	0	0	1	0
Cider (Hain)	1 tbsp	2	0	1	4	—
Red Wine (Regina)	1 oz	4	0	0	0	—
Red Wine (White House)	2 tbsp	4	0	5	2	—
Rice (Nakano)	1 tbsp	0	0	1	0	—
cider	1 tbsp	tr	0	tr	1	—
WAFFLES						
FROZEN						
Apple Cinnamon (Aunt Jemima)	2.5 oz	176	6	616	29	2

FOOD	PORTION	CAL	FAT	SOD	CARB	FIB
Apple Cinnamon (Eggo)	1	130	5	250	18	0
Belgian (Weight Watchers)	1 (1.5 oz)	120	4	220	17	—
Belgian Chef	1	90	2	—	—	—
Belgian Waffles And Sausage (Great Starts)	2.85 oz	280	19	420	21	—
Belgian Waffles Strawberries And Sausage (Great Starts)	3.5 oz	210	8	240	31	—
Blueberry (Aunt Jemima)	2.5 oz	175	5	684	29	1
Blueberry (Downyflake)	2	180	4	570	32	—
Blueberry (Eggo)	1	130	5	250	18	0
Blueberry Batter, as prep (Aunt Jemima)	3.6 oz	204	4	688	39	2
Buttermilk (Aunt Jemima)	2.5 oz	179	6	615	29	1
Buttermilk (Downyflake)	2	190	5	750	32	—
Buttermilk (Eggo)	1	130	5	250	16	0
Homestyle (Eggo)	1	130	5	250	16	0
Hot-N-Buttery (Downyflake)	2	180	6	620	27	—
Minis (Eggo)	4	90	3	190	14	0
Multi-Bran (Nutri-Grain)	1	120	5	220	17	3
Multi-Grain (Downyflake)	2	250	14	500	28	4
Multi-Grain Belgian (Weight Watchers)	1 (1.5 oz)	120	4	200	16	—
Nut And Honey (Eggo)	1	130	5	250	17	0
Oat Bran (Common Sense)	1	110	4	220	16	2
Oat Bran (Downyflake)	2	260	13	650	30	3
Oat Bran With Fruit And Nut (Common Sense)	1	120	5	220	17	2
Original (Aunt Jemima)	2.5 oz	173	6	591	28	2
Plain (Nutri-Grain)	1	120	5	250	18	2
Raisin And Bran (Nutri-Grain)	1	120	5	250	18	2
Regular (Downyflake)	2	120	3	420	20	—
Regular Jumbo (Downyflake)	2	170	4	570	30	—
Rice Bran (Downyflake)	2	210	11	230	25	4
Roman Meal (Downyflake)	2	280	14	680	33	3

FOOD	PORTION	CAL	FAT	SOD	CARB	FIB
Special K (Kellogg's)	1	80	0	120	16	0
Strawberry (Eggo)	1	130	5	250	18	0
Waffle (Kid Cuisine)	3.6 oz	160	3	340	27	—
Waffle With Bacon (Great Starts)	2.2 oz	230	14	710	19	—
Wholegrain Wheat/Oat Bran (Aunt Jemima)	2.5 oz	154	3	676	29	3
buttermilk	1 4-in sq (1.2 oz)	88	3	262	14	1
plain	1 4-in sq) (1.2 oz)	88	3	262	14	1

HOME RECIPE

plain	1 (7 in diam)	218	11	383	25	—

MIX

plain, as prep	1 7-in diam (2.6 oz)	218	10	458	26	1

WALNUTS

Black (Planters)	1 oz	180	17	0	3	—
English Halves (Planters)	1 oz	190	20	0	3	—
black, dried	1 oz	172	16	0	3	1
black, dried, chopped	1 cup	759	71	2	15	—
english, dried	1 oz	182	18	3	5	1
english, dried, chopped	1 cup	770	74	12	22	6

WATER CHESTNUTS
CANNED

Empress Sliced	2 oz	14	0	10	3	—
Empress Whole	2 oz	14	0	10	3	—
La Choy Sliced	¼ cup	18	tr	3	4	tr
La Choy Whole	4	14	tr	2	4	tr
chinese, sliced	½ cup	35	tr	6	9	—

FRESH

sliced	½ cup	66	tr	9	15	—

WATERCRESS
see also CRESS

raw, chopped	½ cup	2	tr	7	tr	tr

WATERMELON

cut up	1 cup	50	1	3	11	1
wedge	⅟₁₆	152	2	10	35	2

SEEDS

dried	1 cup	602	51	28	17	—
dried	1 oz	158	13	28	4	—

FOOD	PORTION	CAL	FAT	SOD	CARB	FIB

WAX BEANS
CANNED

FOOD	PORTION	CAL	FAT	SOD	CARB	FIB
Cut (Owatonna)	½ cup	20	0	—	—	—
Golden Cut Premium (S&W)	½ cup	20	0	385	5	—
Wax Beans (Seneca)	½ cup	20	0	—	—	—

WHALE

FOOD	PORTION	CAL	FAT	SOD	CARB	FIB
raw	3.5 oz	134	3	100	0	—

WHEAT
see BULGUR, BRAN, CEREAL, COUSCOUS, FLOUR, WHEAT GERM

FOOD	PORTION	CAL	FAT	SOD	CARB	FIB
Kamut Grain (Arrowhead)	¼ cup (1.7 oz)	140	1	0	32	5
Seitan Quick Mix (Arrowhead)	⅓ cup (1.4 oz)	150	1	20	14	2
Vital Wheat Gluten Plus Ascorbic Acid (Hodgson Mill)	1 tbsp (0.3 oz)	30	0	0	2	1
sprouted	⅓ cup	71	tr	6	15	—
starch	3.5 oz	348	tr	2	86	—

WHEAT GERM

FOOD	PORTION	CAL	FAT	SOD	CARB	FIB
Arrowhead	3 tbsp (0.5 oz)	50	1	0	10	2
Hodgson Mill	2 tbsp (0.5 oz)	55	1	0	7	4
Kretschmer	¼ cup	103	3	2	12	3
Kretschmer Honey Crunch	¼ cup	105	3	2	15	3
plain, toasted	1 cup	431	12	4	56	—
plain, toasted	¼ cup	108	3	1	14	4
plain, untoasted	¼ cup	104	3	4	15	4
w/ brown sugar & honey, toasted	1 cup	426	9	3	69	—
w/ brown sugar & honey, toasted	1 oz	107	2	1	17	—

WHIPPED TOPPINGS
see also CREAM

FOOD	PORTION	CAL	FAT	SOD	CARB	FIB
Cool Whip Extra Creamy	1 tbsp	13	1	3	1	—
Cool Whip Non Dairy	1 tbsp	11	1	1	1	—
Cool Whip Lite	1 tbsp	9	1	3	1	—
D-Zerta, as prep	1 tbsp	7	1	6	0	—
Diamond Crystal	1 tbsp	4	tr	—	—	—
Dream Whip, as prep	1 tbsp	9	1	4	1	—

FOOD	PORTION	CAL	FAT	SOD	CARB	FIB
Estee Whipped Topping, as prep	1 tbsp	4	tr	0	tr	—
Kraft Real Cream Topping	¼ cup	30	2	5	2	—
Kraft Whipped Topping	¼ cup	35	3	10	2	—
La Creme	1 tbsp	16	1	5	1	—
Pet Whip	1 tbsp	14	1	0	1	—
cream, pressurized	1 cup	154	13	78	7	—
cream, pressurized	1 tbsp	8	tr	4	tr	—
nondairy, powdered, as prep w/ whole milk	1 cup	151	10	53	13	—
nondairy, powdered, as prep w/ whole milk	1 tbsp	8	tr	3	1	—
nondairy, pressurized	1 cup	184	16	43	11	—
nondairy, pressurized	1 tbsp	11	1	2	1	—
nondairy, frzn	1 tbsp	13	1	1	1	—

WHITE BEANS
CANNED

FOOD	PORTION	CAL	FAT	SOD	CARB	FIB
Goya Spanish Style	7.5 oz	130	1	990	29	12
Progresso Cannellini	½ cup	80	tr	220	19	7
white beans	1 cup	306	1	13	58	—

DRIED

FOOD	PORTION	CAL	FAT	SOD	CARB	FIB
regular, cooked	1 cup	249	1	11	45	—
small, cooked	1 cup	253	1	4	46	—

WHITEFISH
FRESH

FOOD	PORTION	CAL	FAT	SOD	CARB	FIB
baked	3 oz	146	6	56	0	—

SMOKED

FOOD	PORTION	CAL	FAT	SOD	CARB	FIB
whitefish	1 oz	39	tr	285	0	—
whitefish	3 oz	92	1	866	0	—

WHITING
FRESH

FOOD	PORTION	CAL	FAT	SOD	CARB	FIB
cooked	3 oz	98	1	113	0	—
raw	3 oz	77	1	61	0	—

WILD RICE

FOOD	PORTION	CAL	FAT	SOD	CARB	FIB
cooked	½ cup	83	tr	3	18	—

WINE
see also CHAMPAGNE, WINE COOLERS

Boone's

FOOD	PORTION	CAL	FAT	SOD	CARB	FIB
Country Kwencher	1 fl oz	24	0	1	3	—
Delicious Apple	1 fl oz	21	0	1	3	—

FOOD	PORTION	CAL	FAT	SOD	CARB	FIB
Sangria	1 fl oz	22	0	1	3	—
Snow Creek Berry	1 fl oz	18	0	tr	3	—
Strawberry Hill	1 fl oz	22	0	1	3	—
Sun Peak Peach	1 fl oz	18	0	1	3	—
Wild Island	1 fl oz	18	0	tr	3	—
Carlo Rossi						
Blush	1 fl oz	21	0	1	1	—
Burgundy	1 fl oz	22	0	1	tr	—
Chablis	1 fl oz	21	0	1	tr	—
Paisano	1 fl oz	23	0	3	tr	—
Red Sangria	1 fl oz	24	0	1	2	—
Rhine	1 fl oz	21	0	1	1	—
Vin Rosé	1 fl oz	21	0	1	1	—
White Grenache	1 fl oz	20	0	tr	1	—
Fairbanks						
Cream Sherry	1 fl oz	42	0	1	4	—
Port	1 fl oz	44	0	1	4	—
Sherry	1 fl oz	34	0	2	2	—
White Port	1 fl oz	44	0	1	4	—
Gallo						
Blush Chablis	1 fl oz	22	0	2	1	—
Burgundy	1 fl oz	22	0	1	tr	—
Cabernet Sauvignon	1 fl oz	22	0	tr	0	—
Chablis Blanc	1 fl oz	20	0	1	tr	—
Chardonnay	1 fl oz	23	0	1	tr	—
Classic Burgundy	1 fl oz	21	0	tr	0	—
French Colombard	1 fl oz	21	0	1	1	—
Hearty Burgundy	1 fl oz	22	0	1	tr	—
Johannisberg Riesling '88	1 fl oz	20	0	1	1	—
Pink Chablis	1 fl oz	20	0	1	1	—
Red Rosé	1 fl oz	23	0	2	1	—
Rhine	1 fl oz	22	0	1	1	—
Sauvignon Blanc '90	1 fl oz	20	0	1	tr	—
White Grenache '92	1 fl oz	20	0	1	1	—
White Grenache New Vintage	1 fl oz	20	0	tr	1	—
White Zinfandel '91	1 fl oz	18	0	1	tr	—
White Zinfandel New Vintage	1 fl oz	18	0	1	tr	—
Zinfandel '87	1 fl oz	23	0	tr	0	—
Sheffield Cellars						
Sherry	1 fl oz	44	0	1	4	—
Tawny Port	1 fl oz	45	0	2	4	—

FOOD	PORTION	CAL	FAT	SOD	CARB	FIB
Vermouth Extra Dry	1 fl oz	28	0	1	1	—
Vermouth Sweet	1 fl oz	43	0	2	4	—
Very Dry Sherry	1 fl oz	32	0	2	1	—
red	3.5 oz	74	0	6	2	—
rose	3.5 oz	73	0	5	2	—
sherry	2 oz	84	0	—	5	—
sweet dessert	2 oz	90	0	5	7	—
vermouth, dry	3.5 oz	105	0	—	1	—
vermouth, sweet	3.5 oz	167	0	—	12	—
white	3.5 oz	70	0	5	1	—

WINE COOLERS
Bartles & Jaymes

FOOD	PORTION	CAL	FAT	SOD	CARB	FIB
Berry	12 fl oz	210	0	0	32	—
Margarita	12 fl oz	260	0	40	46	—
Original	12 fl oz	190	0	10	28	—
Peach	12 fl oz	210	0	5	33	—
Pina Colada	12 fl oz	280	0	0	49	—
Planter's Punch	12 fl oz	230	0	0	36	—
Strawberry	12 fl oz	210	0	0	32	—
Strawberry Daquiri	12 fl oz	230	0	5	37	—
Tropical	12 fl oz	230	0	0	38	—

WINGED BEANS
DRIED

FOOD	PORTION	CAL	FAT	SOD	CARB	FIB
cooked	1 cup	252	10	22	26	—

WOLFFISH
FRESH

FOOD	PORTION	CAL	FAT	SOD	CARB	FIB
atlantic baked	3 oz	105	3	93	0	—

YAM
see also SWEET POTATO
CANNED

FOOD	PORTION	CAL	FAT	SOD	CARB	FIB
Bruce Cut	½ cup	139	1	27	20	—
Bruce Mashed	½ cup	130	1	50	29	—
Bruce Vacuum Pack	½ cup	122	1	30	28	—
Bruce Whole	½ cup	139	1	27	31	—
S&W Candied	½ cup	180	0	355	44	—
S&W Southern Whole In Extra Heavy Syrup	½ cup	139	1	27	31	—
Sugary Sam Golden Cut In Syrup	½ cup	110	0	—	—	—
Trappey's Golden Whole In Heavy Syrup	½ cup	130	0	—	—	—

FOOD	PORTION	CAL	FAT	SOD	CARB	FIB
FRESH						
mountain yam hawaii, cooked	½ cup	59	tr	9	14	—
yam cubed, cooked	½ cup	79	tr	6	19	—
YAMBEAN						
cooked	¾ cup	38	tr	4	9	—
YARDLONG BEANS						
DRIED						
cooked	1 cup	202	1	9	36	—
YEAST						
Fleischmann's Active Dry	1 pkg (¼ oz)	20	0	10	3	—
Fleischmann's Fresh Active	1 pkg (0.6 oz)	15	0	5	2	—
Fleischmann's Household Yeast	½ oz	15	0	5	2	—
Fleischmann's RapidRise	1 pkg (¼ oz)	20	0	10	3	—
baker's, compressed	1 cake (0.6 oz)	18	tr	5	3	2
baker's, dry	1 pkg (¼ oz)	21	tr	—	3	—
baker's, dry	1 tbsp	35	1	—	5	3
brewer's, dry	1 tbsp	25	tr	10	3	—
YELLOW BEANS						
CANNED						
B&M Baked Beans	8 oz	326	7	770	50	—
DRIED						
Bean Cuisine Yellow Eye	½ cup	115	1	5	—	5
cooked	1 cup	254	2	8	45	—
YELLOW EYE BEANS						
CANNED						
B&M Yellow Eye Baked Beans	⅞ cup	290	7	—	—	—
YELLOWTAIL						
FRESH						
baked	3 oz	159	6	42	0	—
YOGURT						
see also YOGURT FROZEN						
All Flavors (Cabot)	8 oz	220	3	120	42	—

FOOD	PORTION	CAL	FAT	SOD	CARB	FIB
All Flavors Ultimate 90 (Weight Watchers)	1 cup	90	0	120	13	—
Amaretto Almond Yo Creme (Yoplait)	5 oz	240	10	—	—	—
Apple (La Yogurt)	6 oz	190	4	—	—	—
Apple Crisp Lowfat (New Country)	6 oz	150	2	85	30	—
Apple Original (Yoplait)	6 oz	190	3	110	32	—
Apples 'n Spice Fat Free (Colombo)	8 oz	190	0	130	39	0
Apricot Fat Free (Colombo)	8 oz	190	0	130	39	0
Banana Custard Style (Yoplait)	6 oz	190	4	95	32	—
Banana Fruit On Bottom (Dannon)	8 oz	240	3	120	43	—
Banana Strawberry Fat Free (Colombo)	8 oz	200	0	130	42	0
Banana Strawberry Low Fat (Colombo)	8 oz	210	4	110	39	0
Bavarian Chocolate Yo Creme (Yoplait)	5 oz	270	11	—	—	—
Black Cherry Low Fat (Colombo)	8 oz	200	4	115	36	0
Black Cherry Lowfat (Breyers)	8 oz	260	3	120	49	—
Black Cherry Lowfat (Light N' Lively)	8 oz	230	2	125	44	—
Black Cherry With Aspartame Cal 70 (Knudsen)	8 oz	70	0	75	12	—
Black Cherry 100 Calorie With Aspartame (Light N' Lively)	8 oz	100	0	100	17	—
Blueberry (Dannon)	8 oz	200	4	160	34	—
Blueberry (La Yogurt)	6 oz	190	4	—	—	—
Blueberry (La Yogurt 25)	8 oz	200	0	—	—	—
Blueberry (Mountain High)	1 cup	220	6	140	31	—
Blueberry Custard Style (Yoplait)	6 oz	190	4	95	32	—
Blueberry Fat Free (Colombo)	8 oz	190	0	130	39	0

FOOD	PORTION	CAL	FAT	SOD	CARB	FIB
Blueberry Fat Free (Yoplait)	6 oz	150	0	95	31	—
Blueberry Fruit Crunch (Friendship)	6 oz	190	4	125	32	0
Blueberry Fruit On Bottom (Dannon)	4.4 oz	130	2	65	23	—
Blueberry Fruit On Bottom (Dannon)	8 oz	240	3	120	43	—
Blueberry Light (Yoplait)	4 oz	60	0	75	9	—
Blueberry Light (Yoplait)	6 oz	80	0	80	13	—
Blueberry Light 100 (Colombo)	8 oz	100	0	140	16	0
Blueberry Low Fat (Colombo)	8 oz	200	4	110	36	0
Blueberry Lowfat (Breyers)	8 oz	250	2	120	48	—
Blueberry Lowfat (Light N' Lively)	4.4 oz	130	1	70	26	—
Blueberry Lowfat (Light N' Lively)	8 oz	240	2	130	46	—
Blueberry Nonfat (Dannon)	6 oz	140	0	105	27	—
Blueberry Nonfat Light (Dannon)	4.4 oz	60	0	70	8	—
Blueberry Nonfat Light (Dannon)	8 oz	100	0	130	17	—
Blueberry Original (Yoplait)	4 oz	120	2	75	21	—
Blueberry Original (Yoplait)	6 oz	190	3	110	32	—
Blueberry Supreme Lowfat (New Country)	6 oz	150	2	90	31	—
Blueberry With Aspartame Cal 70 (Knudsen)	8 oz	70	0	80	11	—
Blueberry With Aspartame Fat Free (Light N' Lively)	8 oz	50	0	60	8	—
Blueberry 100 Calorie With Aspartame (Light N' Lively)	8 oz	90	0	110	15	—
Boysenberry Fruit On Bottom (Dannon)	8 oz	240	3	120	43	—
Boysenberry Lowfat (Knudsen)	8 oz	240	4	135	43	—

FOOD	PORTION	CAL	FAT	SOD	CARB	FIB
Boysenberry Original (Yoplait)	6 oz	190	3	110	32	—
Cappuccino Fat Free (Colombo)	8 oz	180	0	140	35	0
Cherries Jubilee (Yoplait)	5 oz	220	8	—	—	—
Cherry (La Yogurt)	6 oz	190	4	—	—	—
Cherry (La Yogurt 25)	8 oz	200	0	—	—	—
Cherry Custard Style (Yoplait)	6 oz	180	4	95	30	—
Cherry Fat Free (Colombo)	8 oz	190	0	135	39	0
Cherry Fat Free (Yoplait)	6 oz	150	0	95	31	—
Cherry Fruit On Bottom (Dannon)	4.4 oz	130	2	65	23	—
Cherry Fruit On Bottom (Dannon)	8 oz	240	3	120	43	—
Cherry Light (Yoplait)	4 oz	60	0	75	9	—
Cherry Light (Yoplait)	6 oz	80	0	80	13	—
Cherry Lowfat (Knudsen)	8 oz	240	4	135	43	—
Cherry Lowfat (Light N' Lively)	4.4 oz	140	1	70	27	—
Cherry Original (Yoplait)	6 oz	190	3	110	32	—
Cherry Supreme Lowfat (New Country)	6 oz	150	2	90	32	—
Cherry Vanilla (La Yogurt)	6 oz	190	4	—	—	—
Cherry Vanilla Light 100 (Colombo)	8 oz	100	0	120	16	0
Cherry Vanilla Lowfat Swiss Style (Lite Line)	1 cup	240	2	150	45	—
Cherry Vanilla Nonfat Light (Dannon)	8 oz	100	0	130	17	—
Coffee (Friendship)	8 oz	210	3	170	30	0
Coffee & Cream Light 100 (Colombo)	8 oz	100	0	120	16	0
Coffee Lowfat (Dannon)	8 oz	200	3	120	34	—
Cranberry Strawberry Fat Free (Colombo)	8 oz	200	0	120	43	0

FOOD	PORTION	CAL	FAT	SOD	CARB	FIB
Creamy Vanilla Light 100 (Colombo)	8 oz	100	0	130	16	0
Dutch Apple Fruit On Bottom (Dannon)	8 oz	240	3	120	43	—
Exotic Fruit Fruit On Bottom (Dannon)	8 oz	240	3	120	43	—
French Roast Fat Free (Colombo)	8 oz	180	0	140	35	0
French Vanilla Low Fat (Colombo)	8 oz	180	4	130	29	0
French Vanilla Lowfat (New Country)	6 oz	150	2	90	31	—
Fruit Cocktail Fat Free (Colombo)	8 oz	190	0	130	39	0
Fruit Crunch Lowfat (New Country)	6 oz	150	2	90	30	—
Fruit Medley Light 100 (Colombo)	8 oz	100	0	120	16	0
Grape Lowfat (Light N' Lively)	4.4 oz	130	1	70	24	—
Hawaiian Salad Lowfat (New Country)	6 oz	150	2	90	31	—
Juicy Peach Light 100 (Colombo)	8 oz	100	0	140	16	0
Key Lime (La Yogurt)	6 oz	190	4	—	—	—
Lemon Fat Free (Colombo)	8 oz	170	0	150	33	0
Lemon 100 Calorie With Aspartame (Light N' Lively)	8 oz	100	0	150	16	—
Lemon Creme Light 100 (Colombo)	8 oz	100	0	160	16	0
Lemon Custard Style (Yoplait)	6 oz	190	4	95	32	—
Lemon Lowfat (Dannon)	8 oz	200	3	120	34	—
Lemon Lowfat (Knudsen)	8 oz	240	4	135	43	—
Lemon Original (Yoplait)	6 oz	190	3	110	32	—
Lemon Supreme Lowfat (New Country)	6 oz	150	2	90	31	—
Lemon With Aspartame Cal 70 (Knudsen)	8 oz	70	0	125	12	—
Lime Lowfat (Knudsen)	8 oz	240	4	135	43	—
Mandarin Orange Light 100 (Colombo)	8 oz	100	0	120	16	0

FOOD	PORTION	CAL	FAT	SOD	CARB	FIB
Mixed Berries Fruit On Bottom (Dannon)	4.4 oz	130	2	65	23	—
Mixed Berries Fruit On Bottom (Dannon)	8 oz	240	3	120	43	—
Mixed Berries Light 100 (Colombo)	8 oz	100	0	110	16	0
Mixed Berries Lowfat (Dannon)	8 oz	240	3	120	43	—
Mixed Berries Lowfat (New Country)	6 oz	150	2	85	31	—
Mixed Berry (La Yogurt)	6 oz	190	4	—	—	—
Mixed Berry Custard Style (Yoplait)	6 oz	180	4	95	30	—
Mixed Berry Fat Free (Yoplait)	6 oz	150	0	95	31	—
Mixed Berry Lowfat (Breyers)	8 oz	250	2	120	48	—
Mixed Berry Original (Yoplait)	6 oz	190	3	110	32	—
Orange Original (Yoplait)	6 oz	190	3	110	32	—
Orange Supreme Lowfat (New Country)	6 oz	150	2	90	31	—
Peach (La Yogurt)	6 oz	190	4	—	—	—
Peach Fat Free (Colombo)	8 oz	190	0	130	33	0
Peach Fat Free (Yoplait)	6 oz	150	0	95	31	—
Peach Fruit Crunch (Friendship)	6 oz	190	5	125	31	0
Peach Fruit On Bottom (Dannon)	8 oz	240	3	120	43	—
Peach Light (Yoplait)	4 oz	60	0	75	9	—
Peach Light (Yoplait)	6 oz	80	0	80	13	—
Peach Lowfat (Breyers)	8 oz	250	2	120	48	—
Peach Lowfat (Knudsen)	8 oz	240	4	135	43	—
Peach Lowfat (Light N' Lively)	4.4 oz	130	1	65	26	—
Peach Lowfat (Light N' Lively)	8 oz	240	2	120	46	—
Peach Lowfat Blended With Fruit (Dannon)	4.4 oz	130	2	80	24	—
Peach Lowfat Swiss Style (Lite Line)	1 cup	240	14	65	25	—
Peach Melba Low Fat (Colombo)	8 oz	200	4	115	36	0

FOOD	PORTION	CAL	FAT	SOD	CARB	FIB
Peach Nonfat (Dannon)	6 oz	140	0	105	27	—
Peach Nonfat Light (Dannon)	8 oz	100	0	130	17	—
Peach Original (Yoplait)	4 oz	120	2	75	21	—
Peach Original (Yoplait)	6 oz	190	3	110	32	—
Peach With Aspartame Cal 70 (Knudsen)	8 oz	70	0	95	11	—
Peach 100 Calorie With Aspartame (Light N' Lively)	8 oz	100	0	115	16	—
Peaches 'n Cream Lowfat (New Country)	6 oz	150	2	90	31	—
Pina Colada (La Yogurt)	6 oz	190	4	—	—	—
Pina Colada Fruit On Bottom (Dannon)	8 oz	240	3	120	43	—
Pineapple Lowfat (Breyers)	8 oz	250	2	120	50	—
Pineapple Lowfat (Light N' Lively)	4.4 oz	130	1	65	26	—
Pineapple Lowfat (Light N' Lively)	8 oz	230	2	120	47	—
Pina Cola Original (Yoplait)	6 oz	190	3	110	32	—
Pineapple Original (Yoplait)	6 oz	190	3	110	32	—
Pineapple With Aspartame Cal 70 (Knudsen)	8 oz	70	0	125	12	—
Plain (Cabot)	8 oz	140	4	160	16	—
Plain (Friendship)	8 oz	150	3	190	13	0
Plain (Knudsen)	8 oz	200	9	170	16	—
Plain (La Yogurt)	6 oz	140	6	—	—	—
Plain (Mountain High)	1 cup	200	9	140	16	—
Plain Fat Free (Colombo)	8 oz	110	0	170	16	0
Plain Low Fat (Colombo)	8 oz	120	5	150	12	0
Plain Lowfat (Breyers)	8 oz	140	3	170	16	—
Plain Lowfat (Dannon)	8 oz	140	4	125	15	—
Plain Lowfat (Knudsen)	8 oz	160	5	180	17	—
Plain Lowfat (Meadow Gold)	1 cup	160	5	160	16	—
Plain Lowfat Swiss Style (Lite Line)	1 cup	140	2	150	16	—
Plain Nonfat (Dannon)	8 oz	110	0	140	15	—

FOOD	PORTION	CAL	FAT	SOD	CARB	FIB
Plain Nonfat (Weight Watchers)	1 cup	90	0	135	13	—
Plain Nonfat (Yoplait)	8 oz	120	0	160	18	—
Plain Original (Yoplait)	6 oz	130	3	140	15	—
Raspberry (La Yogurt 25)	8 oz	200	0	—	—	—
Raspberries & Cream (Yoplait)	5 oz	230	9	—	—	—
Raspberry Custard Style (Yoplait)	6 oz	190	4	95	32	—
Raspberry Fat Free (Colombo)	8 oz	190	0	130	39	0
Raspberry Low Fat (Colombo)	8 oz	200	4	115	36	0
Raspberry Original (Yoplait)	4 oz	120	2	75	21	—
Raspberry Original (Yoplait)	6 oz	190	3	110	32	—
Raspberry Supreme Lowfat (New Country)	6 oz	150	2	90	31	—
Raspberry Fat Free (Yoplait)	6 oz	150	0	95	31	—
Raspberry Fruit On Bottom (Dannon)	4.4 oz	120	1	65	23	—
Raspberry Fruit On Bottom (Dannon)	8 oz	240	3	120	43	—
Raspberry Light (Yoplait)	4 oz	60	0	75	9	—
Raspberry Light (Yoplait)	6 oz	80	0	80	13	—
Raspberry Lowfat (Knudsen)	8 oz	240	4	135	43	—
Raspberry Lowfat Blended With Fruit (Dannon)	4.4 oz	130	2	80	24	—
Raspberry Nonfat (Dannon)	6 oz	140	0	105	27	—
Raspberry Nonfat (Dannon)	8 oz	200	4	160	34	—
Raspberry Nonfat Light (Dannon)	8 oz	100	0	130	17	—
Raspberry Sundae Style (Meadow Gold)	1 cup	250	4	160	42	—

FOOD	PORTION	CAL	FAT	SOD	CARB	FIB
Red Raspberry 100 Calorie With Aspartame (Light N' Lively)	8 oz	90	0	105	15	—
Red Raspberry Light 100 (Colombo)	8 oz	100	0	140	16	0
Red Raspberry Lowfat (Breyers)	8 oz	250	2	120	48	—
Red Raspberry Lowfat (Light N' Lively)	4.4 oz	130	1	70	24	—
Red Raspberry Lowfat (Light N' Lively)	8 oz	230	2	130	43	—
Red Raspberry With Aspartame Cal 70 (Knudsen)	8 oz	70	0	80	11	—
Red Raspberry With Aspartame Fat Free (Light N' Lively)	8 oz	50	0	60	8	—
Sprinkl'ns All Flavors (Dannon)	1 pkg (4.1 oz)	145	2	95	—	—
Strawberries Romanoff (Yoplait)	5 oz	220	8	—	—	—
Strawberry (Colombo)	8 oz	200	4	110	36	0
Strawberry (La Yogurt)	6 oz	190	4	—	—	—
Strawberry (La Yogurt 25)	8 oz	200	0	—	—	—
Strawberry Banana (La Yogurt)	6 oz	190	4	—	—	—
Strawberry Banana (La Yogurt 25)	8 oz	200	0	—	—	—
Strawberry Banana Fruit Crunch (Friendship)	6 oz	190	4	125	32	0
Strawberry Banana 100 Calorie With Aspartame (Light N' Lively)	8 oz	90	0	100	15	—
Strawberry Banana Custard Style (Yoplait)	4 oz	130	3	60	21	—
Strawberry Banana Custard Style (Yoplait)	6 oz	190	4	95	32	—
Strawberry Banana Fat Free (Yoplait)	6 oz	150	0	95	31	—
Strawberry Banana Fruit On Bottom (Dannon)	4.4 oz	130	2	65	23	—

FOOD	PORTION	CAL	FAT	SOD	CARB	FIB
Strawberry Banana Light (Yoplait)	4 oz	60	0	75	9	—
Strawberry Banana Light (Yoplait)	6 oz	80	0	80	13	—
Strawberry Banana Lowfat (Breyers)	8 oz	250	2	120	50	—
Strawberry Banana Lowfat (Dannon)	8 oz	200	4	160	34	—
Strawberry Banana Lowfat (Knudsen)	8 oz	250	4	135	43	—
Strawberry Banana Lowfat (Light N' Lively)	4.4 oz	140	1	65	29	—
Strawberry Banana Lowfat (Light N' Lively)	8 oz	260	2	120	52	—
Strawberry Banana Lowfat (New Country)	6 oz	150	2	85	31	—
Strawberry Banana Lowfat Blended With Fruit (Dannon)	4.4 oz	130	2	80	24	—
Strawberry Banana Nonfat Light (Dannon)	8 oz	100	0	130	17	—
Strawberry Banana Original (Yoplait)	6 oz	190	3	110	32	—
Strawberry Banana With Aspartame Fat Free (Light N' Lively)	8 oz	50	0	60	8	—
Strawberry Banana With Aspartame Cal 70 (Knudsen)	8 oz	70	0	80	12	—
Strawberry Custard Style (Yoplait)	4 oz	130	3	60	21	—
Strawberry Custard Style (Yoplait)	6 oz	190	4	95	32	—
Strawberry Fat Free (Colombo)	8 oz	190	0	130	39	0
Strawberry Fat Free (Yoplait)	6 oz	150	0	95	31	—
Strawberry Fruit Basket With Aspartame Cal 70 (Knudsen)	8 oz	70	0	90	11	—
Strawberry Fruit Crunch (Friendship)	6 oz	190	5	125	31	0
Strawberry Fruit Cup (La Yogurt)	6 oz	190	4	—	—	—

FOOD	PORTION	CAL	FAT	SOD	CARB	FIB
Strawberry Fruit Cup Lowfat (Light N' Lively)	4.4 oz	130	1	65	26	—
Strawberry Fruit Cup Lowfat (Light N' Lively)	8 oz	240	2	120	47	—
Strawberry Fruit Cup Lowfat (New Country)	6 oz	150	2	85	30	—
Strawberry Fruit Cup Nonfat Light (Dannon)	8 oz	100	0	130	17	—
Strawberry Fruit Cup With Aspartame Fat Free (Light N' Lively)	8 oz	50	0	55	8	—
Strawberry Fruit On Bottom (Dannon)	4.4 oz	130	2	65	23	—
Strawberry Fruit On Bottom (Dannon)	8 oz	240	3	120	43	—
Strawberry Light (Yoplait)	4 oz	60	0	75	9	—
Strawberry Light (Yoplait)	6 oz	80	0	110	13	—
Strawberry Light 100 (Colombo)	8 oz	100	0	140	16	0
Strawberry Lowfat (Breyers)	8 oz	250	2	120	48	—
Strawberry Lowfat (Dannon)	8 oz	200	4	160	34	—
Strawberry Lowfat (Knudsen)	8 oz	250	4	135	45	—
Strawberry Lowfat (Light N' Lively)	4.4 oz	130	1	70	25	—
Strawberry Lowfat (Light N' Lively)	8 oz	240	2	130	45	—
Strawberry Lowfat Blended With Fruit (Dannon)	4.4 oz	130	2	80	24	—
Strawberry Lowfat Swiss Style (Lite Line)	1 cup	240	2	150	46	—
Strawberry Nonfat (Dannon)	6 oz	140	0	105	27	—
Strawberry Nonfat Light (Dannon)	4.4 oz	60	0	70	8	—
Strawberry Nonfat Light (Dannon)	8 oz	100	0	130	17	—
Strawberry Original (Yoplait)	4 oz	120	2	75	21	—

FOOD	PORTION	CAL	FAT	SOD	CARB	FIB
Strawberry Original (Yoplait)	6 oz	190	3	110	32	—
Strawberry Pineapple Orange Fat Free (Colombe)	8 oz	190	0	125	38	0
Strawberry Rhubarb Original (Yoplait)	6 oz	190	3	110	32	—
Strawberry Supreme Lowfat (New Country)	6 oz	150	2	90	30	—
Strawberry 100 Calorie With Aspartame (Light N' Lively)	8 oz	90	0	105	15	—
Strawberry With Aspartame Cal 70 (Knudsen)	8 oz	70	0	85	11	—
Strawberry With Aspartame Fat Free (Light N' Lively)	8 oz	50	0	60	8	—
Tropical Orange (La Yogurt)	6 oz	190	4	—	—	—
Vanilla (La Yogurt)	6 oz	160	4	—	—	—
Vanilla Bean Lowfat (Breyers)	8 oz	230	3	150	41	—
Vanilla Custard Style (Yoplait)	4 oz	130	3	70	20	—
Vanilla Custard Style (Yoplait)	6 oz	180	4	110	30	—
Vanilla Fat Free (Colombo)	8 oz	170	0	150	32	0
Vanilla Lowfat (Dannon)	8 oz	200	3	120	34	—
Vanilla Lowfat (Knudsen)	8 oz	240	4	135	43	—
Vanilla Nonfat (Yoplait)	8 oz	180	0	140	35	—
Vanilla Nonfat Light (Dannon)	8 oz	100	0	130	17	—
Vanilla Original (Yoplait)	6 oz	180	3	120	29	—
Vanilla With Aspartame Cal 70 (Knudsen)	8 oz	70	0	90	11	—
coffee lowfat	8 oz	194	3	149	31	—
fruit lowfat	4 oz	113	1	60	21	—
fruit lowfat	8 oz	225	3	121	42	—
plain	8 oz	139	7	105	11	—
plain lowfat	8 oz	144	4	159	16	—
plain no fat	8 oz	127	tr	174	17	—
vanilla lowfat	8 oz	194	3	149	31	—

FOOD	PORTION	CAL	FAT	SOD	CARB	FIB
YOGURT FROZEN						
see also TOFU YOGURT						
All Flavors Gourmet Yogurt (Bresler's)	5 oz	145	2	—	28	—
All Flavors (Just 10)	1 oz	10	0	14	3	—
All Flavors Lite Yogurt (Bresler's)	5 oz	135	0	—	30	—
Apple Pie (Ben & Jerry's)	½ cup (4 fl oz)	140	3	55	28	0
Banana Strawberry (Ben & Jerry's)	½ cup (4 fl oz)	130	2	30	27	0
Banana Strawberry (Edy's)	3 oz	80	1	40	15	—
Better Than Yogurt Chocolate Fudge (Tofutti)	4 fl oz	120	2	98	25	0
Better Than Yogurt Coffee Marshmallow Swirl (Tofutti)	4 fl oz	100	1	77	24	0
Better Than Yogurt Passion Island Fruit (Tofutti)	4 fl oz	100	1	100	21	0
Better Than Yogurt Peach Mango (Tofutti)	4 fl oz	100	1	102	23	0
Better Than Yogurt Strawberry Banana (Tofutti)	4 fl oz	100	1	92	23	0
Better Than Yogurt Vanilla Fudge (Tofutti)	4 fl oz	120	2	90	24	0
Black Cherry (Breyers)	½ cup (2.7 oz)	140	3	40	25	0
Blueberry (Edy's)	3 oz	80	1	40	15	—
Blueberry (Elan)	4 oz	130	3	50	23	—
Blueberry Cheesecake (Ben & Jerry's)	½ cup (4 fl oz)	130	2	40	26	0
Blueberry Softy (Dannon)	4 oz	110	2	65	21	—
Butter Pecan Softy (Dannon)	4 oz	110	2	65	21	—
Cappuccino Softy (Dannon)	4 oz	110	2	65	21	—
Caramel Almond Praline (Elan)	4 oz	160	4	90	26	—
Cheesecake Softy (Dannon)	4 oz	110	2	65	21	—

FOOD	PORTION	CAL	FAT	SOD	CARB	FIB
Cherry (Edy's)	3 oz	80	1	40	15	—
Cherry Garcia (Ben & Jerry's)	½ cup (4 fl oz)	150	3	40	28	0
Chocolate (Bee-Lite)	4 oz	100	tr	55	23	—
Chocolate (Ben & Jerry's)	1 pop (2.5 fl oz)	150	9	75	17	1
Chocolate (Ben & Jerry's)	½ cup (4 fl oz)	140	3	40	26	0
Chocolate (Breyers)	½ cup (2.7 oz)	150	4	45	25	1
Chocolate (Edy's)	3 oz	80	1	40	15	—
Chocolate (Elan)	4 oz	130	3	50	24	—
Chocolate (Fi-Bar)	1	190	7	160	26	4
Chocolate (Haagen-Dazs)	3 oz	130	3	30	21	—
Chocolate (Sealtest)	½ cup (2.7 oz)	120	2	45	24	tr
Chocolate Almond (Elan)	4 oz	160	6	50	22	—
Chocolate Brownie (Breyers)	½ cup (2.7 oz)	170	5	45	29	1
Chocolate Chip (Edy's)	3 oz	100	1	55	20	—
Chocolate Fudge Brownie (Ben & Jerry's)	½ cup (4 fl oz)	170	4	95	31	1
Chocolate Kissed With Honey	3.5 oz	100	3	50	18	—
Chocolate Kissed With Honey Nonfat	3.5 oz	85	tr	60	19	—
Chocolate Nonfat Softy (Dannon)	4 oz	110	0	65	23	—
Chocolate Shake (Weight Watchers)	7.5 oz	220	1	140	44	—
Chocolate Softy (Dannon)	4 oz	140	2	65	25	—
Chocolate Yogurt Bar (Dole)	1	70	tr	50	13	—
Citrus Heights (Edy's)	3 oz	80	1	40	15	—
Coffee (Elan)	4 oz	130	3	60	22	—
Coffee Almond Fudge (Ben & Jerry's)	½ cup (4 fl oz)	180	7	60	28	0
Coffee Decaffeinated (Elan)	4 oz	130	3	60	22	—
Cookies 'N' Cream (Edy's)	3 oz	100	1	55	20	—
Creamsicle Raspberry (Good Humor)	1 (2.8 oz)	100	1	20	23	0

FOOD	PORTION	CAL	FAT	SOD	CARB	FIB
Dutch Chocolate (Desserve)	4 oz	80	0	62	18	—
Frista Cup (Good Humor)	1 (6.2 oz)	220	5	125	38	1
Golden Vanilla Nonfat Softy (Dannon)	4 oz	100	0	65	22	—
Heath Bar Crunch (Ben & Jerry's)	½ cup (4 fl oz)	170	6	80	29	0
Lemon Meringue Softy (Dannon)	4 oz	110	2	65	21	—
Marble Fudge (Edy's)	3 oz	100	1	55	20	—
Mocha Fudge (Sealtest)	½ cup (2.6 oz)	130	2	45	25	tr
Peach (Breyers)	½ cup (2.7 oz)	140	3	40	24	0
Peach (Elan)	4 oz	130	3	50	23	—
Peach (Haagen-Dazs)	3 oz	120	3	30	20	—
Peach & Vanilla Bar (Haagen-Dazs)	1 bar	100	1	20	18	—
Peanut Butter Softy (Dannon)	4 oz	130	3	70	21	—
Peach Softy (Dannon)	4 oz	110	2	65	21	—
Perfectly Peach (Edy's)	3 oz	80	1	40	15	—
Pina Colada Softy (Dannon)	4 oz	110	2	65	21	—
Plain Softy (Dannon)	4 oz	90	1	60	17	—
Pure Indulgence All Flavors (Dannon)	½ cup	160	6	100	—	—
Raspberry (Ben & Jerry's)	½ cup (4 fl oz)	120	2	35	24	0
Raspberry (Edy's)	3 oz	80	1	40	15	—
Raspberry & Vanilla Bar (Haagen-Dazs)	1 bar (2.5 oz)	90	1	25	19	0
Raspberry Softy (Dannon)	4 oz	110	2	65	21	—
Raspberry Vanilla Swirl (Edy's)	3 oz	80	1	45	15	—
Red Raspberry (Breyers)	½ cup (2.7 oz)	140	4	40	24	0
Red Raspberry Nonfat Softy (Dannon)	4 oz	100	0	60	22	—
Rum Raisin (Elan)	4 oz	135	3	55	25	—
Rum Raisin Nonfat Softy (Dannon)	4 oz	100	0	65	22	—
Strawberry (Borden)	½ cup	100	2	50	19	—
Strawberry (Breyers)	½ cup (2.7 oz)	130	3	40	23	0

FOOD	PORTION	CAL	FAT	SOD	CARB	FIB
Strawberry (Edy's)	3 oz	80	1	40	15	—
Strawberry (Elan)	4 oz	125	3	50	22	—
Strawberry (Fi-Bar)	1	190	7	150	26	4
Strawberry (Haagen-Dazs)	3 oz	120	3	30	21	—
Strawberry (Meadow Gold)	½ cup	100	2	50	19	—
Strawberry Banana (Breyers)	½ cup (2.7 oz)	140	3	40	24	0
Strawberry Banana Softy (Dannon)	4 oz	110	2	65	21	—
Strawberry Banana Yogurt Bar (Dole)	1	60	tr	15	13	—
Strawberry Bar (Dole)	1	70	tr	25	15	—
Strawberry Cheesecake (Breyers)	½ cup (2.7 oz)	160	5	60	26	0
Strawberry Nonfat (Dannon)	6 oz	140	0	105	27	—
Strawberry Nonfat Softy (Dannon)	4 oz	100	0	60	22	—
Strawberry Softy (Dannon)	4 oz	110	2	65	21	—
Toffee Bar Crunch (Breyers)	½ cup (2.7 oz)	160	5	55	26	0
Vanilla (Bee-Lite)	4 oz	110	tr	55	23	—
Vanilla (Breyers)	½ cup (2.7 oz)	140	4	45	24	0
Vanilla (Desserve)	4 oz	70	0	57	16	—
Vanilla (Edy's)	3 oz	80	1	50	15	—
Vanilla (Elan)	4 oz	130	3	60	22	—
Vanilla (Fi-Bar)	1	190	7	150	26	4
Vanilla (Haagen-Dazs)	3 oz	130	3	40	20	—
Vanilla (Sealtest)	½ cup (2.6 oz)	120	2	45	24	0
Vanilla Almond Crunch (Haagen-Dazs)	3 oz	150	5	65	22	—
Vanilla Chocolate Strawberry (Breyers)	½ cup (2.7 oz)	140	4	45	24	0
Vanilla Fudge Twirl (Breyers)	½ cup (2.7 oz)	150	4	45	25	1
Vanilla Kissed With Honey	3.5 oz	100	3	75	17	—
Vanilla Kissed With Honey Nonfat	3.5 oz	85	tr	50	18	—
Vanilla Raspberry Swirl (Breyers)	½ cup (2.7 oz)	140	4	45	24	0
Vanilla Softy (Dannon)	4 oz	110	2	65	21	—

FOOD	PORTION	CAL	FAT	SOD	CARB	FIB
ZABAGLIONE						
see CUSTARD						
ZUCCHINI						
CANNED						
Italian Style (Progresso)	½ cup	50	2	540	8	2
Italian Style (S&W)	½ cup	45	1	467	7	—
italian style	½ cup	33	tr	427	8	—
FRESH						
baby, raw	1 (½ oz)	3	tr	0	1	tr
raw, sliced	½ cup	9	tr	2	2	1
sliced, cooked	½ cup	14	tr	2	4	1
FROZEN						
Big Valley	3.5 oz	12	tr	0	2	—
Breaded Zucchini (Ore/Ida)	3 oz	150	8	340	17	—
Zucchini Sliced (Southland)	3.2 oz	15	0	—	—	—
cooked	½ cup	19	tr	2	4	—

ANNETTE B. NATOW, Ph.D., R.D., and JO-ANN HES-LIN, M.A., R.D., are the authors of seventeen books on nutrition, including *The Fast-Food Nutrition Counter, The Cholesterol Counter, The Fat Counter, The Diabetes Carbohydrate and Calorie Counter, The Fat Attack Plan, The Iron Counter, The Pregnancy Nutrition Counter, The Sodium Counter* and *The Antioxidant Vitamin Counter* (all available from Pocket Books). Both are former faculty members of Adelphi University and State University of New York, Downstate Medical Center. They are editors of the *Journal of Nutrition for the Elderly*, serve as editorial board members for the *Environmental Nutrition Newsletter*, and are frequent contributors to magazines and journals.

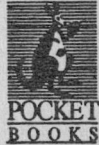